Health Care Transition

Albert C. Hergenroeder
Constance M. Wiemann
Editors

Health Care Transition

Building a Program for Adolescents and Young Adults with Chronic Illness and Disability

Springer

Editors
Albert C. Hergenroeder
Associate Professor, Director of Research
Section of Adolescent Medicine
and Sports Medicine
Department of Pediatrics
Baylor College of Medicine
Texas Children's Hospital
Houston, TX, USA

Constance M. Wiemann
Professor, Chief of Adolescent Medicine
Section of Adolescent Medicine
and Sports Medicine
Department of Pediatrics
Baylor College of Medicine
Texas Children's Hospital
Houston, TX, USA

ISBN 978-3-030-10281-4   ISBN 978-3-319-72868-1 (eBook)
https://doi.org/10.1007/978-3-319-72868-1

Printed on acid-free paper

This Springer imprint is published by the registered company Springer International Publishing AG part of Springer Nature
The registered company address is: Gewerbestrasse 11, 6330 Cham, Switzerland

Preface

Depending on the criteria used, the prevalence of chronic disease in 6–21-year-olds in the USA is 6–30%, affecting one in five families. A generation ago, many of these patients did not survive beyond childhood. Due to advances in medical treatments, 90% of individuals with chronic illness and disability survive childhood, and 750,000 young adults with special health-care needs in the USA transition to adulthood annually. Children with special health-care needs are defined as those who have or are at increased risk for a chronic physical, developmental, behavioral, or emotional condition and who also require health and related services of a type or amount beyond that required by children generally (Newacheck 1998). In this book, we focus on adolescents and young adults with special health-care needs (AYASHCN).

Health-care transition is defined as "the purposeful, planned movement of adolescents and young adults with chronic physical and medical conditions from child-centered to adult-oriented health-care systems" (Blum 1993). We include mental health conditions in this definition. For most AYASHCN who have mild conditions, characterized by no limitation of activity or cognitive impairment, the transition to adulthood appears to be successful. As the complexity of the condition increases, however, health-care transition (HCT) becomes more problematic, resulting in increased morbidity and mortality. Because poor HCT can contribute to this increased risk of morbidity and mortality, many pediatric and professional medical organizations, public health agencies, and advocacy organizations have developed statements or guidelines about the need to develop improved transition planning programs. Children's hospitals are aware that they need formal HCT programs; adult providers recognize the need to develop methods to incorporate young adults with pediatric-onset conditions into their practices; and health-care systems are aware that the transition from pediatric to adult-based care is a particularly important one in managing the health of populations. Despite increased recognition of the importance of HCT from pediatric to adult-based care, evidenced by the number of national conferences and increased peer-reviewed publications on the topic, there has been limited progress in addressing these barriers. There is an emerging yet not established evidence base for best methods in developing HCT programs, and major issues to be answered include defining successful HCT and providing evidence for the predictive validity for actual successful HCT outcomes.

The purpose of this textbook is to provide health-care professionals caring for youth and young adults with chronic illness and disability with a state of the field reference, including the framework, tools, and case-based examples needed to develop and evaluate an HCT planning program that can be implemented regardless of a patient's disease or disability. The editors of this book have been involved in developing HCT programs over the past 17 years. Drawing from their own personal experience as well as the empirical literature, the editors and invited chapter authors provide valuable perspectives on issues to consider in developing HCT programs across a range of health-care settings.

This textbook focuses on how to develop HCT programs regardless of disease or disability. As such, it does not cover condition-specific transition concerns, except as illustrated through case studies. We prefer to think of the transition process as occurring in three phases: preparation, transfer, and engagement of the AYASHCN in the adult health-care system. A process for this course from pediatric to adult-based care is presented in Chap. 1 as the 6 Core Elements of HCT. This process can be applied to any HCT model.

Wherever possible, youth/young adult, caregiver, and both pediatric and adult provider perspectives and voices are represented. The terms children with special health-care needs (CSHCN), youth with special health-care needs (YSHCN), and adolescents and young adults with special health-care needs (AYASHCN) are used throughout the book where appropriate. Many chapters contain brief case examples to illustrate key concepts or address literature gaps. As HCT is a process with overlapping components, there is some overlap among chapters. In addition, we have tried to cross-reference chapters, where appropriate.

This textbook begins with an introductory chapter (Part I) defining HCT describing the urgent need for comprehensive transition planning, the subsequent morbidity and mortality associated with poor transition outcomes, barriers to HCT, and a framework for developing and evaluating health-care transition programs. Part II focuses on the anatomic and neurochemical changes that occur in the brain during adolescence and young adulthood, the impact of these changes on cognitive function and behavior, and the ways in which cognitive function and behavior influence AYASHCN management of their illness during transition. The HCT perspectives of important participants in the HCT transition process—youth/young adults, caregivers, and both pediatric and adult providers—are presented in Part III, as well as changes in insurance and additional financial barriers experienced as youth age into young adulthood. Part IV presents ten chapters each addressing an aspect of developing HCT programs, from establishing administrative structures and processes to preparing, transferring, and tracking AYASHCN as they leave the pediatric setting to their successful acceptance into the adult health-care system. A successful transition from the perspective of five key stakeholders in the transition process—patients, caregivers, pediatric providers, adult providers, and third-party payors—is presented in Part V. Issues of HCT finance are covered in two chapters (Part VI). Part VII explores special issues in HCT, such as HCT and the medical home, the international perspective on transition, legal issues in HCT, and transitioning youth with medical complexity or cognitive/intellectual disabilities. The chapters in this section that represent relatively new topics in HCT include the hospitalist's and dentist's perspectives on HCT and the increased role of pharmacists and palliative care. Models of HCT programs are presented in Part VIII, including a case study of a hospital-based transition planning program and an overview of a variety of programmatic models currently operating in the field, as well as the state of the field in terms of evidence to support best practice. A single concluding chapter forms Part IX.

In all, there are 37 chapters from 63 authors representing 46 medical centers in North America and Europe.

It is important to note that as of the writing of this textbook, the infrastructure of HCT finance is currently being threatened by repeal of the ACA, with proposed dramatic reductions in Medicaid and CHIP payments upon which many AYASHCN depend for life-sustaining therapies.

Houston, TX Albert C. Hergenroeder
Houston, TX Constance M. Wiemann

Contents

Contributors

Sarah Ahrens, M.D. Department of Medicine, University of Wisconsin School of Medicine and Public Health, Madison, WI, USA

Rosemary Alexander, Ph.D. Texas Parent to Parent, Austin, TX, USA

Ana Catalina Alvarez-Elias, M.D., M.Sc. Hospital Infantil de Mexico Federico Gomez, Universidad Nacional Autonoma de Mexico, Mexico City, Mexico

Sick Kids, The Hospital for Sick Children, University of Toronto, Toronto, ON, Canada

Khush Amaria, Ph.D., C.Psych. Division of Adolescent Medicine and Department of Psychology, Good 2 Go Transition Program, Hospital for Sick Children, Toronto, ON, Canada

Beth E. Anderson, Ph.D. Social Care Institute for Excellence, London, UK

Marilyn Augustine, M.D. Division of Endocrinology and Metabolism, University of Rochester Medical Center, Rochester, NY, USA

Cecily L. Betz, Ph.D., R.N. Department of Pediatrics, University of Southern California (USC), Keck School of Medicine, Los Angeles, CA, USA

USC University Center for Excellence in Developmental Disabilities, Children's Hospital Los Angeles, Los Angeles, CA, USA

Rebecca Boudos, L.C.S.W. Chronic Illness Transition Program, Ann and Robert H. Lurie Children's Hospital of Chicago, Chicago, IL, USA

Laura G. Buckner, M.Ed., L.P.C. Texas Center for Disability Studies, The University of Texas, Austin, TX, USA

Jonathan Burton, B.Pharm. Right Medicine Pharmacy, University of Stirling, Stirling, UK

Isabel Yuriko Stenzel Byrnes, L.C.S.W., M.P.H. Social Worker and Patient Advocate, Redwood City, CA, USA

Roisin Campbell, M.Sc. Pharmacy Department, Musgrave Park Hospital, Belfast, UK

Mary R. Ciccarelli, M.D. Indiana University School of Medicine, Indianapolis, IN, USA

Ryan J. Coller, M.D., M.P.H. Department of Pediatrics, University of Wisconsin School of Medicine and Public Health, Madison, WI, USA

Division of Hospital Medicine, Pediatric Complex Care Program, Madison, WI, USA

Allan Colver, M.A., M.D., M.B.B.S. Institute of Health and Society, Newcastle University, Newcastle, UK

Mallory Cyr, M.P.H. Mallory Cyr, LLC, Denver, CO, USA

Gail Dovey-Pearce, D.Clin.Psych. Northumbria Healthcare NHS Foundation Trust, North Shields, UK

Ellen Roy Elias, M.D. Departments of Pediatrics and Genetics, University of Colorado School of Medicine, Special Care Clinic, Children's Hospital Colorado, Aurora, CO, USA

Kimberly Espinoza, D.D.S., M.P.H. Department of Oral Medicine, University of Washington School of Dentistry, Seattle, WA, USA

Cynthia Fair, L.C.S.W., M.P.H., Dr.P.H. Department of Public Health Studies, Elon University, Elon, NC, USA

Maria Ferris, M.D., M.P.H., Ph.D. Healthcare Transition Program, University of North Carolina at Chapel Hill, Chapel Hill, NC, USA

Emily M. Fredericks, Ph.D., C.S. C.S. Mott Children's Hospital, Ann Arbor, MI, USA

University of Michigan Medical School, Ann Arbor, MI, USA

Angelo P. Giardino, M.D., Ph.D. Texas Children's Hospital, Houston, TX, USA

Academic General Pediatrics, Department of Pediatrics, Baylor College of Medicine, Houston, TX, USA

Nicola J. Gray, Ph.D. Green Line Consulting Limited, Manchester, UK

James Harisiades, M.P.H. Office of Child Advocacy, Ann and Robert H. Lurie Children's Hospital of Chicago, Chicago, IL, USA

Ian S. Harris, M.D. Department of Medicine, Division of Cardiology, Adult Congenital Heart Program, University of California—San Francisco, San Francisco, CA, USA

Laura C. Hart, M.D., M.P.H. Cecil G. Sheps Center for Health Services Research, University of North Carolina at Chapel Hill, Chapel Hill, NC, USA

Albert C. Hergenroeder, M.D. Section of Adolescent Medicine and Sports Medicine, Department of Pediatrics, Baylor College of Medicine, Texas Children's Hospital, Houston, TX, USA

Janet Hess, Dr.P.H. Department of Pediatrics, Morsani College of Medicine, University of South Florida, Tampa, FL, USA

Ellen F. Iverson, M.P.H. Division of Adolescent and Young Adult Medicine, Department of Pediatrics, Keck School of Medicine, University of Southern California and Children's Hospital Los Angeles, Los Angeles, CA, USA

Jill Ann Jarrell, M.D., M.P.H. Section of Pediatric Palliative Care, Department of Pediatrics, Baylor College of Medicine, Texas Children's Hospital, Pavilion for Women, Houston, TX, USA

Marybeth R. Jones, M.D., M.S.Ed. Division of General Pediatrics, University of Rochester Medical Center, Rochester, NY, USA

Tammy I. Kang, M.D., M.S.C.E. Section of Pediatric Palliative Care, Department of Pediatrics, Baylor College of Medicine, Texas Children's Hospital, Pavilion for Women, Houston, TX, USA

David Kanter, M.D., M.B.A., C.P.C. Medical Coding, MEDNAX Services, Inc, Fort Lauderdale, FL, USA

CPT Editorial Panel, American Academy of Pediatrics, Fort Lauderdale, FL, USA

Miriam Kaufman, B.S.N., M.D. Division of Adolescent Medicine, Good 2 Go Transition Program, Hospital for Sick Children, Toronto, ON, Canada

Mary Ellen Kleinhenz, M.D. Department of Medicine, Division of Pulmonary, Critical Care, Allergy and Sleep, Adult Cystic Fibrosis Program, University of California—San Francisco, San Francisco, CA, USA

Alice A. Kuo, M.D., Ph.D. Division of Internal Medicine and Pediatrics, UCLA Department of Medicine, Los Angeles, CA, USA

Jennifer Lail, M.D. Chronic Care, James M. Anderson Center for Health Systems Excellence, Cincinnati Children's Hospital Medical Center, Cincinnati, OH, USA

Complex Care Center, Division of General Pediatrics, Cincinnati, OH, USA

Erica Lawson, M.D. Department of Pediatrics, Division of Rheumatology, University of California, San Francisco, CA, USA

Kristin Liabo, Ph.D. University of Exeter, Exeter, UK

Debra Lotstein, M.D., M.P.H. Department of Anesthesia and Pediatrics, Keck School of Medicine, University of Southern California, Los Angeles, CA, USA

Comfort and Palliative Care Division, Los Angeles, CA, USA

Janet Ma, M.D. Division of Internal Medicine and Pediatrics, UCLA Department of Medicine, Los Angeles, CA, USA

Janet E. McDonagh, M.D. Paediatric and Adolescent Rheumatology, Centre for Musculoskeletal Research, Faculty of Biology, Medicine and Health and NIHR Manchester Musculoskeletal Biomedical Research Unit, University of Manchester, Manchester, UK

Manchester University NHS Trust, Manchester Academic Health Science Centre, Manchester, UK

Margaret A. McManus, M.H.S. The National Alliance to Advance Adolescent Health, Washington, DC, USA

Got Transition, Washington, DC, USA

Teresa Nguyen, M.P.H. Got Transition, Washington, DC, USA

Kitty O'Hare, M.D. Division of General Medicine, Department of Medicine, Brigham and Women's Hospital, Harvard Medical School, Boston, MA, USA

Division of General Pediatrics, Department of Medicine, Boston Children's Hospital, Harvard Medical School, Boston, MA, USA

Megumi J. Okumura, M.D., M.A.S. Departments of Pediatrics and Medicine, Divisions of General Pediatrics and General Internal Medicine, University of California, San Francisco, CA, USA

James Passamano, J.D. Sufian and Passamano, LLP, Houston, TX, USA

Martha Perry, M.D. General Pediatrics and Adolescent Medicine, University of North Carolina at Chapel Hill, Chapel Hill, NC, USA

Laura Pickler, M.D., M.P.H. Family Medicine and Clinical Genetics, University of Colorado, Children's Hospital Colorado, Aurora, CO, USA

Alexandra M. Psihogios, Ph.D. Division of Oncology, The Children's Hospital of Philadelphia, Philadelphia, PA, USA

Brett W. Robbins, M.D. Division of Adolescent Medicine, University of Rochester Medical Center, Rochester, NY, USA

Sophie Rupp, B.A. Department of Public Health Studies, Elon University, Elon, NC, USA

Nathan Samras, M.D., M.P.H. Division of Internal Medicine and Pediatrics, UCLA Department of Medicine, Los Angeles, CA, USA

Kathy Sanabria, M.B.A., P.M.P. American Academy of Pediatrics, Elk Grove, IL, USA

Gregory Sawicki, M.D., M.P.H. Division of Respiratory Diseases, Department of Medicine, Boston Children's Hospital, Harvard Medical School, Boston, MA, USA

Lisa A. Schwartz, Ph.D. Division of Oncology, The Children's Hospital of Philadelphia, Philadelphia, PA, USA

Perelman School of Medicine of the University of Pennsylvania, Philadelphia, PA, USA

Parag Shah, M.D., M.P.H. Chronic Illness Transition Program, Ann and Robert H. Lurie Children's Hospital of Chicago, Chicago, IL, USA

Division of Hospital Based Medicine, Department of Pediatrics, Northwestern University Feinberg School of Medicine, Chicago, IL, USA

Niraj Sharma, M.D., M.P.H. Division of General Medicine, Department of Medicine, Brigham and Women's Hospital, Harvard Medical School, Boston, MA, USA

Division of General Pediatrics, Department of Medicine, Boston Children's Hospital, Harvard Medical School, Boston, MA, USA

Swaran P. Singh, M.B.B.S., M.D., D.M., F.R.C.P. University of Warwick, Coventry, UK

Amy Sopchak, J.D. Sufian and Passamano, LLP, Houston, TX, USA

Claire Stansfield, M.Sc. University College London, London, UK

Beth Sufian, J.D. Sufian and Passamano, LLP, Houston, TX, USA

Gregg Talente, M.D., M.S. Department of Medicine and Pediatrics, University of South Carolina School of Medicine, Columbia, SC, USA

Ahmet Uluer, D.O. Division of Pulmonary Medicine, Department of Medicine, Brigham and Women's Hospital, Harvard Medical School, Boston, MA, USA

Division of Pulmonary Medicine, Department of Medicine, Boston Children's Hospital, Harvard Medical School, Boston, MA, USA

Laura J. Warren Texas Parent to Parent, Austin, TX, USA

Stacey Weinstein, M.D. Division of Internal Medicine and Pediatrics, UCLA Department of Medicine, Los Angeles, CA, USA

Patience H. White, M.D., M.A. Departments of Medicine and Pediatrics, George Washington School of Medicine and Health Sciences, Washington, DC, USA

Got Transition, Washington, DC, USA

Constance M. Wiemann, Ph.D. Section of Adolescent Medicine and Sports Medicine, Department of Pediatrics, Baylor College of Medicine, Texas Children's Hospital, Houston, TX, USA

Roberta G. Williams, M.D. Department of Pediatrics, Keck School of Medicine, University of Southern California and Children's Hospital Los Angeles, Los Angeles, CA, USA

Jason Woodward, M.D., M.S. Cincinnati Children's Hospital Medical Center, Cincinnati, OH, USA

Part I

Introduction

1 Introduction: Historical Perspectives, Current Priorities, and Healthcare Transition Processes, Evidence, and Measurement

Patience H. White and Margaret A. McManus

Health-Care Transition in the United States

Historical Perspectives and Current National Organization Priorities

C. Everett Koop, MD, considered one of the most influential surgeon generals in American history, played a pivotal role in establishing transition as a national priority. In 1989, he convened a surgeon general's conference, "Growing Up and Getting Medical Care: Youth with Special Health Care Needs." In his opening remarks, Dr. Koop noted: "Our transition concerns are not amendable to a quick fix. A basic underlying defect in the system has to do with the lack of a transition protocol for healthy adolescents from pediatric to adult services." [1]. In his closing remarks, Dr. Koop's call to action addressed the need for collaborative efforts to develop transition guidelines for professionals, address financial barriers, and conduct new research.

P. H. White, M.D., M.A. (✉)
Departments of Medicine and Pediatrics, George Washington School of Medicine and Health Sciences, Washington, DC, USA

Got Transition, Washington, DC, USA
e-mail: PWhite@thenationalalliance.org

M. A. McManus, M.H.S.
The National Alliance to Advance Adolescent Health, Washington, DC, USA

Got Transition, Washington, DC, USA

The Maternal and Child Health Bureau (MCHB), under the leadership of Dr. Merle McPherson, was charged with implementing the surgeon general's call to action. A series of state and national efforts were undertaken in the 1990s, including establishing a set of core outcomes for state Title V programs for children with special needs, one of which was on transition: "Youth with special health care needs (YSHCN) will receive the services necessary to make transitions to adult life, including adult health care, work and independence." [2]. Starting in the 1990s and continuing to present time, MCHB has funded a series of special projects and a national center on transition. Also during this time, the National Survey of Children with Special Health Care Needs was funded, with questions for parents of YSHCN about receipt of transition support.

Professional statements on transition were first introduced by the Society of Adolescent Medicine (SAM) in 1993 in response to significant advances in medical science and associated improvement in survival among children with severe chronic illness [3]. A well-cited definition of transition was introduced in SAM's statement: "Transition is defined as the purposeful, planned movement of adolescents and young adults with chronic physical and medical conditions from child-centered to adult-oriented health-care systems." [3]. In addition, four key elements associated with transition success were identified: (1) professional and environmental support for promoting adolescent development of new skills in autonomy and independence, (2) decision-making

A. C. Hergenroeder, C. M. Wiemann (eds.), *Health Care Transition*,
https://doi.org/10.1007/978-3-319-72868-1_1

and consent for adolescents to take on a greater role in their own health care, (3) family support to encourage and support adolescent independence, and (4) professional sensitivity to the psychosocial issues of disability, including shared responsibility between pediatric and adult professionals to assure that care is continuous.

In 2002, the American Academy of Pediatrics (AAP), the American Academy of Family Physicians (AAFP), and the American College of Physicians (ACP) published a consensus statement on health-care transition for young adults with special health-care needs [4]. This policy statement defined six steps needed to "maximize lifelong functioning and potential through the provision of high-quality, developmentally appropriate health care services that continues uninterrupted as the individual moves from adolescence to adulthood." [4]. These steps called for (1) ensuring that all YSHCN have an identified provider with responsibility for transition planning; (2) identifying core transition knowledge and skills as part of physician training and certification; (3) preparing up-to-date medical summaries; (4) developing written transition plans starting at age 14; (5) applying the same guidelines for primary and preventive care for all youth and young adults, including those with special needs; and (6) ensuring access to affordable and continuous health insurance coverage.

Current Health-Care Transition Priorities and National Professional HCT Efforts

Health-care transition is one of the Healthy People 2020 national objectives [5]. Specifically, Healthy People calls for increasing the proportion of YSHCN whose health-care provider has discussed transition planning from pediatric to adult health care. Health-care transition is also an MCHB Title V national performance priority: to increase the proportion of youth with and without special health-care needs who receive the services necessary to make transitions to adult care [6]. As many as 32 state Title V programs have elected to focus on transition as a priority [7]. MCHB continues to support a national resource center on health-care transition, called Got Transition [8], and numerous training and special projects that incorporate health-care transition. The Substance Abuse and Mental Health Services Administration (SAMHSA), too, has established a "Healthy Transitions" grant program, to support state interventions for 16–25-year-olds with serious mental health conditions [9]. In addition, the Centers for Medicare and Medicaid Services (CMS) includes care transitions in its Medicaid health home option for individuals with chronic conditions [10]. Another important national effort is the National Committee on Quality Assurance's patient-centered medical home recognition requirements that incorporate pediatric-to-adult transitions [11]. All of these efforts demonstrate growing national attention on health-care transition.

In 2011, the AAP, AAFP, and ACP released a joint clinical report that, for the first time, went beyond a general statement on transition and offered specific guidance for primary and specialty care on practice-based transition supports using an age-based algorithm for all youth with a component for YSHCN that begins in early adolescence and continues into young adulthood [12]. This clinical report defined six practice-based steps, including (1) discussing an office transition policy with youth and parents, (2) developing a transition plan with youth and parents, (3) reviewing and updating the transition plan and preparing for adult care, (4) increased engagement of youth in self-care and decision-making in preparation for an adult approach to care starting at age 18, (5) incorporating transition planning in chronic care management and addressing age-appropriate transition issues, and (6) ensuring transition completion. Further, the clinical report recommended that transition planning begin between ages 12 and 14 and that transfer out of pediatric care should take place between 18 and 21. Finally, the clinical report emphasized the importance of communication between pediatric and adult providers as well as timely exchange of current medical information. The 2011 clinical report served as the framework and set the stage for the current HCT quality improvement process called the Six Core Elements of Health Care Transition, discussed below [13]. This 2011 clinical report is currently being updated jointly by the AAP, AAFP, and ACP and will likely be released in 2018.

Snapshot of Chronic Conditions in Adolescents and Young Adults in Transition

According to the National Survey of Children's Health, in 2011/2012, an estimated 25% of 12–17-year-olds had a special health need [14]. Comparable special-needs prevalence estimates for the young adult population are not available. Related literature on the chronic condition prevalence rate in the young adult population is at least 30%, with an estimated 5% of this population having a disability that affects their daily functioning [15, 16]. The Institute of Medicine, in their 2014 report on the health of young adults, described young adults as "surprisingly unhealthy" as a result of risky behaviors that peak in this age group, onset of mental health conditions, unintentional injury, substance abuse, and sexually transmitted diseases [16]. The Society of Adolescent Health and Medicine, in its new position statement on young adult health, described this period as one in which "unmet health needs and disparities in access to appropriate care, health status and mortality rates are high." [17].

Recognizing these vulnerabilities and the significance of adolescence and young adulthood in terms of establishing a healthy foundation for adulthood, it is concerning that their utilization of health services is so low. In 2015, 27% of young adults had no usual source of care, and as many as 45% made no doctor visit in the past year. This lack of connection to care, although not as dramatic, is evident with mid-adolescents—8% of 15–18-year-olds were without a source of care, and 25% made no doctor visit compared to 4% of 10–14-year-olds without a source of care and 18% without a doctor visit [18]. Although youth and young adults with chronic conditions have higher utilization rates than those without [18], still there is a sizeable population without access to and regular use of health care. Clearly, the implications of these utilization patterns suggest the urgency of outreach and facilitated access as part of all transition interventions.

Health-Care Transition Needs of Youth and Young Adults

National surveys reveal that the majority of youth with special health-care needs (YSHCN) and young adults are not receiving health-care transition counseling. According to the 2009/10 National Survey of Children with Special Health Care Needs, 60% of YSHCN are not receiving needed transition support [19]. This nationally representative survey measured receipt of transition counseling by using responses to four specific measures and their follow-up questions:

1. Doctors have discussed shift to adult provider, if necessary.
2. Doctors have discussed future health needs, if necessary.
3. Doctors have discussed future insurance needs, if necessary.
4. Caretakers report that the child has usually or always been encouraged to take responsibility for his/her health-care needs.

YSHCN least likely to receive needed transition preparation were male; Hispanic; Black; with low to moderate income; with emotional, behavioral, or developmental conditions; without a medical home; and publicly insured or uninsured [20]. The newest national survey results from the 2016 NSCH survey showed even fewer youth received transition services than previously reported. This new internet survey of parents of youth ages 12 through 17 reported that YSHCN (84%) are not receiving recommended HCT preparation and an even greater proportion of youth without special needs (86% of non-YSHCN) also failed to receive recommended transition preparation. These survey results also reveal major gaps in YSHCN having time alone with their health-care providers during the preventive care visit and in receiving anticipatory guidance related to privacy and consent changes that happen at age 18 as well as the eventual shift to an adult provider. In addition, these data show that about 30% of YSHCN are not actively working with their provider to gain self-care skills [20].

According to the 2007 Survey of Adult Transition and Health, 76% of young adults, aged 19–23, reported not receiving transition counseling services [21]. This national survey sample is of young adults whose parents were interviewed when their youth were 14–17, as part of the 2001 National Survey of Children with Special Health Care Needs. Receipt of transition counseling in this survey used the following three measures:

1. Doctors have discussed how their needs would change with age.
2. Doctors have discussed how to obtain health insurance as an adult.
3. Meeting with adults at school or somewhere else to set goals for what you would do after high school and make a plan to achieve them (called a transition plan).

The main factors associated with not receiving transition counseling were not having a personal doctor or nurse and problems with provider-patient communications.

Table 1.1 Barriers: youth and families' perspectives [22–24]

• Hard to leave long-standing pediatric provider(s)
• Lack of information about transition process
• Difficult to find adult specialty doctors/adult support systems
• Not prepared for adult care
• Lack of communication/coordination between pediatric and adult providers/systems

Table 1.2 Barriers: pediatric and adult clinicians' perspectives [25–31]

• Poor communication and coordination between pediatric and adult providers/systems
• Hard to let go of long-standing relationships
• Low levels of youth/young adults' knowledge of their own health, privacy and consent issues, how to use health care
• Limited adult health system infrastructure support – Inadequate care coordination support – Little information on community resources – Poor access to adult mental health clinicians
• Adult clinicians' lack of knowledge/training in pediatric-onset diseases, young adult health and communication
• Adult clinicians' preference for consultation support from pediatric colleagues
• Little time and low payment for HCT activities

Much has been written about disease-specific barriers experienced by youth, young adult, family, and clinicians (see Tables 1.1 and 1.2) as well as adverse outcomes associated with lack of structured transition support. These barriers are discussed throughout the book, in nearly every chapter, and from a variety of personal, professional, and systems perspectives. Most commonly youth and families are anxious about leaving their long-standing pediatric clinicians, the lack of information regarding the transition process, and poor communication between pediatric and adult clinicians. Pediatric providers express concern about the lack of adult clinicians available and their training in the care of youth with pediatric-onset chronic illnesses. Recent adult provider surveys, however, show that many adult clinicians are interested in learning from their pediatric colleagues and are willing to care for young adults with pediatric-onset diseases if improved communications and infrastructure support can be provided especially for those youth with medically complex diseases [32].

Many studies show the adverse impacts from lack of health-care transition support in terms of medical complications [33, 34], limitations in health and well-being [35, 36], lack of treatment and medication adherence [34, 37], discontinuity of care [38], consumer dissatisfaction [35, 39], and higher emergency room, hospital utilization, and higher costs of care [34, 40, 41]. For example, in a review of transition for youth with diabetes, delayed first appointments in adult care, increased hospitalizations, and worsening A1C levels were seen in the transition period [42]. In studies of transition for youth with HIV, youth had poor medication adherence and worsening disease with lower CD4 counts during transition to adult providers [43]. Other studies report young adults with sickle cell disease transferring from pediatric clinics had increased episodes of pain and higher mortality [44] and youth with transplants had higher rates of rejection and allograft loss immediately following transfer [45].

The Six Core Elements of HCT Quality Improvement Process and Evidence for Structured HCT Interventions

With the 2011 AAP/AAFP/ACP Clinical Report as a framework, a new quality improvement structured transition process, called the Six Core Elements of Health Care Transition, was developed and tested between 2011 and 2013 in learning collaboratives launched in Washington DC, Massachusetts, Colorado, New Hampshire, and Wisconsin (Fig. 1.1). These learning collaboratives utilized the evidence-based quality improvement methodology from the National Initiative for Children's Healthcare Quality and pioneered by the Institute for Healthcare Improvement. This work demonstrated that the Six Core Elements approach and tools were feasible to use in both primary and subspecialty clinical settings and resulted in measurable improvements in the transition process [46].

The Six Core Elements of HCT define the basic components of health-care transition support that any practice, health-care system, transition model, or program can use to develop a successful transition process that includes the three key components of HCT: preparation, transfer, and integration into adult care. Clinicians/systems can choose to implement all or only a few of the core elements, and they can also customize the sample tools to fit their patient population needs and resources. Using a quality improvement process allows flexibility to determine how much support youth will require to attain needed skills related to self-care and health system utilization. Patients with medically complex conditions, developmental disabilities, and mental health conditions will likely require more time and system support. Patients who have more family support and resources, greater self-management skills, or less complex disease will likely require less system support.

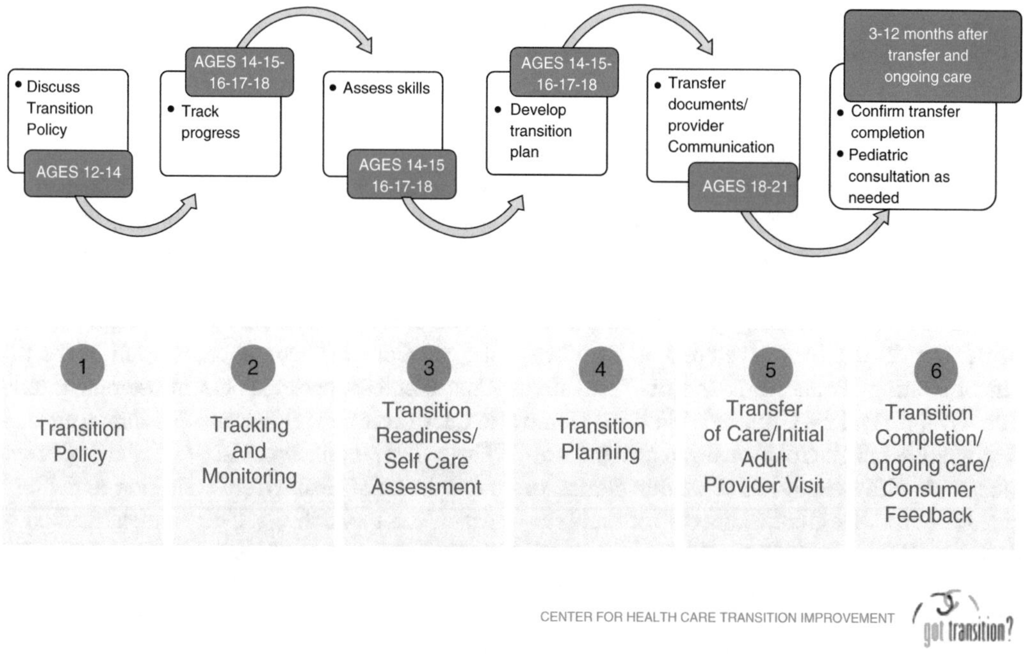

Fig. 1.1 Six Core Elements of Transition-Transitioning Youth to an Adult Health Care Provider Version [8]

The Six Core Elements approach includes packages and sample tools for different settings: (1) for those youth who are leaving a pediatric, med-peds, or family physician practice to move to an adult provider (called "Transitioning Youth to Adult Health Care"), (2) for those who will be transitioning to an adult model of care but not changing providers (called "Transitioning to an Adult Approach to Care without changing providers") for use by family medicine and med-peds providers, and (3) for those who are integrating into an adult practice (called "Integrating Young Adults into Adult Health Care") for use by internal medicine, family medicine, and med-peds providers accepting transfer of young adults. A side-by-side display comparing the three packages can be found at http://gottransition.org/resourceGet.cfm?id=206.

The Six Core Elements quality improvement approach has been successfully customized and utilized in different settings and models of care, including many American College of Physicians subspecialty societies [47], a DC Medicaid-managed care organization [48], and several integrated care systems in both primary and subspecialty care settings, such as Henry Ford Health System, Walter Reed Medical Center, Cleveland Clinic, the University of Rochester Medical System [49], and Kansas City Mercy Children's Hospital (for all their pediatric departments) [50]. Got Transition, with their system partners, published a tip sheet "Starting a Transition Improvement Process Using the Six Core Elements of Health Care Transition" that summarizes the key initial steps for a health-care quality improvement process [51]. Due to requests from many primary care practices, Got Transition developed a tip sheet "Incorporating Pediatric-To-Adult Transition into NCQA Patient-Centered Medical Home Recognition" [52]. Got Transition also has collaborated with school-based health clinics to customize the Six Core Elements for their student population, including utilizing the readiness assessment results for building self-care skills in health education classes [53]. In addition, with a med-peds residency education program that utilized the Six Core Elements and combines quality improvement with improving transition care [54].

In a 2017 systematic review of evaluation studies conducted between 1995 and 2016, Gabriel et al. [55] identified 43 transition studies that found significant positive effects of structured transition interventions. Almost all of these studies examined youth with a single chronic condition. Using the triple aim framework of population health, consumer experience, and costs of care, the authors discovered statistically significant positive outcomes in 28 studies. Positive population health outcomes were most often reported in terms of adherence to care, improved patient-reported health and quality of life, and development of self-care skills. Additional positive outcomes in the systematic review included improved experience of care, increased ambulatory care visits, less time between the last pediatric and initial adult visit, and lower emergency room and hospital use. Many different HCT models were used in these evaluation studies, but descriptive information about these interventions was limited, which precluded associating significant positive outcomes with particular models.

Health-Care Transition Process and Outcome Measurement

An essential part of the transition process is measuring transition performance among individual clinicians/practices and networks/systems in terms of both process and outcome. For example, if one measures implementation progress using the Six Core Elements process, each of the Six Core Elements packages has measurement tools to track transition implementation improvements. There are two options: (1) the "Current Assessment of Health Care Transition Activities," which is a qualitative self-assessment method to determine the level of health-care transition support available, and (2) the "Health Care Transition Process Measurement Tool," which is an objective scoring method for assessing implementation of the Six Core Elements. Each can be completed at the beginning of a quality improvement (QI) process to provide as a baseline and then periodically to assess progress.

A useful framework for measuring outcomes is based on the triple aims of population health, consumer experience, and utilization and costs (see also Chaps. 23, 24, and 25) [56]. To measure population health, several variables can be considered, including self-care skills, adherence to care (e.g., medications and drug blood levels), continuity of care, disease-specific measures (e.g., A1C levels), mortality, and quality of life (QoL) [55]. The latter variable is a difficult indicator of the transition impact because the health-care transition process may be a minor component affecting the young adult's QoL. Consumer experience can be measured with the "Consumer HCT Feedback Survey" that is a part of the Six Core Elements packages. The questions are mainly based on the questions from the National Survey of Children with Special Health Care Needs and the ADAPT survey [57]. There are only a few studies measuring consumer feedback, and many are disease-specific, such as the "Mind the Gap Scale" for youth with arthritis [58]. There is little data from surveys of clinician experience of a structured transition process in the literature. One study used a structured interview format to obtain provider experience with the Six Core Elements approach [46]. To measure utilization and cost, variables include the outpatient, inpatient and emergency room use, time lapse between pediatric and adult health visits, and their associated costs [55]. Other chapters add to the discussion of patient and family experiences and outcomes (see Chaps. 4, 5, 19, 26, 35, and 36).

Health-Care Transition Interventions and Models of Care

As mentioned previously, the 2011 AAP/AAFP/ACP Clinical Report and the Six Core Elements of HCT, which address planning, transfer, and integration into adult care, can be utilized in many different interventions and models of transition care. There is no consensus regarding recommended HCT models, and it is likely that many models of care will be needed to reflect the complexity of the population transitioning with, for example, more support being needed for the more complex youth and young adult population. There are several chapters in this text that provide the reader with current opinions on various transition interventions, models, and measures (see Part IV, Chaps. 9–18; Part VII, Chaps. 26–28; and, Part VIII, Chaps. 35 and 36).

Conclusion

Now is the time to improve the transition from pediatric adult-based care for youth with and without special needs. There is increased need and interest from health-care systems, primary and specialty care practices, hospitals, public health programs, and national organizations. Many transition improvements are being undertaken. The Six Core Elements offer a process that can be successfully adapted and implemented in a variety of settings and models. This introduction has covered the history and current experience around HCT and the latter is covered in greater detail in the following chapters.

References

1. Magrab PR, Millar HEC, editors. Surgeon General's conference: growing up and getting medical care: youth with special health care needs. Jekyll Island, GA: Office of the Surgeon General; 1989.
2. McPherson M, Weissman G, Strickland BB, van Dyck PC, Blumberg SJ, Newacheck PW. Implementing community-based systems of services for children and youths with special health care needs: how well are we doing? Pediatrics. 2004;113:1538–44.
3. Blum RW, Garell D, Hodgman CH, Jorissen TW, Okinow NA, Orr DP, et al. Transition from child-centered to adult health-care systems for adolescents with chronic conditions. A position paper of the Society for Adolescent Medicine. J Adolesc Health. 1993;14:570–6.
4. American Academy of Pediatrics, American Academy of Family Physicians, American College of Physicians-American Society of Internal Medicine. A consensus statement on health care transitions for young adults with special health care needs. Pediatrics. 2002;110:1304–6.

5. HealthyPeople.gov. Disability and Health. https://www.healthypeople.gov/2020/topics-objectives/topic/disability-and-health/objectives. Accessed 29 Jun 2017.
6. Lu MC, Lauver CB, Dykton C, Kogan MD, Lawler MH, Raskin-Ramos L, et al. Transformation of the title V maternal and child health services block grant. Matern Child Health J. 2015;19:927–31.
7. McManus M, Beck D. Transition to adult health care and state title V program directions: a review of 2017 block grant applications. Washington, DC: Got Transition; 2017.
8. Got Transition. Got Transition Home Page. http://www.gottransition.org. Accessed 29 Jun 2017.
9. Substance Abuse and Mental Health Services Administration (SAMHSA). Healthy Transitions Grant Information. https://www.samhsa.gov/nitt-ta/healthy-transitions-grant-information. Accessed 29 Jun 2017.
10. Centers for Medicare & Medicaid Services. Health Homes for Enrollees with Chronic Conditions. www.cms.gov/smdl/downloads/SMD10024.pdf. Accessed 29 Jun 2017.
11. National Committee for Quality Assurance (NCQA). NCQA PMCH Standards and Guidelines. http://www.ncqa.org/programs/recognition/practices/patient-centered-medical-home-pcmh/getting-recognized/documents. Accessed 29 Jun 2017.
12. American Academy of Pediatrics, American Academy of Family Physicians, American College of Physicians, Transitions Clinical Report Authoring Group, Cooley WC, Sagerman PJ. Supporting the health care transition from adolescence to adulthood in the medical home. Pediatrics. 2011;128:182–200.
13. Got Transition. Six Core Elements of Health Care Transition. http://www.gottransition.org/resources/index.cfm. Accessed 29 Jun 2017.
14. Data Resource Center for Child & Adolescent Health. How Many Children in the United States Have Special Health Needs. http://childhealthdata.org/browse/survey. Accessed 29 Jun 2017.
15. Brault MW. Americans with disabilities: 2010. https://www.census.gov/library/publications/2012/demo/p70-131.html. Accessed 29 Jun 2017.
16. Institute of Medicine and National Research Council of the National Academies. Investing in the health and well-being of young adults. Washington, DC: The National Academies Press; 2014.
17. Society for Adolescent Health Medicine (SAHM). Young adult health and well-being: a position statement of the Society for Adolescent Health and Medicine. J Adolesc Health. 2017;60:758–9.
18. Spencer D, McManus M, Thiede Call K, Turner J, Harwood C, White P. Health care coverage and access among children, adolescents, and young adults, 2012–2015: implications for future health reforms. J Adolesc Health. In press.
19. McManus MA, Pollack LR, Cooley WC, McAllister JW, Lotstein D, Strickland B, et al. Current status of transition preparation among youth with special needs in the United States. Pediatrics. 2013;131:1090–7.
20. U.S. Department of Health and Human Services, Health Resources and Services Administration, Maternal and Child Health Bureau. Frequently asked questions: 2016 National Survey of Children's Health. https://mchb.hrsa.gov/data/national-surveys/data-user. Accessed 8 Jan 2018.
21. Sawicki GS, Whitworth R, Gunn L, Butterfield R, Lukens-Bull K, Wood D. Receipt of health care transition counseling in the National Survey of adult transition and health. Pediatrics. 2011;128:e521–9.
22. Bregnballe V, Boisen KA, Schiotz PO, Pressler T, Lomborg K. Flying the Nest: a challenge for young adults with cystic fibrosis and their parents. Patient Prefer Adherence. 2017;11:229–36.
23. Heath G, Farre A, Shaw K. Parenting a child with chronic illness as they transition into adulthood: a systematic review and thematic synthesis of parents' experiences. Patient Educ Couns. 2017;100:76–92.
24. Rutishauser C, Sawyer SM, Ambresin AE. Transition of young people with chronic conditions: a cross-sectional study of patient perceptions before and after transfer from pediatric to adult health care. Eur J Pediatr. 2014;173:1067–74.
25. White P, McManus M, Alblan M, et al. Adult Physician Perspectives on Transition from Pediatric to Adult Health Care. Poster presented at the 16th Annual Chronic Illness and Disability Conference, Houston, TX, October 1–2, 2015.
26. Garvey KC, Wolpert HA, Rhodes ET, Laffel LM, Kleinman K, Beste MG, et al. Health care transition in patients with type 1 diabetes: young adult experiences and relationship to glycemic control. Diabetes Care. 2012;35:1716–22.
27. Nehring WM, Betz CL, Lobo ML. Uncharted territory: systematic review of providers' roles, understanding, and views pertaining to health care transition. J Pediatr Nurs. 2015;30:732–47.
28. Okumura MJ, Kerr EA, Cabana MD, Davis MM, Demonner S, Heisler M. Physician views on barriers to primary care for young adults with childhood-onset chronic disease. Pediatrics. 2010;125:e748–54.
29. Peter NG, Forke CM, Ginsburg KR, Schwarz DF. Transition from pediatric to adult care: internists' perspectives. Pediatrics. 2009;123:417–23.
30. Szalda DE, Jimenez ME, Long JE, Ni A, Shea JA, Jan S. Healthcare system supports for young adult patients with pediatric onset chronic conditions: a qualitative study. J Pediatr Nurs. 2015;30:126–32.
31. Telfair J, Alexander LR, Loosier PS, Alleman-Velez PL, Simmons J. Providers' perspectives and beliefs regarding transition to adult Care for Adolescents with sickle cell disease. J Health Care Poor Underserved. 2004;15:443–61.
32. White P, Cuomo C, Johnson-Hooper T, et al. Adult Provider Willingness to Accept Young Adults into

Their Practice: Results from Three Integrated Delivery Systems. Poster presented at the 17th Annual Chronic Illness and Disability Conference, Houston, TX, October 27–28, 2016.
33. Logan J, Peralta E, Brown K, Moffett M, Advani A, Leech N. Smoothing the transition from paediatric to adult services in Type 1 diabetes. J Diabetes Nurs. 2008;12:328–38.
34. Cadario F, Prodam F, Bellone S, Trada M, Binotti M, Trada M, et al. Transition process of patients with type 1 diabetes (T1dm) from Paediatric to the adult health care service: a hospital-based approach. Clin Endocrinol. 2009;71:346–50.
35. Chaudhry SR, Keaton M, Nasr SZ. Evaluation of a cystic fibrosis transition program from pediatric to adult care. Pediatr Pulmonol. 2013;48:658–65.
36. Maslow G, Adams C, Willis M, Neukirch J, Herts K, Froehlich W, et al. An evaluation of a positive youth development program for adolescents with chronic illness. J Adolesc Health. 2013;52:179–85.
37. Annunziato RA, Baisley MC, Arrato N, Barton C, Henderling F, Arnon R, et al. Strangers headed to a strange land? A pilot study of using a transition coordinator to improve transfer from pediatric to adult services. J Pediatr. 2013;163:1628–33.
38. Wojciechowski EA, Hurtig A, Dorn L. A natural history study of adolescents and young adults with sickle cell disease as they transfer to adult care: a need for case management services. J Pediatr Nurs. 2002;17: 18–27.
39. McDonagh JE, Southwood TR, Shaw KL, British Society of P, Adolescent R. The impact of a coordinated transitional care Programme on adolescents with juvenile idiopathic arthritis. Rheumatology (Oxford). 2007;46:161–8.
40. Gilmer TP, Ojeda VD, Fawley-King K, Larson B, Garcia P. Change in mental health service use after offering youth-specific versus adult programs to transition-age youths. Psychiatr Serv. 2012;63: 592–6.
41. Robertson LP, McDonagh JE, Southwood TR, Shaw KL, British Society of Paediatric Adolescent Rheumatology. Growing up and moving on: a multicentre UK audit of the transfer of adolescents with juvenile idiopathic arthritis from paediatric to adult centred care. Ann Rheum Dis. 2006;65: 74–80.
42. Wafa S, Nakhla M. Improving the transition from pediatric to adult diabetes healthcare: a literature review. Can J Diabetes. 2015;39:520–8.
43. Wiener LS, Kohrt BA, Battles HB, Pao M. The HIV experience: youth identified barriers for transitioning from pediatric to adult care. J Pediatr Psychol. 2011;36:141–54.
44. Majumdar S. The adolescent with sickle cell disease. Adolesc Med State Art Rev. 2013;24:295–306, xv.
45. Lochridge J, Wolff J, Oliva M, O'Sullivan-Oliveira J. Perceptions of solid organ transplant recipients regarding self-care management and transitioning. Pediatr Nurs. 2013;39:81–9.
46. McManus M, White P, Barbour A, Downing B, Hawkins K, Quion N, et al. Pediatric to adult transition: a quality improvement model for primary care. J Adolesc Health. 2015;56:73–8.
47. American College of Physicians. Condition-Specific Tools. https://www.acponline.org/clinical-information/high-value-care/resources-for-clinicians/pediatric-to-adult-care-transitions-initiative/condition-specific-tools. Accessed 29 Jun 2017.
48. McManus M, White P, Pirtle R, Hancock C, Ablan M, Corona-Parra R. Incorporating the six Core elements of health care transition into a Medicaid managed care plan: lessons learned from a pilot project. J Pediatr Nurs. 2015;30:700–13.
49. Jones MR, Robbins BW, Augustine M, Doyle J, Mack-Fogg J, Jones H, et al. Transfer from pediatric to adult endocrinology. Endocr Pract. 2017;23(7):822–30.
50. Hickam T, White P, et al. Implementing a nationally recognized pediatric-to-adult transitional care approach in a major children's hospital. Health Soc Work. 2018. https://doi.org/10.1093/hsw/hlx049/4744462.
51. White P, Cooley WC, McAllister JW. Starting a transition improvement process using the six Core elements of health care transition. Washington, DC: Got Transition; 2015.
52. Harwood C, McManus M, White P. Incorporating pediatric-to-adult transition into NCQA patient-centered medical home recognition. Washington, DC: Got Transition; 2017.
53. White P, Caskin A, Aramburu MG, Harwood C, McManus P. Adapting the Six Core Elements of Health Care Transition for Use in a School-Based Health Clinic and School Health Education. Poster presented at the 18th Annual Chronic Illness and Disability Conference, Houston, TX, October 4–6, 2017.
54. Volertas SD, Rossi-Foulkes R. Using quality improvement in resident education to improve transition care. Pediatr Ann. 2017;46:e203–6.
55. Gabriel P, McManus M, Rogers K, White P. Outcome evidence for structured pediatric to adult health care transition interventions: a systemic review. J Peds. 2017;188:263–269.e15.
56. Prior M, McManus M, White P, Davidson L. Measuring the "triple aim" in transition care: a systematic review. Pediatrics. 2014;134:e1648–61.
57. Sawicki GS, Garvey KC, Toomey SL, Williams KA, Hargraves JL, James T, et al. Preparation for transition to adult care among Medicaid-insured adolescents. Pediatrics. 2017;140(1):e20162768.
58. Shaw KL, Southwood TR, McDonagh JE, British Society of P, Adolescent R. Development and preliminary validation of the 'Mind the gap' scale to assess satisfaction with transitional health care among adolescents with juvenile idiopathic arthritis. Child Care Health Dev. 2007;33:380–8.

Part II

The Adolescent and Young Adult: A Developmental Perspective

The Anatomical, Hormonal and Neurochemical Changes that Occur During Brain Development in Adolescents and Young Adults

2

Allan Colver and Gail Dovey-Pearce

Case Study

At age 17, Jessica Platt was admitted to an adult ward in a UK hospital with an illness requiring admission for some days. She was distressed by the lack of understanding staff appeared to have of her situation. She undertook her own research and wrote a pamphlet. One of its pages is reproduced here; note especially the clarity of the middle paragraph Fig. 2.1.

The full pamphlet and background are available at: https://sites.google.com/site/yph-sig/networking/the-blog/participationinactionteensinhospital. Reprinted with permission from Jessica Platt.

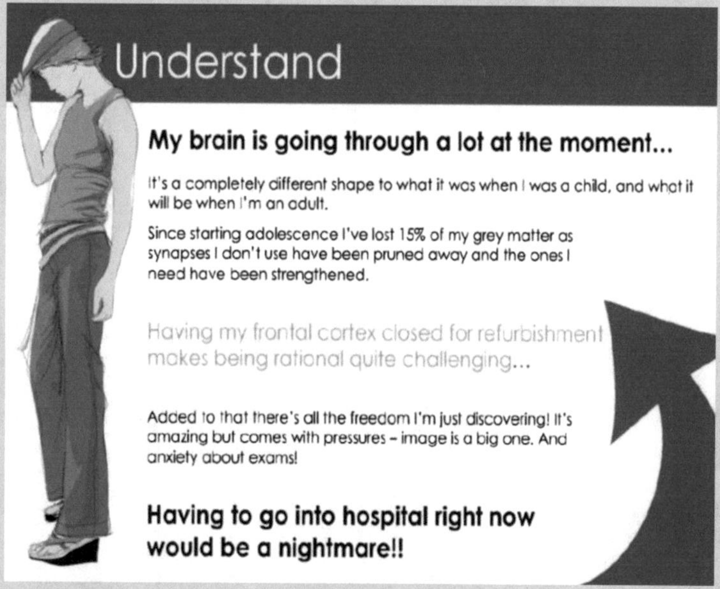

Fig. 2.1 Adolescent Brain Pamphlet

A. Colver, M.A., M.D., M.B.B.S. (✉)
Institute of Health and Society, Newcastle University, Newcastle, UK
e-mail: allan.colver@ncl.ac.uk

G. Dovey-Pearce, D.Clin.Psych.
Northumbria Healthcare NHS Foundation Trust, North Shields, UK

A. C. Hergenroeder, C. M. Wiemann (eds.), *Health Care Transition*,
https://doi.org/10.1007/978-3-319-72868-1_2

Anatomical, Hormonal and Neurochemical Changes

By age 6 years, the brain is at 95% of its peak volume [2]. Total cerebral volume peaks at 14.5 years in males and 11.5 years in females.

Cortical Grey Matter

Grey matter consists of neurones, synapses and unmyelinated axons. In the adolescent brain, there is a gradual increase in grey matter followed by reduction—the so-called inverted U [2, 3]. The sensory and motor regions mature first, followed by the remainder of the cortex, which follows a posterior to anterior loss of grey matter with the last area to change being the superior temporal cortex (Fig. 2.2) [2]. Histological studies, mainly in animals, show that there is a massive synaptic proliferation in the prefrontal area in early adolescence, followed by a plateau phase and subsequent reduction and reorganisation. Longitudinal imaging studies in humans have recently confirmed histological studies. It is the rarely used synaptic connections that are assumed to be pruned, leading to a more efficient and specialised brain [3, 4]. This prefrontal region is the site of executive control of short- and long-term planning, emotional regulation, decision-making, multi-tasking, self-awareness, impulse control and reflective thought (see Table 2.1, below). It is important to realise that when the posterior cortices for vision and sensory-motor control are approaching the end of their inverted U trajectories at about age 10–13 years (i.e. synaptic proliferation stopped some time ago and pruning is almost complete), the prefrontal cortex is still in a state of massive synaptic proliferation.

Table 2.1 Prefrontal cortex functions

The prefrontal cortex is the site of:
• Executive control of short- and long-term planning
• Emotional regulation
• Decision-making
• Multi-tasking
• Self-awareness
• Impulse control
• Reflective thought

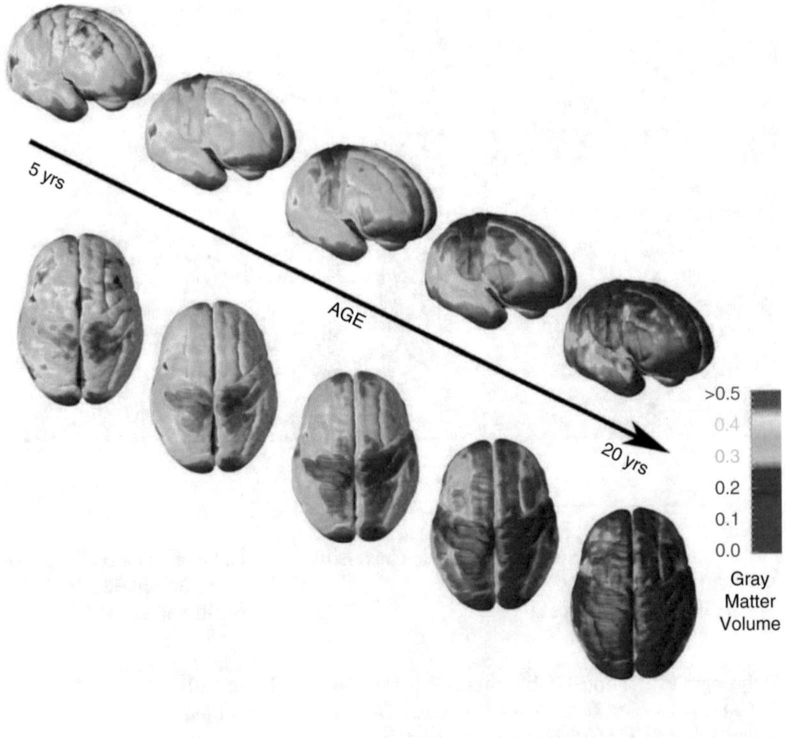

Fig. 2.2 Right lateral and top views of the dynamic sequence of grey matter maturation over the cortical surface. The side bar shows a colour representation in units of grey matter volume. Fifty-two scans from thirteen subjects each scanned four times at approximately 2-year intervals. Reprinted with permission from [2]

Sub-Cortical Grey Matter

The basal ganglia or nuclei are the striatum (caudate nucleus and putamen), ventral striatum (nucleus accumbens), globus pallidus, subthalamic nucleus and substantia nigra. These nuclei are involved in transmission circuits which control movement and higher-order cognitive and emotional functioning. The limbic system, consisting of the hippocampus, amygdala, septic nuclei and limbic lobe, is closely involved in emotional regulation, reward processing, appetite and pleasure seeking.

Due to their small size, accurate visualisation of these regions is more difficult than for cortical grey matter; however, the caudate nucleus follows a similar 'inverted U' shape trajectory and limbic structures develop sooner than the basal ganglia [2].

White Matter

White matter tracts between the prefrontal cortex and subcortical structures develop in a steady but non-linear manner [1], with more rapid development of functional tracts in early adolescence and levelling off in young adulthood. The changes reflect a mixture of ongoing myelination and increased axonal diameter. In contrast to grey matter changes, the white matter increases occur in all lobes of the brain simultaneously [5, 6]. Recent studies, using diffusion tensor imaging, show that this increase in myelination and axon density in white matter tracts between the prefrontal cortex and basal ganglia continues to develop throughout adolescence [1, 7].

Pubertal Hormones

Grey matter changes in the same sequence in boys and girls, but girls' grey matter peaks about 1 year before that of boys [8]. This difference corresponds with pubertal maturity, suggesting brain development and puberty may be interrelated [9]. The behavioural changes of adolescence correspond to the timing of puberty, not chronological age, as do the gender differences in mental health problems such as depression.

Although there are many associations between pubertal hormone levels, behaviours and grey and white matter changes, it is difficult to know if these are causative. Studies need first to control for age, sex and onset of puberty before examining if there are residual associations with pubertal hormone levels. Until recently the causal effects of pubertal hormones on brain structure and function were thought to occur only in the perinatal and late gestation periods; effects in adolescence were thought at most to sensitise certain brain structures. However, recent developments in the field are challenging this view and are reviewed by Schulz [10]. Studies in rodent models suggest there might be a causal link. Studies which involve castration or oophorectomy at various ages and injection of pubertal hormones show that sexually dimorphic (i.e. different in male and female) behaviours are influenced by the presence of pubertal hormones during adolescence, whether these come from the gonad or are administered by injection [10]. Further, there is evidence of sexual dimorphism in aspects of brain structure maturation in the limbic, basal ganglia and frontal cortex systems [10]. Extrapolated to humans, this might indicate the pubertal hormones determine to some extent the patterns of adolescent brain maturation, rather than just facilitating changes generated independently. There is now some evidence for this in humans. Striatal volumes are unrelated to puberty stage or testosterone level, but larger grey matter volumes in the limbic system in both sexes are associated with later stages of puberty and higher levels of circulating testosterone. The sensitivity of the limbic system to testosterone is sexually dimorphic, and this may be responsible for the greater risk of anxiety and depression in girls [11]. There are also associations between white matter microstructure and sex and pubertal level—and a small residual effect of pubertal hormones [12].

Neurotransmitters

Dopamine is the neurotransmitter involved in priming and firing reward-seeking circuits and in reinforcing learning. There are two significant dopaminergic pathways, the mesolimbic from the midbrain to the limbic structures and the mesocortical from the midbrain to the frontal cortex [13]. Both primates and rodents exhibit increases in functionally available dopamine during adolescence as compared to other life periods and the brain's sensitivity to dopamine [14]. Dopamine receptors increase in the striatum and prefrontal cortex in adolescence and then decline, but this is not due to underlying pubertal hormone levels [15]. This elevation of dopamine levels affects the efficiency with which synaptic signalling can regulate behaviour in an adaptive manner. The neuro-circuitry of reward seeking is thought to be determined by dopamine signals received by the nucleus accumbens [14, 16].

Oxytocin is the hormone commonly known for its role in a variety of social behaviours, including social bonding in maternal behaviour and hostility to those outside a person's core social group [17]. Oxytocin can also act as a neurotransmitter and may play an important role during adolescence [18]. Pubertal hormone levels are strongly correlated with oxytocin-mediated neurotransmission in the limbic areas [19, 20] where there is proliferation of oxytocin receptors during adolescence. These changes in oxytocin transmission may explain why adolescents show heightened responses to emotional stimuli in comparison to children and adults [21].

Endocannabinoids are substances produced from within the body that activate cannabinoid receptors. Although endocannabinoids are intercellular signallers, they differ in numerous ways from dopamine. For instance, they use retrograde signalling between neurons. This allows the postsynaptic cell to control its own incoming synaptic traffic. The ultimate effect on transmission depends on the nature of the more conventional anterograde transmission by other neurotransmitters. So, as is often the case when the anterograde excitatory neurotransmitter is dopamine, the retrograde signalling by the endocannabinoids exercises inhibitory modulation. This is a relatively new field of enquiry which is likely to influence how we understand the development of emotional behaviour [22, 23].

Summary

New imaging techniques show unequivocal changes in the white and grey matter of the brain which take place between 11 and 25 years of age and increased dopaminergic activity in the prefrontal cortices, the striatum and limbic system and the pathways linking them. The brain is dynamic, with some areas developing faster and becoming more dominant until other areas catch up. These changes represent a period of 'pruning, re-wiring and insulation' that sees predominant neural circuits surviving and becoming more efficient. This happens first in primary systems (such as motor and sensory) in early adolescence, with executive systems (memory, planning, emotional regulation, decision-making and behavioural inhibition) only maturing in young adulthood. Broadly, changes start in **functional units** of the brain (such as limbic system, basal ganglia, prefrontal cortex) and progress to changes in **functional networks** as white matter steadily increases. Changes in the neurotransmitters and their receptors, especially dopamine, facilitate these processes. The importance of pubertal hormones in brain maturation is still uncertain. These points are summarised in Table 2.2.

Plausible mechanisms link these changes to the cognitive and behavioural features of adolescence. The changing brain may generate abrupt behavioural change with the attendant risks; but it also produces a brain which is flexible and able to respond quickly and imaginatively. Ideally, the young person's immediate environment and wider society set a context that allows adolescent exuberance and creativity to be bounded in relative safety, thus allowing them to experiment and explore the opportunities available to them, in order to develop their sense of self and make decisions about their future. Whilst these changes apply to all young people, there are additional

Table 2.2 The adolescent brain—all you need to know

• It is certain that the brain changes much during adolescence
• The changes continue from 11 to 25 years
• Pubertal hormones are probably not the main determinant of change

challenges for young people with chronic illness and disability in the context of their transition to adulthood, who need to learn to manage their health condition during this dynamic phase of life. Further, their health care providers need to understand how to facilitate this.

References

1. Lebel C, Beaulieu C. Longitudinal development of human brain wiring continues from childhood into adulthood. J Neurosci. 2011;31(30):10937–47.
2. Lenroot RK, Giedd JN. Brain development in children and adolescents: insights from anatomical magnetic resonance imaging. Neurosci Biobehav Rev. 2006;30(6):718–29. PubMed PMID: WOS:000241208800002. English.
3. Casey BJ, Jones RM, Hare TA. The adolescent brain. Ann N Y Acad Sci. 2008;1124:111–26. PubMed PMID: 18400927. Pubmed Central PMCID: 2475802.
4. Giedd JN. The teen brain: insights from neuroimaging. J Adolesc Health. 2008;42(4):335–43.
5. Giedd JN, Castellanos FX, Rajapakse JC, Kaysen D, Vaituzis AC, Vauss YC, et al. Cerebral MRI of human brain development—ages 4–18. Biol Psychiatry. 1995;37:657.
6. Sowell ER, Peterson BS, Thompson PM, Welcome SE, Henkenius AL, Toga AW. Mapping cortical change across the human life span. Nat Neurosci. 2003;6(3):309–15. PubMed PMID: 12548289.
7. Hasan KM, Sankar A, Halphen C, Kramer LA, Brandt ME, Juranek J, et al. Development and organization of the human brain tissue compartments across the lifespan using diffusion tensor imaging. Neuroreport. 2007;18(16):1735–9. PubMed PMID: WOS:000250329300020. English.
8. Giedd JN, Blumenthal J, Jeffries NO, Castellanos FX, Liu H, Zijdenbos A, et al. Brain development during childhood and adolescence: a longitudinal MRI study. Nat Neurosci. 1999;2(10):861–3. PubMed PMID: 10491603.
9. Blakemore SJ, Burnett S, Dahl RE. The role of puberty in the developing adolescent brain. Hum Brain Mapp. 2010;31(6):926–33. PubMed PMID: 20496383. Pubmed Central PMCID: 3410522.
10. Schulz KM, Sisk CL. The organizing actions of adolescent gonadal steroid hormones on brain and behavioral development. Neurosci Biobehav Rev. 2016;70:148–58. PubMed PMID: 27497718. Pubmed Central PMCID: PMC5074860.
11. Neufang S, Specht K, Hausmann M, Gunturkun O, Herpertz-Dahlmann B, Fink GR, et al. Sex differences and the impact of steroid hormones on the developing human brain. Cereb Cortex. 2009;19(2):464–73. PubMed PMID: WOS:000262518800021. English.
12. Herting MM, Maxwell EC, Irvine C, Nagel BJ. The impact of sex, puberty, and hormones on white matter microstructure in adolescents. Cereb Cortex. 2012;22(9):1979–92. PubMed PMID: 22002939. Pubmed Central PMCID: PMC3412439.
13. Wahlstrom D, Collins P, White T, Luciana M. Developmental changes in dopamine neurotransmission in adolescence: behavioral implications and issues in assessment. Brain Cogn. 2010;72(1):146–59. PubMed PMID: 19944514. Pubmed Central PMCID: PMC2815132.
14. Berridge KC, Robinson TE. What is the role of dopamine in reward: hedonic impact, reward learning, or incentive salience? Brain Res Rev. 1998;28(3):309–69. PubMed PMID: WOS:000078202000003. English.
15. Andersen SL, Thompson AP, Krenzel E, Teicher MH. Pubertal changes in gonadal hormones do not underlie adolescent dopamine receptor overproduction. Psychoneuroendocrinology. 2002;27(6):683–91.
16. Braams BR, van Duijvenvoorde AC, Peper JS, Crone EA. Longitudinal changes in adolescent risk-taking: a comprehensive study of neural responses to rewards, pubertal development, and risk-taking behavior. J Neurosci. 2015;35(18):7226–38. PubMed PMID: 25948271.
17. Insel TR, Fernald RD. How the brain processes social information: searching for the social brain. Annu Rev Neurosci. 2004;27:697–722. PubMed PMID: 15217348.
18. Sannino S, Chini B, Grinevich V. Lifespan oxytocin signaling: maturation, flexibility, and stability in newborn, adolescent, and aged brain. Dev Neurobiol. 2017;77(2):158–68. PubMed PMID: 27603523.
19. Chibbar R, Toma JG, Mitchell BF, Miller FD. Regulation of neural oxytocin gene expression by gonadal steroids in pubertal rats. Mol Endocrinol. 1990;4(12):2030–8. PubMed PMID: 2082196.
20. Insel T, Young L, Witt D, Crews D. Gonadal steroids have paradoxical effects on brain oxytocin receptors. J Neuroendocrinol. 1993;27:697–722.
21. Kirsch P, Esslinger C, Chen Q, Mier D, Lis S, Siddhanti S, et al. Oxytocin modulates neural circuitry for social cognition and fear in humans. J Neurosci. 2005;25(49):11489–93. PubMed PMID: 16339042.
22. Lee TT, Gorzalka BB. Evidence for a role of adolescent Endocannabinoid signaling in regulating HPA Axis stress Responsivity and emotional behavior development. Int Rev Neurobiol. 2015;125:49–84. PubMed PMID: 26638764.
23. Vanderschuren LJ, Achterberg EJ, Trezza V. The neurobiology of social play and its rewarding value in rats. Neurosci Biobehav Rev. 2016;70:86–105. PubMed PMID: 27587003. Pubmed Central PMCID: PMC5074863.

The Relationships of Adolescent Behaviours to Adolescent Brain Changes and their Relevance to the Transition of Adolescents and Young Adults with Chronic Illness and Disability

3

Allan Colver and Gail Dovey-Pearce

Introduction

> *I would there were no age between ten and three-and-twenty, or that youth would sleep out the rest; for there is nothing in the between but getting wenches with child, wronging the ancientry, stealing, fighting.*—William Shakespeare: The Winter's Tale

This famous quotation appears to side with the difficulties which adolescents may present, but Shakespeare is sympathetic to adolescents in Romeo and Juliet—his one play that over the centuries has never gone out of fashion. Romeo and Juliet are young, aged 16 and 13 years. Shakespeare looks at them in wonder and love, even as they show typical adolescent behaviours of peer reinforcement, novelty seeking, impulsivity and not looking far ahead. They meet at a party, are attracted to each other, immediately realise their families are enemies but the same night are talking outside Juliet's bedroom and within a few days are married secretly.

A. Colver, M.A., M.D., M.B.B.S. (✉)
Institute of Health and Society, Newcastle University, Newcastle, UK
e-mail: allan.colver@ncl.ac.uk

G. Dovey-Pearce, D.Clin.Psych.
Northumbria Healthcare NHS Foundation Trust, North Shields, UK

The teenage years are marked by certain indisputable biological realities. In terms of the personal and social aspects of adolescence, anthropological and historical research has demonstrated that what it means to be young varies between cultures and over historical periods [1, 2] and what is widely understood as 'normal adolescence' is socially constructed [3]. In current Western societies, we understand adolescents to be steadily acquiring autonomy in all areas of life, shifting their focus from the developmental tasks of childhood, such as friendships and school, to more adult goals, such as career and intimate relationships [4]. With the process influenced by internal and external factors, adolescents commonly explore a variety of experiences and experiment with different behaviours, in order to develop their sense of self and make decisions about their future. In the current economic climate, many people moving through adolescence and on into young adulthood now return or continue to live at home in their 20s; and increased life expectancy may persuade young people to spend more time exploring places, jobs and relationships. As young people pursue college education, career choices, marriage and childbirth later in life, life decisions may be delayed, and role exploration and experimentation continue to the mid-20s. Arnett [5] argues that following adolescence there is a distinct phase of 'emerging

A. C. Hergenroeder, C. M. Wiemann (eds.), *Health Care Transition*,
https://doi.org/10.1007/978-3-319-72868-1_3

adulthood' with its own internal psychological states and external behaviours. Young people do not work their way steadily through a list of tasks [4]; rather they move flexibly between them.

In summary, adolescents need to achieve four developmental tasks:

- Consolidate their identity.
- Achieve independence from their parents.
- Establish adult relationships outside their families.
- Find a vocation.

While some clinicians seek to understand their adolescent patients and can empathise with the challenges they face, others may feel out of their comfort zone, may be upset by their interpretation of what an adolescent has said (or not said) and may even be irritated by adolescents. Understanding how different the adolescent's brain is to their own may help child and adult clinicians relate better to adolescents and thereby promote their health.

It is tempting to 'blame the brain' for behaviours that occur more in adolescence and do not fit with our understanding of what constitutes acceptable child and adult behaviour. However, there is not clear demarcation as behaviours such as risk-taking and novelty seeking are not the sole preserve of young people, and in being open to a wider social network and paying more attention to the perspectives of others, young people can make creative contributions to society.

While focusing on the neurobiological changes of the adolescent brain, this chapter will also consider the social context within which young people in Western societies develop their sense of self and make decisions about their future. We will consider if there is any concordance between these internal processes and the changes occurring in the adolescent brain.

Possible Links Between Adolescent Behaviour and Brain Changes

Evolutionary perspectives suggest that adolescent brain change is needed to prime adaptive behavioural changes during adolescence. For instance, increased sociability may be linked to the search for a reproductive partnership [6]. However, multiple other factors will influence the behavioural, social and psychological changes of adolescence, and few would argue with Lenroot and Giedd that 'Although the brain is the physical substrate for cognition and behavior, relationships between the size of a particular brain area and these functions are rarely straightforward' [7].

The new neurobiological evidence enhances our understanding of how young people are primed to seek new experiences and take risks. The adolescent brain's neurobiological mechanisms provide scaffolding to support young people in their move towards adulthood [4]. However, many other mechanisms dependent on social experience and internal psychological processes are relevant. For example, whether the drive to seek social reward leads to building relationships with new people or inhibitory social anxiety, due to sensitivity to the views of others, will depend upon socially mediated experiences such as how they were parented and internal psychological processes such as personality development and the development of resilience.

Risk-Taking and Novelty Seeking

Novelty seeking is a striking feature of adolescence, and it is hypothesised that it may be an important part of our evolution, contributing to the search for different sources of food and mates [8]. However, novelty seeking also renders adolescents more susceptible to harm. Boys in particular experience higher rates of serious injuries than children or young men in their late 20s [9]. Examples of risky behaviours that can be noted in adolescence, such as experimenting with alcohol and substance use and sexual behaviours, are not due to adolescent ignorance or perceived invincibility as adolescents in fact evaluate risks in the same way as adults, even tending to overestimate risk [10, 11]. As outlined above, developmental theorists suggest that young people need to explore a range of situations, behaviours and experiences, in order to understand the options available to them, consolidate their view of themselves and have an experiential framework that informs their decision-making about their future [4, 5]. The primacy of social feedback is a further driver for novelty seeking and risk-taking behaviour in group situations. Some novelty is presented rather than sought. Opportunities to drive a car or to be excited sexually as a result of pubertal hormones are not available until adolescence. The novelty of these activities is then further heightened by the enhanced dopamine reward system (Chap. 2).

Increased risk-taking in adolescents is associated with the drive to try something new [12] and is thus intertwined with their novelty seeking behaviour. Risk-taking is exaggerated in adolescence, relative to children and adults [13, 14]. Impulse control is largely dependent on the ability to suppress irrelevant thoughts and actions in order to focus on the goal in question, especially when there are appealing distractions [15, 16]. Impulse control improves in an almost linear course with age and is associated with activation of the prefrontal cortex [18]. Why does impulse control not take over to regulate risk-taking in adolescence? Although the frontal cortex continues to develop, a **temporary imbalance** develops during adolescence between the frontal cortex and the basal ganglia and limbic system [19] where neurotransmitter changes promote novelty and reward seeking behaviours. In particular, the nucleus accumbens of the basal ganglia and the amygdala of the limbic system outrun the development of the prefrontal cortex. This results in powerful novelty seeking behaviour and strong emotional responses to social inclusion and exclusion [13, 20].

Changes in dopaminergic activity (Chap. 2) in the subcortical grey matter render the neural circuits hypersensitive to reward and novelty at a time when the prefrontal cortex has not changed sufficiently to deal with this large, sudden subcortical drive. This may not be a steady state; adolescents understand risks well and regulate well much of their behaviour. But they sometimes make poor decisions, often in exciting or stressful situations and especially in the presence of peers—so called hot cognition when the primacy of some thoughts, impulses and potential outcomes dominate others that are available to the adolescent. The increase in activation of the nucleus accumbens and amygdala when making risky choices is more pronounced when emotional information is also being processed [13, 20]. It is important for parents, teachers and clinicians to understand this. Toddler tantrums are now understood, and parents learn to respond calmly, not assigning a motivation or intent to the tantrum. Similarly, for adolescent behaviours which might appear rude or confrontational or irrational, we must try to understand when behaviour might indeed be conscious boundary-pushing or when it might actually be more about the young person's attempts to manage the internal and dynamic changes and challenges as described above. The challenge for the adults is to not assign to the behaviours motivations or intentions that are not there.

Social Behaviour

Adolescents become more sociable, form more complex social relationships and are more sensitive to peer acceptance and rejection than younger children [21, 22]. Adolescents find such peer relationships more rewarding than adults do [23, 24]. It is postulated that there is a 'social brain' (Fig. 3.1) [26]. In order to study parts of the brain that might be associated with understanding other people and making decisions accordingly, functional magnetic resonance imaging (fMRI) has been performed at the same time as young people undertake tasks involving empathy [27], theory of mind [28], facial processing [29, 30] and being influenced by acceptance and rejection of peers [31]. In these tasks, regions of the brain identified (as shown in Fig. 3.1) were much more active in adolescents than in younger children or in 25-year-olds. While some of the tasks, such as jointly attending to something with another person or facial processing, operate from about 4 years of age, they mature further during adolescence. The more complex aspects of social cognition and their associated brain networks continue to develop across adolescence and into early adulthood.

As many of the sites and circuits for social information processing are changing rapidly during the adolescent years, it is postulated

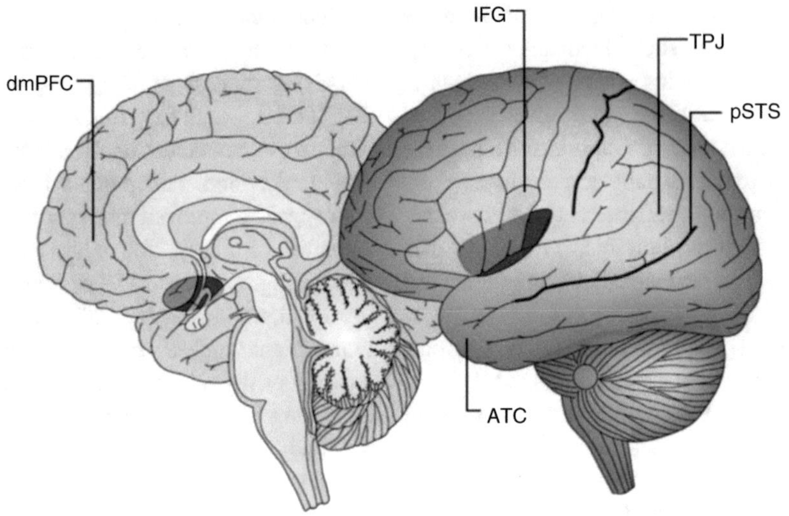

Fig. 3.1 The social brain. Adapted from Blakemore. The dorsal medial prefrontal cortex (dmPFC) and temporoparietal junction (TPJ) are involved in thinking about mental states; the posterior superior temporal sulcus (pSTS) is involved in observing faces and biological motion; the anterior temporal cortex (ATC) is involved in applying social knowledge; and the inferior frontal gyrus (IFG) is involved in understanding the actions and emotions of others. Reprinted by permission from Macmillan Publishers Ltd: Nature Reviews Neuroscience [25], copyright 2008

that adolescence may represent a sensitive period for the long-term organisation of social behaviour [32].

These interactions help develop social skills away from the home environment, but it is not clear how peer approval comes to dominate over other spheres of social approval. Socialising may also have disadvantages, and several studies show adolescents are hypersensitive to peer rejection as compared to children or adults [21]. The ability to regulate the psychological distress caused by social ostracism develops through adolescence into adulthood [33].

Social science and psychology have demonstrated the effects of past stress on social behaviours. Children who were very deprived or abused handle adolescence with much more difficulty. Their behaviours are more extreme and persist longer and are more likely to be bound into a vicious circle of drug or alcohol dependency and more likely to manifest mental illness, anxiety and depression especially. Also such young people are less able to cope with peer rejection. Studies using fMRI show that the quality of parenting influences how the adolescent brain responds to peer feedback in terms of neural circuitry and connectivity: negative parenting attenuates basal ganglia reactivity to peer acceptance, and positive parenting attenuates basal ganglia reactivity to peer rejection [34]. Deprivation and physical abuse in infancy are associated with increased limbic system (amygdala) reactivity in human teenage subjects. Using resting-state fMRI, adolescents with a history of child maltreatment or trauma exhibit weaker connectivity between the amygdala and the prefrontal cortex, corresponding to the weakened responses to peer acceptance such young people demonstrate [34].

Case Study

Clinicians should remember that adolescents themselves are learning about the changes taking place in their brains. They should also remember that most of the students they teach are still in adolescence.

This Vimeo video (which can be viewed on the web) only lasts 3 min but is a powerful account of the insights young people have into their own adolescence. It was made by an adolescent group in London working with a neuroscientist. In the first half of the video, the young man says 'You say to me' and recounts how the adult world views young people. In the second half, the young man says 'I say to you' and presents the alternative account from the young people's world.

https://vimeo.com/68216338

Sleep

Sleep is the period when the brain regenerates and reorganises after the day. Electrical connectivity is converted into synaptic changes and pruning also occurs. This happens during slow-wave sleep, with babies and adolescents showing the greatest amount of slow-wave sleep. The greater slow-wave activity in the adolescent sleep cycle and the need for adequate sleep result from the greater synaptic plasticity of the adolescent brain.

The suprachiasmatic nucleus of the hypothalamus contains an endogenous circadian mechanism that regulates a number of daily rhythms, including the timing of sleep and activity. Even when rested during holiday periods, adolescents show a delay to the start of their sleep cycle as compared to the preadolescent. This delay is associated with pubertal stage but is not due to the influence of pubertal hormones on the circadian rhythm. Thus, young people do naturally need go to bed later.

A recent study [35] suggests that in human adolescents, the amount of sleep over some years is correlated with grey matter volume in the hippocampus. Using diffusion tensor imaging, other investigators found that sleep variability over 3 weeks correlated with white matter integrity. This supports the conclusion that lack of sleep affects learning, memory and emotional responses [36]. Adolescents need more sleep but usually have less sleep than preadolescents, as Fig. 3.2 shows. Few schools have adapted sufficiently to allow adolescents the 9 h of sleep per night they need during the week [17].

Relevance to Healthcare and Transition of Adolescents and Young Adults with Chronic Illness and Disability

This chapter and the previous one point to developmental changes with implications relevant to all adolescent and young adult (AYA) healthcare but especially important for those with chronic illness and disability where there is the need for regular healthcare and transfer of care between paediatric and adult services. Healthcare providers need to get it right for AYA, as their formative experiences of utilising services and building working relationships with healthcare professionals will set the foundation for health decisions and behaviours in

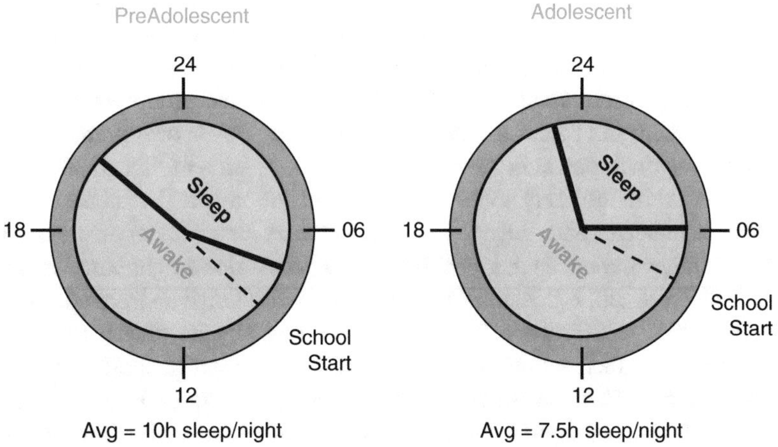

Fig. 3.2 The sleep cycle. Reprinted with permission from [37]

adulthood. Adolescents are learning to value and understand relationships outside of the family. They need, in their hesitating ways, to form relationships and value structures outside the family, and this must happen in healthcare settings. AYA expect staff consistency and civility in order to develop a trusting partnership. They value good communication skills such as being approachable, avoiding problem-saturated talk, asking questions in an easy-to-answer way, shaping the discussion by using analogies in keeping with their interests and acknowledging that they will have their own views and perspectives [38, 39]. It may not come easily to healthcare professionals, but if they are to engage with their adolescent patients, they must employ tactics that adolescents are programmed to value. This does not mean the healthcare professionals should try to be 'cool' and youthful; rather they should be open, use more facial expression and take an interest in the young person as well as their illness.

AYA want healthcare professionals to talk directly to them, even if other people are in the consultation; this requires healthcare professionals to have the skills to manage the agenda of both the young person and the parent/carer, while still keeping to time. It also requires understanding of privacy and confidentiality legislation and guidance so that appropriate boundaries are in place in the consultation. Gradually introducing into the consultation time alone with the adolescent is important, but this should be done responsively. This means that one 14-year-old might prefer a parent in the room for all but a few minutes of individual time, while another 14-year-old might come straight in by themselves. Equally, there will be those in their early 20s who might want their parent in the room.

AYA are more likely to be able to attend to their healthcare and engage with healthcare teams if they have had other positive experiences of looking ahead, articulating their choices and experiencing self-direction. This could be within the context of their schoolwork or their hobbies, for example. Their health and wellbeing decisions will also feel more relevant if considered in this wider context. An example would be considering diabetes self-care with the goal of staying well to attend training sessions and keep a place on the football team, rather than a detailed discussion of national targets for blood glucose control. Thus, healthcare professionals need to be as interested in the other life choices of the young person as in their health goals.

As well as seeking health advice about their condition, AYA need support for other areas of their life with health connotations and might feel unsure about how appropriate this is or how to achieve this with the time pressure of the healthcare consultation. It will improve a young person's ability to ask questions if health professionals open up lines of discussion to indicate that the healthcare professionals are interested in health and wellbeing in the widest sense (sexuality, mental health, weight, exercise, etc.). The HEADSSS (Home, Education, Activity, Drugs, Sex, Suicide, Safety) instrument is useful in this respect [40].

The adolescent brain is more flexible, excitable, original and adjustable than the adult brain and needs to find its own way of incorporating new behaviour, rather than being imposed upon by anxious healthcare professionals. Imposing one's own views of good healthcare on an AYA may produce a defiant reaction and understandable non-compliance. It may also stop the AYA from experimenting with different approaches to their health and healthcare management. Adolescents need graded opportunities for self-management and risk-taking.

Peer support can be very helpful if it validates a decision; but being with peers may also lead to decisions influenced more by the social context and group pressures rather than the young person's own preferences. Given the earlier discussion of 'hot cognition', adolescents should not be asked to make key decisions at times of excitement or stress. Managing one's own condition might come more easily from peer interaction than from educational programmes delivered by healthcare professionals. Some AYA might want support from a peer of their choice (e.g. asking for an accompanying friend to join the consultation). Peer support can also mean support from other AYA using the same healthcare service, and there is mounting evidence to support this, for example, from experience of residential camps for those with diabetes [41, 42] and from promotion of social forums for those with chronic renal problems [43]. However, social reinforcements may work positively for some young people but not for others. Peer support and group-based activities should always be an option for the young person to consider, rather than something with which they have to engage (see Chap. 4).

Finally, there are two organisational factors healthcare professional should consider. First, incorporating training in adolescent health into professional training is essential and does not yet happen routinely in the U.K. or the U.S.A. Good examples of training resources are European training in effective adolescent care and health [44] and National Health Service (NHS) E-learning for Health, adolescent health module [45]. Second, healthcare professionals are well placed to help buffer young people from the potentially overwhelming demands of the healthcare system [46]. Professionals can advocate for young people across an organisation, using recent guidance, to ensure that systems work well to support young people (UK guidance [47] and Australian guidance [48]).

Conclusion to Chaps. 2 and 3

We hope you have found these chapters exciting and informative. Adolescence can be regarded as the most profitable period of life from a socio-evolutionary perspective. Insights from neuroscience help us to understand and appreciate adolescence. However, there is a constant interaction between the brain and behaviour. Behaviours may themselves change the brain just as much as preprogrammed maturation of the brain influences social behaviour.

The neuroscience is still at an early stage of development. Even the algorithms to compute brain volumes and activation of brain regions during resting-state and functional MRIs are the subject of uncertainty and debate. Our theories of regulatory mechanisms within neurocircuits are new and likely to look simplistic 20 years from now. And we know little about how brain injury might influence brain maturation and adaptation in chronic illnesses such as diabetes [49], post head injury [50] or cerebral palsy [51, 52].

References

1. Pollock L. Forgotten children: parent–child relations from 1500 to 1900. Cambridge: Cambridge University Press; 1983.
2. O'Day R. The family and family relationships, 1500–1900: England, France and the United States of America. Basingstoke: Macmillan; 1994.
3. Allen D. 'Just a typical teenager': the social ecology of 'normal adolescence'–insights from diabetes care. Symb Interact. 2012;36:40–59.
4. Roisman GI, Masten AS, Coatsworth JD, Tellegen A. Salient and emerging developmental tasks in the transition to adulthood. Child Dev. 2004;75(1):123–33. PubMed PMID: 15015679. eng.
5. Arnett J. Emerging adulthood. A theory of development from the late teens through the twenties. Am Psychol. 2000;55(5):469–80.
6. Savin-Williams RC, Weisfeld GE. In: Adams GR, Montemayor R, Gullotta TP, editors. An ethological perspective on adolescence. Newbury Park, CA: Sage Publications; 1989.
7. Lenroot RK, Giedd JN. Brain development in children and adolescents: insights from anatomical magnetic resonance imaging. Neurosci Biobehav Rev. 2006;30(6):718–29. PubMed PMID: WOS:000241208800002. English.
8. Kelley AE, Schochet T, Landry CF. Risk taking and novelty seeking in adolescence: introduction to part I. Ann N Y Acad Sci. 2004;1021:27–32. PubMed PMID: 15251871.
9. Steinberg L. A social neuroscience perspective on adolescent risk-taking. Dev Rev. 2008;28(1):78–106. PubMed PMID: 18509515. Pubmed Central PMCID: 2396566.
10. Millstein SG, Halpern-Felsher BL. Perceptions of risk and vulnerability. J Adolesc Health. 2002;31(1 Suppl):10–27. PubMed PMID: 12093608.
11. Reyna VF, Farley R. Risk and rationality in adolescent decision-making: implications for theory, practice, and public policy. Psychol Sci Public Interest. 2006;7:1–44.
12. Steinberg L. Cognitive and affective development in adolescence. Trends Cogn Sci. 2005;9(2):69–74. PubMed PMID: 15668099.
13. Ernst M, Nelson EE, Jazbec S, McClure EB, Monk CS, Leibenluft E, et al. Amygdala and nucleus accumbens in responses to receipt and omission of gains in adults and adolescents. NeuroImage. 2005;25(4):1279–91. PubMed PMID: 15850746.

14. Galvan A, Hare T, Voss H, Glover G, Casey BJ. Risk-taking and the adolescent brain: who is at risk? Dev Sci. 2007;10(2):F8–F14. PubMed PMID: 17286837.
15. Casey BJ, Tottenham N, Fossella J. Clinical, imaging, lesion, and genetic approaches toward a model of cognitive control. Dev Psychobiol. 2002;40(3):237–54. PubMed PMID: 11891636.
16. Cauffman E, Shulman EP, Steinberg L, Claus E, Banich MT, Graham S, et al. Age differences in affective decision making as indexed by performance on the Iowa gambling task. Dev Psychol. 2010;46(1):193–207. PubMed PMID: 20053017.
17. Minges KE, Redeker NS. Delayed school start times and adolescent sleep: a systematic review of the experimental evidence. Sleep Med Rev. 2016;28:86–95. PubMed PMID: 26545246. Pubmed Central PMCID: PMC4844764.
18. Casey B, Trainor R, Orendi J. A developmental functional MRI study of prefrontal activation during performance of a go–no-go task. J Cogn Neurosci. 1997;9:835–47.
19. Casey BJ, Jones RM, Hare TA. The adolescent brain. Ann N Y Acad Sci. 2008;1124:111–26. PubMed PMID: 18400927. Pubmed Central PMCID: 2475802.
20. Monk CS, McClure EB, Nelson EE, Zarahn E, Bilder RM, Leibenluft E, et al. Adolescent immaturity in attention-related brain engagement to emotional facial expressions. NeuroImage. 2003;20(1):420–8. PubMed PMID: 14527602.
21. O'Brien SF, Bierman K. Conceptions and perceived influence of peer groups: interviews with preadolescents and adolescents. Child Dev. 1988;59(5):1360–5. PubMed PMID: 3168646.
22. Kilford EJ, Garrett E, Blakemore SJ. The development of social cognition in adolescence: an integrated perspective. Neurosci Biobehav Rev. 2016;70:106–20. PubMed PMID: 27545755.
23. Spear LP. The adolescent brain and age-related behavioral manifestations. Neurosci Biobehav Rev. 2000;24(4):417–63.
24. Douglas LA, Varlinskaya EI, Spear LP. Rewarding properties of social interactions in adolescent and adult male and female rats: impact of social versus isolate housing of subjects and partners. Dev Psychobiol. 2004;45(3):153–62. PubMed PMID: 15505797.
25. Blakemore SJ. The social brain in adolescence. Nat Rev Neurosci. 2008;9(4):267–77. PubMed PMID: 18354399. PMID: 18354399.
26. Blakemore SJ. Development of the social brain in adolescence. J R Soc Med. 2012;105(3):111–6. PubMed PMID: 22434810.
27. Decety J, Michalska KJ. Neurodevelopmental changes in the circuits underlying empathy and sympathy from childhood to adulthood. Dev Sci. 2010;13(6):886–99. PubMed PMID: 20977559.
28. Burnett S, Sebastian C, Cohen Kadosh K, Blakemore SJ. The social brain in adolescence: evidence from functional magnetic resonance imaging and behavioural studies. Neurosci Biobehav Rev. 2011;35(8):1654–64. PubMed PMID: 21036192.
29. Haxby JV, Hoffman EA, Gobbini MI. Human neural systems for face recognition and social communication. Biol Psychiatry. 2002;51(1):59–67. PubMed PMID: 11801231.
30. Golarai G, Ghahremani DG, Whitfield-Gabrieli S, Reiss A, Eberhardt JL, Gabrieli JD, et al. Differential development of high-level visual cortex correlates with category-specific recognition memory. Nat Neurosci. 2007;10(4):512–22. PubMed PMID: 17351637. Pubmed Central PMCID: 3660101.
31. Sebastian CL, Tan GC, Roiser JP, Viding E, Dumontheil I, Blakemore SJ. Developmental influences on the neural bases of responses to social rejection: implications of social neuroscience for education. NeuroImage. 2011;57(3):686–94. PubMed PMID: 20923708.
32. Blakemore SJ, Mills KL. Is adolescence a sensitive period for sociocultural processing? Annu Rev Psychol. 2014;65:187–207. PubMed PMID: 24016274.
33. Sebastian C, Viding E, Williams KD, Blakemore SJ. Social brain development and the affective consequences of ostracism in adolescence. Brain Cogn. 2010;72(1):134–45. PubMed PMID: WOS:000274128400014. English.
34. Tottenham N, Galvan A. Stress and the adolescent brain: amygdala-prefrontal cortex circuitry and ventral striatum as developmental targets. Neurosci Biobehav Rev. 2016;70:217–27. PubMed PMID: 27473936. Pubmed Central PMCID: PMC5074883.
35. Taki Y, Hashizume H, Thyreau B, Sassa Y, Takeuchi H, Wu K, et al. Sleep duration during weekdays affects hippocampal gray matter volume in healthy children. NeuroImage. 2012;60(1):471–5. PubMed PMID: 22197742.
36. Telzer EH, Goldenberg D, Fuligni AJ, Lieberman MD, Galvan A. Sleep variability in adolescence is associated with altered brain development. Dev Cogn Neurosci. 2015;14:16–22. PubMed PMID: 26093368. Pubmed Central PMCID: PMC4536158.
37. Hummer DL, Lee TM. Daily timing of the adolescent sleep phase: insights from a cross-species comparison. Neurosci Biobehav Rev. 2016;70:171–81. PubMed PMID: 27450579.
38. Lugasi T, Achille M, Stevenson M. Patients' perspective on factors that facilitate transition from child-centered to adult-centered health care: a theory integrated metasummary of quantitative and qualitative studies. J Adolesc Health. 2011;48(5):429–40. PubMed PMID: 21501800. PMID: 21501800.
39. Fegran L, Hall EO, Uhrenfeldt L, Aagaard H, Ludvigsen MS. Adolescents' and young adults' transition experiences when transferring from paediatric to adult care: a qualitative metasynthesis. Int J Nurs Stud. 2014;51(1):123–35. PubMed PMID: 23490470.
40. Modern Medicine Network. HEADSSS 3.0. 2014. http://contemporarypediatrics.modernmedicine.com/resource-center/heeadsss3-0.
41. Wang YC, Stewart S, Tuli E, White P. Improved glycemic control in adolescents with type 1 diabetes

mellitus who attend diabetes camp. Pediatr Diabetes. 2008;9(1):29–34. PubMed PMID: 18211634.
42. Carlson KT, Carlson GW Jr, Tolbert L, Demma LJ. Blood glucose levels in children with type 1 diabetes attending a residential diabetes camp: a 2-year review. Diabet Med. 2013;30(3):e123–6. PubMed PMID: 23157253.
43. Harden PN, Walsh G, Bandler N, Bradley S, Lonsdale D, Taylor J, et al. Bridging the gap: an integrated paediatric to adult clinical service for young adults with kidney failure. BMJ. 2012;344:e3718. PubMed PMID: 22661725.
44. EuTeach. European training in effective adolescent care and health. http://www.unil.ch/euteach/home.html.
45. NHS Health Education England. Adolescent health module E-learning for Health. 2017. http://www.e-lfh.org.uk/home/.
46. Dovey-Pearce G, Hurrell R, May C, Walker C, Doherty Y. Young adults' (16-25 years) suggestions for providing developmentally appropriate diabetes services: a qualitative study. Health Soc Care Community. 2005;13(5):409–19. PubMed PMID: 16048529.
47. Royal College of Paediatrics and Child Health. You're Welcome. 2017. http://www.yphsig.org.uk/resources-1/service_development.
48. The Royal Children's Hospital Melbourne. Engaging with and assessing the adolescent patient. Clinical Practice Guidance. http://www.rch.org.au/clinical-guide/guideline_index/Engaging_with_and_assessing_the_adolescent_patient/.
49. Gaudieri PA, Chen R, Greer TF, Holmes CS. Cognitive function in children with type 1 diabetes: a meta-analysis. Diabetes Care. 2008;31(9):1892–7. PubMed PMID: 18753668. Pubmed Central PMCID: 2518367.
50. Baillargeon A, Lassonde M, Leclerc S, Ellemberg D. Neuropsychological and neurophysiological assessment of sport concussion in children, adolescents and adults. Brain Inj. 2012;26(3):211–20. PubMed PMID: 22372409.
51. Parkes J, White-Koning M, Dickinson HO, Thyen U, Arnaud C, Beckung E, et al. Psychological problems in children with cerebral palsy: a cross-sectional European study. J Child Psychol Psychiatry. 2008;49(4):405–13. PubMed PMID: 18081767.
52. Woolfson L. Family well-being and disabled children: a psychosocial model of disability-related child behaviour problems. Br J Health Psychol. 2004;9(Pt 1):1–13. PubMed PMID: 15006197. PMID: 15006197.

Part III

Personal and Professional Perspectives on Healthcare Transition

4 Healthcare Transition from the AYASHCN's Perspective

Isabel Yuriko Stenzel Byrnes

When an Illness Is Life-Limiting

Looking forward to a future is a prerequisite in health-care transitioning. Transition starts at diagnosis, as parents start to imagine the future. When Ana and I were first diagnosed, my parents began to grieve and cope with fears about our early deaths. My mother expressed feeling overwhelmed by the caregiving burdens and not being able to even imagine how we'd handle this as we grew up. Over time, my parents felt more competent in managing our treatments and focused on ways to control aspects of the illness. Fear of our early deaths diminished, but what remained motivated our family to live a normal and positive life as possible, not knowing how long it would last.

I learned about the possibility of my mortality at 10, when a hospital friend with CF died. The anxiety and fear of dying drove me to do take my health needs seriously, so I could have a future. With much adherence and effort, I outlived my prognosis. This accomplishment fueled my sense of agency.

The most important word for those with life-limiting conditions is *possibility*. I wish someone had talked to me when I was an anxious teenager and told me to believe in all of the possibilities of my life. Yes, dying young was a real possibility. Yet growing up, going to college, falling in love, getting married, getting a lung transplant, and having a career were also all possibilities. I just had to work very, very hard doing my medical treatments and have some hope, grace, and luck.

One of my friends with CF explained our situation as follows:

> *You are planning on taking two trips: one to the North Pole, and one to Hawaii. You have to pack your suitcases to be prepared for both climates. So pack your down jacket and your bikini. In other words, plan your life journey with the possibility of living a full life, and plan your other journey with the possibility of death. We learn to live and cope with challenges imposed by illness with full awareness that "anything could happen."*

This philosophy allowed me to live in both denial and confrontation of my reality. If we prepare to take ownership of our medical care as children and teens, then we will not be caught off guard when we survive. We will be confident in managing our health needs as we pursue adulthood. What a celebration! If, sadly, we do in fact die, we have embraced life with hope and optimism, which enhances the quality of our lives.

HCT as a Normative Event

It is normal for all children to move from preschool to high school as they grow. We become comfortable with a classroom of friends, but inevitably, we move on to the next class and meet new teachers and peers. We say goodbye, gain trust,

I. Y. Stenzel Byrnes, L.C.S.W., M.P.H.
Social Worker and Patient Advocate,
Redwood City, CA, USA
e-mail: isabear27@gmail.com

A. C. Hergenroeder, C. M. Wiemann (eds.), *Health Care Transition*,
https://doi.org/10.1007/978-3-319-72868-1_4

and become settled in the next classroom. It is a normal developmental process, then, for adolescents and young adults with special health-care needs (AYASHCN) to move from a pediatric health-care team, one with whom we feel familiar and comfortable, to an adult care team who can care for our childhood illnesses and also better address adult health care needs. It *is* important for adult patients to see providers trained in adult medicine. A tragic example of this is my sister Ana's extreme gastrointestinal pain that developed in her late 30s. A pediatrician may have attributed this to normal CF issues, but sadly, she was ultimately diagnosed with colon cancer: a curse that seems to afflict older adults with CF.

Parents naturally teach their children to take on more responsibility as they grow; each new task mastered fosters self-esteem. My parents had the wisdom to pair normative developmental tasks with illness-related tasks. For example, when I was old enough to brush my teeth without a reminder, I was old enough to take my pancreatic enzymes at meals by myself. When I was old enough to call a friend on the phone, I was old enough to order my medication. When I was old enough to wash dishes, I was old enough to sterilize my nebulizers. When I was old enough to drive on freeways, I was old enough to drive to medical appointments by myself. With each success, my parents learned to trust me; with each mistake, they learned to supervise a bit more. This is typical for all parenting.

Moving away from home is a normal rite of passage. In high school, like all my friends, my great focus was getting into a good college. Then Ana and I were accepted into a university 400 miles from home. Living away from my parents, then, meant that Ana and I would be completely responsible for our health-care needs. By 18, we had to be prepared.

Promoting Autonomy in Disease Management by Family and Health-Care Providers

Every parent's goal is to raise their child to become self-sufficient, to make smart decisions for their lives, and to be happy. Learning to gain autonomy with a health condition can be an *opportunity* to facilitate growth. AYASHCN have the potential to learn resilient traits such as accelerated maturity, taking responsibility, acceptance of prognosis, gaining control, redefining normality, finding social support, and enhancing problem-solving [1]. These traits can foster success in academics, sports (when appropriate), and hobbies and eventually in a work environment.

Autonomy in disease management is gained gradually, as parents, teachers, friends, and health-care providers all participate in supporting a child's learning. Promoting autonomy starts with the family. It is not unusual for parents to feel protective, guilty, and responsible for their ill child's survival [2]. Without any choice, a parent (usually a mother) becomes a case manager, nurse, and expert in her child's disease. The parent retains the power in the family when it comes to medical care. Sometimes, this mother can struggle to relinquish this power to the patient. I have met a 40-year-old with a congenital heart defect whose mother still put her pills out for her. Recently, a mother of a teenager with CF shared:

I'm so scared that when my son leaves for college, he'll undo all the hard work I've put into raising him to be as healthy as he is, and I'll have no control over him.

When a teen leaves the home, the parents face the loss of a deeply dependent relationship, loss of their role, and loss of purpose. I had friends who became nonadherent in college and their health deteriorated permanently; they had to learn the hard way why treatments were important. Relinquishing control is one of the hardest things a parent of an AYASHCN can do. I met a mother of a CF child who exclaimed to me her epiphany:

I finally realized my daughter was the one with CF, and that I didn't have the disease. It was up to her to learn how to live with her CF. I could do everything I could to manage her CF, but ultimately she's the one who has to manage her CF.

As a young child, I had many opportunities to practice owning my health care. I remember the first time I had to go to the nurses' station to take my pills, around kindergarten. I was self-conscious and angry that I had to be singled out. Eventually, I exerted my autonomy by either skipping these pills or by fourth grade, I packed my own pills in my lunch bag so I could take them myself.

Sleepovers at friends' homes were other opportunities to manage my health needs away from my parents. My mother allowed us to have an active role in the decision-making process: did we want to do our treatment before we went to Jenny's house, or did we want to do our treatment at Jenny's house, with Jenny? By 10 and 12, respectively, my mother sent Ana and me off to spend a week with our grandmothers. My parents sent a letter of instruction to our grandmothers about our treatments and instructed us to "teach" our grandmothers about what we needed for our therapies. My mother packed our pills and told these surrogate parents to make sure we took them. This open communication helped to ensure that all parties were informed about what needed to be done for us to stay healthy.

Another milestone was when I spent the night in the hospital by myself for the first time. I was 5, and my mom said she had to go home to take care of my sister and brother. I remember being terrified. Yet, I learned to use the call button and ask the nurse for the bedpan. Today, many children's hospitals have a bed for a parent in the child's room. The parent provides comfort and familiarity. However, this also sends a message that the child needs a spokesperson and isn't safe alone with only nurses to care for her.

Establishing the habit of adherence was essential to teach autonomy. My parents taught us that treatments were nonnegotiable. When we were 5, my dad told us, "Every treatment you miss is one day less of your life." He drilled into us the importance of choice and consequence. Also, my father installed a battery in our family van, so we could do treatments on the road. Adherence required creativity. As teens, my parents joked that we could get tattoos and piercings, dye our hair, or do anything else to our bodies, but we could not skip our treatments.

My mother became a respiratory therapist when my sister and I were in grade school. As a working mom now, she needed us to help out with housework as well as our own treatments. As twins, Ana and I encouraged each other to be compliant. We'd compete over who could tolerate longer chest percussion or who'd cough up more mucus. During high school, my older brother drove us in the family van to school, and we'd go to the van each lunch break and do a treatment.

Health-care providers also fostered our autonomy. As teens, our pediatrician drew pictures of lung alveoli to describe atelectasis and other disease processes, so we became knowledgeable about our disease. We learned why we needed our treatments and IV antibiotic "tune-ups." Education motivated us.

Ana and I learned to become self-reliant from disappointments as well. While hospitalized, we often pushed the call button when the IV machine was beeping. Unfortunately, sometimes it took over 30 minutes for a nurse to respond. Anxious about clotting my IV, I learned to turn the alarm off and release saline to flush my line. Frustration led to problem-solving and autonomy.

Most AYASHCN do not have a sibling who shares the same health challenges. Ana and I developed an enmeshed relationship, which allowed us to separate from our parents. In an effort to spare our parents from the burden of our care, we started to do chest percussion for each other at age 12. We took charge of our treatments when we moved away to college. When Ana and I were seniors in college, our clinic coordinator started to assign different exam rooms for each of us. At first, we were resistant and angry. The coordinator said we needed to differentiate and learn to speak up for ourselves, without the crutch of the other twin in the room. This was the first step in helping us gain true autonomy from each other.

The Role of Parents

Parents create a family culture, with unspoken or spoken themes [3]. Themes might include empowerment, anger, victimization, blaming, overprotectiveness, or enmeshment. These themes will influence how a child learns to own her illness and how the child ultimately transitions to independence.

In my family, themes such as striving for normalcy, yearning for control, and self-sufficiency helped us develop self-esteem based on what was normal: our studies, our love of nature, creativity, pets, and friends. These "normal" things gave our lives meaning and purpose. They helped to define my identity. My parents had "The Serenity Prayer" framed on the wall at home; they believed in controlling as much as they could around our health and surrendering the rest. We were constantly planning, problem-solving, and strategizing how to maintain our health: from doing up to five treatments a day to researching clinical trials and to asking our doctor for new medical devices. We incorporated treatments into our daily routine: early in the morning, we'd head to our parents' bedroom for therapy, and after dinner we'd lay over their laps in the living room during the nightly news for chest percussion. My father's German and mother's Japanese cultures valued self-sufficiency. When we missed weeks of school, my parents didn't believe in IEPs (Individual Education Plans). They encouraged us to call our friends for the homework assignment, and my father tutored us in math and science.

My parents expressed gratitude that we had so many opportunities and such good medical care to take care of ourselves. My parents believed in "no pain, no gain" and that raising us took sacrifice. Each lunch hour in junior high school, my father would drive 20 minutes to our school parking lot to help us do a treatment. He passed this duty onto my brother when we made it to high school.

And because no family is perfect, my mother was plagued with depression when we were teens, mostly caused by marital distress and our worsening health. She would work, come home, and go to bed. This forced us kids to make dinner, pack our own lunches, and initiate treatments on our own. Inadvertently, she was preparing us to take responsibility. Ultimately, she worked through her depression.

Though my mother experienced anticipatory grief over losing us, some denial guided her to teach us to become self-sufficient. When Ana and I were 12, my mother taught us the tedious task of washing our nebulizers every night. I used to cry and plead for her to do it for me. While it was hard for her to see me upset, she did not give in. She insisted this was a chore that was required when I grew up. This chore expanded to include learning how to clean a toilet, do laundry, and so on, so I could function as a young adult living on my own. I had no privileges as a sick child!

When I left home for college, I remember my father's stern command, "Enjoy your time at Stanford. Remember, first comes health. Then comes your studies. Then comes everything else." My mother's worries led her to call a cystic fibrosis nonprofit agency close to our college to see what kind of support they could offer us. Soon, we were invited to homes of CF families and developed a close-knit community of friends. This relieved my mother's fears tremendously.

Shortly after we arrived at college, we attended a cystic fibrosis specialist for the first time. When the doctor reviewed our lung capacities and BMI, she stated, "I can't believe your parents would send such sick daughters away from home for college!" We were taken aback by her comment but also knew that my parents believed that in some way quality of life was as important as quantity.

My medications were all changed at my new clinic at college. Soon, my parents no longer knew what meds I was on. Throughout my young adult years, when my mother would call us, her questions always focused on health: did we do our treatments, how were we feeling, how much sleep did we get, what medications are helping, and so on. Over the years, I felt my parents didn't really know about *my life*, except that I was alive. I now encourage young parents I meet to ask about their child's interests, friends, and what they did lately, before they ask about health.

As independent as my sister and I were in college, we never fully gained independence from our parents, until we got married or started working. We remained on our parents' insurance under the medically disabled dependent program. My parents would visit when one of us was hospitalized. They helped us financially throughout college and graduate school, because we didn't have the energy to work part time and earn extra income. Every school break, we'd return home and resume having our parents help us with treatments. My parents assured us that they would always be there and that we could even return home if our health worsened. This could be a reality for many AYASHCN.

The Role of Peers/Support Groups

It is normal for adolescents to shift their attachment focus from parents to peers. A transformative event in my life was attending cystic fibrosis summer camp. At 11, I learned there were children like me, all facing the burden of learning how to manage their medical care. At camp, we learned that there were trusted adult counselors who could do treatments for us and supervise our medications. The education at camp helped me gain mastery over my disease. I also saw kids with CF who didn't do their treatments, and over the years those kids didn't return. We held annual memorials for the kids who died the prior year. This reality motivated me more than anything else that in order to survive, I *had* to be adherent. Camp also exposed me to older adults with CF who took their treatments seriously. They became my role models and showed me the positive possibilities for my future.

CF camp taught me how to accept CF as part of who I was. Owning my CF and incorporating CF into my identity helped me speak up for my needs for the rest of my life. If I resisted CF, denied or dismissed it, I could never fully advocate for myself. CF camp made me feel special rather than different. Some good things came out of having this disease. My CF peers helped me let go of shame.

My many months in the hospital exposed me to other sick children who became my friends. I met kids who had diabetes, cancer, kidney disease, and sickle cell anemia. I learned that other kids have to deal with different challenges. But I also saw kids who didn't take care of themselves and overheard many angry lectures from their parents and health-care providers.

Like any teenager, I had a strong need to fit in and belong. While I fit in academically with my healthy peers, my frequent absences, violent coughing episodes, and being a late bloomer made me painfully self-conscious. Yet, my illness became a weeding tool, and I attracted compassionate friends who could understand my medical needs. They asked questions and showed me that I didn't have to waste energy hiding my medication or holding in my cough. Some visited me in the hospital. My friends would help with chest percussion or ward off smokers at the mall. As we entered adulthood, friends expressed gratitude that Ana and I taught them about appreciating life. They helped me practice telling others about my CF and trusting that some people are capable of embracing it. Eventually, I tested this practice with dating and was lucky to find a husband who could handle my health needs and love me for who I am. I have been happily married for 19 years.

In summary, providers can encourage families to get involved with disease communities and camps. Hospitals can provide support groups for families to create a safe place to learn to own the disease. Online peer-to-peer support for digitally minded teens and young adults can be invaluable. Providers can educate children and their parents how to speak openly about their health condition to peers and schools. Positive relationships are healing and life prolonging.

Promoting Self-Efficacy with Treatments

Self-efficacy is the extent or strength of one's belief in one's own ability to complete tasks and reach goals. Self-efficacy begins at a young age. As a child, I discovered that if I didn't take my enzymes, I would have a stomachache. My brother would make fun of the smell in the bathroom. That was enough to instill the habit of taking my enzymes.

As my disease progressed, I was overcome with fear of dying. I developed an anxiety disorder that remained unrecognized and untreated. My parents were emotionally ill-equipped to help me cope. Eventually, I harnessed my anxiety to motivate me to do more treatments religiously. Ultimately, increasing the frequency of treatments helped me stay out of the hospital. I felt empowered that I could "overcome" CF. New antibiotics and medications became available that helped me stay well. Then my drive to keep up with treatments was fueled by the hope that new medications and a cure would be around the corner. We joined a clinical trial as young adults, and this dramatically improved our lung capacity. Clearly, self-efficacy is cultivated when there are positive results from our efforts.

Advice for Parents

Many parents of CF children have asked me when to tell their child about the life-threatening nature of the disease. They fear that if a child learns she can die of the disease, she will lose hope and grow anxious. A child knows innately that their condition is serious. And with today's digital world, it's easy to find out the hard way about a prognosis online. I am an advocate of offering honest, developmentally appropriate information to children. Generalizing human vulnerability by saying, *We all will die someday. That's why I eat healthy and exercise. Just like doing your treatments, taking care of myself will let me be strong for as long as possible.* Offering an outlet for emotions, such as a support group, camp, or therapist, or having family discussions about how the child feels about her disease and her future, is important.

Setting goals and fostering a sense of self-worth will help motivate AYASHCN to live with optimism and hope. Unaddressed depression and anxiety will impact adherence [4]. Including healthy siblings is important, because the prognosis will impact them as well. My brother worried about losing his sisters, told the neighbors we were dying, and turned to drugs and alcohol as a teen to cope. Ultimately, offering supportive resources to AYASHCN to promote resilience is as important as medication itself. With this support, the child will find her own way to learn to regulate her own emotions around the disease.

School

School is the most normal experience of childhood; it exposes kids to academics, sports, music, and clubs that provide the foundation for self-esteem and self-efficacy. My parents encouraged my sister and me to focus on what *was* working. School gave us the chance to be good at something, which allowed our identities to encompass more than just being sick kids. Our teachers encouraged us and praised our academic achievements. Some teachers came to our hospital room to administer tests. Our academic successes played a significant role in helping us feel respected, responsible, and capable of self-efficacy.

There can be a limit to self-efficacy. As our disease progressed, we increased the frequency and duration of our treatments. Sometimes our hands bled from doing hours of chest percussion. When my sister started working at a hospital, she coordinated with a respiratory therapist to give her chest percussion during lunch break. But eventually, the striving to *do more* no longer offered positive outcomes. We felt like failures. My parents' motto rang true: "Do your best, that's all you can do." We finally acknowledged what a cruel disease we had.

Promoting Self-Advocacy

One benefit of having a chronic condition is learning how to express one's thoughts and feelings. This is the underpinning of self-advocacy. As I grew older, I gained body awareness and could read the slightest change in symptoms. I learned to articulate any concerns to my providers. By 15, my doctor met me alone with my sister in the exam room, while my mother waited outside. He would ask what was *really* going on. Of course, we hated to be hospitalized and wished we could pretend all was well. But our clinical numbers (lung function, weight loss) were the evidence. My mother would join at the end of the visit to affirm our reports and express her concerns but only after we had the chance to discuss ours.

By early adulthood, my illness, as well as my health-care providers, taught me how to express basic feelings: "I think, I feel, I need, I want…." This was a breakthrough for me. My mother's Japanese culture taught me to not burden others and to be passive. But this approach would shorten my life. If I didn't speak up for my health needs, no one else would. Even my twin couldn't feel what I was feeling; she couldn't speak up for me.

Self-advocacy starts at an early age. Learning how to tell people the name of your disease and what it affects is a milestone. This empowerment means the child is no longer a victim but an educator and ambassador for her disease. A number of my younger friends with CF did "show and tell" in grade school, sharing about their illness. A vibrating vest has a coolness factor when classmates can try on the device. It takes practice to become accustomed to saying, "I have [this condition] and that's why I need to do [my inhaler before soccer practice]." In some cases, a fundraiser like a walk is an opportunity for kids to speak up to their peers, neighbors, and friends, as a conversation starter about their illness. I remember overcoming my embarrassment and inviting my friends to join a fundraiser called "Bowl for Breath." They enthusiastically joined. Telling others about your illness is a requirement in adulthood, when we need to request accommodation in the workplace, health care, housing, or travel.

Self-advocacy often develops in response to emotions. As a teen, I would get angry when nurses came into my hospital room asking when did we "catch" CF (CF is genetic). One resident said, "You have CF? At your age, you're supposed to be dead!" We faced much ignorance and carried tremendous anger. I felt a strong desire to educate everyone about CF. Fear also fueled my self-advocacy. As a young adult, I was scared of being disliked by my providers. I thought that if I upset them, they wouldn't take good care of me. As a teenager, a nurse was going to inject an antibiotic into my IV line. She dropped the syringe, without the cap on, picked it up, and prepared to insert it into my line. Terrified of infection, I exclaimed, "No! Please get another needle!" I made the nurse upset, but my fear fueled my outspokenness. Similarly, I was terrified of multiple needle sticks when the nurse had to start an IV. It took time to learn to be assertive to tell the nurse what vein to use.

This advocacy continued in college, when we visited the Disabled Students Services office. It was a relief that our college offered accommodations. Ana and I asked to room together, and for a private bathroom in the dorm room, to avoid infections. We overcame shame and joined the Disabled Students Speaker's Bureau to educate students about living with a serious illness. As much as we wanted to be normal, having CF was *not* normal, and we had to accept this and advocate for special services.

Readiness to Transition

All children have their own pace in transitioning. I do not believe there should be an absolute age for transitioning, such as 21 years. Factors that may impact transitioning include emotional maturity, intellectual functioning, disease awareness and acceptance, family dynamics, and self-esteem. I've met 25-year-olds with CF who would rather play video games than do their treatments; and I've met 16-year-olds with CF who are fully independent, take their high school equivalency test, and start working. Culture matters too; my parents came from countries where children earned independence at a younger age than in America. In Japan, it is not uncommon for 6-year-olds to take the train by themselves. So, by 8, my mother encouraged us to walk to school, to take the bus, and to learn how to manage our medication at school by ourselves. And because of my mother's accent and English difficulties, she asked us to speak up for ourselves and for her at a young age.

Socioeconomic status (SES) can ease the transition to independence. Ana and I were privileged; at 18, my uncle bought Ana and me a car to share. This gave us the freedom to go to the doctor by ourselves. SES can impact going away for college. AYASHCN may have to continue living with their parent for longer than their healthy peers. Some CF friends had to return home after college because of inability to work full time. Medical expenses can impose significant financial burden for many AYASHCN. It's important to recognize that "success" as an AYASHCN does not mean true independence from family members. AYASHCN should always be validated, encouraged, and praised for any incremental steps toward self-reliance.

The physical condition of the patient impacts the ability to transition. It can be difficult when a parent sends a sick teen away to college, and their health deteriorates significantly. I have lost several friends to CF during college. The parents were racked with guilt for letting their child go despite severe illness. Over time, they could make peace with the fact that they allowed their child to pursue their dreams, despite the outcome, and the young adult truly lived.

When my sister was 24, we were encouraged to see an adult provider. At this time, her lung capacity was roughly 25% and she was evaluated for a lung transplant. She felt abandoned by her pediatric team, and by sending her off to an inexperienced adult pulmonologist, she shared, "They were giving up on me." It would've been more appropriate to wait until after her transplant to transition to an adult provider or transition earlier like age 21 when her health was still stable. It is not appropriate to transition a patient when they are in crisis.

Addressing Mental Health, Substance Use, and Reproductive Health Issues

I appreciated having *normal* teen and young adult issues addressed by my providers. I hated when they only cared about my chest! My illness impacted me physically and emotionally, so having providers who took my mental health seriously was important to me.

My mental health was not addressed by my pediatrician, though he provided words of encouragement and a caring presence. The inpatient social worker spent the time to ask Ana and I how we were coping with our illness. We opened up to her, more than to our parents. She helped us see that we could hate CF but didn't have to hate ourselves. Our social worker also counseled my mother through her depression, and I was glad my mom was getting support. Much later, I learned that the number one predictor of a child's coping with their illness is the coping skills of the parents [5].

After college, the social worker continued to be our primary mental health resource. It helped to learn how certain medications worsened anxiety and tools to cope with anxiety. When my sister reached end stage and needed a transplant, I grieved losing her as a sister and caregiver—along with my own declining health. Both of us cried at nearly every clinic visit. My doctor prescribed an antidepressant in my late 20s. There was no stigma; most of my CF (and many non-CF) peers were using antidepressants. And my social worker suggested I see a psychotherapist. Writing a memoir became a therapeutic outlet as well.

My peers with CF impacted my mental health significantly. They taught me to *be stronger than your illness*. They taught me the motto, *Do your 'I hates' first.* Endure what's uncomfortable, so you feel accomplished afterward. However, the cost of belonging was witnessing numerous losses. One after another, our CF friends died. The grief exacerbated my anxiety and depression.

Rebellion is one way to deal with the intense emotions associated with illness. Rebellion can lead to self-loathing, unreasonable anger at others, and nonadherence. Providers can help AYASHCN find healthy ways to rebel against their situations. What helped me was the use of profanity and body art, expressing myself in art and writing, my spirituality, complaining to people closest to me, and directing my frustrations toward healthy distractions.

It was part of a routine psychosocial assessment to ask about use of drugs, alcohol, smoking, or other rebellious behaviors. My providers made no assumptions about how I looked or what I was like and asked about these behaviors. My providers educated me on the dangers of alcohol interacting with some medication. I witnessed plenty of substance use in my CF peers. I never got involved in drinking, smoking, or drugs, because I valued an intact mind and didn't have the luxury of experimenting with anything that hurt my body. For some, getting drunk was a way to escape CF, at least for a bit. Their friends used substances, so they wanted to fit in. Soon, these behaviors became a habit. And for some, their habits shortened their life or made them ineligible for transplantation.

Since I was a teenager, my providers also assessed my sexual development and activity. Since I had no development until my late teen years, I wasn't shown the embarrassing Tanner stage pictures until I was around 17. I had terrible body image and couldn't imagine anyone wanting to date me. I was 22 when I met my first boyfriend. I was put on birth control shortly after I started dating, to regulate my periods, but also for other benefits! Right after my wedding to this boyfriend, I lost my parents' insurance and was now on my husband's insurance. The first thing my new adult doctor asked about was whether I was planning to get pregnant. He then told me that pregnancy could exacerbate my lung condition, so I (and my husband) accepted that we'd be childless. In sum, it's important to not make any assumptions about AYASHCN. It is a myth in the health-care world that young people with serious health issues are asexual. I knew a friend with 11% lung capacity who was still having sex! Sexuality is an outlet for pleasure and a way to befriend even an ill body.

Finding an Adult Provider

Access to competent adult providers is critical for all AYASHCN. My sister and I were part of the early generation where adult CF care providers were not yet established. We visited and fired a number of adult providers who, while well-intentioned, did not have training on how to care for us. Several said CF patients are knowledgeable and can tell them what they needed. True for me, but I still needed a doctor.

The week we drove to college for freshmen orientation, my mother joined us to visit a local adult pulmonologist. This doctor introduced herself by asking, "So, how can I help you?" We were turned off by her lack of acknowledgment that we had long medical history and required significant medical guidance. This clinic was not a Cystic Fibrosis Center, accredited by the Cystic Fibrosis Foundation. This adult pulmonologist had not heard of the national CF conference for providers. I found a reliable pediatric care team much farther away and stayed with them through college until my mid-20s.

This pediatric team developed an "adult program" incrementally. Initially, the core pediatric team joined one adult pulmonologist. This gradual transition offered the familiarity of my pediatric team with the introduction of a new adult pulmonologist. The team reassured Ana and me that this doctor was competent. By then, I was the expert of my own body. But I was struggling with new issues like bowel obstructions, diabetes, and massive hemoptysis and was scared. I needed someone who could care for increasingly complicated disease.

Part of my gradual transition meant that when I needed to be hospitalized, I was admitted to the adult hospital. This is when I missed the pediatric nurses the most; they were friendlier than the adult providers. Hand-holding didn't exist in the big adult hospital. Over time, both CF care teams worked hard to train the staff to provide the kind of care that CF patients were used to in the pediatric system. Even adult gynecologists, endocrinologists, gastroenterologists, lab technicians, RTs and PTs, and primary care doctors were trained to care for CF adults.

It took almost a decade after I moved to college to find a fully functional CF adult care team. My pediatric team coordinated the transfer of care so the adult team knew my history before I showed up at clinic. I appreciated having an adult-trained nurse, social worker, nutritionist, respiratory therapist, and internist/pulmonologist devoted to all of my care needs. The entire team attended the national CF conference, making me feel confident that they knew what they were doing. But working with young adults within a family system took practice. Family boundaries are important for adults. One of my CF friends in college shared that her adult doctor called her mother back home to see if this student was taking her medication, since her lung capacity was declining. My friend angrily confronted this doctor. It's important that providers treat their patients as adults and respect their confidentiality unless explicit permission was given to share their health information with their parents.

Nowadays, there are more systematic processes for transitioning. At specific ages, young patients are educated in advance about transition goals and are expected to meet those goals [6]. Young adults are introduced to their adult providers ahead of transition, with the familiar pediatric team present. This meet-and-greet opportunity breaks the ice and gives the patient a chance to interview the provider and get a sense of their personality and expertise.

Terminating the Relationship with the Pediatrician

Saying goodbye is one of life's most normal and yet difficult rituals. Termination with our pediatrician happened organically, when we moved away for college. For a year or two, during school break we'd return to our pediatrician for a "tune-up." Gradually, Kaiser developed a coordinated CF Center, and we were transferred to the new program. We kept in touch with Christmas cards until my pediatrician died 3 years ago. I never imagined I'd outlive him. I will never forget how my pediatrician encouraged Ana and me to lead a normal life and apply for college, despite our advanced disease. He told us, "Follow your dreams." I will forever be grateful for his blessing.

The pediatric team who cared for Ana and me during our young adult years became a family we never wanted but learned to love. They witnessed the toughest years of end-stage disease, supporting us through many tears and triumphs. They saw my sister through her transplant.

When it came time for my transplant, I had already transferred to the adult team. I deteriorated into respiratory failure and was intubated. No one was sure if lungs would become available. I was touched to hear later that my pediatric team came to my bedside, while I was sedated, to say goodbye. They *really* cared. And then, when lungs were offered and I survived, they all returned to celebrate with me.

In summary, one piece of wisdom I've learned in 45 years is to question the American value of "independence." An AYASHCN will feel like a failure if she can never achieve the desired independence. But no human being is truly independent. We are all *interdependent*. It really does take a village to raise a young person, especially an AYASHCN. From parents to teachers, to counselors, to friends, to an illness community, and to the pediatric and adult care teams, all work together to guide and encourage self-management in the young patient. The goal of transitioning should not be independence, but developmentally appropriate self-management of health-care needs. AYASHCAN should be encouraged to find ways to feel satisfied with a sense of independence within a dependent situation with peers, partners, and, in some cases, still parents. No matter what, leaving a pediatric care team is a coming of age experience and a cause for celebration. This transition is part of a success story.

Isabel dedicates this chapter to the memory of her twin Anabel Stenzel, whose reciprocal caregiving allowed her to transition and survive to middle age, while sharing an extraordinary life. For more about the Stenzel twins' story, see The Power of Two: A Twin Triumph over Cystic Fibrosis (Missouri, 2014) and their documentary film, www.thepoweroftwomovie.com.

References

1. Jamieson N, Fitzgerald D, Singh-Grewal D, et al. Children's experiences of cystic fibrosis: a systematic review of qualitative studies. Pediatrics. 2014;133:1683–97. https://doi.org/10.1542/peds.2014-0009.
2. Pelentsov LJ, Laws TA, Esterman AJ. The supportive care needs of parents caring for a child with a rare disease: a scoping review. Disabil Health J. 2015;8:475–91. https://doi.org/10.1016/j.dhjo.2015.03.009.
3. Fogarty JA. The grieving child: comprehensive treatment and intervention strategies. Tucson, AZ: The American Academy of Bereavement, Carondelet Health Care; 1988.
4. Smith B, Modi A, Quittner A, Wood B. Depressive symptoms in children with cystic fibrosis and parents and its effects on adherence to airway clearance. Pediatr Pulmonol. 2010;45:756–63.
5. Quittner AL, Goldbeck L, Abbott J, et al. Prevalence of depression and anxiety in patients with cystic fibrosis and parent caregivers: results of the international depression epidemiological study across nine countries. Thorax. 2014;69:1090–7.
6. Towns SJ, Bell SC. Transition of adolescents with cystic fibrosis from paediatric to adult care. Clin Respir J. 2011;5:64–75. https://doi.org/10.1111/j.1752-699X.2010.00226.x.

5 Healthcare Transition from the Family Perspective

Laura G. Buckner

Hearing About Health Care Transition (HCT)

Many family members report first learning about HCT when their child becomes "of age."

Vignette

18-year-old Amanda and her mother, Leslie, come for Amanda's annual checkup. The office is a multi-specialty clinic, and Amanda has been receiving services there with several providers for most of her childhood and adolescence. After so many years of these regular visits, mother and daughter enjoy comfortable relationships with the doctors, nurses, and support staff and converse easily with them as they move through Amanda's routine appointments. Upon completion of her annual checkup, Amanda and her mother approach the front desk to set up Amanda's next appointment. There they are told Amanda has aged out: this was her last appointment.

Leslie is surprised but recovers quickly and says, "Oh, OK. Who do we need to see from now on?" She is met by blank looks. Leslie is an experienced mom who has encountered many medical concerns with her daughter, and she faces those blank looks with great aplomb. It's only later, after consulting by phone with Amanda's primary clinic physician, she is dismayed and panicked to learn there is no recommendation for Amanda's healthcare transition. The situation becomes more serious when they are unable to get new prescriptions for Amanda's medications because they do not yet have an adult provider for Amanda. Leslie posts a message to an online support group for advice and learns many other families are reporting similar experiences. Few can offer any helpful advice.

Leslie reaches out to her personal networks and finds a primary care physician willing to take Amanda into her practice, despite her lack of knowledge or experience with Amanda's conditions. It takes months to find

L. G. Buckner, M.Ed., L.P.C.
Texas Center for Disability Studies, The University of Texas, Austin, TX, USA
e-mail: Laura.buckner@utexas.edu

A. C. Hergenroeder, C. M. Wiemann (eds.), *Health Care Transition*,
https://doi.org/10.1007/978-3-319-72868-1_5

and establish relationships with the specialists Amanda requires. The applications for Social Security and vocational rehabilitation services stall. A medical emergency in the midst of this lengthy transition could be devastating. Amanda and her parents experience tremendous anxiety in the interim.

The pediatric provider is troubled when Leslie calls and asks, "Why didn't you tell us she would have to leave your clinic at the age of 18?" The reality, as the pediatric provider knows, is there are no adult providers with the knowledge, skill set, and willingness to accept young adults with childhood-onset conditions that she is aware of. The pediatrician realizes it's time to develop an intentional process of preparing patients and their families for HCT.

Why HCT Is Important

The transition from pediatric to adult-based healthcare seems simple, from the eyes of the parent whose child has no significant healthcare issues. Initially, the typically developing and healthy young adult might obtain healthcare through the college health clinic, an urgent care clinic, or the emergency room. They likely begin engaging adult healthcare providers as the need emerges; for example, a young woman needing birth control might select a gynecologist. These adult patients make their medical decisions and maintain the privacy of those decisions. Typically developing young adults and their families often address the transition to adult-based care as the need arises. Teaching them to take on the responsibilities of setting and keeping appointments, asking questions, managing prescription medications, and taking care of any annual medical exams is a natural and collaborative experience.

But for adolescents and young adults with special healthcare needs (AYASHCN), the transition is not simple. A well-planned and well-executed transition to adult-based care is essential. The disease or disorder already compromises their health and places them at increased risk of developing more significant health concerns in adulthood. That risk rises dramatically when knowledgeable adult providers are not available. For many such patients, the family is faced with replacing many pediatric specialists, a daunting and—for some—near impossible process.

Vignette

Gabe's mom, Cristin Lind, struggled to explain this complicated network and came up with "Gabe's Care Map©" (see Fig. 5.1) [1]. She shared it with a group of primary care physicians and says, "They got it." There was a multitude of providers and organizations involved in Gabe's life, and his family was juggling them all! In 2012, the Huffington Post published an article about Gabe's Care Map, and Cristin's simple attempt to explain the complexity of her son's support needs took on a life of its own. Today, Ms. Lind and her pediatrician are further developing the practice of care mapping. More information is on Ms. Lind's website (https://durgastoolbox.com/caremapping/). Care mapping can be a useful tool in the transition process for families, young adults, and their providers.

Transition isn't a new concept, and it occurs elsewhere besides the healthcare system. Federal special education law requires public schools to address a student's transition from public school during the student's annual Individualized Education Program (IEP) meetings. The transition planning must begin before the age of 16 (some states begin as early as age 14). Remarkably, many families

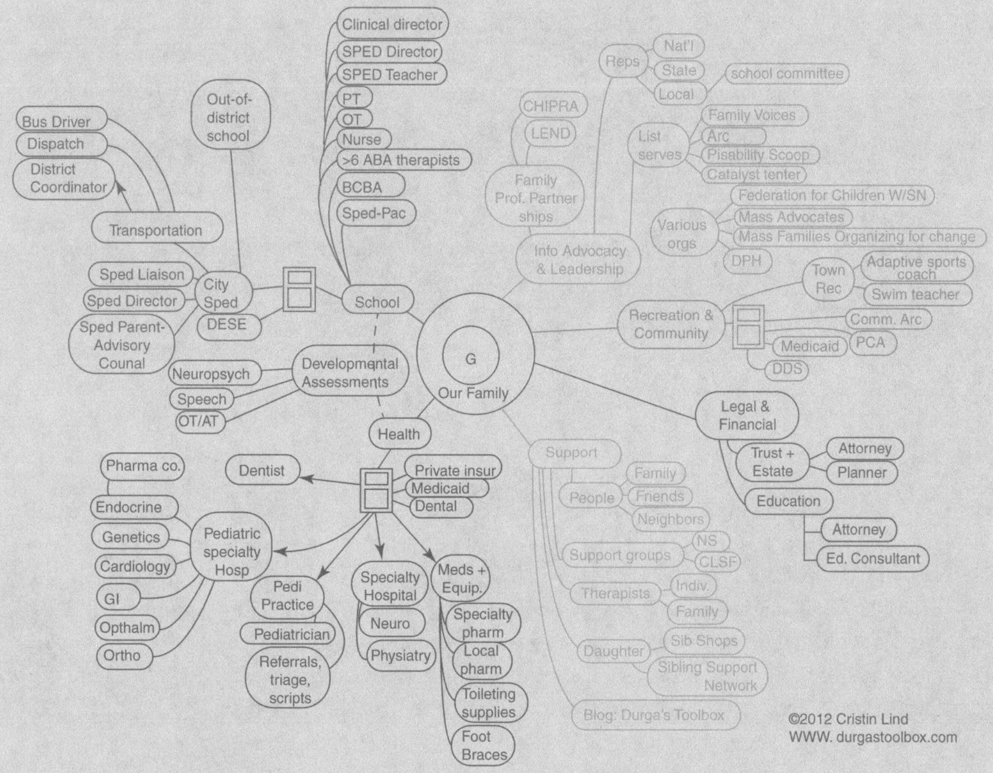

Fig. 5.1 Gabe's Care Map

are uninformed about the next steps when their student ages out of special education services (somewhere between the ages of 18 and 22, depending on the IEP). How can they be so unprepared? Explanations include families are overwhelmed by the daily needs of their loved one, the network of services and providers they are managing, and fears for their child's future. Families are trying to survive, to get through today. The necessary preparations for the future end up on their back burners, until the day arrives and no preparations are in place. They have reached the cliff.

As unprepared as families often are for the transition from public school services, they are equally unprepared for the changes occurring as their young adult transitions from pediatric to adult-based healthcare. Parents think doctors will prepare us parents and lead the way. We don't know to initiate the conversation about the transition, and even if we did, we are too terrified to ask. We count on our providers to guide and support us through.

Families address multiple transitions simultaneously for their AYASHCN, listed in Table 5.1, below.

While some young adults will experience changes in their healthcare at age 18, changes can occur again at the age of 21–22. For some, they will no longer be able to receive services at their pediatric hospital. Depending on the state's Medicaid system, some Medicaid benefits become limited after the age of 21. Consider Norah, who needed her wisdom teeth removed at the age of 22. Norah was receiving Medicaid care, which had always been sufficient for her needs. They were dismayed to learn Norah's Medicaid benefits excluded dental care at the age of 22. Had they removed her wisdom teeth before her 22nd birthday, Medicaid would have covered the costs.

Table 5.1 Multiple transitions that families are undergoing during HCT

• Departing public school special education services (an entitlement)
• Applying for state vocational rehabilitation services (eligibility-based)
• Applying for Medicaid (eligibility-based) (see Chaps. 8 and 25)
• Researching and meeting new health insurance eligibility requirements (see Chap. 8)
• Dealing with managed care, PPO, or HMO (finding approved providers, checking the prescription formulary, etc.)
• Filing an initial application (or redetermination) for the Social Security Administration's supplemental security income (eligibility-based) (see Chap. 8)
• Addressing legal protections (possible guardianship, medical power of attorney, supported decision-making, HIPAA release, living will) (see Chap. 30)
• Obtaining long-term services and supports for those with significant support needs (eligibility-based and often wait-listed, sometimes for years)

We want these AYASHCN to manage their own healthcare to the greatest extent possible. But building self-management skills takes time. Developmental readiness must be considered. For example, adolescence probably isn't the best time to suddenly turn over medication management. A measured, methodical approach to teaching self-management skills, as the patient is ready, is vital. Helping parents understand what they can do to assist in the process is invaluable.

Transition planning is a process, not an event. Good transition planning—in the school, the home, and the doctor's office—requires significant time, intentional planning, development of self-management and self-advocacy skills, and clear, honest communication. Without it, AYASHCN can face potentially dire consequences to their health and well-being.

Special Considerations for AYASHCN with Cognitive Delay

Patients with intellectual disabilities are going to require more time and preparation on the part of the medical team and the family. Understanding how the individual communicates, what kinds of support they need in the medical environment, and ways to ease anxieties goes a long way toward a successful clinic visit. Are there specific parts of an exam that are troublesome for the patient? What helps? How can the practice accommodate those needs? For patients who don't use words, what do their behaviors communicate? Some families are prepared to provide this information; others may need prompting questions or conversations to help the healthcare provider uncover these details. Taking the time to discover those details is crucial to the eventual transition to adult-based healthcare (see Chaps 17, 22, and 32).

Presume competence! We may never know what some individuals with intellectual disabilities understand due to their inability to express themselves verbally. The provider may need to look to family member(s) to help communicate, yet providers should address the patient directly, as they would any other patient, and include them in all conversations about their health concerns. A danger for people with intellectual disabilities is others' misperceptions about their ability to speak for themselves with support. A presumption of incompetence or lack of capacity can result in preventing the patient from developing skills necessary for managing their personal health. Knowledge of their condition, understanding its issues, self-management skills, self-advocacy, and self-efficacy are at risk, and the danger for poor health outcomes escalates.

One example of underestimating individuals with intellectual disabilities is the perception of guardianship as the only option (see Chap. 30). Guardianship is a critical support for some, but it should be the last option rather than the first (and only) option. It is an expensive process, requiring the assistance of an attorney and a court. Although courts are instructed to design guardianships to encourage the development or maintenance of maximum self-reliance and independence of the incapacitated person, it's not uncommon for courts to create full guardianships. Full guardianship removes the rights of the individual to make even the simplest of decisions for themselves, such as the right to decide where they want to live and work and how they want to spend their days. Families think their only option is guardianship (it's the one option they hear about from education and medical professionals, among others) and end up spending money and removing their young adult's personal and civil rights unnecessarily. Reversing guardianship can be a challenging and costly process.

Alternatives to guardianship include durable power of attorney, medical power of attorney, and HIPPA release. A new and practical solution available to some individuals and their families is supported decision-making. This measure provides a legal means for an individual to choose a trusted individual or team of people who can provide support to the person without taking over their right(s) to decision-making. Guardianship is substituted decision-making: the guardian makes decisions for the individual. Supported decision-making provides for autonomy and self-direction while offering necessary guidance and support. Supported decision-making is not yet a legally available option in every state; more information on supported decision-making (including states in which it is an option) can be found online at http://supporteddecisionmaking.org/.

Look to the family to support their emerging young adult with an intellectual disability—they have valuable knowledge and experience—but not at the expense of ignoring the patient.

Vignette

A neurologist was explaining the results of a sleep study showing sleep apnea to my son, David (who can present as competent but has significant intellectual disabilities). He explained that airways become constricted during sleep. I could see the information was going over my son's head. I stopped the doctor and said to David, "David, when you are using the water hose at home, what happens if it gets kinked?" David explained how the water starts trickling from the hose or even stops completely. I told David, "That's what the doctor is saying is happening to the 'hose' in your nose and throat, the hose that carries oxygen to your lungs and helps you breathe while you're sleeping." "Oh!" David said. He asked "So there's a kink in my air hose? That's why I'm not sleeping like I'm supposed to?" The doctor said, "That's brilliant. Mind if I steal it?" Family members are well-versed in what their young adult understands and how they communicate. Direct your communication to the patient, but invite the family to assist if needed. Other forms of assistance from the physician's office are listed in Table 5.2, below.

Some parents hold high expectations for their child despite the intellectual disability. They will welcome conversations about transition and efforts to encourage self-efficacy and self-advocacy, despite their reasonable anxieties and concerns.

Others, being cautious and protective, will find your efforts harder to understand and support. They've spent years advocating for their child's services, often with a multitude of providers. They're aware of their child's vulnerabilities, and the future is frightening. Their protectiveness can negatively affect their and the providers' perception of their child's abilities.

Table 5.2 Other forms of assistance that the physician's office could provide to assist with HCT

• Translating or helping to explain medical information
• Clarifying treatment options as they relate to the individual's personal preferences and needs
• Taking extra time for discussion, questions, and decision-making
• Assisting with setting up and keeping appointments
• Helping with managing medications (refills, dosing) or other treatment regimens
• Easing fears or anxieties in the healthcare environment
• Assisting with decision-making
• Assisting with documentation for insurance claims, medical records

Well-meaning families can limit their young adult's autonomy and privacy by speaking for them, making all their healthcare and other service decisions, and assuming their child is incapable of assisting or of having an opinion. This scenario happens for AYASHCN without cognitive delay, but it is more frequent for those with intellectual disabilities.

Cultural understandings and expectations can complicate HCT. Healthcare providers should familiarize themselves with and be respectful of cultural norms around chronic illness and disability, self-efficacy, and self-advocacy. A conversation about the family's expectations for their young adult's life beyond childhood can help healthcare professionals provide culturally competent HCT guidance.

When family members take charge of all their young adult's decisions, without consulting them or encouraging their autonomy or self-advocacy, the healthcare provider(s) may follow the parents' lead, further disempowering the patient. Physicians have an opportunity to present an expectation of autonomy, self-advocacy, and self-efficacy, by looking to the adolescent or young adult first and consulting family members secondarily. Meeting with the adolescent alone for some part of the visit helps set that expectation. Letting the parent(s) know the provider is following standard clinical practice should help the parents understand this as part of the HCT process.

Whether they see their young adult as competent and capable of making decisions or not, their child will legally be considered an adult at age 18. Providers should help family members prepare for this reality. The family will need to put legal protections in place if their young adult needs support for decision-making and consent. The provider will need to have this conversation more than once and ask questions about the patient's and the family's plans.

Transition Planning in a Clinical Setting

A parent may say "He's going to live with us for the rest of his life" and consider the matter of transition to adulthood settled. The sad secret many parents harbor but will never say aloud is their hope the child will die before they do. This thought can be paralyzing. Rather than taking a proactive approach by teaching self-advocacy skills and building strong circles of support, some families simply ignore the inevitability of not being able to care for their AYASHCN. What's a healthcare provider to do in the face of such resistance? Begin the conversation early and revisit it annually. Families need a road map (see Chaps. 4, 16, and 26). Having a transition policy for your practice, posting it in a visible space, and reviewing it together with families will help keep HCT a priority. Physicians should provide timelines and assure patients and their family members they will be supported through the process. But there's more to your role.

The American Academy of Pediatrics, American Academy of Family Physicians, and American College of Physicians-American Society of Internal Medicine state, "After the age of majority, all youth deserve to be treated as adults and to experience an adult model of care," even when they require decision-making support or are under legal guardianship.

Your patient's experience of being treated as an adult and experiencing an adult model of care requires preparation. Adult care assumes that the patient knows how to set and keep appointments, understands their health condition(s), is experienced in managing their health condition(s) including any medication or other necessary regimens, and is prepared to discuss their health management with the adult provider. The necessary knowledge and skills must be taught, practiced, and experienced before they enter adult care. Show them small steps they can take toward transition, e.g., having their child introduce themselves and present their health insurance card when checking in for an appointment or having the young person write their name and address on the check-in forms. The provider taking the lead at every opportunity, and beginning early, can help patients learn self-advocacy and self-efficacy.

Person Centered Thinking© [2] offers a model which proposes the difference between what is important to the person and what's important for them (see Table 5.3). Because of their training, health care professionals (and often family members as well), tend to focus on what's important for the person (health and safety), and pay less or no attention to what's important to them (the things that bring the person happiness, contentment, satisfaction, fulfillment or comfort). Nobody wants to live a life focused on their health and safety only, even when there are significant health concerns. We know people are more likely to do what's important for them (things related to their health and safety) when they can see a connection between that and something that's important to them. For example, David is more likely to pay attention to his low-sodium diet and kidney health if he can see its connection to his love of running. He is more inclined to use his CPAP machine when he understands how it impacts his ability to get a good night's sleep and wake up on time for work. Patients often do what's important for their health and safety if these behaviors improve or are connected to the things that matter most (important to them). Patient's self-efficacy and adherence to their treatment can be improved by hooking it to what's important to them. Training for healthcare providers in eliciting important information is needed. More information about person-centered practices can be found here: http://tlcpcp.com.

Table 5.3 Person-centered thinking—the balance of health and safety with quality of life

• Developed and taught by the learning community for person-centered practices [2]
• Defines health and safety as "important for" the person
• Defines anything that helps the person feel satisfied, content, happy, fulfilled, or comforted as "important to" the person
• AYASHCN often experience lives focused on what's important for them, without enough consideration for what's important to them
• People naturally desire balance between doing what's important for them and having what's important to them
• People are more likely to do what's important for them when they can connect it to what's important to them
• Patient self-efficacy and adherence to treatment increase when what's important for them is "hooked" or connected to something important to them
• http://www.tlcpcp.com/

Patients and families who have undergone an organized, well-defined transition process report better outcomes in their adult-based healthcare experiences. They express gratitude for well-written care summaries, referrals to knowledgeable adult providers when possible, time spent ensuring as much stability as possible before ending the relationship, and a warm sense of closure between the patient, family, and provider. The time taken for these measures may mean the difference between the patient successfully navigating the transition to adult-based care and having a poor health outcome. The website—www.gottransition.org—provides one resource for patients, families, and healthcare providers to organize the process. Their resources specific to healthcare professionals include six core elements of transition:

1. Transition policy
2. Transition tracking and monitoring

3. Transition readiness
4. Transition planning
5. Transfer of care
6. Transfer completion

Unfortunately, most AYASHCN and their families report seeing none of these elements before leaving their pediatric-based care. It's no wonder so many find themselves facing an abyss!

Promoting Self-Efficacy

Self-efficacy is essential for young patients to succeed in managing their health problems as they transition. The concept of self-efficacy theorizes that people must believe in their capacity to achieve their goals before they can work toward those goals. In terms of healthcare, patients must first have confidence in their ability to manage their health. Confidence comes from gaining knowledge and skills, having repeated opportunities for practice, and experiencing success. These points are summarized in Table 5.4.

Learning from others in a similar situation can aid in attaining self-efficacy, for the patient and family member(s). As young parents, we knew our son would need a lot of help to get through school, and we wanted him to have an inclusive education with his non-disabled peers (not the usual route for students with intellectual disabilities). Although I have a degree in special education, I doubted my ability to be his advocate for a different educational path. I associated myself with other parents whose kids were older than mine and who were successfully navigating the path I wanted to take. They supported and encouraged me and walked alongside me providing resources, knowledge, experience, and insight. They built my self-efficacy, and soon I was not only successfully teaming with my son's school professionals to create an inclusive education program for him but mentoring others to do the same. Years after his graduation, one of my mentors told me "You know, I wasn't sure it would work for your son." I was floored. "I believed you!" I said. "And that's why it worked for you and your son," she replied. "It worked because you believed you could make it work." I had gained confidence and self-efficacy followed.

Table 5.4 Promoting self-efficacy

• Patients must believe in their capacity to achieve their goals before they can work toward those goals
• Confidence in one's ability to manage their own health is critical
• Confidence is built through gained knowledge, practiced skills, and experienced success

Associating with people on a similar journey, others who have navigated various systems and gained hands-on expertise can be an empowering experience. Can your practice help patients and their families link with others? Family members and individuals involved in support organizations are quick to share their learning, offer support, and are eager to learn from others on the same path. One caution: If there is a significant difference between the families in terms of the HCT outcomes, these efforts can backfire. The person who is experiencing success may feel guilty or uncomfortable with the person who is having more difficulty. On the other hand, the person experiencing less success may feel the more successful person sets an expectation they can't reach. When my son was small, our neurologist gave my name (with my permission) to another parent whose son (several years older than mine) was diagnosed with the same disease as my son. The conversation started out fine. The other mom asked if my son was talking yet. "Yes, he's begun using some words," I said. "What about your boy?" I asked. A silence ensued on the other end of the phone until she finally choked out, "No, he can't talk at all." We never spoke again, despite living 15 minutes apart. I felt sad and a little guilty. I can't imagine what she felt.

Some parent support organizations provide a parent-matching program in which they connect families dealing with similar circumstances. A critical component of an effective matching program is training for the families engaged in the match, better preparing them to answer questions and provide support without falling into the kind of situation I found myself described above. Another underutilized but valuable resource can be adults living with similar conditions or concerns.

There are other methods to build patient self-efficacy into your practice, and they are discussed in other sections of this book (see Chaps. 5, 13, 19, and 20). Assessing self-efficacy skills, and encouraging patient and family to practice the undeveloped ones, builds capacity and confidence. One doctor routinely assigns homework to his patients based on this assessment, attempting to build the patient's skills throughout their adolescent years in his care.

Technology

Technology may help AYASHCN and families improve their self-efficacy. Apps on our phones, iPads, smart watches, and computers may provide ways to manage details of daily living. For example, a patient who cannot tell time can set timed reminders on his phone for medication reminders or appointment alerts on his calendar. The Medical ID app (available for IOS and Android platforms) provides readily accessible medical ID information on the patient's cell phone, especially in an emergency. Apps for tracking blood glucose levels, carbohydrate intake, and medication doses can assist with diabetes management. Many healthcare providers and clinics have moved to electronic communication, permitting patients to access records and communicate with their physician(s) electronically. Creative families have assisted a loved one in their home via the computer, providing everything from medication and schedule reminders to walking their adult child through a recipe.

Our son has intellectual disabilities as well as significant medical issues including kidney disease. He was a competitive varsity-level distance runner in high school and still enjoys running today. His nephrologist and dietitian talked with him about the importance of a low-sodium diet. But when we showed him a fitness and diet tracking app on his phone and helped him understand what his target sodium numbers should be, the sodium in his diet took on a new level of importance. The app also tracked his distance running, connecting what is important for him (low-sodium diet) to what's important to him (his love of running).

Promoting Self-Advocacy

Teaching self-advocacy skills—the practice of speaking for oneself, asking questions, making one's decisions, understanding one's rights and responsibilities, and asking for help and support—is crucial to successful transition. Self-advocacy is not an all-or-nothing practice. Family members and others in their circle of support can help the young adult to apply self-advocacy skills. Parents who work to support and empower their young adult's self-advocacy often report surprise at their child's growth and capabilities as they have an opportunity to do so.

Some families will resist promoting self-advocacy skills, whether it be from their fears, misperceptions of their child's capacity, or their own poor self-advocacy skills. Cultural norms and expectations can contribute to the resistance.

Most family members will view you, the patient's healthcare provider, as the expert. The provider can present self-advocacy opportunities and model family members' roles. Addressing yourself to your patient before the family member is a great start. Speaking to the patient—asking questions of the patient and giving time for the answer—sets the expectation of self-advocacy. Patients and their family members will come to expect it and prepare for it.

The same goes for making choices and decisions. First, ask open-ended questions to the patient. What do they think about the medication they are taking? Is it helping? How do they know it is helping? What are they pleased about in terms of their health and healthcare? What concerns do they have? Avoid closed-ended questions: those that can be answered with a "yes" or "no." Ask open-ended questions that open the door to conversation. And then listen. The provider's actions are as much about modeling the presumption of the patient's competence and self-advocacy as they are about hearing what the patient says.

Talking with your patient(s) about their health condition(s), answering their questions, and asking them what they understand about it prepare them to have those same conversations with adult care providers who will expect those kinds of discussions.

The Role of Parents in Preparing for HCT

Parents' roles and responsibilities begin years before the subject of transition is broached. Transition planning begins at birth. Parenting is all about preparing our kids for what life will throw their way, from disagreements on the kindergarten playground to the drama of junior high and the rigors of high school. Our child's health concerns and disabilities complicate our task.

Honest discussions about the child's diagnosis and medical condition, adapted for the child's age and ability to comprehend, create an essential foundation. Making the diagnosis and medical concerns an ongoing conversation provides the opportunity for the young person to learn important details about their condition, the necessary measures to manage the condition, and provides the opportunity to ask questions or address concerns. These kinds of conversations through the years can serve as a basis for the later development of more advanced self-efficacy and self-advocacy skills. In hindsight, the 27 years we've spent talking openly about David's condition, cursing it at times, shedding tears, and teaching him to address his concerns head on, have resulted in a young man who faces significant health problems with optimism, courage, and hope.

For some parents, however, this kind of conversation is too uncomfortable. Parents naturally want to protect their children, and shielding them from the painful truths of their condition(s) may seem easier in the short run. Unfortunately, our failures to honestly address the issues set the young person up for discomfort and avoidance in later years, potentially leading to serious health consequences. As parents, we must provide models of courage, competency, and honesty as we help our children face the realities of their medical concerns or disabilities and prepare them to manage the resulting issues. Don't underestimate the value of your support. Our kids tend to rise to the level of our expectations.

Transition readiness assessment tools used in the clinic can provide the patient, parents, and provider with an assessment of transition readiness (see Chap. 13). Transition planning tools can then be used over time to improve self-efficacy in tasks for adolescents and young adults to practice and gain competency as they prepare for the transition. Parents can use transition planning tools as a series of steps, tackling the tasks and providing instruction and encouragement, while gently encouraging their young person to take on more responsibility. Parents may be surprised at how competent their child can be with the right opportunity and support.

Finding an Adult Provider

It's happened; the time has come to leave the safety and security of the pediatrician's office and move into the world of adult-based care. Where to begin?

Parents say getting a referral from their pediatric-based care providers—who they have come to know, rely upon, and even love—is golden. We trust pediatric providers' recommendations.

Unfortunately, many family members report getting no such help. Whether it's a lack of time, knowledge, resources, or connections, families find themselves out there on the bridge to nowhere, trying to create their own bridges. They make call after call, only to learn the provider they're calling doesn't take their insurance, doesn't take Medicaid, isn't taking new patients, or doesn't feel he has the necessary knowledge or experience to treat their child. Without proper transition planning, this exercise in frustration can happen while there is a high need for continued medical care. The young adult has "aged out" of the pediatric clinic and must find adult-based care in a hurry. The risk of time lost, money wasted, and mistakes made is high.

How can the healthcare professional help? Get networked. Know who can do what you do in the adult system, develop a relationship with the person/clinic, and offer your referrals and recommendations.

Parents' Recommendations

A mom whose daughter has multiple physical health issues and developmental disabilities offered this recommendation to other families:

> Figure out what is your child's most critical medical need or what medical specialty is most important and find that physician first. It's preferable if you can find one already in a medical home system or electronic records system. Then build relationships with the other specialists you need who are already involved in that system if possible. If that's not feasible, find your most important specialist first and then try to find a network that includes the other providers you need in one system, so you only deal with one specialist out of the system.

The only danger with this strategy is if, for some reason, the patient can no longer access the medical home or networked system (e.g., change in insurance), they run the risk of losing the entire network. It's important to pay attention to coverage that can change at 18, 21, and again at 26 or even with PPO or MCO provider lists.

Another parent suggests: "Identify your current providers. Create a list of potential adult providers for each specialty. Ask each current provider 'If this were your child, who would you seek out for adult care?'" Other recommendations from parents are listed in Table 5.5.

Terminating the Relationship with the Pediatrician

For many of us, the child's pediatrician has been a constant in a sea of change, through the ups and downs of our lives. He/she has helped us through crisis. It's possible they have been there since our child was diagnosed. They have been our rock. For us—patient and family—ending our relationship with the pediatrician is hard.

Make our goodbyes easier by making sure everyone knows it's coming well in advance. Having a plan and clear timelines ensures nobody is surprised when the last appointment comes. Knowing where we will go for our young adult's health care, and having a thorough medical summary to take with us, eases our anxiety. Assuring us the pediatrician is still there if the adult provider needs a consult is comforting.

Lastly, pediatricians, give us time to thank you for the role you've played in our lives and to say goodbye. We're eternally grateful and will never forget you and what you've done for us. Thanks. A summary of parents' wishes for assistance from their pediatric provider is presented in Table 5.6.

Table 5.5 Other recommendations from parents of AYASHCN who have transitioned their AYASHCN to adult care

• "Network with other parents of individuals with special healthcare needs"
• "Get as much help from the pediatric doctor as possible"
• "Make an appointment to get to know the new doctor and for them to get to know your child. If you don't like the doctor, keep looking"
• "Do your own research. Ask questions!"
• "Start early!"

Table 5.6 Parents' HCT wish list

• Inform us about transition and then ask the question "What can we do to help you and your son/daughter make a successful transition?"
• Recognize it's one of the more stressful times for us as family members
• Help me by sharing what you know about my child with a medical summary, prepared for the new doctors
• Give me timelines, give me recommendations, and give me referrals
• We always hear the term "talk with your doctor," but sometimes it takes a lot for families to ask their questions
• Work with us as a team instead of leaving it all up to the parent
• Have patience with us. None of this is easy
• Show interest
• Give parents information on networking
• Prepare to work with the increasing population of special needs of young adults
• Be willing to consult with the new provider if necessary
• Support family through the transition to help make sure adult physicians are acutely aware of child/adult needs. It can be overwhelming for parents to change doctors for medically complex children. We are fearful that child's medical history won't be fully reviewed or understood. Communication and support are critical.
• The hardest thing was leaving our pediatric providers because of our emotional connection to them. They had been with us for 22 years!

References

1. "Gabe's Care Map" used with permission from author Cristin Lind.
2. Establishing a Healthcare Transition program for Adolescents and Young Adults with Chronic Illness and Disability includes person-centered concepts, principles, and materials used with permission from The Learning Community for Person Centered Practices. Find out more at http://tlcpcp.com.

6 Healthcare Transition from the Pediatric Provider's Perspective

Cecily L. Betz

Healthcare transition (HCT) planning is a relatively new field of practice and research that has emerged to address the complex needs and issues associated with the "aging out" of adolescents and young adults with special healthcare needs (AYASHCN). The "aging out" of AYASHCN involves the transition from adolescence to emerging adulthood and beyond and transfer from pediatric to adult healthcare. The challenges associated with the extended survival rates of AYASHCN have been discussed in scholarly publications and in clinical forums since the late 1980s [1]. Why then, three decades later, has the vision of creating linkages between the pediatric and adult systems of care to ensure the smooth and uninterrupted provision of care not been realized [2–5]? What issues and challenges account for the evident discomfort, reluctance, and competency deficits among healthcare professionals within these two systems of care [6–8]?

This chapter will examine the challenges of developing a competent pediatric provider workforce to provide HCT services, followed by a presentation of strategies that could facilitate the transfer of care to adult care providers. A summary of the barriers and strategic approaches for successful resolution is presented in Table 6.1. The chapter will conclude with an analysis of the practice implications for pediatric care providers.

Table 6.1 HCT barriers and strategies to overcome barriers

Barriers	Strategies
• Provider's lack of training and experience with providing healthcare transition services	• Provider training that includes consulting with interdisciplinary colleagues about resources and referrals; access online HCT training programs
• Lack of institutional structure and resources to support the provision of HCT services or development of HCT programs	• Infrastructure support for HCT planning that includes institutional HCT champions; accessing resources as presented in Tables 6.2 and 6.3
• AYASHCN and family reluctance to transfer care	• Generate revenue for services by consulting finance officer and acquire knowledge of CPT Codes
• Provider reluctance to facilitate transfer of care	• Create partnerships with adult providers/ organizations; refer to Table 6.4

C. L. Betz, Ph.D., R.N.
Department of Pediatrics, University of Southern California (USC), Keck School of Medicine, Los Angeles, CA, USA

USC University Center for Excellence in Developmental Disabilities, Children's Hospital Los Angeles, Los Angeles, CA, USA
e-mail: cbetz@chla.usc.edu

A. C. Hergenroeder, C. M. Wiemann (eds.), *Health Care Transition*,
https://doi.org/10.1007/978-3-319-72868-1_6

Barriers Encountered by Healthcare Providers

Lack of Training

One of the most frequently reported barriers by providers on both sides of the service divide is lack of training resources and opportunities. Although both pediatric and adult service providers share a need for training, their learning requirements differ. Pediatric providers cite the dearth of training to foster not only their understanding of HCT planning service models but also their acquisition of the knowledge and skills necessary to become a competent provider to provide HCT services [16–19].

The learning needs of pediatric providers are not relegated only to preparation beginning in early adolescence and the transfer of care in emerging adulthood. Provider needs also include acquiring skills and knowledge to conduct specialized HCT-focused assessment and intervention based upon an interdisciplinary model of care facilitated by service coordination and referral as well as an understanding the realm of adult services. Pediatric providers are now expected to learn about HCT frameworks of care as well as adult service systems of care, including employment such as job development and training, rehabilitation, postsecondary education, housing, transportation, disability services, and community living supports and services. Pediatric providers involved in HCT planning need to be knowledgeable of the range of available adult services in order to be proficient and competent with service coordination and referrals for transition and adult services based upon the AYASHCN's interests, needs, and preferences. For example, a HCT service coordinator's knowledge of the publicly financed vocational training programs (i.e., Department of Vocational Rehabilitation, state's Workforce Investment Act workforce system, Job Corps) available in the AYASHCN's community can greatly benefit the AYASHCN who might otherwise enroll in a costly proprietary vocational program and, upon completion, accumulate significant loan debt.

In contrast, the learning needs of adult care providers are based upon their lack of experience and clinical training in providing care to adults with childhood-acquired chronic conditions (for additional information on adult provider learning needs, refer to Chap. 7 "Healthcare Transition from the Adult Provider's Perspective") [7, 20–22]. To date, few medical and interdisciplinary training specialty programs integrate HCT for AYASHCN into didactic and clinical training [23, 24]. There are areas of specialty practice that have raised these issues associated with clinical practice, professional training, and research. For example, in 2005 the American College of Cardiology issued a position statement entitled *Training in Transition of Adolescent Care and Care of the Adult with Congenital Heart Disease* related to training of cardiologists to meet the growing population of adults with congenital heart disease (ACHD) [25]. In this document, ACHD curriculum and training competencies are identified to provide care to ACHD. Other examples of guidelines for the care of adults with childhood-acquired conditions are listed in Table 6.2.

Lack of Structure for HCT Planning

For pediatric and adult providers of care for AYASHCN, limited training and informational resources exist within institutional settings [8, 18, 26]. There are a number of reasons for this. Foremost, limited institutional resources have been directed to generate a HCT infrastructure for training, ongoing technical assistance, and service support. Children's medical centers and other pediatric healthcare institutions have a myriad of clinical care priorities associated with their organizational mission, and the financial constraints make it difficult to direct or allocate funding for a HCT infrastructure. Relatively few HCT experts are available within institutions to provide consultation to colleagues. Although increased attention has been directed to this growing HCT service needs, the widespread adoption of HCT programs has yet to be realized. Available HCT resources that can be accessed on publicly-funded or foundation-supported websites may not be appropriate/applicable for repli-

Table 6.2 Examples of adult care guidelines

American Academy of Pediatrics (AAP), American Academy of Family Physicians (AAFP), and American College of Physicians (ACP)	AAP, AAFP, and ACP (2011). Supporting the healthcare transition from adolescence to adulthood in the medical home [9]
American College of Physicians	Guidelines and Tools Developed for Pediatric-to-Adult Health Care Transitions Initiative [10]
Autism	National Institute for Health and Clinical Excellence (NICE) (2012). Autism: recognition, referral, diagnosis, and management of adults on the autism spectrum. London (UK): National Institute for Health and Clinical Excellence (NICE) [11]
Cystic fibrosis	Cystic fibrosis adult care: consensus conference report [12]
Complex care	Pediatric Complex Care Association. Children and Young Adults with Medical Complexity: Serving an Emerging Population [13]
Sickle cell disease	National Heart, Lung, and Blood Institute. Evidence-Based Management of Sickle Cell Disease: Expert Panel Report, 2014 [14]
Spina bifida	Centers for Disease Control and Prevention. Living with spina bifida [15]

cation in a specific institutional setting. Available instructional materials for AYASHCN and their families will need to be adapted for local community application. Lastly, as described in greater detail later, HCT programs that are reliant on extramural support may be difficult to sustain beyond the funding period [23].

Service Reimbursement

A major impediment with the implementation of HCT service programs and the access to adult healthcare services is the lack of or inadequate reimbursement for services [8, 17, 23]. For patients enrolled in State Medicaid programs, the rate of reimbursement is 61% of the Medicare rate [27]. Furthermore, the time interval for receiving payments for the provider's care is excessively long. Given the low reimbursement rates for beneficiaries enrolled in the State Medicaid programs, access to specialty medical care is problematic [28]. A number of reimbursement options (based upon CPT and fee for service [FFS] codes) have been recommended to obtain reimbursement from public and private payers; however, institutional approval and mechanisms for enabling charges by the financial managers is needed [29].

Other HCT programs have been initiated with the support of extramural funding from governmental agencies and nonprofit foundations. Typically, the infusion of funds for HCT program startups are based upon a specific period of time and funder requirements. However, the key to success with seed funding to develop and implement HCT program is program sustainability. It is a challenge, and, to date, few programs have been successful.

AYASHCN and Family Reluctance to Transfer Care

Many studies have been conducted examining AYASHCN's and family members' (primarily parents) perspectives on HCT, with emphasis on the transfer of care [30, 31]. These studies have included perspectives prior to and following the transfer of care and identify two major concerns. First is leaving their primary and specialty care pediatric providers. These relationships are formed over what may be an unpredictable course of the healthcare need/disability. Leaving behind the shared history and lived experience of this unique relationship with pediatric providers is difficult as the feelings of confidence, security, and expectations will end, and new relationships with unknown adult providers will need to be established. Second is parental and AYASHCN concerns with locating adult providers center around issues of competence, convenience, and a different model of care wherein an integrated model of care available in pediatrics is likely not available [30, 31]. Furthermore, as the payment for services model changes with enrollment in a new insurance plan, particularly a public plan, accessing providers who will accept patients with low rates of reimbursement is difficult.

Provider Reluctance to Facilitate Transfer of Care

Pediatricians' are attached to their patients [17, 26, 32, 33]. Pediatricians are concerned about the competencies and potentially restrained attitudes of adult providers to receive adults with childhood-acquired chronic conditions. Adult providers lack comfort in providing services to some AYASHCN as they have not received the training needed to address the needs of this new specialty population. Adult providers who have received adults with chronic conditions into their practice report that AYASHCN were not well prepared to assume responsibilities for their care.

Lack of Identified Adult Providers for Transferring Care

Challenges exist in locating adult providers who are available to receive AYASHCN into their practices [23, 32]. Pediatric and adult professional organizations have raised this issue in policy-related, position statements and clinical guidelines documents [17, 34].

Potential Strategies to Overcome HCT Barriers

Provider Training

Resources for learning about transition and adult community-based resources for AYASHCN and their families exist within a number of major pediatric medical centers. Interdisciplinary providers within large pediatric hospitals can be consulted for HCT planning. Social workers are excellent resources for locating community-based resources connected with transportation, conservatorship, respite support, access to healthcare, youth employment programs, and other postsecondary education and training programs. Physical therapists can provide assistance with referrals to orthotists, durable medical equipment, assistive devices, and adaptive recreational programs. Registered dieticians can be of assistance with issues regarding accessing community programs needed for the range of feeding concerns. Occupational therapists can provide assistance with referrals for services and supports needed to acquire skills and supports for activities of daily living (ADLs). These are just a few examples of the scope of practice that interdisciplinary colleagues can bring to the development and implementation of a HCT program. Other institutional resources available include the hospital attorney, financial counselors, and information technology (IT) personnel.

There are online training resources and websites that can be accessed for instructional purposes (see Table 6.3).

Infrastructure Support for HCT Planning

Realization of the training needed to become an effective and competent HCT provider is manifest as the proliferation of peer-reviewed literature on the topic; its prominence at national professional and consumer-driven conferences as evident with the annual Chronic Illness and Disability Conference, Transition from Pediatric to Adult Care sponsored by the Baylor College of Medicine and Texas Children's Hospital; and the policy-making and standards of practice promulgated by pediatric and interdisciplinary professional organizations such as the American Academy of Pediatrics, American College of Physicians, and Society of Pediatric Nurses. Institutional efforts to provide HCT training and resources need champions to move this effort forward. Colleagues from other institutions who have created a sustainable HCT infrastructure may be helpful. Reaching out to HCT networks and resources, such as the

Table 6.3 Online training resources and websites

Got Transition. This website, funded by the Health Resources and Services Administration, contains extensive resources on HCT. Its focus is on the Six Core Elements, which identify the basic elements needed for HCT
Website link: http://www.gottransition.org/resources/
University of Illinois at Chicago's Division of Specialized Care for Children. Specialized Care for Children. A number of transition tools and resources are available on this site, which can be useful models for developing tools specific to the institutional/practice setting
Website link: http://dscc.uic.edu/browse-resources/transition-resources/
American College of Physicians, Pediatric to Adult Care Transitions Initiative. The aim of the HCT toolkit is to assist adult providers with resources to assist them to provide HCT services
Website link: https://www.acponline.org/clinical-information/high-value-care/resources-for-clinicians/pediatric-to-adult-care-transitions-initiative
American Association on Health and Disability. This website contains a page specifically focused on HCT resources for providers entitled *Healthcare Transition Resources: Providers*. It contains numerous resource links to other websites that provide instructional assistance
Website link: https://www.aahd.us/best-practice/healthcare-transition-resources-providers/
University of Florida, Education and Health Care Transition Graduate Certificate. This is an online HCT training program for healthcare professionals and educators. The focus of the training is the integration of health issues/needs in the educational setting
Website link: https://education.ufl.edu/education-healthcare-transition/
The Hospital for Sick Children (Toronto, Canada), Good 2 Go Transition Program. This Canadian HCT program offers numerous resources that have application for replication in other international settings. Foremost among resources developed is the Passport for Health, a prototype for assisting consumers with self-management needs
Website link: http://www.sickkids.ca/good2go/
The National Youth Transition Center. This website is a youth-driven website to provide assistance, support, and resources to facilitate the employment of youth with disabilities. Many important issues relevant to long-term planning are presented on the website. Excellent resource for adolescents and emerging adults with special healthcare needs
Website link: http://www.thenytc.org/
Society for Adolescent Medicine and Health. Transition to Adult Health page. On this page, resources are available to links on other topics connected with HCT such as mental health and sexual and reproductive health
Website link: http://www.adolescenthealth.org/Resources/Clinical-Care-Resources/Transition-to-Adult-Care.aspx
Illinois Chapter, American Academy of Pediatrics. An online HCT program (15 CME) for pediatricians to learn the details about HCT planning, including the prominent features of the service model
Website link: www.illinoisaap.org
The Health Services for Children with Special Needs, Health Care Transition for Adolescents and Young Adults, An Online Video CME Series. This one CME unit provides content on the Six Core Elements of Health Care Transition
Website link: https://www.hscsnlearning.org/transition/

Health Care Transition Research Consortium, *Got Transition*, and others, listed in Tables 6.2, 6.3 and 6.4, are recommended.

HCT Service Reimbursement

It will be necessary to confer closely with institutions' financial (billing and coding) experts to explain the HCT service description and its match with the transition-related CPT codes. An excellent resource for reference is *2017 Coding and Reimbursement Sheet for Transition from Pediatric to Adult Health Care* located on the Got Transition website [29].

AYASHCN and Family Reluctance to Transfer Care

There are a number of strategies that can be employed to potentially mitigate AYASHCN's and their parents' concerns associated with transferring to adult providers. First, informing about the even-

Table 6.4 Strategies for finding adult providers

1.	Find an internist/primary care provider (health home) prior to the transfer of care period who can make service referrals to specialty providers
2.	Create a community-based partnership with an adult medical center/managed care organization
3.	Confer with the community-based Department of Rehabilitation, Workforce Investment Act agency, as some local offices compile lists of community providers who provide specialized and primary care services to adults with childhood-acquired conditions
4.	Access condition-specific websites (i.e., spina bifida) as they may have listings of adult clinics/providers that are available
5.	Contact the local Center for Independent Living (CIL), a grassroots advocacy organization for adults with disabilities that are directed by and staffed with individuals with disabilities. Many of the CILs maintain lists of community-based providers and agencies that are disability-sensitive and competent
6.	Access the Internet sites and/or download apps that will assist in locating physicians such as WebMD and Yelp
7.	Network with other consumers to learn by "word of mouth" providers who are recommended
8.	Contact the human resources representative within the parent's/consumer's employment setting; speak with the health insurance agent
9.	Consult with the individual designated as the HCT coordinator will be developing a resource list of health providers/agencies available in the community

tual transfer of care can be initiated early on, even with the first encounter to introduce the concept of HCT planning [9, 35]. In that way, the eventual transfer of care is introduced as a future event that is a natural component of the transition into adulthood. Advanced planning and discussion enable review of the issues and needs the AYASHCN and family have as well as their input and engagement in the process of transfer when it finally occurs.

Provider Reluctance to Facilitate Transfer of Care

Fostering linkages with adult provider services and facilitating communication between both groups of providers will be advantageous in overcoming the hesitation with referrals. Several models have been reported that have been effective in facilitating the transfer of care to adults [2, 3, 17]. These models include clinic appointments conducted jointly with both pediatric and adult providers, preparatory visits to the adult clinic or with the adult provider prior to the transfer of care, or having the pediatric provider attend the first visit with the adult provider [2, 3, 5, 17, 23]. As presented in Table 6.4, a number of recommendations to locate adult providers are provided. Additional content on facilitating linkages with adult providers is discussed in the next section.

Communicating with the adult provider who is to take over the patient's care. Communication with the adult provider should begin well ahead of the transfer of care as a means of avoiding the potential discontinuities and/or lapse in care [9].

A widely accepted recommendation and standard of practice advocated is the transmission of the AYASHCN's medical records using a medical summary [9, 23, 36]. The AYASHCN's medical summary could contain the following information: (a) demographic information such as address, phone number, date of birth, and family composition, (b) allergies including adverse reactions to medical procedures typically conducted (i.e., voiding cystourethrogram [VCUG]), (c) list of medications including dosage and frequency, (d) listing of current providers including the contact information of phone number and email address, (e) previous hospitalizations with reasons for admission, (f) previous/recent emergency/urgent care visits, (g) dates of most recent laboratory and diagnostic tests conducted and results, and (h) provider comments about adherence to daily treatment needs. Examples of HCT medical summaries can be found in Table 6.5 (also see Chap. 15). For additional information on strategies to facilitate the transfer of care to adult providers, refer to Chap. 10 where strategies on engaging with adult providers to receive AYASHCN as patients are discussed.

Table 6.5 Medical summary templates

Organization	Medical summary title	Website link
American College of Cardiology	Pediatric to Adult Care Transitions Tools Medical Summary & Emergency Care Plan for Young Adults with Congenital Heart Disease	http://www.acc.org/~/media/Non-Clinical/Files-PDFs-Excel-MS-Word-etc/Membership/Sections-Councils/Adult-Congenital-Pediatric/F16327_CHD_MEDICAL_SUMMARY.PDF?la=en
American College of Rheumatology	Medical Summary and Emergency Care Plan: Juvenile Idiopathic Arthritis	https://www.rheumatology.org/Portals/0/Files/Medical-Summary-JIA.pdf
American Society of Hematology	General Hematology Clinical Summary	http://www.hematology.org/Clinicians/Priorities/Transitions/5577.aspx
American Society of Hematology	Sickle Cell Disease Clinical Summary	http://www.hematology.org/Clinicians/Priorities/Transitions/5579.aspx
Got Transition	Sample Medical Summary and Emergency Care Plan Six Core Elements of Health Care Transition 2.0	http://www.gottransition.org/resourceGet.cfm?id=227
HealthIT.gov	Transition of Care Summary	https://www.healthit.gov/providers-professionals/achieve-meaningful-use/menu-measures/transition-of-care
Hospital for Sick Children	Health Passport	http://www.sickkids.ca/Good2Go/For-Youth-and-Families/Transition-Tools/MyHealth-Passport/Index.html
New England Consortium of Metabolic Programs	Medical Health Summary	http://newenglandconsortium.org/for-families/transitioning-teens-to-young-adults/transition-toolkit/medical-health-summary/
Southeast Texas Medical Associates	Hospital Care Summary	http://www.setma.com/Medical-Home/transition-of-care-one-form-of-care-coordination
University of Chicago	Transition Summary	http://transitioncare.uchicago.edu/files/2011/06/Portable-Medical-Documents.pdf

HCT as an Expected Outcome in a Pediatric Practice

The necessity of HCT as a service specialty for AYASHCN is acknowledged by many professional organizations, such as the American Academy of Family Physicians (AAFP), American Academy of Pediatrics (AAP), American College of Physicians (ACP) Society of Adolescent Health and Medicine, Society for Paediatric Endocrinology, and Society of Pediatric Nurses. The Agency for Healthcare Research and Quality indicates that 21 clinical guidelines for practice have been published [23]. Table 6.2 displays information on clinical guidelines for adults with childhood-acquired conditions.

The first review of literature on HCT based upon 43 studies was published spanning 21 years (1982–2003). Since then the HCT literature has proliferated with systematic reviews and evidence to guide practice and identify relevant outcomes of care. The outcomes of optimal HCT include successful referrals to adult providers, condition stability, rates of emergency department visits, and hospitalizations [2, 5, 37–39]. Challenges associated with the measurement of HCT outcomes include tracking AYASHCN who enter into new systems of care, moving to new communities of choice, and changes with modes of contact (i.e., cell phone, land lines, and incorrect addresses). Coupled with the logistic difficulties with tracking is the availability of fiscal and personnel resources to enable tracking. For many programs, long-term follow-up is not possible due to the limitations with resources. However, it may be feasible to devise methods for tracking that can be integrated into the systems of care as found with managed care organizations that provide both pediatric and adult care (i.e., Kaiser Permanente), institutional support allocated for time-limited tracking, and the inevitability of the creation of partnerships with community-based adult providers and organizations. Successful HCT is the ultimate outcome of pediatric care for AYASHCN and their families.

Case Example

A major pediatric medical center decides to develop a HCT infrastructure to serve as a HCT resource and support to specialty programs. The process of establishing a policy is described in Chap. 11 and the process of establishing a HCT program is described in Chap. 9. The hospital's vice president for patient care services (VP-PCS) was chosen to champion this HCT initiative. The VP-PCS convened a task force, composed of several interdisciplinary providers interested in starting HCT services. A task force is organized that is selected together with the hospital's parent advocate. The task force conducted a needs assessment and identified many issues: identifying that adult providers' patients can be transferred once their eligibility for services is terminated; acquiring HCT training including adult-oriented community services, developing instructional resources for AYASHCN and their families, and generating revenue for HCT services.

A strategic plan involving a larger group of stakeholders was formed to discuss execution of the strategic plan. The strategic plan includes (a) allocation of fiscal resources to support this effort, (b) implementation of a HCT provider training program, (c) creation of transfer procedure to adult providers, (d) formation of linkages with adult providers for the transfer of care, and (e) setup mechanism for service reimbursement.

A HCT expert was hired to provide consultation. The consultation included a Grand Rounds HCT presentation, consultation with individual specialty teams, and meeting with members of the strategic planning team and task force. The consultant recommendations included review of other institutionally based HCT efforts, examples of other successful transfer of care models, HCT documents and resources that can be accessed and replicated, and reimbursement models effectively used in other settings.

A strategic plan was written. Implementing the various components of the plan, including training, forming the community-based partnerships, and protocols, was analogous to HCT planning in the clinical setting, described in other chapters.

As the HCT field has evolved, more models of care are being developed, tested, and disseminated. Those who have undertaken HCT programmatic efforts are now sharing their knowledge. This accumulation of clinical experience and expertise is paving the way for others to learn from their experience to hopefully avoid the pitfalls of the past and strategize future planning more effectively.

Numerous HCT resources and supports exist to facilitate the development of new HCT services. These resources have been named throughout this chapter. Clinical guidelines to direct service providers with the development of the HCT delivery model are available for application to the practice setting. Although significant advances have been made in the field of HCT that have effected progress in clinical practice and research, one best practice has not been established nor will it be. Rather structures and processes from other programs will need to be adopted and evaluated for each institution.

References

1. Magrab PR, Miller, H.E.C., editor Surgeon's General's Conference: Growing up and getting medical care: Youth with special health care needs. A summary of conference proceedings. Surgeon's General's Conference: Growing up and getting medical care: Youth with special health care needs A summary of conference proceedings; 1989 March 13–15, 1989; Jekyll Island, Georga: National Center for Networking Community Based Services. Georgetown University Child Development Center.
2. Betz CL, O'Kane LS, Nehring WM, Lobo ML. Systematic review: Health care transition practice service models. Nurs Outlook. 2016;64(3):229–43. PubMed PMID: 26992949.
3. Bloom SR, Kuhlthau K, Van Cleave J, Knapp AA, Newacheck P, Perrin JM. Health care transition for youth with special health care needs. J Adolesc Health. 2012;51(3):213–9. PubMed PMID: 22921130. English.

4. Campbell F, Biggs K, Aldiss SK, O'Neill PM, Clowes M, McDonagh J, et al. Transition of care for adolescents from paediatric services to adult health services. Cochrane Database Syst Rev. 2016;4:CD009794. PubMed PMID: 27128768.
5. Chu PY, Maslow GR, von Isenburg M, Chung RJ. Systematic Review of the Impact of Transition Interventions for Adolescents With Chronic Illness on Transfer From Pediatric to Adult Healthcare. J Pediatr Nurs. 2015;30(5):e19–27. PubMed PMID: 26209872. Pubmed Central PMCID: NIHMS710745.
6. Nehring WM, Betz CL, Lobo ML. Uncharted Territory: Systematic Review of Providers' Roles, Understanding, and Views Pertaining to Health Care Transition. J Pediatr Nurs. 2015;30(5):732–47. PubMed PMID: 26228310.
7. Okumura MJ, Heisler M, Davis MM, Cabana MD, Demonner S, Kerr EA. Comfort of general internists and general pediatricians in providing care for young adults with chronic illnesses of childhood. J Gen Intern Med. 2008;23(10):1621–7. PubMed PMID: 18661191.
8. Okumura MJ, Kerr EA, Cabana MD, Davis MM, Demonner S, Heisler M. Physician views on barriers to primary care for young adults with childhood-onset chronic disease. Pediatrics. 2010;125(4):e748–54. PubMed PMID: 20231189.
9. American Academy of Pediatrics, American Academy of Family Physicians, American College of Physicians, Transitions Clinical Report Authoring G, Cooley WC, Sagerman PJ. Supporting the health care transition from adolescence to adulthood in the medical home. Pediatrics. 2011;128(1):182–200. PubMed PMID: 21708806.
10. American College of Physicians. Guidelines and Tools Developed for Pediatric-to-Adult Health Care Transitions Initiative. 2016. https://www.acponline.org/acp-newsroom/guidelines-and-tools-developed-for-pediatric-to-adult-health-care-transitions-initiative.
11. National Institute for Health and Clinical Excellence (NICE). Autism: Recognition, referral, diagnosis and management of adults on the autism spectrum. London (UK): National Institute for Health and Clinical Excellence (NICE); 2012. 57, Clinical guideline, no. 142. https://www.guideline.gov/summaries/summary/37864.
12. Yankaskas JR, Marshall BC, Sufian B, Simon RH, Rodman D. Cystic fibrosis adult care: Consensus conference report. Chest. 2004;125(1 Suppl):1S–39S.
13. Pediatric Complex Care Association. Children and Young Adults with Medical Complexity: Serving an Emerging Population. 2016. http://pediatriccomplexcare.org/wp-content/uploads/2016/03/PCCA-CMSWhitePaper012716.pdf.
14. National Heart Lung, and Blood Institute. Evidence-Based Management of Sickle Cell Disease: Expert Panel Report, 2014. 2014. https://www.nhlbi.nih.gov/health-pro/guidelines/sickle-cell-disease-guidelines.
15. Centers for Disease Control and Prevention. Living with Spina Bifida. 2016. https://www.cdc.gov/ncbddd/spinabifida/adult.html.
16. Al-Yateem N. Child to adult: transitional care for young adults with cystic fibrosis. Br J Nurs. 2012;21(14):850–4. PubMed PMID: 23252167. English.
17. Camfield PR, Gibson PA, Douglass LM. Strategies for transitioning to adult care for youth with Lennox Castuat syndrome and related disorders. Epilepsia. 2011;5(Suppl. 5):21–7.
18. Collins SW, Reiss J, Saidi A. Transition of care: what is the pediatric hospitalist's role? An exploratory survey of current attitudes. J Hosp Med. 2012;7(4):277–81. PubMed PMID: 22125023.
19. McDonagh JE, Southwood TR, Shaw KL, Bristish Paediatric Rheumatology G. Unmet education and training needs of rheumatology health professionals in adolescent health and transitional care. Rheumatology. 2004;43(6):737–43.
20. LoCasale-Crouch J, Johnson B. Transition from pediatric to adult medical care. Adv Chronic Kidney Dis. 2005;12(4):412–7. PubMed PMID: 16198281.
21. Patel MS, O'Hare K. Residency training in transition of youth with childhood-onset chronic disease. Pediatrics. 2010;126(2):S190–S3.
22. Suris JC, Akre C, Rutishauser C. How adult specialists deal with the principles of a successful transition. J Adolesc Health. 2009;45(6):551–5.
23. McPheeters M, Davis AM, Taylor JL, Brown RF, Potter SA, Epstein RA. Transition care for children with special health needs. Technical brief No. 15. Rockville, MD: Agency for Healthcare Research and Quality Prepared by the Vanderbilt University Evidence-based Practice Center under Contract No. 290–2012–00009-1; 2014.
24. Peter NG, Forke CM, Ginsburg KR, Schwarz DF. Transition from pediatric to adult care: internists' perspectives. Pediatrics. 2009;123(2):417–23.
25. Murphy DJ Jr, Foster E, American College of Cardiology Foundation, American Heart Association, American College of Physicians Task Force on Clinical Competence. ACCF/AHA/AAP recommendations for training in pediatric cardiology. Task force 6: training in transition of adolescent care and care of the adult with congenital heart disease. J Am Coll Cardiol. 2005;46(7):1399–401. PubMed PMID: 16198870.
26. Fernandes SM, Khairy P, Fishman L, Melvin P, O'Sullivan-Oliveira J, Sawicki G, et al. Referral patterns and perceived barriers to adult congenital heart disease care: Results of a survey of U.S. pediatric cardiologists. J Am Coll Cardiol. 2011;60(23):2411–8.
27. Ubel P. Why Many physicians are reluctant to see Medicaid patients. Forbes. 2013;
28. American Medical Association. Report of the Council on Medical Service. Chicago, Illinois; 2016.
29. McManus MM, R. Practice Resource-No.2, 2017 Coding and Reimbursement Tip Sheet for Transition from Pediatric to Adult Health Care Washington, D.C: Got

Transition and American Academy of Pediatrics. 2016. http://www.gottransition.org/resourceGet.cfm?id=353.
30. Betz CL, Nehring WM, Lobo ML. Transition Needs of Parents of Adolescents and Emerging Adults With Special Health Care Needs and Disabilities. J Fam Nurs. 2015;21(3):362–412. PubMed PMID: 26283056.
31. Betz CL, Lobo ML, Nehring WM, Bui K. Voices not heard: a systematic review of adolescents' and emerging adults' perspectives of health care transition. Nurs Outlook. 2013;61(5):311–36. PubMed PMID: 23876260.
32. Fernandes S, Fishman L, O'Sullivan-Oliveira J, Ziniel S, Melvin P, Khairy P, et al. Current practices for the transition and transfer of patients with a wide spectrum of pediatric-onset chronic diseases: Results of a clinician survey at a free-standing pediatric hospital. Int J Child Adolesc Health. 2012;3:507–15.
33. Gilliam PP, Ellen JM, Leonard L, Kinsman S, Jevitt CM, Straub DM. Transition of adolescents with HIV to adult care: Characteristics and current practices of the adolescent trials network for HIV/AIDS interpretation. J Assoc Nurses AIDS Care. 2011;22(4):283–94.
34. Clarizia NA, Chahal N, Manlhiot C, Kilburn J, Redington AN, McCrindle BW. Transition to adult health care for adolescents and young adults with congenital heart disease: Perspectives of the patient, parent and health care provider. Can J Cardiol. 2009;25(9):e317–e22.
35. Betz CL, Smith KA, Van Speybroeck A, Hernandez FV, Jacobs RA. Movin' On Up: An Innovative Nurse-Led Interdisciplinary Health Care Transition Program. J Pediatr Health Care. 2016;30(4):323–38. PubMed PMID: 26483330.
36. Society of Pediatric (SPN). SPN Position Statement: Transition of Pediatric Patients into Adult Care. Chicago, Illinois: Society of Pediatric Nurses; 2016. p. 9.
37. Coyne B, Hallowell SC, Thompson M. Measurable Outcomes After Transfer From Pediatric to Adult Providers in Youth With Chronic Illness. J Adolesc Health. 2017;60(1):3–16. PubMed PMID: 27614592.
38. Lotstein DS, McPherson M, Strickland B, Newacheck PW. Transition planning for youth with special health care needs: results from the National Survey of Children With Special Health Care Needs. Pediatrics. 2005;115(6):1562–8. PubMed PMID: 2009019696.
39. Prior M, McManus M, White P, Davidson L. Measuring the "triple aim" in transition care: a systematic review. Pediatrics. 2014;134(6):e1648–61. PubMed PMID: 25422015.

Healthcare Transition from the Adult Provider's Perspective

7

Nathan Samras, Janet Ma, Stacey Weinstein, and Alice A. Kuo

Vignette

As an internal medicine physician, you are happy to see a 21-year-old new patient, Emily, on your schedule this morning because these visits are usually straightforward. Your heart rate speeds up as your medical assistant tells you that she has Turner syndrome, and you try to remember what you learned about this condition in medical school.

Emily is accompanied by her mother who tells you about her history of Turner syndrome, hypothyroidism, bicuspid aortic valve, moderate aortic regurgitation, and menstrual irregularity. She has not seen her general pediatrician for the past 2 years but has seen her pediatric endocrinologist and pediatric cardiologist over the past 6 months. Unfortunately she does not have any medical records, but she knows she is taking oral contraceptives and levothyroxine.

Emily's mother asks many questions about her daughter's health and sometimes answers questions that were specifically directed to the patient. The involvement of the mother in the patient visit is surprising to you. As you try to answer the multiple questions, they both then ask you about resources for patients and families for Turner syndrome as an adult. You feel unprepared and a little overwhelmed.

Introduction

The case of a new patient such as Emily is not rare nor is the internist's perception that this patient has "drifted" to your office from pediatric care rather than being part of a carefully planned and executed handoff [1]. While there are many pediatricians and pediatric subspecialists who continue to provide care long past the traditional age of 18 years often because of a lack of transition resources, in 2002, the American Academy of Pediatrics, the American Academy of Family Physicians, and the American College of Physicians-American Society of Internal Medicine recommended that adults with special health-care needs be cared for by adult-focused primary care physicians [2, 3].

Eighteen million adolescent and young adult patients are transitioning to adult care annually

N. Samras, M.D., M.P.H. (✉) • J. Ma, M.D.
S. Weinstein, M.D. • A. A. Kuo, M.D., Ph.D.
Division of Internal Medicine and Pediatrics, UCLA Department of Medicine, Los Angeles, CA, USA
e-mail: nsamras@mednet.ucla.edu

A. C. Hergenroeder, C. M. Wiemann (eds.), *Health Care Transition*,
https://doi.org/10.1007/978-3-319-72868-1_7

according to the U.S. Census Bureau, and 18–25% of these patients have chronic medical or mental health conditions including genetic disorders like Turner syndrome [4–6]. Modern medical care has enabled more than 90% of children with special health-care needs to reach adulthood, yet many internists and adult subspecialists are not comfortable taking care of conditions that are more common in the pediatric population [7, 8]. This may stem from the lack of exposure to less common conditions or a lack of knowledge of guidelines and resources to care for these patients.

Though many chronic conditions have consensus guidelines on the care of patients with conditions such as Turner syndrome, some of the rarer conditions may not, leading to potential increased discomfort and lack of confidence once these patients reach adulthood [9]. Even for specialists who are familiar with consensus guidelines, such as adult gastroenterologists (GI) who take care of patients with inflammatory bowel disease, research has shown that adult GI providers are often uncomfortable with these adolescents and young adults with special health-care needs (AYASHCN) because they lack training in adolescent medicine [10, 11]. Pediatricians compared to internists are less comfortable treating the chronic conditions of hypertension, diabetes, depression, and chronic pain, and therefore young adults with complex health needs who also have these conditions may be transitioned out of a pediatrician's office prematurely [12]. The provider's discomfort may be exacerbated by the need for additional training in reproductive health, vocational training, and complex care coordination [13].

This textbook provides resources to help pediatric providers develop transition programs to equip AYASHCN with the self-management skills needed to navigate within the adult health-care system. Unfortunately 22% of children with special health-care needs (CSHCN) between 12 and 17 years of age report that their doctor does not usually or always encourage adolescents to take responsibility for their care, and only 31% received all the needed guidance for the transition to adult health care [8]. Even if such guidance occurs, the adult provider must still be prepared to receive these young adults and complete the transition process appropriately.

This chapter will discuss some of the common concerns of adult health providers assuming care for AYASHCN and then describe how transition care is analogous to high-quality primary care, with which most adult physicians are familiar. These concerns often involve provider and health system-related issues such as lack of provider competency or confidence in care for these patients, lack of training in many childhood conditions and adolescent related issues, lack of communication between pediatric and adult providers, as well as time and reimbursement-related concerns [14, 15]. There are additional concerns related to the youth themselves and their stage of human development, such as patient maturity and readiness to transition, psychosocial needs, and parental/family involvement [14].

Lack of Internists Trained to Care for This Population

There are more than 30 million young adults between 18 and 24 years old in the United States, and approximately 25–30% of this population has special health-care needs [6, 15, 16]. Although 80–90% of internists believe that primary care of AYASHCN should be provided by adult health-care providers after transition, not enough internists across multiple disciplines are comfortable doing so [5, 12]. The challenge in finding interested providers worsens for patients with developmental disabilities and complex health or mental health conditions [15]. The current primary care shortage in the United States is expected to worsen over time as an aging population grows [17]. Dual-trained internal medicine-pediatrics physicians appear to be ideal providers for this population, but this specialty is not able to care for the entire population of AYASHCN with fewer than 10,000 practicing internal medicine-pediatrics physicians in the United States [1].

In addition to requiring primary care, AYASHCN are not the same as healthy young adults and often need subspecialty care. Unfortunately there is a lack of qualified or interested adult subspecialists available to provide specialty services for this population [1, 12]. It takes time for the primary care physician to build a network with the few adult subspecialists who are available. Mental health providers are especially needed for AYASHCN who have unique challenges during the transition period, but many internists have difficulty identifying high-quality behavioral health providers for these young adults and who also accept insurance [18].

Internists are often not comfortable taking care of young adults with complex medical and mental health conditions because of insufficient training in internal medicine residency for child-onset medical conditions [12]. Pediatricians have frequently cited concerns about finding appropriately trained and interested adult providers for their complex patients, especially ones with developmental or intellectual disabilities [15]. This difficulty can be decreased by maximizing communication between the internist and pediatrician during the transition period to communicate salient aspects of disease-specific care. Often this care is not just specific to a medical treatment plan but involves multidisciplinary treatment teams, and the primary care medical home model discussed later in this chapter is one of many that has flexibility to coordinate this care. In addition, internists who have experience caring for larger populations of patients with the same condition (e.g., cystic fibrosis) can improve provider comfort and confidence [12].

AYASHCN Lack Adequate Preparation for Transition

At Emily's visit, her mother reports that she orders refills and picks up Emily's medicines. The mother also makes all of her medical appointments. At the appointment today, Emily appears to be indifferent about her health issues. Her mother reveals that Emily has a history of depression 4 years ago treated with an antidepressant for about 2 years and then weaned off when her mood seemingly improved. When asked how Emily's mood is now, the mother replies, "It's all right, I guess."

Although our patient Emily seems indifferent to her care, she may never have been guided to be more independent in these health administrative tasks. Emerging adult patients should be encouraged to take on more adult responsibilities regarding their health, which may require a more prolonged and deliberate transition process that extends from the pediatric or adolescent provider into the adult office. This may involve reminders, input, and guidance from their parents or other family health advocates, with assistance in processing information and in reinforcing recommendations. Providers and family can be integral in this guided decision-making process [1]. Adult health providers may be surprised by young adults' continued dependence on parental guidance, but they should work with them and their parents to help the young adult develop more self-care skills and responsibilities [15].

Although the transfer of care from pediatric to adult care may occur at a defined age such as 18 or 21 years old, the psychosocial development of adolescent and young adult patients occurs at a later age. The young adult stage of life represents a distinct developmental stage, similar to how we view adolescence, that is termed "emerging adulthood" [19]. This period spanning from approximately ages 18 to 25 is marked by a transition to independence—involving identity exploration, instability, self-focus, feeling in between, and possibilities [15, 19].

Health-related decision-making during emerging adulthood includes engaging in riskier behaviors, decreased frequency of seeking care despite elevated health risks, and less adherence to provider recommendations. These may be due to multiple neurodevelopmental and psychosocial factors that are often underappreciated by the adult provider (see Chaps. 2 and 3 for a full discussion of brain development and its impact on behavior).

Beyond the neurodevelopmental perspective, emerging adults as a group are demographically heterogeneous, and their social circumstances may have a significant impact on their health and ability to assume greater responsibility in their care. Within this age group, 40% are not enrolled in college, and only 40% have full-time jobs [15, 20]. Patients may be away at school, may be living at home with parents, or may have initially left the home and are now returning. They may be unmarried but living with romantic partners or roommates in a variety of living arrangements [15]. Understanding their social circumstances is crucial to guide young adults through the process of improving their self-care.

Understanding the Life Course Health Development of the Emerging Adult

Young adults and emerging adults are perceived to be healthier than their adolescent or adult counterparts. However, their overall morbidity and mortality are worse compared to their adolescent counterparts [21]. According to the Institute of Medicine, young adults are surprisingly unhealthy, possibly related to the risky behaviors in this age group, the onset of serious mental health conditions, unintentional injury, substance abuse, and sexually transmitted infections [22]. In addition to these health risks, young adults' utilization of health services including primary or preventive care is significantly lower than adolescents and adults over the age of 25, while their emergency room use is higher. In 2014, 25% of young adults in the United States were without a usual source of medical care [23]. Their adherence to recommendations decrease, and the medical complications are increased even when they do receive health care [15].

The internist may view the young adult visit as a straightforward encounter. A routine primary care visit of a healthy young adult female may consist of checking blood pressure and performing a routine pap smear [15]. However this routine visit does not address risk factors that could affect current and future adult health.

The Life Course Health Development model can frame the care of the emerging adult patients where the person's childhood years impact their lifelong physical and mental health conditions [24]. Many chronic adult conditions such as hypertension, diabetes mellitus type 2, and dyslipidemia may have developed because of risk factors or a lack of protective factors in a person's early life during critical periods of development [24]. For example, weight gain in young adulthood leads to complications from obesity in later adulthood [25]. Substance use often starts in adolescence but peaks in young adulthood and can lead to addiction and related complications [26]. Interventions in the adolescent and young adult years can alter a person's health in later years; therefore all primary care providers should recognize risk factors and attempt to address risky behaviors, which may prevent certain chronic diseases [15, 24].

Poor Coordination Between Pediatricians and Internists

One of the internist's biggest frustrations for bringing AYASHCN into their practice is the lack of medical records, medication reconciliation, transition plan, and recommendations from the AYASHCN's pediatrician [1, 27]. In addition, integrating an AYASHCN for the first time into adult practices can be difficult when patients and family have had long-term relationships with their pediatric providers. There is evidence that post-transition access to care is improved if patients and families meet adult providers before this transfer [28]. A transition policy in the health system can help set expectations that transition for all youth is a normal process (see Chaps. 16–17). Adult providers should make time to establish trust with the whole family during the initial meetings, often prioritizing this rapport over discussion of specific medical details or treatment plans. A similar process exists in taking geriatric patients into an adult practice and can be considered as a reference when seeing young adults. This relationship building does not need to wait until the first face-to-face meeting. A process that starts months ahead of time may help foster a stronger initial therapeutic relationship during the first meeting between the patient, family, and adult provider. Internists should be ready to establish a line of communication with the previous pediatric provider prior to the initial visit either in person or over the phone. This helps the flow of important medical information and also provides reassurance to the patient and family that crucial social or cultural information has been communicated. The immediate post-transfer period is also an important time for the adult and pediatric providers to communicate information that may not be readily apparent from written records and to provide recommendations or assistance with future care [1].

Time Alone with Physician Without the Parents Present

Although the integration of all caregivers into the transition process is important, most AYASHCN also need to have opportunities for independent interactions with their adult provider, which may be difficult if the caregivers have been advocating for the patient during all prior appointments. The transition of an emerging adult into increasing adult roles and responsibilities is unlikely to be completed at age 18, and adult providers should be cognizant of providing opportunities both for parental input and for patient independence with the understanding of all parties—patients, caregivers, and providers—of how much independence the patient will have in their health care in the future. In studies looking at transition from the patient perspective, adult provider characteristics such as decision-making opportunities and time alone with the health-care provider without parents, in addition to providers' social skills and bedside manner, impact satisfaction with their transition experience [29].

It may be challenging for parents to give up some of decision-making authority even if the young adult patients desire more autonomy. This concern may be more acute when meeting a new adult provider with whom the family has not yet established enough trust and rapport to cede some of that control [15]. In early visits during the establishment of care, adult providers may want to balance both the involvement of the parents to provide crucial health information and time alone with the patient to foster trust and independence [29].

Time to Care for Complex Patients

The care of medically complex patients usually requires more time than a typical follow-up visit for a nonmedically complex youth. A survey of pediatricians and internists indicated concern that the young adults and their parents often expect an unusually long amount of time during the visit and more frequent attention overall [29]. This is reported more frequently from pediatricians than internists [12]. With many health systems focusing on relative value unit-based productivity, medically complex patients can affect a provider's productivity metric, making it a financial liability for practices to care for high volumes of these patients. There are mechanisms to accurately bill for the extra time for medical evaluation and care coordination that may resolve this discrepancy between time and reimbursement (see Chap. 25) [15].

Medical Home Model

Several health-care system initiatives are already in place for patients of many ages, which can help meet the goals of caring for both young adults and the more complex AYASHCN. For example, the Patient-Centered Medical Home (PCMH) model includes three interrelated processes—preventive care, acute illness management, and chronic disease management—and has six standards applicable to all primary care patients regardless of their health status or complexity [1, 30]:

(a) Patient-centered access
(b) Team-based care
(c) Population health management
(d) Care management and support
(e) Care coordination and care transitions
(f) Performance measurement and quality improvement

In prior comparative studies, the PCMH model had a small to moderate positive effect on preventive care services and patient satisfaction, along with a modest reduction in emergency room visits, although not hospitalizations [31].

Providing high-quality transition services via an integrated and comprehensive model may one day become the standard of care of any primary care practice. The World Health Organization also supports a paradigm shift to build an integrated health-care system. Their goals include patient- and family-centered care, focus on preventive medicine, and supporting patients with community resources [32].

The care coordination in the PCMH model is especially important in the care of AYASHCN. There are evidence-based guidelines for chronic care management that involve written care plans and close care coordination between a multidisciplinary team of providers [1]. A co-management partnership with subspecialists includes a shared medical summary and written care plans that have been prepared together with the patient and family members to synchronize care across all providers. Care coordination can improve patient self-management skills, empowering the AYASHCN to communicate with the provider or care coordinator by telephone, electronic media, or in person clinic visits when health needs arise, and these health literacy and self-care skills should be monitored on a regular basis, with support offered if necessary [1]. A registry may be helpful to track the transition process for AYASHCN (see Chap. 12).

Training in Adolescent Medicine and Mental Health

Increased experience with adolescent medicine and a focus on the psychosocial needs surrounding this emerging adult period of time of 18–25 years old are crucial [1, 15]. Internal medicine, family medicine, and pediatrics residents should have additional training in adolescent medicine during residency, with emphasis on the need for mental health support for this population. For AYASHCN, the family has typically played a big role in their health care, and the patient and the caregivers have to adjust to new roles relating to independent decision-making for the AYASHCN. To ease this adjustment and maximize the PCMH model, the internist should employ a family-centered model when appropriate to include all caregivers to maximize coordination of care while minimizing stress for the whole family, as well as discussing specific resources for behavioral health when those needs arise [1].

The adolescent "HEADSS" screening approach (home, education/employment, activities, drugs/diet, sexuality, suicidality) has been shown to be an effective mechanism to screen for psychosocial needs in this population [33]. The HEADSS approach is the standard of care to screen for adolescent psychosocial stressors. The HEADSS history may reveal drug and alcohol abuse, poor eating habits, lack of exercise, sexual risk behavior, and untreated depression or anxiety which will impact future health if not addressed appropriately at the right time [17]. Adult providers can easily use the HEADSS approach without significant additional training. They can act on the information provided to encourage the young adult patient to make wise health-care decisions that will have long-lasting impact on their health [1].

The vignette suggests that addressing Emily's underlying mood issues is essential in order to help manage her self-care skills, independence, and apparent lack of interest in her care. Young adults have higher rates of mental health issues compared to their adolescent and older adult counterparts, with higher rates of suicidal ideation, plan, and attempts [34]. Forty-six percent of young adults in college report psychiatric diagnoses in the last year [2]. This data underscores the importance of prevention and screening in this age group as 75% of mental health disorders present prior to age 25 [34]. While addressing mental health issues can seem daunting to address in primary care, surveys on provider attitudes indicate that adult health-care providers were overall more comfortable addressing mental health issues in the office than pediatricians, with pediatricians reporting more barriers due to insufficient mental health and social work support [12]. The adult primary care provider is uniquely positioned to screen for mental health problems with tools such as HEADSS, intervene, and have a large impact on many aspects of these patients' health care and overall health outcomes.

Disability and End-of-Life Issues

Internists report discomfort caring for young adults with severe disabilities because of lack of specific training, but they can draw on their experience caring for elderly patient with chronic disabilities and end-of-life issues to help guide them with the care of the transitioning young adult patient. Identification of the patient advocate, caregiver, legal guardian, and medical decision-maker is essential to the initial visit. An advanced directive from previous pediatric documentation should be verified with the patient and family, or discussion of an advanced directive should be initiated if one has not yet been completed (see Chap. 30).

Difficulty Accessing Health Care as an Adult

In addition to psychosocial, developmental, and familial/relationship barriers to adult care for AYASHCN, young adults also face structural and systems challenges in accessing adult health care. Both young adults and providers have concerns about the patient's access to health insurance during this transition period [15, 35]. Childhood insurance programs subsidized through the government can end as patients reach adulthood, such as Medicaid, SHIP, and Title V. Marketplace plans that enable patients to stay within the same health-care system that may have cared for their complex condition throughout childhood may be financially inaccessible. Expansions in the health-care safety net through Medicaid may enable these patients to be insured, but due to Medicaid's lower reimbursement rates, they may have fewer options for adult primary care or specialty providers who have more experience caring for medically complex patients. Reducing Medicaid would have a deleterious effect on AYASHCN.

Patients with disabilities have less employment opportunities that may limit access to employee-based health insurance, and young adults are also more likely to take part-time or unpaid work early in their career, which may not come with full health-care benefits. Many parents are themselves uninsured or under-insured which negates the benefit of recent changes to health-care laws to enable young adults to stay on their parents' insurance through age 26. College-based insurance plans may be inaccessible for young adults attending a 2-year community or city colleges or vocational programs [36]. The current health-care legislative landscape poses potential future challenges to accessing adult health insurance and care for AYASCHN, including lifting bans on lifetime caps and protections for preexisting conditions.

Changes in federal law with the Patient Protection and Affordable Care Act (ACA) of 2010 have improved health insurance options for young adults, enabling not only coverage of dependents to age 26 but also have improved portability of insurance, improved access to coverage through health exchanges, and the exclusion of preexisting conditions as criteria to provide coverage that has been a consistent issue within this specific patient population [1]. However, many young adults either have low levels of health insurance literacy or are unaware of their benefits or undervalue these benefits [37], with fewer than 25% of young adults aware of Medicaid expansion and less than a third of young adults being aware of health insurance marketplaces [35]. Young adults are less likely to schedule preventive health visits despite their coverage under the current law [15]. Variability in coverage through Title V, Medicaid, Supplemental Security Income, and Social Security Disability Income among states can make it difficult for patients and providers to navigate [1].

Access challenges are not limited to insurance alone; AYASHCN may have accessed additional resources through pediatrics such as care coordination that may be scarcer in adulthood. Youth with intellectual and developmental disabilities have fewer options for daytime programs with educational and recreational components than programs available through the K-12 school system for children. Allied health professionals such as physical therapy, occupational therapy, and speech therapy are more available for developmentally disabled children than adults. Social workers and case managers may also be less available in the adult health-care setting. Custodial issues such as guardianship or conservatorship and residential placement can limit access.

At the time of this writing, the debate regarding health care may lead to changes in the current law, and subsequently patients should be aware of but not dependent on the ACA protections as described previously. Patients should be encouraged to pursue employment options that include commercial insurance coverage that is advantageous to high-risk people, often in the form of large group plans with pooled risk [1]. Additional reimbursement and dedicated payment plans are also needed for providers taking care of transitional care patients, as this is a major concern for providers to receive payment for the added time and complexity to take care of them [15].

Social Determinants of Health

Medical care for all patients can be improved if the provider is aware of their social determinants of health, and this is particularly important in underserved populations and AYASHCN [38]. Access to care, provider availability, local public health and community resources, and insurance coverage impact the quality of care, and the pediatric to adult transition process is heavily influenced by medical, psychosocial, environmental, socioeconomic, and other factors [1]. Although internists may initially consider this a unique barrier to the transitioning population, the techniques to assess and respond to this aspect of an individual's health, for example, through the PCMH model, are the same as in all ages. It is not a matter of lack of training but rather a difference in focus and time allocation to ensure that the social determinants of health are addressed in developing treatment plans.

Key Steps for Accepting AYASHCN

As discussed, the adult provider has many models to facilitate caring for AYASHCN, such as creating a transition policy statement, using a standardized transition readiness assessment tool, communicating and collaborating with patients' pediatric providers, obtaining all necessary medical records, focusing on team based care, knowing and utilizing care coordinators and local resources, setting goals with the patient/family, and maintaining a continuously updated individualized comprehensive health-care plan [15, 22]. The Six Core Elements of Transition is one commonly used structure (see Chap. 1). These and other topics will be further expanded upon in Chap. 17.

Other models of facilitating entry into adult care for AYASHCN are discussed elsewhere in this textbook (e.g., see Chap. 36). The recognition of the importance of successful transition care has grown. With the implementation of the ACA, the Centers for Medicare and Medicaid Services (CMS) has implemented an amendment to improve transitional care services, which many states had adopted by the end of 2015. The ACA has also increased attention and focus on advanced primary care initiatives, accountable care organizations, and additional reimbursement for transition-related services [15].

Ideally health-care systems should have dedicated payments to support multidisciplinary chronic disease management for AYASHCN [1]. Chapters 23–25 address billing and reimbursement for HCT. Additional education, research, and health-care reform are essential to support adult and pediatric providers participating in transition care for AYASHCN. Although the best methods to support transition are still emerging, the continuing medical education resources on the "Got Transition" website (gottransition.org) and American College of Physicians (ACP) resources on caring for adults with child onset conditions are helpful to practicing providers and institutions who want to implement transition care processes or procedures [15]. Though many supports and services are already available for providers caring for transition patients, additional support from the health-care systems level will help transition care be an aspect of high-quality primary care that is accessible to all AYASCHN.

Conclusion

As the changing epidemiology of young adults with chronic conditions originating in childhood continues to progress, the number of these individuals surviving into adulthood necessitates a reexamination of health-care delivery systems and how to provide appropriate care. Adult primary care and specialty providers need more education and support to care for this growing population. Although evidence-based best practices need to be established, resources have been developed to help adult providers feel more comfortable with these patients. With some guidance and support to adult providers, the capacity to care for young adults with chronic conditions originating in childhood will improve, leading to better health care outcomes for this group.

References

1. American Academy of Pediatrics. Supporting the health care transition from adolescence to adulthood in the medical home. Pediatrics. 2011;128(1):182–200.
2. American College Health Association National College Health Assessment Reference Group Data Assessment Fall. 2009. www.acha-ncha.org/docs/ACHA-NCHA_Reference_Group_Report_Fall2009.pdf. Accessed 27 Oct 2017.
3. American Academy of Pediatrics, American Academy of Family Physicians, American College of Physicians-American Society of Internal Medicine. A consensus statement on health care transitions for young adults with special health care needs. Pediatrics. 2002;110(6 Pt 2):1304–6.
4. U.S. Census Bureau, Current population survey, 2013.
5. Blum RW. Overview of transition issues for youth with disabilities. Paediatrician. 1991;18:101–4.
6. National Survey of Children's Health. Child and adolescent health measurement initiative. http://childhealthdata.org/learn/NSCH. Accessed 27 Oct 2017.
7. Sakakibara H. Transition of women with turner syndrome from pediatrics to adult health care: current situation and associated problems. Front Pediatr. 2017;5:28.
8. Youth with Special Health Care Needs Receive the Services Necessary to Make Transitions to Adult Health Care. NS-CSHCN CHARTBOOK 2009-2010. Illustrated Findings from the National Survey of Children with Special Health Care Needs. mchb.hrsa.gov/cshcn0910/core/pages/co6/co6tahc.html. Accessed 27 Oct 2017.
9. Gravholt CH, et al. Clinical practice guidelines for the care of girls and women with turner syndrome: proceedings from the 2016 Cincinnati international turner syndrome meeting. Eur J Endocrinol. 2017;177(3):G1–G70.
10. Sebastian S, et al. The requirements and barriers to successful transition of adolescents with inflammatory bowel disease: differing perceptions from a survey of adult and paediatric gastroenterologists. J Crohn's Colitis. 2012;6(8):830–44.
11. Hait EJ, et al. Transition of adolescents with inflammatory bowel disease from pediatric to adult care: a survey of adult gastroenterologists. J Pediatr Gastroenterol Nutr. 2009;48(1):61–5.
12. Okumura MJ, et al. Comfort of general internists and general pediatricians in providing Care for Young Adults with chronic illnesses of childhood. J Gen Intern Med. 2008;23(10):1621–7.
13. Trivedi I, Keefer L. The emerging adult with inflammatory bowel disease: challenges and recommendations for the adult gastroenterologist. Gastroenterol Res Pract. 2015;2015:260807.
14. Peter NG, et al. Transition from pediatric to adult care: internists' perspectives. Pediatrics. 2009;123(2):417–23.
15. Pilapil M, et al. Care of adults with chronic childhood conditions: a practical guide. Alexandria, VA: Society of General Internal Medicine; 2016.
16. United States Census Bureau. Age and sex composition: 2010. 2010 census briefs. www.census.gov/prod/cen2010/briefs/c2010br-03.pdf. Accessed 27 Oct 2017.
17. The Complexities of Physician Supply and Demand: Projections from 2014 to 2025. Association of American Medical Colleges. www.aamc.org/download/458082/data/2016_complexities_of_supply_and_demand_projections.pdf. Accessed 27 Oct 2017.
18. McLaren S, et al. 'Talking a different language': an exploration of the influence of organizational cultures and working practices on transition from child to adult mental health services. BMC Health Serv Res. 2013;13:254–64.
19. Arnett JJ. Emerging adulthood. A theory of development from the late teens through the twenties. Am Psychol. 2000;55(5):469–80.
20. U.S. Census Bureau. Current population survey. 1999. www.census.gov/prod/2001pubs/p23-205.pdf. Accessed 27 Oct 2017.
21. Park MJ, et al. The health status of young adults in the United States. J Adolesc Health. 2006;39(3):305–17.
22. Institute of Medicine and National Research Council. Investing in the health and well-being of young adults. Washington, DC: The National Academies Press; 2015.
23. Center for Disease Control. Health, United States, 2015, with special feature on racial and ethnic health disparities. www.cdc.gov/nchs/data/hus/hus15.pdf. Accessed 27 Oct 2017.
24. Halfon N, et al. The handbook of life course health development science. New York, NY: Springer International Publishing; 2017.
25. Dummer TJ, et al. Targeting policy for obesity prevention: identifying the critical age for weight gain in women. J Obes. 2012;2012:934895.
26. Hingson RW, et al. Age at drinking onset and alcohol dependence: age at onset, duration, and severity. Arch Pediatr Adolesc Med. 2006;160(7):739–46.
27. Hunt S, Sharma N. Pediatric to adult-care transitions in childhood-onset chronic disease: hospitalist perspectives. J Hosp Med. 2013;8(11):627–30.

28. Bloom SR, et al. Health care transition for youth with special health care needs. J Adolesc Health. 2012; 51:213–9.
29. Sonneveld HM, et al. Gaps in transitional care: what are the perceptions of adolescents, parents and providers? Child Care Health Dev. 2012;39:69–80.
30. Defining the Patient Centered Medical Home, U.S. Department of Health & Human Services. pcmh.ahrq.gov/page/defining-pcmh. Accessed 27 Oct 2017.
31. Ferrante JM, et al. Principles of the patient-centered medical home and preventive services delivery. Ann Fam Med. 2010;8(2):108–16.
32. World Health Organization. Innovative care for chronic conditions, building blocks for action. http://www.who.int/chp/knowledge/publications/icccglobalreport.pdf. Accessed 27 Oct 2017.
33. Goldenring JM, Rosen DS. Getting into adolescent heads: an essential update. Contemp Pediatr. 2004;21(1): 64–90.
34. U.S. Department of Health and Human Services. Substance Abuse and Mental Health Services Administration. Results from the 2010 National Survey on Drug Use and Health: Summary of National Findings. www.samhsa.gov/data/sites/default/files/NSDUHNationalFindingsResults2010-web/2k10ResultsRev/NSDUHresultsRev2010.pdf. Accessed 27 Oct 2017.
35. Long SK, et al. The health reform monitoring survey: addressing data gaps to provide timely insights into the affordable care act. Health Aff (Millwood). 2014;33(1):161–7.
36. Postolowski C, et al. Helping students understand health care reform and enroll in health insurance. 2013. www.clasp.org/resources-and-publications/files/ACA-Toolkit_Helping-Students-Understand-Health-Care-Reform-and-Enroll-in-Health-Insurance.pdf. Accessed 27 Oct 2017.
37. Dauner KN, Thompson J. Young adult's perspectives on being uninsured and implications for health reform. Qual Rep. 2014;19(4):1.
38. Barr VJ, et al. The expanded chronic care model: an integration of concepts and strategies from population health promotion and the chronic care model. Hosp Q. 2003;7(1):73–82.

8 Healthcare Insurance Changes as Youth Become Young Adults

Beth Sufian, James Passamano, and Amy Sopchak

Important Issues

Discuss Changes Before Turning 18

The medical team and the young adult's family may not realize that AYASHCN have limited options for access to health insurance. It is important to make sure AYASHCN and their families receive accurate information regarding the law and effective strategies for maintaining or obtaining health insurance coverage or government benefits.

Disclaimer
The following information is general in nature and is not meant to be legal advice. Nothing in this chapter should be considered to be legal advice regarding a specific individual's situation.
There is no guarantee that the information in this chapter has not changed between the time it was drafted and the time the chapter was published. Please check to see if laws related to the Affordable Care Act, Medicaid, Social Security or COBRA.

B. Sufian, J.D. (✉) • J. Passamano, J.D.
A. Sopchak, J.D.
Sufian and Passamano, LLP, Houston, TX, USA
e-mail: bsufian@sufianpassamano.com

Changes to coverage due to age are complicated. The medical team should not expect the young adult to navigate the changes alone and should include the family in discussions about options for health insurance coverage. The medical team should familiarize itself with the age limits for programs that are available in their state.

Track Government Program Eligibility in the Medical Chart

It is helpful if the pediatric medical team notes in a patient's chart if a young adult receives Supplemental Security Income ("SSI") benefits or is eligible for other government programs. This will remind the medical team to alert the patient and family before eligibility changes occur when the patient turns 18 years of age.

Different Eligibility Criteria for Different Programs

Different government programs have different eligibility criteria for individuals over the age of 18. For example, Social Security benefit eligibility changes once a person reaches the age of 18. Many AYASHCN lose their SSI benefits because they do not realize that they will have to meet a new adult medical eligibility standard and different non-medical eligibility criteria when they turn 18.

A. C. Hergenroeder, C. M. Wiemann (eds.), *Health Care Transition*,
https://doi.org/10.1007/978-3-319-72868-1_8

In addition, the Supplemental Nutrition Assistance Program (SNAP), which provides food stamps, will have different eligibility guidelines for persons over the age of 18 as will assistance from the Housing and Urban Development agency.

Employer Based Health Insurance

Employer based health insurance policies offer an option for coverage if the young adult works for an employer who provides coverage. The young adult may also have health insurance coverage through a parent or guardian who works for an employer who offers health insurance coverage.

Social Security Benefits

Supplemental Security Income (SSI)

SSI is a program that provides a monthly cash benefit and Medicaid coverage. A person must meet certain low income and medical requirements in order to receive SSI benefits. A child must live in a household that meets the SSI low income and assets criteria set out by the Social Security Administration (SSA) in regulations. Once a child turns 18, SSA only considers the young adult's income and assets when determining if he meets the SSI non-medical criteria.

Social Security Disability Insurance (SSDI)

SSDI provides a monthly benefit and Medicare coverage and does not have an asset limit. Sometimes AYASHCN transition to adult care between the ages of 21 and 26. These adults may have worked enough to be eligible for SSDI benefits. If their health requires them to stop work or reduce their work hours to part time hours they may be eligible for SSDI.

The SSDI applicant or recipient cannot be engaged in substantial work activity at the time the application for SSA benefits is filed. In 2017, an applicant for SSDI benefits cannot be making more than $1170 a month from part time work. This dollar amount changes each year and is $1170 before taxes are taken out of the work earnings check. A person who is self-employed has a different earnings cut off in order to be eligible for and stay eligible for SSDI benefits.

A person who has never worked will NOT be eligible for SSDI benefits. Often people tell the young adult that he should enroll in "Full Disability benefits". There is no such thing as "Full Disability". If a young adult has never worked he is not eligible for SSDI benefits. The Social Security representative checks eligibility for both SSI and SSDI and only one application needs to be filed.

Medicare coverage begins after receipt of the actual SSDI benefit for 24 months plus the 5 month SSDI waiting period. Medicare will not start until 29 full months from the month the person became unable to engage in full time work.

To prevent a lapse of coverage the individual can COBRA her employer based insurance for 29 months until Medicare starts. See COBRA section below. A person may also choose to purchase an insurance policy on either the Federal Healthcare Exchange, a state Healthcare Exchange, from an insurance agent or directly from an insurance company.

SSA Medical Criteria

A diagnosis of a chronic illness does not automatically make a person eligible for Social Security benefits. A person applying for SSI or SSDI benefits must meet certain medical criteria. The medical criteria are called "The Social Security Medical Listing".

Social Security Medical Listing

Children and adults with chronic illness can determine if they meet a Social Security Medical Listing by going to www.ssa.gov and looking for the SSA Blue Book. The SSA Blue Book lists medical conditions and the criteria a person must meet for SSA medical eligibility.

The SSA Medical Listing for children is usually different from the SSA Medical Listing for adults with the same medical condition. This means that when a child transitions to adulthood at the age of 18 the medical eligibility criteria for Social Security benefits may be different than when the child first became eligible for benefits. Medical criteria for some conditions includes things such as how many hospital stays the person had in the year prior to applying for Social Security benefits or if the person must use supplemental oxygen or has low lung function.

Showing Medical Equivalence

An adult who does not meet one of the listed medical criteria will have to show that her condition is as severe as one of the listed criteria. SSA assesses whether a person has a certain medical condition and also considers the degree of severity of symptoms.

It has become increasingly difficult to obtain a finding of disability by SSA if a person is advocating she meets the SSA medical criteria because her condition is as severe as the listed medical criteria found in the SSA regulations. Therefore, the person will need detailed medical records to substantiate her claim.

Many at SSA are skeptical of using one letter from a physician as the basis for a finding that the person is unable to engage in substantial work activity. A letter can be sent to outline how the applicant meets the medical criteria but the SSA representative or judge will want to see medical records for the year prior to applying for benefits.

Medical Records

The SSA will base its decision about medical eligibility on the medical records it receives to support a finding the person meets the SSA Medical Listing for their condition or that their medical condition is as severe as the Social Security listed medical criteria. Medical records that contain information that documents how the young adult's medical limitations prevent engagement in full time work are helpful.

Typically the SSA will only consider medical records from the year prior to the application date. However, there are certain circumstances that will result in SSA needing additional medical records for a longer period of time. The SSA will request medical records from medical providers but often the records are not sent. Many advocates suggest the applicant provide medical records to SSA. It is helpful to keep a copy of the medical records sent to SSA.

If there are obstacles to obtaining medical records at certain institutions the medical team members can meet with their medical records department to determine a system that makes medical records available quickly when needed for an SSA application or SSA review. Without medical records the application for benefits is likely to be denied or if SSA is conducting a Continuing Disability Review the lack of medical records could result in termination of benefits.

Appealing a Denial of Benefits

If the applicant meets the medical and work requirements but his initial application is denied he can file an appeal. Filing an appeal allows the applicant to accrue benefits while the appeal is pending. A person whose benefits are terminated after a review must appeal the termination within 10 days of receipt of the notice of termination in order to continue receiving benefits while the appeal is pending. Otherwise, if the person appeals after 10 days but before 60 days are up the person can appeal but will not receive benefits during the appeal.

Benefit Review at Age 18

A person who has received SSI benefits as a child and then reaches his 18th birthday, will have his eligibility reviewed by Social Security.

The young adult will have to show that she still meets the SSA medical criteria, income and asset requirements at that time. Some families receive SSA review paperwork and do not think they need to complete it because their child has SSI benefits. Failure to complete the SSI 18 year-old review paperwork will result in termination of SSI benefits.

SSI benefits can provide access to insurance coverage for AYASHCN. Access to SSI benefits should be protected unless the young adult is able to work full time at a job that provides health insurance coverage. Loss of SSI benefits can lead to loss of Medicaid making it difficult to access medical care.

SSI Issues Specific to the Transitioning Adult

Income Criteria

An adult applying for SSI benefits must meet the medical, income and asset criteria. An adult age 18 or older, will not have his parent's income and assets counted when SSA determines if the applicant meets the SSA income and asset criteria.

During the application process the adult cannot be engaged in work activity that results in earnings that would result in the SSI benefit being zero.

In most cases, for every $2 a person makes from work activity $1 is deducted from the SSI benefit amount. If work earnings result in the SSI check being reduced to zero in one month then the person will lose his SSI and lose his Medicaid. The fact the person will not have access to health insurance coverage does NOT mean the Medicaid coverage will continue. The Medicaid coverage stops if the SSI stops. In 31 states the person may apply for Medicaid separately but in 19 states there will be no way the young adult can obtain Medicaid coverage.

Case Example

Max works part time and makes $300 in one month, Max's SSI check will be reduced by $150 dollars. If Max is enrolled in a SSI-related work program then his SSI benefit may not be reduced.

SSI Work Programs

SSI has two work programs that may allow the SSI recipient to work and not loose SSI or Medicaid. The PASS program allows the SSI recipient to save money for a work goal. The PASS program requires the SSI recipient meet with an SSA representative and come up with a written plan for what will be done with the money saved.

The other SSI work program is called Section 1619b which allows the SSI recipient to work and make a certain amount of money and still keep Medicaid but stop receiving the SSI monthly cash benefit. SSA representatives will have more information on these programs.

Household Expense Deduction

When the transitioning young adult with chronic illness lives with her parents, the amount of money the parents are contributing to the support of the young adult will be counted by SSA as income to the adult. Without an agreement to pay her portion of household expenses, the SSI benefit will be reduced by one third to account for parental support. If another family member or a boyfriend or girlfriend is paying for household expenses then the SSI benefit will also be reduced by one third to account for the support.

However, if the adult who is applying for SSI benefits has a valid written agreement to pay her share of household expenses, there should not be a reduction in the SSI benefit amount. The written agreement is submitted to the SSA when the application for benefits is submitted. The written agreement must contain specific language in order for the agreement to be valid. An applicant can discuss the elements of a valid loan agreement with a SSA representative.

Eligible for Both SSDI and SSI

Some AYASHCN may have worked a short amount of time before becoming unable to work and may be eligible for a small SSDI benefit. These individuals are often called "Dual Eligibles". The SSI benefit amount will be reduced by the SSDI benefit amount received.

Case Example

Isabella is eligible to receive an SSDI benefit of $200 and so can also receive an SSI benefit of $530. The 2017 SSI base benefit amount is $730. A small number of states supplement the base SSI amount with state funds so the monthly SSI amount is higher. Dual Eligibles will be eligible for SSDI and Medicare after meeting a 24 month waiting period for Medicare. The Dual Eligible recipient will also be eligible for SSI benefits and so will receive Medicaid coverage upon approval for the SSI program.

Table 8.1 The medical team should be concerned about the following AYASHCN who

Has a chronic illness
Has Medicaid
Does not have SSI
Lives in a state that has not expanded Medicaid to low income adults

Medicaid Eligibility

Children and Medicaid

In most states, children under the age of 18 who live in a household that meets certain low income guidelines may be eligible for Medicaid even if the child is not eligible for SSI. Many children who have a chronic illness rely on Medicaid for the provision of health insurance coverage.

SSI Benefits and Medicaid Coverage

In 39 states, SSI benefit approval automatically qualifies a child or adult for Medicaid coverage. In 11 states, once the SSI application has been approved, a separate application for Medicaid must be filed. The 11 states that require a separate application are: Connecticut, Hawaii, Illinois, Indiana, Minnesota, Missouri, New Hampshire, North Dakota, Ohio, Oklahoma and Virginia. Notice of SSI approval in these 11 states will instruct the SSI recipient on where to file the Medicaid application.

Assessing Young Adult Need for Medicaid

The medical team should start discussing other health insurance options with the family and the young adult at least 3 months before the 18th birthday.

Adult Eligibility for Medicaid

Once the child turns 18 she may be eligible for Medicaid as a low income adult if she lives in one of the 31 states that expanded Medicaid coverage under the ACA. However, if she lives in one of the 19 states that did not expand Medicaid to low income adults then she will have to receive SSI benefits in order to obtain Medicaid coverage. Search for "Medicaid Expansion" to see if a specific state has expanded Medicaid. Table 8.1 lists those AYASHCN who health care providers should be concerned about in terms of losing coverage.

There are efforts in Congress to end the Medicaid expansion for low income adults. The outcome of this effort is unknown at the time of publication. Medical teams, AYASHCN and their families should follow the news regarding efforts to repeal the ACA which includes ending the ACA Medicaid Expansion.

State Programs[1,2]

Children with Special Healthcare Needs Programs (CSHCN)[3]

CSHCN state programs offer health insurance to children that have certain medical conditions. These programs have higher income eligibility guidelines than Medicaid and tend to be a payor of last resort. In some states CSHCN programs may provide insurance coverage to some transitioning AYASHCN.

Often there are waiting lists for CSHCN. The medical team should determine if there is a waiting list for CSHCN in their state. In some states it could be years before the young adult could become eligible for CSHCN due to long waiting lists.

[1] 42 U.S.C. 423.

[2] 42 U.S.C. 1382.

[3] 42 U.S.C.701 (a)(1)(D).

State Children's Health Insurance Program[4]

The State Children's Health Insurance Program (SCHIP) provides Medicaid coverage to children whose household income exceeds the Medicaid guidelines. Coverage under SCHIP is limited to children under the age of 18 (or in some states under 19). AYASHCN should determine what type of health insurance coverage will be available to them before SCHIP coverage ends.

The Affordable Care Act

At the time of publication of this chapter, the Affordable Care Act (ACA) offers the option of purchasing health insurance coverage on a Healthcare Exchange and the possibility of obtaining premium subsidies to help with the cost of the health insurance policy.

Individuals with disabilities may be able to work full time. Some may find that their employer offers health insurance to employees. Under the ACA and the Health Insurance Portability and Accountability Act (HIPAA) the person cannot be excluded from coverage. Under HIPAA if the employer offers health insurance to employees then the employer must offer the insurance to all employees. If the employer does not offer insurance coverage then the person can purchase coverage on the ACA Healthcare Exchange which can be found at www.healthcare.gov.

Pre-Existing Condition Clauses[5]

The ACA abolished pre-existing condition clauses in health insurance policies sold in the United States. Prior to the ACA pre-existing condition clauses were used to deny coverage for an individual health insurance policy if the applicant had expenses related to a health condition that was treated or diagnosed within 6 months prior to enrollment on the policy.

As long as the mandates of the ACA are in effect a person cannot be denied the ability to purchase a health insurance policy due to a pre-existing condition.

Limiting Age of 26

The ACA provides that all dependents must be allowed to stay on their parent's health insurance policy until the dependent reaches the age of 26 years old.

The dependent child can be married or employed and still continue on their parents health insurance policy. Age is the governing factor not being a full time student. There is no requirement that the child be receiving Social Security benefits in order to continue until the age of 26 as a covered dependent.

Caps on Coverage

The ACA prohibits individual and group health plans from placing a lifetime limit on the aggregate dollar value of coverage and placing annual limits on overall plan coverage. Insurers can still exclude certain services from coverage or place a limit on the amount the insurer will pay for a certain service. There are 45 services that are considered essential services under the ACA and these services cannot be limited or excluded under a health insurance plan.

Health Insurance Exchanges

A Health Insurance Exchange is a government operated internet site that offers eligible health insurance plans in the state where the citizen resides. A Health Insurance Exchange can offer health insurance plans to small businesses. There is a federal Health Insurance Exchange website www.healthcare.gov. A few states operate their own Healthcare Exchanges.

A person is not required to purchase a health insurance plan through a Healthcare Exchange but in order to receive a government subsidy to

[4] 42 U.S.C. 1397bb.

[5] 42 U.S.C. 1181.

Table 8.2 Changes in circumstances that will allow a special enrollment period for purchasing a health insurance policy on a Healthcare Exchange

Moving to another state
A change in income
A loss of health insurance
A change in family size

help pay for health insurance premiums the policy must be purchased through a Healthcare Exchange. The Healthcare Exchange will have an income and family size calculator to determine the amount of premium subsidy a person will receive.

Special Enrollment Period

A person can enroll outside the open enrollment period if she had health insurance coverage during the Healthcare Exchange open enrollment period but had a change in circumstance after the close of the open enrollment period. Typical changes in circumstances that will allow a person a special enrollment period and the opportunity to purchase a health insurance policy on a Healthcare Exchange are listed in Table 8.2.

State Insurance Law: Continued Coverage if Child Is Incapable of Self Support

According to the mandates of the ACA, private health insurance policies only have to provide coverage for dependent children up to their 26th birthday.

AYASHCN who reach the age of 26 may qualify for an extension of benefits under a state law that provides for a continuation of coverage if the dependent child is incapable of self-support due to a mental or physical condition. After proof is submitted to the insurance company that provides evidence the dependent child is incapable of self-support, the health insurance coverage is extended until the dependent is able to self-support.

If the employer is contributing to premium payments the employer will typically be required to continue to contribute to premium payments.

Case Example

Jacquie is covered under her mother's employer based policy. The mother contributes $100 toward the premium and her employer pays the other $400. Jacquie turns 26 and reaches the limiting age on the policy. Jacquie's treating physician certifies in writing that she is incapable of self-support due to her chronic condition. The employer will then continue to pay the $400 portion of the premium.

The following states do not have a state law that extends coverage to AYASHCN incapable of self-support: Alabama, Alaska, Kansas, Maine, Oklahoma and Oregon. Sometimes insurance companies in these states may offer an extension of coverage for a dependent who is incapable of self-support due to a physical or mental condition but in these states there is no legal duty to do so.

Table 8.3 lists steps typically taken in order to apply for an extension of benefits due to inability

Table 8.3 Steps to apply for an extension of benefits due to the inability to self-support

1.	Obtain a form from the health insurance company prior to the young adult reaching the limiting age on the policy.
2.	The treating physician must certify in writing that the young adult is incapable of self-support due to their medical condition.
3.	The insurance company can request information about income the young adult has earned from work activity.
4.	The young adult who makes enough money from work activity to support himself will most likely not be able to extend coverage under his parent's policy.
5.	Some state laws allow an insurance company to determine the amount a person can make that will be considered self-support based on cost of living in the state. Most state laws do not have dollar limit to be considered a person who is incapable of self-support.
6.	The insurance company can require re-certification every year showing the young adult is still unable to self-support due to medical condition and has not made enough money in the prior year to self-support.
7.	The young adult must be unmarried.

Table 8.4 Examples of COBRA qualifying events and the duration of the extension period

Qualifying Event	Duration of Extension Period
Termination, resignation or layoff	18 months
Death of policyholder	36 months
Divorce or separation from policyholder	36 months
Adult becomes eligible for SSDI benefits	29 months
Child reaches a limiting age under the policy	36 months

to self-support. A young adult who is not eligible for an extension of coverage based on his inability to self-support can extend coverage under COBRA for 36 months. However, under COBRA, the policyholder must pay the full premium amount. See Section below on COBRA.

COBRA Extension of Benefits[6]

For employers with 20 or more employees, the Consolidated Omnibus Budget Reconciliation Act of 1985 (COBRA) provides a continuation of health insurance coverage if a qualifying event takes place. The coverage under the policy remains the same. The COBRA extension period varies depending on the qualifying event. Examples of qualifying events and the duration of extended coverage are in Table 8.4, above.

Under COBRA the employee pays the full premium. It is a good idea to save money in the event coverage must be extended under COBRA. COBRA sets out certain time limits for notice and enrollment.

The employer has up to 14 days after employee notifies employer of a qualifying event to provide a COBRA election notice. The employee then has 60 days to decide whether to elect COBRA continuation coverage. The employee has 45 days after the day of the COBRA election to pay the initial premium. Failure to pay the premium results in cancellation of the policy with no possibility of reinstatement. COBRA can provide a way to continue good insurance coverage.

[6]26 U.S.C. 54.4980B-0.

Conclusion

Transitioning AYASHCN face many challenges when determining how to best access health insurance coverage to cover medical treatment and medications. Knowledge of the choices and planning for changes in coverage due to reaching a limiting age for Medicaid coverage or private health insurance is crucial to make sure that AYASHCN have access to coverage for treatment.

The ACA has provided coverage and peace of mind to AYASHCN and their family members. At the time of publication it is unclear whether Congress will repeal the ACA and its mandates for access to health coverage for all Americans. If the ACA is repealed access to health insurance coverage will be difficult. AYASHCN will have to carefully plan their life choices so that they are sure they have access to health insurance coverage.

Hopefully Congress will take steps to strengthen the ACA and continue to provide funds for Medicaid. A variety of health coverage options allows AYASHCN who are transitioning to adult care with more choices for their future.

Additional Resource

- To obtain your state's Department of Insurance contact information go to www.naic.org/state_web_map.htm.
- To review policies offered on the Healthcare Exchange go to www.healthcare.gov
- The Social Security Administration's website has information on the different SSA programs and application procedures at www.ssa.gov.
- To request a phone interview to apply for Social Security benefits call SSA at 1-800-772-1213. An application may also be completed on line at www.ssa.gov or at a local Social Security office but only for those applying for Social Security Disability Insurance benefits.

- A list of the SSA medical criteria can be found at www.ssa.gov/disability/professionals/bluebook.
- For a list of Medicaid eligibility income guidelines by state go to http://www.statehealthfacts.org/comparetable.jsp? ind = 203&cat = 4
- For more information about each state's SCHIP program please visit http://www.insurekidsnow.gov
- The Department of Labor has information on COBRA at www.dol.gov/ebsa/faqs/faq_consumer_cobra.html

Part IV

Developing a Healthcare Transition Program

9 Establishing the Administrative Structure and Support for a Healthcare Transition Program

Mary R. Ciccarelli and Jason Woodward

Case Vignette

Joy is a 22-year-old female with a history of lumbosacral myelomeningocele who presents to the children's hospital emergency room for symptoms of a urinary tract infection. She is unable to tell you her urologist's name or follow-up plan. She has a small pressure ulcer on one heel and states her wheelchair needs some repairs. Your institution's pediatric multidisciplinary spina bifida clinic has created an upper age limit of 21 for pediatric care. When you review the last clinic note, it mentions transitioning to adult care without specific plans. When you ask about primary care, she says she has not seen her pediatrician in 3 years. You call the pediatric urology team to schedule follow-up and are told she is too old for their clinic. You wonder what can be done at your institution to improve the transition of care for the growing number of young adults with chronic conditions who are still receiving intermittent services.

Healthcare transition (HCT) programs are designed to create processes to guide the progress and movement of youth from pediatric to adult healthcare. When individuals work to establish a transition program regardless of the scope or size, attention must be paid to the design and accuracy in the implementation of the model, as well as the subsequent performance of the model to deliver efficacy in its outcomes. If we wish to implement a transition program with desired outcomes and fidelity to a specific model, then a systematic approach to development, growth, and sustainability of the program is critical. Longer-range multifaceted strategies and plans are necessary. Implementation science (IS) can be a useful approach to study the methods to promote integration of transition evidence into healthcare practice. Logic models create a clear visual representation of the intervention and evaluation plans and the relationships among the available resources, the planned activities, programmatic aims, and intended outcomes. Figure 9.1 creates the skeleton for building out a visual representation of a program [1].

The six stages of IS are described as *exploration and adoption, installation, initial implementation, full operation, innovation, and sustainability* (see Fig. 9.2) [2]. We will use the visual framework of IS and a logic model to discuss an organized approach in the development of an administrative structure for transition programs.

M. R. Ciccarelli, M.D. (✉)
Indiana University School of Medicine, Indianapolis, IN, USA
e-mail: mciccare@iupui.edu

J. Woodward, M.D., M.S.
Cincinnati Children's Hospital Medical Center, Cincinnati, OH, USA

A. C. Hergenroeder, C. M. Wiemann (eds.), *Health Care Transition*,
https://doi.org/10.1007/978-3-319-72868-1_9

Logic Model Template				
INPUT/ RESOURCES	**ACTIVITIES**	**OUTPUT**	**OUTCOMES**	**IMPACT/ AIMS**
Funding, personnel, equipment, supplies	**Processes of program**, i.e. transition services to be delivered	**Process measures**, i.e. number of patients served	**Performance measures: Short term**, i.e. patients have transition planning / **intermediate term**, i.e. transition completion for patients served	**Long term outcomes**, i.e. improved health indicators in young adults with chronic illness

Fig. 9.1 Logic model template

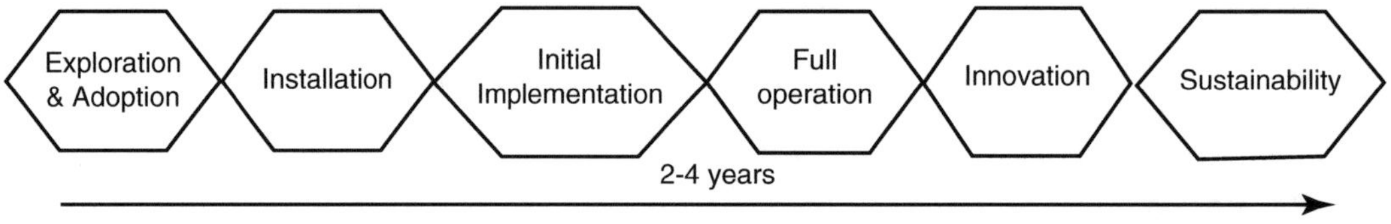

Fig. 9.2 Stages of implementation science

Exploration *is the process of identifying the need for an intervention, assessing the proposed innovation, and examining its potential fit within the system. Readiness factors that are key include the system's motivation for change, resources, and organizational climate.* Logic model contributions during this stage should yield a summary of the input and impact strategies. In these early stages of design and development, we will discuss three components: assessment, marshaling, and then feasibility [3].

Initial assessment requires that planners look at the institutional current state and its surrounding environment. The following list of items may be used to help in organizing your approach: the people to be served, the nature of the service, the potential variability or distortions to the service, controllability of the process, cost, personnel, space and equipment, intersecting agencies, local and central government, private sector, special interest groups, and the media [4]. One can consider exploring the three concentric circles of the setting and environment: those of the core program, the organization, and surrounding influential components [2]. This could include assessing the key personnel's skills or training needs (core components), understanding the institution's strategic plan or stated goals and priorities (organizational components), and reviewing state Title V priorities or state and federal funding initiatives (influence factors). It is important at this early stage of planning to consider the staff time and support needed to complete a needs assessment and evaluate the organization and community's readiness for change and identify funding streams to support this initial work.

The marshaling of interest must focus on the readiness of the organization and/or community to move forward with the work. No community, regardless of its size, has an easy time implementing a program to address a complicated issue like the pediatric to adult HCT. Testing of an organization's readiness to institute an innovation can begin first with asking questions and collecting descriptive data including critical incidents related to the topic of concern. It is pertinent to perform a review of what related or complementary HCT programs already exist. Also consider processes, activities, or policies which impact transition. Sometimes the potential of these complementary programs or processes to support HCT to adult care may only be recognized by those doing the assessment but may provide important insight into the organization's readiness and potential key collaborators. It is also valuable to map out a list of possible useable resources and funding for the program.

Large organizations are complex with many goals, which at times can be conflicting. Nonaligned leadership priorities are an issue that can stand in the way of successful implementation of worthwhile and valuable programs [5]. Considering the issues which are most important to the host organization as well as to the potential funders plays a significant role in fostering institutional support and shaping the discussions of planning, preparation, and first steps of initiation. A children's hospital's interest or need for program development could be focused on the desire to decrease the number of adults admitted to their facility in order to maintain room for pediatric patients. Alternatively, the institution may be more focused on the need to develop policies and procedures to share the care of subpopulations of young adults between a combination of both adult and pediatric providers. State Title V agencies may wish to improve their performance on transition statewide across all youth as one of their national performance measures. Adult health systems may be focused on capturing more covered lives for their accountable care organizations by moving aging youth into their practices.

Local contextual conditions about the patients and families to be served shape the planning for complex healthcare interventions. Features which can have impact range from demographics (age range of transferring youth, diagnostic mix) and socioeconomic indicators (ethnicity, family constituency, urban vs. rural residence, income level) to current level of utilization of community resources. If the health system already has an understanding of the patients they serve, then operationalizing changes becomes easier. In large organizations, this awareness may be quite variable between leaders, sections of service delivery, and even at the level of individual providers and other personnel, resulting in different viewpoints that will alter the needed work in aligning and marshaling support for program development.

Key informants provide the necessary information to assess and propel forward the community readiness. They are persons who are likely to know about the problem or issue of concern, but not necessarily leaders or decision-makers. Seek those who have community knowledge of current efforts and the problem (barriers and gaps in transition). Think inclusively about how to include the appropriate leadership (appointed leaders and influential community members). Input from youth, young adults, and families is critical to understanding the experience of service recipients in healthcare transition [6]. While national data comparisons are useful, demonstrating the alignment or disparity through these consumers' local experiences can be illuminating for the development of transition services in their specific environment. When collecting a transition working group, attention should be given to the range of potential constituents and stakeholders. Table 9.1 demonstrates a group representative of the different perspectives collected for the program design to address HCT of youth with epilepsy [7].

Effective planning requires an analysis that takes into account issues which will both help and hinder the forward progress. A SWOT (Strengths, Weaknesses, Opportunities, Threats) analysis is a strategic planning tool to sort the information into factors which could positively or negatively affect the project [8]. It synthesizes the current state and environmental scan into categories of internal organizational strengths and

Table 9.1 Multidisciplinary transition working group representing perspectives for youth with epilepsy

• Pediatric and adult epileptologists
• Psychiatrists
• Academic and community family doctors
• Community neurologists
• Pediatric and adult epilepsy programs nurses and social workers
• Adolescent medicine physicians
• Complex care team of physicians, nurses, and social workers
• Lawyer
• Occupational therapist
• Community epilepsy agencies
• Patients with epilepsy
• Parents of patients with epilepsy and severe intellectual disability
• Project managers

weakness and external community opportunities and threats and promotes a more comprehensive understanding of the current state. The internal factors of strengths and weaknesses typically encompass finances, facilities, and equipment, manpower and current processes. The external factors of opportunities and threats take into account economic, environmental, political trends, and regulations. Table 9.2 is a SWOT example from an osteogenesis imperfecta transition program analysis [9].

Attitudes, resources, and political climate vary across communities, as do stages of readiness to take on a new innovation such as transition services. Consensus and support can evolve once there is adequate forward momentum. Community/institutional readiness has interesting parallels to the individual stages of behavior change model of Prochaska and DiClemente. The first stages in the community readiness model are no awareness, denial, and vague awareness [10]. Just as strategies to address individual person's readiness for change vary, so do the strategies to address the varying stages of community readiness. The act of conducting a community readiness assessment has been shown to improve awareness of the issue in leaders and stakeholders. Ongoing exposure of a community to a program also tends to increase in the community readiness at a stepwise and somewhat predictable rate [11]. If the community is not yet ready for planning, then corrective work must first be accomplished. When the predominant stage of readiness is "no awareness," then individual meetings to provide information to leaders and community members is an appropriate approach. Clear information about local examples and incidents can address denial. Advertising and surveys can advance a community's belief that they can do something about the issue during the "vague awareness" stage. During "preplanning," developers might use targeted further education of organizational and community leaders and focus group to begin to outline concrete ideas and potential strategies. Information from outside sources should be sought to support this strategizing. The American Academy of Pediatrics, American Academy of Family Physicians, and American College of Physicians have created and updated consensus documents and recommendations for transition [12]. The American College of Physicians' Council of Subspecialty Societies initiated a project to develop specialized toolkits to facilitate more effective transition and transfer of young adults into the adult healthcare setting [13]. This work has been performed in collaboration with Got Transition (GT)/Center for Health Care Transition Improvement [14], a cooperative agreement between the Maternal and Child Health Bureau and the National Alliance to Advance Adolescent Health, Society of General Internal Medicine (SGIM), and Society of Adolescent Health and Medicine (SAHM).

Installation *prepares the new program prior to actually beginning the delivery of patient services with attention given to budgets, human resources, facilities, and policies.* Preparation provides the existing data, such as specific statistics and costs to the system/organization that would be associated with both maintenance of

Table 9.2 Sample SWOT analysis

Strengths
• Program closely linked to care coordination, led by interprofessional team
• Transition definition included pediatric to adult medical care, school to work, and dependent to independent living
• Allowed time to assess patient readiness up to age 21
• Monitoring of program and collection of evaluative data
Weaknesses
• Institutional changes, i.e., more diagnostic focused, new EHR, and reduced transition focus
• Conflict between recruitment into transition program and research participation
• Insufficient transition tools and gaps in implementation
Opportunities
• Multisite transition model employing cross-site pediatrics to adult system personnel
• User evaluations, including second-generation users
Threats
• Dissatisfaction of adult hospital care team
• Patient dissatisfaction with changes in service delivery between adult and pediatric sites

the current state and anticipated results of enacting the innovation. Key elements that may be designed to support an effective transition to adult-centered healthcare have been described to include the means to provide preparation of involved parties, support flexible timing, utilize care coordination and/or transition clinic visits, and engage interested adult-centered healthcare providers. Mentors and peer groups are also noted as potential strengths [15]. Additional elements required should be based on the local needs assessment and program's stated goals. Influential leaders can help with generating further awareness and support via organized education and advocacy, i.e., grand rounds and stakeholder retreats. During this phase, the analysis of feasibility is critical to verify that the institution has the necessary infrastructure to support and sustain whatever model of program is forming within the delineated strategic plan. The logic model focuses on the specific design of activities and their intended outputs and outcomes. There is not yet a consensus unifying model of transition care that can be recommended for adoption. Rather the design should reflect national principles and the locally desired aims and intended impact through application of the local existing and intended inputs and resources. The complexity of the whole process of pediatric to young adult transition demands system-level solutions. As in all transfers of care, providers need to align across multiple settings, collaboration needs to occur across various sectors and systems, and facilitated communication (including record sharing) is required. In most settings, capacity building is also necessary for successful programs. Therefore it is essential that the goals and objectives of the transition program are clearly stated prior to or as this discussion of activities and needed inputs occurs. There will likely need to be prioritization of objectives and intended outcomes to be able to prioritize essential resources during the initial piloting phase.

Transition system design calls for a new, flexible approach to funding [16]. Budgets can potentially have income from multiple funding sources across the spectrum of federal, state, and local government programs and contracts, foundation grants, healthcare payers special programs, traditional billing for services at the individual patient level, healthcare or academic institution initiatives, and/or community organizations. When approaching funders, the planners should be ready to discuss the needed resources to accomplish specific objectives while paying attention to aligning these proposals with the funder's mission and goals. Once again, the logic model is a succinct and effective tool to use in presentations. Funders desire clarity around what the funds would be purchasing, i.e., specific benefits and how outcomes and progress will be measured. Funders typically expect an appraisal of specific sustainability designs as they consider approving use of their money for a proposal [17].

Governmental initiatives are one important and viable option. Internationally, Australia in 2008 and England in 2008 created governmental transition strategies for youth with disabilities. Both countries acknowledged the need for specific funding for at least the piloting of programs and noted that episode-based funding was less likely to promote ongoing program success. Both also highlighted the need for cross-sectoral collaboration beyond the health system to also incorporate both education and social services, especially for youth with complex conditions [13].

In the United States, the Maternal and Child Health (MCH) Title V Program has a history of calling for programs for pediatric to adult transition. MCH initiated a major transformation process over the past few years in which transition is one of their national performance measures. In 2017, a total of 32 state Title V agencies selected the delivery of services necessary for youth to make transitions to adult care as one of their focused goals. MCH has adopted a measurement framework that involves key stakeholders, including youth, young adults, and parents/caregivers as well as pediatric and adult clinicians, healthcare plans and payers, and public health programs [18]. Almost two-thirds of state Title V programs (20 of 32) reported participating in interagency efforts. Numerous agencies or departments were participating in state collaborations, including education, developmental disability, rehabilitation, behavioral health,

Medicaid, and Social Security Administration offices.

The U.S. Cystic Fibrosis Foundation is a pertinent example of a funding organization which has been proactive in addressing HCT. They created organizational incentives to urge institutions to better prepare for the increasing numbers of young adults in need of specialized adult-oriented care. They created specialized clinical fellowships for physician providers and mandated establishment of adult programs [19].

Healthcare insurance payments can come in the form of special payer programs or at the level of billing for health-related services to individual patients. Provider payment models for care coordination, population health, and other services vary by level of implementation nationally. HCT, particularly for those patients with more complexity, can be seen as a subtype of population health and care coordination programs. Health-based risk adjustment capitated payment models may be preferred to any existing fee-for-service models in supporting care coordination [20] (see Chaps. 23 and 24). However, there are still limited existing analyses for capitated payments as they relate to the transition of youth or young adults with special healthcare needs. A number of institutions have created smaller pilot programs using department or institutional funds to test transition service delivery models.

Beyond finances, resources include aspects of the project which are available and dedicated to or used by the program. They include human resources and talent (e.g., administrative and program staff, parents, peers, etc.), organizational tools (e.g., committees, board members, electronic health records, data collection and tracking tools, etc.), community contributions (e.g., partnerships, business volunteers, workshops, etc.), and supplies (e.g., equipment, office space, books and materials, transportation, etc.). From a logic model perspective, activities are what the program does with the resources that are an intentional part of the program. The goals of the program should direct the activities, which then suggest the needed staff and other resources.

Details of transition program activities include decisions which run across a number of domains: format, setting, periodicity, patient inclusion, and so forth. Programs can focus on activities such as self-management preparation, acclimation of youth and caregivers to adult care models, creation of networks across pediatric and adult health systems, methods to navigate the transfer, and/or interactive means of communication of health information. Programs can be seated within a single primary care practice, a specific diagnosis-based subspecialty, a multispecialty program, a hospital/health system, or within a state program. Many transition pilots create processes which are more comprehensive beyond just a healthcare focus. Chronologically young adults face accompanying life transitions from school to work and family to independent living. Programs can be housed in health systems or government-based settings, i.e., Medicaid or Title V, or even community-based advocacy groups such as in a parent-to-parent network and center for independent living or as a vocational rehabilitation service.

Categorizing patients into their complexity of needs may be one way to help determine setting, as well as resource needs. The primary and/or shared ownership of the transition process may occur in the primary care medical home team for teens who have no specific chronic health conditions. They need help with a summary of their history, transfer to an adult provider, and continuation of their healthcare financing, as well as basic skills to take care of their own health and to navigate the health system when they need episodic care. Those youth with a single chronic condition diagnosis may most effectively receive services through either their primary care or principle specialist. They need to address all the same issues as their peers without chronic conditions, but they also may need more information about their specific condition and treatment, how to maintain surveillance over their current state of health and potential changes in their health and skills in system navigation that are further expanded. Those youth with medical complexity and multiple conditions are the group most likely to need a more expanded approach to preparation and planning, perhaps with specially tailored transition navigators and coordinators and/or multidisciplinary teams. Payer case managers could divide patients into their appropriate groups for different levels of services. Health systems could use navigators and/or care coordinators for these different levels of need. In our experience, the details of the planned activities and subpopulations of patients are particularly important to determining staffing and appropriate setting, as the time and skills required for transition planning activities have not been well-described and may require more staff time than typically allocated by other care coordination models.

Crowley provided a systematic review of HCT interventions and categorized them as the following: directed at the patient (educational programs, skills training), staffing (identified transition coordinators, joint clinics run by pediatric and adult physicians), and service delivery (separate young adult clinics, out of hours phone support, enhanced follow-up) [21]. Self-management supports can use creative methods. The Maestro Project is an example of self-management programming that encourages socialization with peers and relationships with health professionals by using several methods of service delivery including a comprehensive website, a bimonthly newsletter, a monthly evening drop-in group, and educational events [22]. Personally controlled health records (PCHRs) are a type of patient-controlled electronic application that can support both monitoring and support systems for adolescents who are facing the navigation of complex social, developmental, and healthcare transitions. An electronic web-based collection of a patient's comprehensive medical history can be created to create a portable reference for critical medical information. It can also be designed to include information beyond classic medical records with additions such as personal characteristics, real-time patient data entry, and exchange with others, used in a way that integrates all this information across sites of care in a manner that is readily accessible to and controlled by the individual [23].

The next steps in programmatic installation success require getting the transition service providers into place. Key core components for team instillation are (Fig. 9.3) personnel must be well-selected, appropriately trained, and regularly assessed for adherence to the desired model; the

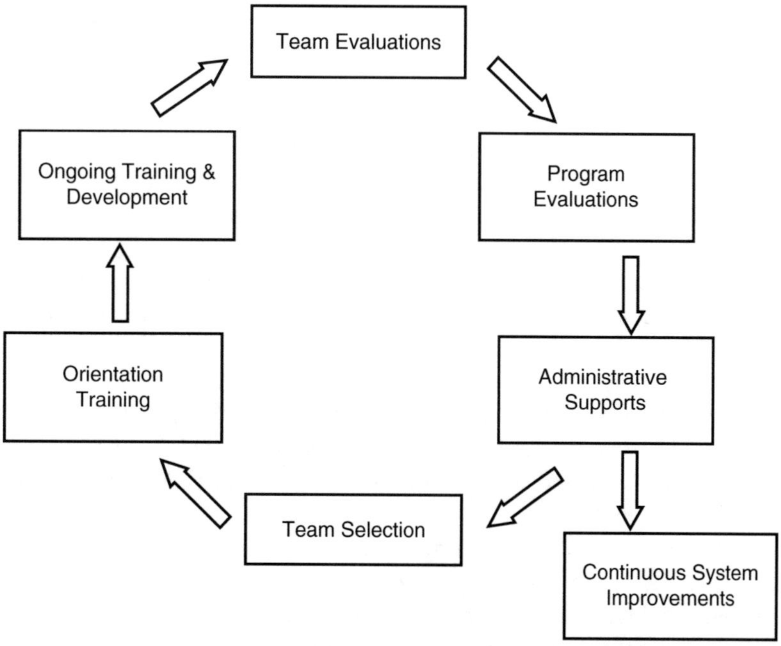

Fig. 9.3 Core components during implementation phase [2]

organizational infrastructure must provide the necessary oversight to training and evaluation processes; program consumers (i.e., youth and families) must be fully involved in the process and evaluation; and institutional administration and governmental policies need to encourage or support the work [2]. Well-designed hiring of staff for HCT programs requires attention and alignment of the program principles with the behavioral and experiential fit of the hires [24]. Our experience has been that ideal transition program staff are passionate about transition, prefer collaborative work, are adaptable to change, and enjoy challenges and continuous improvement.

Hiring staff for the first time, at the startup of a program, is somewhat different from later filling of ongoing positions. Experienced and mission-driven individuals can help with program improvements and evolution. Rationales exist which can assist with decisions around the type of manpower to seek. A social worker's knowledge of resources and systems and understanding of culture, relationships, and family dynamics can allow for unique collaboration with the healthcare team, family, and community supports in transition programs [25]. Pediatric nurses have important roles as transition coordinators, consultants, or direct service providers to ensure health-related needs are met as relates to continuous healthcare financing and services and access to community services and health-related adaptations are incorporated into day-to-day life [26]. In addition during inpatient stays, nurses are likely to have pivotal roles in HCT discussions and planning [27]. When care involves different medical, social, and psychological aspects, a transdisciplinary team model has potential strengths in transition program design for both cross-training potential and overlapping of role responsibilities in order to provide cohesive and integrated transition service plans [28]. Another way to afford cross-training is through sharing of employees between agencies, such as those with needed expertise, like MCH Title V programs, centers for independent living or parent-to-parent networks. When the goal is a shared transition plan of care, one can recognize the value in staff who represent the following disciplines: patient advocates, nursing, medicine, and social work [29]. Mental health service providers are another key discipline for a number of subgroups of patients, i.e., those with or at significant predictable risk of mental health service needs. Programs tailored for young adults demonstrate the importance of employment of staff experienced with this age group, who can focus on independent-living skills, age-appropriate social skills, relationships and dating, family supports, roommates, educational and vocational services, and peer specialists [30]. Larger organizations will have specific hiring rules and human resources systems while still allowing for interviewing to focus on desired key behavioral traits. Skills, personal qualities, commitment to or passion for transition, and/or demographic characteristics for alignment with population to be served may all be factors used in selection.

The training and professional development of staff are both an initial and continuous process, whether for a program of one staff or a larger team. Content areas for a transition program will likely include expertise in existing national transition toolkits, youth and young adult development, the biopsychosocial model of care, family dynamics, adherence and motivational counseling, healthcare financing, principles of decision-making, activated self-advocacy, and health system navigation. Other skill sets may be home, community, education, and work supports for individuals with special needs, quality improvement methods, and research data collection and management.

Initial implementation *moves all the planning into service delivery. It tests the service delivery plan against the originally referenced evidence, principles, and policies, using process observations and cycles of improvements.* In-service training and regular updates are important during initiation. Apprenticeships, workshops, and tours of collaborating community or government organizations are all possible orientation methods. Particularly when developing novel programs, seeking expertise in similarly goaled programs may help form a community of professionals who can learn together in a learning collaborative.

Program evolution is a necessary component in new innovations. Use of evaluation dashboards and continuous quality improvement methods are critical to oversight, feedback, and success. Initial design may not hold true in the hands of actual users. Patient demographics and needs may lead to shifts and modifications in the processes. In one program, after the team was hired, policies were piloted, and the initial consultative ambulatory transition service was launched, it evolved to focus more specifically on the needs of youth with significant neurocognitive disabilities based on heavy utilization of the program by this specific subpopulation. Team members needed skill development in service specific to this group of patients. Feedback from patients, families, and primary care providers helped structure medical summaries for improved clarity. Collaborations with community organizations targeted specific needs of the population receiving services. Needs for additional funding sources and collaborators were identified given the shift in patient characteristics [28].

Quality improvement methodology is essential at this stage of development to support needed adaptations to the service delivery and guide successful program evolution. Frameworks such as the PDSA (Plan-Do-Study-Act) can be employed to encourage regular measurements for tests of change and program enhancements. For successful implementation of quality improvement work, regular meetings of the staff or others providing program support are often helpful and can ensure fidelity to the proposed service delivery model, development of needed changes, and assessment of relevant outcomes. Youth and families' feedback is very important while establishing programs to better serve them. As much as possible, data should be used to drive proposed changes or growth in services.

Full implementation *takes the new innovation and further integrates it across the organization. It expands the program to full staffing and full patient loads and stabilizes standard practices. It is a process which usually takes 2–4 years to achieve.* During this stage of "stabilization," evaluation data, progress reports, and program modifications should be shared locally and disseminated beyond the area of service delivery.

As programs mature, design efficiencies can be considered. When in actual performance settings, the appropriate caseloads for team members are more realistically refined. The range of time to completion of complex tasks can be better reviewed. Theories used in program creation may or may not hold true and therefore need modification or replacement. Over time, the HCT program may also experience turnover in staff from initial developers to those who are now hired as sustainers. Attention to properly engaging and training new hires remains important for program fidelity.

There is an obligation across those who work in the still evolving field of transition to share their work with others for replication, comparison, and refinement. Organizations such as the International Health Care Transition Research Consortium is one such working group, with an annual conference and monthly conference calls to share emerging and best HCT practices. Peer-reviewed submissions are needed in both pediatric and adult care forums to advance the work and create more clearly defined standards.

Innovation *adapts and adjusts to particulars of program expansion while still maintaining sufficient fidelity to the model and originating principles.* Service agreements, directories, and databases evolve during "expansion." If not already systematized, it is preferable that the quality of the work and processes now reach beyond individually based accountability or team-based informal agreements, to systematic processes and continuous improvement as the main characteristics whereby the transition staff learns by evaluating their function, leading to improvements, and teamwork provides synergistic value [29].

Upon gaining more experience and skill in transition service delivery, teams may find other ways to edit and refine use of the electronic health record. Recent advancements in technology have led to the development of an eHealth Enhanced Chronic Care Model which inserts a complete feedback loop between the patient and the professional team [31]. Considerations for transition would include how to better use medical summaries and transition assessments and plans, as well

Logic Model of transition program for youth with intellectual disability			
ACTIVITIES	**SHORTER TERM OUTCOMES**	**LONG TERM OUTCOMES**	**IMPACT**
Building personal capacity Enhancing skills and employability Providing formal supports Engaging Community	Inclusive activities Mobilized community resources Increased community participation Appropriate supports Increased individual choice & control	Meaningful participation Increased income Fulfilling relationships Employment Continuing learning Reduced challenging behaviors Healthier lifestyles	Reduced dependence on traditional services Mainstream participation Community contributions Positive family relationships Enhanced quality adjusted life years

Fig. 9.4 Sample logic model of transition program for youth with intellectual disability

as measurement and documentation of transition program graduation criteria. Various methods of co-management and communication between patient and caregivers, primary care, and other providers may be trialed and tailored to the preferences of the different practices [32]. Other educational tools for youth, families, and providers may be developed. External evaluation further fuels modifications and improvements. McAnaney used a logic model approach (Fig. 9.4) to digest formative evaluations by consumers and staff of transition programs [33]. This evaluative approach can challenge the staff to look critically and systematically at their planned work and intended results, leading to well-reasoned modifications and advancements.

Sustainability *requires attention to long-term funding, facilities, staff turnover, governance, and incorporation in the larger system of care. Full program maturation is generally realized over 5–10 years.* Funding resources should be diversified during this "professionalization" phase. Expansion may occur beyond the original program to new localities. Train the trainer services may be used as a way to further export successful work. Fixsen recommends that essential implementation outcomes are changes in professionals' behavior, organizational structure and culture, and in relationships with program consumers, stakeholders, and systems partners [2].

Actually reaping the rewards of changing the organizational culture to sustain an effective system for the transition of youth from pediatric to adult services takes time. All three phases of the transition chronology must be in place: the preparation for transition, supporting structures during transfer, and engagement into adult healthcare. *The Wall Street Journal Guide to Management* recommends that successful institutionalization of culture change requires that involved parties understand the "why" of the change, the resources are appropriately shifted to where they are needed, and the providers and staff, as well as the institutional leadership, have the motivation to want the change [34]. It is critical that successful pediatric health systems incorporate into their mission and culture the concept that effective health care transition is the necessary culmination of pediatric care [35].

References

1. W.K. Kellogg Foundation Evaluation Handbook. In: W.K. Kellogg Foundation. 2010. https://www.wkkf.org/resource-directory/resource/2010/w-k-kellogg-foundation-evaluation-handbook. Accessed 22 Oct 2017.
2. Fixsen DL, Naoom SF, Blasse KA, Friedman RM, Wallace F. Implementation research: a synthesis of the literature. Tampa, FL: University of South Florida, Louis de la Parte Mental Health Institute, The National Implementation Research Network (FMHI Publication #231); 2005.
3. Adelman HS, Taylor L. On sustainability of project innovations as systemic change. J Educ Psychol Consult. 2003;14:1–25.
4. Chase G. Implementing a human service program: how hard will it be? Public Policy. 1979;27:385–434.
5. Rosenheck RA. Organizational process: a missing link between research and practice. Psychiatr Serv. 2001;52:1607–12.

6. Reiss JG, Gibson RW, Walker LR. Health care transition: youth, family, and provider perspectives. Pediatrics. 2005;115:112–20.
7. Andrade DM, Bassett AS, Bercovici E, et al. Epilepsy: transition from pediatric to adult care. Recommendations of the Ontario epilepsy implementation task force. Epilepsia. 2017;58:1502–17.
8. Renault V Section 14. SWOT analysis: strengths, weaknesses, opportunities, and threats. In: Chapter 3. Assessing community needs and resources|Main Section|Community Tool Box. http://ctb.ku.edu/en/table-of-contents/assessment/assessing-community-needs-and-resources/swot-analysis/main. Accessed 22 Oct 2017.
9. Dogba MJ, Rauch F, Wong T, Ruck J, Glorieux FH, Bedos C. From pediatric to adult care: strategic evaluation of a transition program for patients with osteogenesis imperfecta. BMC Health Serv Res. 2014;14:489.
10. Edwards RW, Jumper-Thurman P, Plested BA, Oetting ER, Swanson L. Community readiness: research to practice. J Community Psychol. 2000;2:291–307.
11. Kostadinov I, Daniel M, Stanley L, Gancia A, Cargo M. A systematic review of community readiness tool applications: implications for reporting. Int J Environ Res Public Health. 2015;12:3453–68.
12. American Academy of Pediatrics; American Academy of Family Physicians American College of Physicians; Transitions Clinical Report Authoring Group, Cooley WC, Sagerman PJ. Supporting the health care transition from adolescence to adulthood in the medical home. Pediatrics. 2011;128:182–200.
13. Pediatric to Adult Care Transitions Initiative. In: Pediatric to Adult Care Transitions Initiative| Resources for Clinicians|ACP. https://www.acponline.org/clinical-information/high-value-care/resources-for-clinicians/pediatric-to-adult-care-transitions-initiative. Accessed 24 Oct 2017.
14. Got Transition/Center for Health Care Transition Improvement. Six Core Elements of Health Care Transition 2.0. In. GotTransition.org, a program of the National Alliance to Advance Adolescent Health. 2014. http://www.gottransition.org/resourceGet.cfm?id=206. Accessed 22 Oct 2017.
15. Binks JA, Barden WS, Burke TA, Young NL. What do we really know about the transition to adult-centered health care? A focus on cerebral palsy and spina bifida. Arch Phys Med Rehabil. 2011;88:1064–73.
16. Hepburn CM, Cohen E, Bhawra J, Weiser N, Hayeems RZ, Guttmann A. Health system strategies supporting transition to adult care. Arch Dis Child. 2015;100:559–64.
17. Funding Guide|Identifying and Accessing Funding Opportunities. In: County Health Rankings & Roadmaps. University of Wisconsin Population Health Institute. http://www.countyhealthrankings.org/roadmaps/funding-guide/identifying-and-accessing. Accessed 22 Oct 2017.
18. McManus M, Beck D. Transition to Adult Health Care and State Title V Program Directions: A Review of 2017 Block Grant Applications. Report 3 Got Transition/Center for Health Care Transition Improvement, The National Alliance to Advance Adolescent Health. 2017. http://www.gottransition.org/resourceGet.cfm?id=431.
19. Tuchman LK, Schwartz LA, Sawicki GS, Britto MT. Cystic fibrosis and transition to adult medical care. Pediatrics. 2010;125:566–73.
20. Field MJ, Jette AM, editors, Institute of Medicine (US) Committee on Disability in America (2007) The future of disability in America. National Academies Press, Washington, DC.
21. Crowley R, Wolfe I, Lock K, McKee M. Improving the transition between paediatric and adult healthcare: a systematic review. Arch Dis Child. 2011;96:548–53.
22. Van Walleghem N, Macdonald CA, Dean HJ. Evaluation of a systems navigator model for transition from pediatric to adult care for young adults with type 1 diabetes. Diabetes Care. 2008;31:1529–30.
23. Weitzman ER, Kaci L, Quinn M, Mandl KD. Helping high-risk youth move through high-risk periods: personally controlled health records for improving social and health care transitions. J Diabetes Sci Technol. 2011;5:47–54.
24. Rabinowitz P Section 1. Developing a plan for staff hiring and training. In: Chapter 10. Hiring and training key staff of community organizations | Main Section | Community Tool Box. http://ctb.ku.edu/en/table-of-contents/structure/hiring-and-training/develop-a-plan/main. Accessed 22 Oct 2017.
25. Shanske S, Arnold J, Carvalho M, Rein J. Social workers as transition brokers: facilitating the transition from pediatric to adult medical care. Soc Work Health Care. 2012;51:279–95.
26. Betz CL. Facilitating the transition of adolescents with developmental disabilities: nursing practice issues and care. J Pediatr Nurs. 2007;22:103–11.
27. van Staa A, Sattoe JN, Strating MM. Experiences with and outcomes of two interventions to maximize engagement of chronically ill adolescents during hospital consultations: a mixed methods study. J Pediatr Nurs. 2015;30:757–75.
28. Ciccarelli MR, Brown MW, Gladstone EB, Woodward JF, Swigonski NL. Implementation and sustainability of statewide transition support services for youth with intellectual and physical disabilities. J Pediatr Rehabil Med. 2014;7:93–104.
29. Vyt A. Interprofessional and transdisciplinary teamwork in health care. Diabetes Metab Res Rev. 2008;24:S106–9.
30. Embrett MG, Randall GE, Longo CJ, Nguyen T, Mulvale G. Effectiveness of health system services and programs for youth to adult transitions in mental health care: a systematic review of academic literature. Adm Policy Ment Health. 2016;43:259–69.
31. Gee PM, Greenwood DA, Paterniti DA, Ward D, Miller LM. The eHealth enhanced chronic care model: a theory derivation approach. J Med Internet Res. 2015;17:e86.

32. de Jong CC, Ros WJ, Leeuwen MV, Schrijvers G. How professionals share an E-care plan for the elderly in primary care: evaluating the use of an E-communication tool by different combinations of professionals. J Med Internet Res. 2016;18:e204.
33. McAnaney DF, Wynne RF. Linking user and staff perspectives in the evaluation of innovative transition projects for youth with disabilities. J Intellect Disabil. 2016;20:165–82.
34. How to change your Organization's culture. In: The wall street journal guide to management: building a workplace culture, adapted from The WSJ Complete Small Business Guidebook. New York:Three Rivers Press, 2009. http://guides.wsj.com/management/innovation/how-to-change-your-organizations-culture/. Accessed 22 Oct 2017.
35. Hergenroeder AC, Wiemann CM, Bowman VF. Lessons learned in building a hospital-wide transition program from pediatric to adult-based health care for youth with special health care needs (YSHCN). Int J Adolesc Med Health. 2016;28:455–8.

10 Mobilizing Pediatric Providers

Kathy Sanabria, James Harisiades,
Rebecca Boudos, and Parag Shah

Mobilizing Pediatric Providers

Due to advances in medicine, pharmacology, and technology, adolescents and young adults with special healthcare needs (AYASHCN) are now living into adulthood. Pediatric providers are in an important position to guide AYASHCN through the transition to adult care. Helping youth with their transition to adult care requires knowledge of best practices and resources as well as commitment from practitioners to facilitate healthcare transition (HCT) planning. Got Transition has established guidelines for practices outlining the services they should be providing to ensure better transitions for their patients [1]. These guidelines include elements such as identifying patients most in need of support during their transition, creating medical summaries, conducting transition assessments, and ensuring a good handoff to their adult counterparts. Providers must have dedicated time to learn how to use the guidelines and work with patients and families to implement them. In addition, it takes time to plan practice-specific workflows and create useful tools. Mobilizing and incentivizing providers to facilitate interest and commitment to accomplishing these tasks is challenging, but essential.

Through two case examples (one within a regional children's hospital through the establishment of a Chronic Illness Transition Program and the other at a state level through a local chapter of the American Academy of Pediatrics [AAP]), this chapter illustrates pediatric provider roles and their importance to HCT processes and explores ideas to help motivate and mobilize providers to engage patients in HCT planning.

Case Example #1: Establishment of a Transition Program at a Regional Hospital
(See Table 10.1)
Organizing a hospital-wide transition program and mobilizing providers begins with environmental assessment and information gathering. At one tertiary care center, information on the importance and process of implementing

K. Sanabria, M.B.A., P.M.P.
American Academy of Pediatrics,
Elk Grove, IL, USA

J. Harisiades, M.P.H.
Office of Child Advocacy, Ann and Robert H. Lurie Children's Hospital of Chicago, Chicago, IL, USA

R. Boudos, L.C.S.W.
Chronic Illness Transition Program, Ann and Robert H. Lurie Children's Hospital of Chicago,
Chicago, IL, USA

P. Shah, M.D., M.P.H. (✉)
Chronic Illness Transition Program, Ann and Robert H. Lurie Children's Hospital of Chicago,
Chicago, IL, USA

Division of Hospital Based Medicine, Department of Pediatrics, Northwestern University Feinberg School of Medicine, Chicago, IL, USA
e-mail: pshah@luriechildrens.org

A. C. Hergenroeder, C. M. Wiemann (eds.), *Health Care Transition*,
https://doi.org/10.1007/978-3-319-72868-1_10

Table 10.1 Key features of local hospital initiative to establish a healthcare transition program

• Created a champion with protected time
• Formed multidisciplinary, inclusive, steering committee
• Integrated tools into EMR
• Initiated innovative projects incubator with mini-grants

transitioning into practice was gathered by a small group of champions. These initial champions were self-motivated providers who embraced the topic and were passionate about improving care and strengthening pathways to adulthood for AYASCHN. Their drive was inspired by professional and personal experiences. These champions learned from presentations at the Pediatric Academic Societies, the medical literature, site visits, and consultations with leaders of established programs at other children's hospitals. One of these members reported directly to the hospital president and made the case for the importance of establishing a transition program as a leading children's hospital. This top executive-level buy-in was significant in securing institution endorsement for the program and mobilizing champions and leaders for its implementation.

Identification and engagement of a physician leader for the transition program was the first step in formalizing the program, which was further solidified with the appointment of a social worker to serve as the transition program coordinator. These were selected by a committee through an open application process. Working together, the physician leader and transition program coordinator have been the driving force around broader physician engagement with division-specific champions and clinical integration of the transition program within the medical center.

Start-up funding was also essential to launching the transition program to attract physician leaders and support the first phases of practice integration. As described above, funding from a hospital auxiliary provided the support to pilot four initial demonstration projects (in spina bifida, nephrology, cardiology, and hepatology). These demonstration projects helped to mobilize champions in each of the aforementioned divisions. The request for proposals (RFP) for funding support was structured but intentionally open-ended to encourage physicians (and their teams) to exercise creativity, innovation, and adaptation based on their unique models of care. Sustained support from a family foundation interested in the program has secured protected time for the transition program coordinator, and budgeted time allocation for the medical director has provided longitudinal stability since program start-up.

The process of provider engagement has been incremental, starting with efforts to orient and educate physicians about transitioning. Several vehicles were utilized, including Grand Rounds and other institution-wide learning structures, resident noon conferences, targeted presentations to primary and subspecialty care divisions, continuing medical education (CME) courses, and articles in medical center publications. Complementing these physician-focused strategies were educational interventions for nurses, social workers, and other staff, including pastoral care and family life specialists. This contributed to educational reinforcement within and across multidisciplinary teams. Moreover, it acculturated transitioning within the medical center, which encouraged broader engagement and participation among physician-led teams. Over time, program expansion, institutional infrastructure accommodations, and more extensive physician recruitment evolved. Several strategies contributed to this momentum. These are described next.

Steering Committee

A steering committee comprised of hospital-wide stakeholders in HCT was formed to help motivated providers become champions and leaders within their departments. It was a centralized forum to facilitate strategic planning, information exchange, progress updates from participating transition clinics, and presentations from community organizations and partners. Physicians actively participate along with social workers, nurses, and psychologists. Consisting of representatives from over 20 divisions, the steering committee meets quarterly and provides an open forum for consensus building and discussions of quality and process improvement. Steering committees can be useful in providing a place for motivated providers to get a start in building a transition program within their departments.

Transition Clinic

A transition clinic led by the medical director and transition program coordinator was created to help providers in the hospital with patients with complex transition needs. The addition of this service has further bolstered physician engagement by introducing an assessment of transition readiness, coordination of transfer of care to adult providers, and assessment of social needs and services, facilitating efforts to discuss HCT with patients, and providing a resource to navigate the transition process.

Electronic Medical Record Integrations

To create an infrastructure that makes it easier for providers to perform some of the recommended interventions, the transition champions created medical summaries, transition orders, and transition assessment tools within the electronic medical record (EMR). This streamlined access to concise and consolidated information in the EMR software to document patient progress through HCT preparation and planning. These electronic enhancements have supported greater ease and ability of physicians to integrate transition planning into their clinics and therefore increased physician engagement.

Mini-grants on Completion of Transfer to Adult Providers

To recruit new champions and leaders, an RFP for mini-grants to address strategies for enhancement and evaluation of the transfer of care process and development of adult provider relationships was issued by the Office of Child Advocacy (using Endowment Fund monies) to all transition program participants. In response, notably, these projects involved both the hospital pediatric providers and adult providers to whom patients would be transferred. This has resulted in an increased interest from various providers to engage in the transition process, along with program enhancements such as joint clinics for both pediatric and adult physicians at Lurie Children's prior to transfer of care and improved methods for streamlined transfer of most salient information for first patient visit to the adult provider.

Case Example #2: A Statewide Transition Initiative (See Table 10.2)
This example describes successes and challenges for engaging providers in a statewide transition improvement project, led by the state chapter of the AAP [2]. The aim of the *Transition Care Project* was to improve HCT by providing training, resources, and technical assistance to both pediatric and adult primary care providers and using a quality improvement approach to encourage and implement HCT services in their practices. Practices were assisted in building self-management skills in adolescents, developing written transition policies, preparing and maintaining medical summaries, and assisting providers to think about and incorporate transition planning into their encounters.

Recruitment

Multiple strategies were utilized for recruitment, including promoting the project to chapter members via a direct mail and email invitation, reaching out to professional contacts at teaching

Table 10.2 Key features of statewide transition improvement project

• Professional contacts used for initial recruitment
• MOC credit available to promote interest
• Quality improvement metrics to help motivate

institutions, contacting providers within the regional medical district, and contacting practices that had previously participated in a successful project with the chapter. Ultimately, five self-selecting pediatric practices signed formal agreements to participate in pilot testing; the agreement included a small stipend to support pilot activities. A lead physician at each site was identified and served as champion and determined which care teams and staff members would be required to participate. Ancillary staff members, including clerical and front desk staff, were also strongly encouraged to participate. Participants included 18 physicians, 3 nurse practitioners, 10 nurses, and 4 social workers. Each pilot site then selected the key clinical activities (KCAs) most important for their practice. The project leaders identified continuing medical education (CME) and maintenance of certification (MOC) Part 4 credit as potentially effective tools to incentivize physicians' and allied health professionals' participation and motivate continued engagement. The addition of CME and MOC credit helped to mobilize providers and increase the rate of performing these activities as shown in the tables below.

Table 10.3 identifies three practices that had multiple participating providers working together on the same KCAs selected by those practices. Tracking these KCAs engaged providers further in these transition initiatives.

Table 10.3 Transitioning youth results by practice

	Mean change in chart review score, baseline to cycle 3[a]		
Key clinical activity (KCA)	Practice 1 ($n = 5$)	Practice 2 ($n = 2$)	Practice 5 ($n = 5$)
Written transition policy	6.0*	7.5	8.6*
Assess healthcare and transition readiness skills	6.2*		
Identify adult provider		5.5	5.8*
Discuss insurance, benefits, social services	2.6		
Portable medical summary			5.2*

*Paired t-test statistically significant, $p < 0.05$
[a]Cycle 3 was 24 weeks after baseline

Project findings indicate that it is possible for a variety of medical practices to mobilize providers to improve their care for transitioning patients, given a combination of incentives and tools implemented within a team-based care setting. Between 2012 and 2016, 32 pediatric providers and their practices have participated in the training for MOC Part 4 credit. In addition, the training and resources are being utilized by health systems, and online course resources for patients and families are available for free.

Roles for Pediatric Providers (See Table 10.4)

The Champion

Each service or clinic needs a transition champion who has dedicated time and authority to oversee the planning and implementing of HCT programs and is genuinely interested and invested in their success. This individual sets the direction of the program, mobilizes others with specific knowledge and experience, and keeps the program moving forward, especially when barriers are encountered. A champion with authority would be uniquely positioned to facilitate participation from providers who are not as invested in the development of transition tools but must be involved at the implementation level in order for transition best practices to be delivered to all patients. In Case 1, this would include the medical director and the transition program coordinator, and in Case 2, this would include leaders of the statewide chapter of the AAP.

Table 10.4 Key types of providers

Providers	Key elements
Champion	• Set the direction of the program • Mobilize others • Needs to have authority • Keeps program moving through barriers
Leaders	• Bring specific expertise • Develop more specific tools
Implementers	• Majority of providers • Will need to be motivated

The Leaders

Since constructing a transition program requires the development of tools, policies, and workflows, mobilizing a variety of providers to provide oversight and expertise to address these specific tasks is also essential. These providers can bring their unique areas of expertise to develop specific transition tools and processes, such as how to conduct a transition assessment, how to work with the EMR to develop a medical summary, or how to maintain a registry. In Case 1, these may include members of the steering committee and recipients of the mini-grant program, and in Case 2, this would include the leaders at each of the pilot sites.

The Implementers

In order for a transition program to be successful, providers who are not directly involved in the development of transition tools and programs must still be motivated to use them (see Chap. 14 for additional strategies to promote HCT planning behaviors). Ultimately the goal is for transitioning to become a routine part of pediatric practice for all providers.

Supporting and Motivating Providers

Structural Support (See Table 10.5)

Structure describes the context in which care is delivered, including hospital buildings, staff, financing, and equipment [3]. Funding is perhaps the most challenging issue in establishing and sustaining a transition program. Funding for protected physician and staff time, particularly at the program leadership level, is critical to developing infrastructure [4]. In addition to academic pursuits of research and government funding, philanthropic and "donor-centric" funding from foundations, corporations, groups, and individuals with interest in transitioning should be pursued. In larger medical centers or settings, a foundation within the institution may be approached to provide support for donor identification, cultivation, and grant submissions. Parents of AYASCHN can sometimes be instrumental in connecting to funding sources. Case 1 describes how start-up of the medical center's transition program was financed by a hospital auxiliary and a child advocacy endowment fund established as part of a capital campaign. Sustained support from a family foundation interested in the program has secured protected time for the transition program coordinator. Integration of protected time within organizational administrative budgets is also significant, particularly in ensuring sustained physician leadership for the program, and allows for investment in long-term endeavors.

Table 10.5 Structural supports

• Obtain funding for protected time for champions and leaders
• Use internal, foundation, and family funding resources
• Establish plan for long-term funding

Barriers and Facilitators

In mobilizing pediatric providers, one must consider the most common barriers pediatricians report that prevent them from providing transition services. Time, reimbursement, a steep initial learning curve, and uncertainty about the effectiveness of the program are some of the barriers to engaging pediatric providers in formal HCT programs [5, 6]. Competing priorities for provider time can also limit interest and availability to implement the program. These time constraints can be partially addressed by creating an operational infrastructure that maximizes ease and efficiencies to support provider engagement. Moreover, this also maximizes the capacity to extract provider talent and energy to advance innovation and program development.

Pediatricians also report difficulty identifying adult-oriented providers and obtaining reimbursement for transition services and time spent performing recommended transition interventions (see also Chaps. 6 and 21) [6, 7]. Pediatric providers lack familiarity with the adult service system, community resources, guardianship,

Table 10.6 Overcoming barriers

• Optimizing workflows and tools to make transition interventions easier to implement are critical in overcoming time barriers
• Ideas include
– Developing lists of adult providers
– Creating billing resources
– Integrating HCT planning tools into the EMR
– Coordinating support from interdisciplinary providers such as social workers, case managers, psychologists, and resource navigators

and insurance options for young adults with disabilities [7]. To mitigate these barriers and increase the likelihood that providers will actively participate in HCT programming, it is important to identify or create these resources and educate physicians and other practice members about their availability (see Table 10.6). This may involve developing lists of adult providers, resources, and information about billing, integrating transition planning tools into the EMR, and establishing support mechanisms from interdisciplinary providers such as social workers, case managers, psychologists, and resource navigators [8].

Highlight HCT Outcomes and Effectiveness

The implementers described above are more willing to perform interventions when their effectiveness is known or plans to be studied [5]. The effectiveness of various transition efforts to highlight when motivating providers include improvements in patient knowledge, self-confidence, and transfer rates. (See Chaps. 19–23 for different perspectives on defining successful transition.) It is also important to identify metrics—structure, process, and outcomes—that can be used to track, monitor, and evaluate HCT program activities, such as described in Case Example #2 and further elaborated in Chap. 14 [9–11]. Examples of structural outcomes include establishment of any of Got Transition's six core elements. Process outcomes could include improved patient knowledge, self-confidence, and transition readiness (see Chap. 13) [12, 13]. Finally, desired endpoints could include transition experience, successful transition to adult care, and increased quality of life (see Chap. 36).

Mobilizing Providers in the Absence of Adult Providers

While adult providers may be difficult to find or not necessary given the scope of practice for the pediatric provider (such as dually certified med-ped providers or family medicine providers), implementing transition processes in the pediatric setting should still continue. This includes creating tools described above, cultivating transition champions, and incorporating an adult model of care. Motivating providers to conduct these tasks can often be difficult in the absence of identified adult providers and need for transfer. Pediatric providers must understand how the adult model of care differs from the pediatric model and the importance of developing disease self-management and self-advocacy skills in transitioning AYASHCN (see Chap. 15). Motivating providers in these settings to implement this model will require champions, leaders, and motivators as described above.

Conclusion

Mobilizing and motivating pediatric providers to perform optimal transition-related interventions are often difficult due to lack of knowledge, time constraints, and lack of belief in the efficacy of these interventions on the part of the provider. In addition, creating a transition program within a practice or institution requires the time and effort of many providers. A transition champion with authority is essential, along with dedicated leaders, to initiate, maintain, and improve HCT programs and changes in workflows moving forward. To influence the behavior of most providers, the aforementioned barriers must be addressed. We have presented two examples of ways in which these barriers were addressed in different settings and at different levels. Delivering education, constructing an infrastructure that simplifies HCT interventions, providing incentives such as CME and MOC credit, and tracking quality measures can help keep providers motivated and help mobilize new providers.

References

1. Six Core Elements of Health Care Transition. 2017. www.gottransition.org.
2. Sanabria KE, Ruch-Ross HS, Bargeron JL, Contri DA, Kalichman MA. Transitioning youth to adult healthcare: new tools from the Illinois transition care project. J Pediatr Rehabil Med. 2015;8(1):39–51. PubMed PMID: 25737347.
3. Donabedian A. Evaluating the quality of medical care. 1966. Milbank Q. 2005;83(4):691–729. PubMed PMID: 16279964. Pubmed Central PMCID: PMC2690293.
4. White PCW, McAllister J. Starting a transition improvement process using the six Core elements of health care transition. Washington, DC: National Alliance to Advance Adolescent Health; 2015.
5. Lau R, Stevenson F, Ong BN, Dziedzic K, Treweek S, Eldridge S, et al. Achieving change in primary care--causes of the evidence to practice gap: systematic reviews of reviews. Implement Sci. 2016;11:40. PubMed PMID: 27001107. Pubmed Central PMCID: PMC4802575.
6. Okumura MJ, Kerr EA, Cabana MD, Davis MM, Demonner S, Heisler M. Physician views on barriers to primary care for young adults with childhood-onset chronic disease. Pediatrics. 2010;125(4):e748–54. PubMed PMID: 20231189.
7. McManus M, Fox H, O'Connor K, Chapman T, MacKinnon J. Pediatric perspectives and practices on transitioning adolescents with special needs to adult health care. Washington, DC: National Alliance to Advance Adolescent Health; 2008. Report No.
8. Wiemann CM, Hergenroeder AC, Bartley KA, Sanchez-Fournier B, Hilliard ME, Warren LJ, et al. Integrating an EMR-based transition planning tool for CYSHCN at a Children's hospital: a quality improvement project to increase provider use and satisfaction. J Pediatr Nurs. 2015;30(5):776–87. PubMed PMID: 26209173. Epub 2015/07/26. eng.
9. McManus M, White P, Pirtle R, Hancock C, Ablan M, Corona-Parra R. Incorporating the six Core elements of health care transition into a Medicaid managed care plan: lessons learned from a pilot project. J Pediatr Nurs. 2015;30(5):700–13. PubMed PMID: 26239121.
10. Jones MR, Robbins BW, Augustine M, Doyle J, Mack-Fogg J, Jones H, et al. Transfer from pediatric to adult endocrinology. Endocr Pract. 2017;23:822–30. PubMed PMID: 28534683.
11. McManus M, White P, Barbour A, Downing B, Hawkins K, Quion N, et al. Pediatric to adult transition: a quality improvement model for primary care. J Adolesc Health. 2015;56(1):73–8. PubMed PMID: 25287984. Epub 2014/10/08. eng.
12. Cadario F, Prodam F, Bellone S, Trada M, Binotti M, Trada M, et al. Transition process of patients with type 1 diabetes (T1DM) from paediatric to the adult health care service: a hospital-based approach. Clin Endocrinol. 2009;71(3):346–50. PubMed PMID: 19178523.
13. Chu PY, Maslow GR, von Isenburg M, Chung RJ. Systematic review of the impact of transition interventions for adolescents with chronic illness on transfer from pediatric to adult healthcare. J Pediatr Nurs. 2015;30(5):e19–27. PubMed PMID: 26209872. Pubmed Central PMCID: PMC4567416.

11 Developing Transition Policies, Procedures, or Guidelines

Roberta G. Williams and Ellen F. Iverson

Vignette

A 22-year-old patient with myelomeningocele and hydrocephalus with an obstructed ventriculoperitoneal shunt is seen in the emergency department of a free-standing children's hospital where, 8 years ago, his shunt had been revised by a pediatric neurosurgeon. He has been followed as an outpatient by pediatric neurology, neurosurgery, and a multidisciplinary spina bifida team. Emergency department staff and nurse supervisor question the plan for admission because of his adult age. This is just one of many examples of stressful encounters and complex decisions that must be made when young adult patients present to a children's hospital. These situations are difficult at best because appropriately trained providers may not be available within adult institutions or programs. This patient and family made a rational decision to seek emergency care in a pediatric center, reasoning that providers will be more experienced in managing emergent care related to his condition. However, the decision to do so can create confusion and stress among pediatric emergency department staff unless there is a clearly articulated hospital policy about the upper bounds of age for admission.

Policies and Guidelines on Transition and Transfer

Over the past two decades, there has been growing concern about the formidable challenges faced by young adults with complex healthcare needs who are migrating from pediatric systems of care to adult providers and adult healthcare systems. Mounting evidence of increased morbidity and mortality, avoidable hospitalizations and ED visits and gaps in care in these years have compelled leaders in healthcare policy, practice, and research to better understand the underlying contributors of these trends. This evidence drew a harsh spotlight on the glaring absence of policy and practice guidelines to ensure the establishment of adult-oriented care as patients emerge into young adulthood. This is complicated by the limitations of properly trained providers as young adults with special healthcare needs leave their pediatric teams

R. G. Williams, M.D. (✉)
Department of Pediatrics, Keck School of Medicine, University of Southern California and Children's Hospital Los Angeles, Los Angeles, CA, USA
e-mail: rwilliams@chla.usc.edu

E. F. Iverson, M.P.H.
Division of Adolescent and Young Adult Medicine, Department of Pediatrics, Keck School of Medicine, University of Southern California and Children's Hospital Los Angeles, Los Angeles, CA, USA

A. C. Hergenroeder, C. M. Wiemann (eds.), *Health Care Transition*,
https://doi.org/10.1007/978-3-319-72868-1_11

familiar with childhood-acquired conditions and transfer to adult care systems often ill-prepared to support young adults with complex medical conditions. On the other hand, some providers in a children's hospital may not feel comfortable dealing with adult medical and psychosocial issues. As a result, there is often lack of consensus about the age of transfer. Hospital policies vary widely because of geographic differences in available resources and there are often different policies within the same institution for different patient groups due to the special circumstances of their disease as well as provider resources.

In 2002, the American Academy of Pediatrics, the American Academy of Family Physicians, and the American College of Physicians-American Society of Internal Medicine released the consensus report highlighting the emerging evidence that young adults face grave risks to their health and well-being in these years of transition [1]. From this report arose the genesis of a framework for transition care, policy, and guidelines for institutions and providers. Pediatric tertiary care institutions charged with caring for children and adolescents living with an enormously varied array of chronic conditions, rare diseases, and disabilities face challenges in developing and enforcing policy about the age of transfer to adult health systems because of differing patient needs and provider availability.

Obstacles in Adult Care Provision Within a Children's Hospital

State regulations are specific about the age range of patients within pediatric nursing credentials. Likewise, there are regulations regarding the certification of physicians who provide oversight of nurse practitioners and physician assistants. Pediatric facilities can operate within these bounds by establishing an adolescent/young adult service with medicine-pediatric providers in the primary or subspecialty role. In the absence of specialized inpatient services, advanced planning is needed to define the special circumstances for admission that will satisfy state and local regulatory requirements.

Developing a Hospital-Wide Admission Policy Regarding Age of Transfer

As adolescents with complex chronic medical conditions approach adulthood, decisions must be made about transfer to adult primary care and identifying appropriate, qualified adult subspecialists with experience managing pediatric acquired conditions. There is wide variation in the age at transfer of chronically ill pediatric patients to adult providers and hospitals. This is determined by local resources, benefit guidelines and limitations, beliefs about when transfer should take place, and professional relationships. The limited access to appropriately trained adult providers and facilities for patients with chronic and rare disease is well documented. As a result, there is increasing pressure on children's facilities to care for young adults.

Programs covered by Title V services commonly transfer patients to an adult program when these services expire. Patients age out of these benefits at 18–21 years of age, varying by state. Title V benefits provide for nurse managers, social workers, and dietitians—the type of wrap-around services that define the medical home. Therefore, to transfer patients prior to the expiration of these services would deny them these services that are not generally available in adult programs. Exceptions to this are some adult programs for cystic fibrosis, congenital heart disease, and cancer. It is no surprise, then, that many pediatric subspecialty programs will continue to care for patients until they reach the age at which these benefits expire.

As documented by Goodman et al. [2], adult admission to children's hospitals, although still a minority, is the fastest-growing age group [1]. Indeed, many children's hospitals are debating whether the upper age limits for admission are 18, 21, 25, 30, or undefined. In some institutions, the higher age cutoff is limited to certain large programs such as oncology or cardiology. Until there is a consensus based on defined quality measures, there will continue to be locally determined policies that are influenced by state credentialing, age limit for state healthcare coverage, and financial factors. This intensifies the need for a proactive, deliberative process to guide transfer policies, particularly for free-standing children's hospitals.

Development of consensus around transfer policies must take into account the marked differences within multiple subspecialties and provider types. Moreover, there are different opportunities and constraints, depending upon the institutional structure, whether a free-standing pediatric hospital or a pediatric program imbedded within a general hospital. In this chapter, we will discuss the process of developing both transition policies at the institutional level and guidelines at the subspecialty level as well as transfer procedures that vary locally. Along the way, we have had some successes and have encountered obstacles. Geographical, economic, and workforce factors vary widely across the country, so that this specific example may not be relevant to all programs.

Table 11.1 Needs assessment questions for assessing current transfer practices by medical divisions providing chronic care

Is there a current policy for age of transfer?
Is there a mechanism for coordination with insurance and other payers related to transfer to adult providers?
What is the practice consistency among the group?
What are present internal resources for adolescents and young adults (AYA) to support transition and transfer?
Do you currently partner with adult primary care providers?
Do you currently partner with adult subspecialty providers?
What are the age limits and changes necessary for Medicaid, SSI, Title V, or other coverage?
What specific institutional resources are required for care of young adults (e.g., nursing and physician certification)?
What is the likelihood of hospitalization, surgery, or ICU care for young adults in your patient cohort?
What other subspecialty services are commonly required for your patients?
What is the role of primary care and who provides the central coordination function?
Are there age limits of certification among the team of providers in your program?
Does the natural history of the disease predict stability at age 18–21?

Developing a Hospital Transition/Transfer Policy at a Free-Standing Children's Hospital

At Children's Hospital Los Angeles (CHLA), we initiated the process of policy development by undertaking an extensive exploration of transfer practices of each medical division that provides longitudinal care for chronic patients, asking the questions in Table 11.1.

Responses were accumulated and discussed among a panel of physicians, nurses, and social workers with broad representation from subspecialty programs that included critical care and emergency medicine - providers that might be called upon to care for young adult patients. This proved illuminating as several patterns emerged. Some patient groups had conditions that are familiar to adult providers, for example, certain types of renal disease, and specific cancers. Such patients were typically transferred at an earlier age. However, many disease groups are unfamiliar to adult medicine, and these were typically retained by the pediatric program until a later age. There were some marked differences of transfer age within the same subspecialty, for example, cystic fibrosis patients have a smooth, standard transfer to an associated adult program, whereas ventilator-dependent pulmonary patients had more limited access to an appropriate adult facility and were transferred later and at opportunistic times. Patients for whom organ transplant is anticipated would be more likely to remain in pediatric care, where the transplant list is more favorable. Also, patients with developmental delay experience additional hurdles in securing the services of adult providers and tend to remain under pediatric care longer than those who have the capacity to live independently.

Next, we cataloged locally available adult healthcare resources for each patient group, for both privately and publically insured patients. Discussions with a broad range of constituents ensued—including intensive care and emergency medicine physicians and staff, hospital administration, human resources, patients, and families. We also reviewed and discussed state regulations for practice limits and practice certification. Several themes emerged. Many intensive care faculty and staff were uncomfortable with the prospect of providing care to adult patients. This sentiment was shared by other nursing personnel who concentrate on the care of infants. Consultative services that were overburdened with pediatric patients resisted the idea of accepting an adult patient at the expense of a longer wait list for children. The same idea was expressed for inpatient services that are chronically short on available beds.

We held initial discussions about the upper limits age for inpatient admission as well as recommendations of age to transfer outpatients to an adult provider in order to define general principles around age of transfer as well as potential mitigating circumstances. A Transition Council was formed as a forum consisting of physicians, nurses, and social workers belonging to all subspecialty groups caring for patients with chronic illness as well as young adult patients and families. In addition, the Council included adult subspecialists with medicine-pediatrics training and a career interest in diseases originating in childhood. These colleagues were invaluable in providing perspective on the available resources and communication needs of the receiving physician at the time of transfer. The diversity of experience offered by the Transition Council was critical in building a complete picture of the obstacles encountered during the transfer process. The principle issues developed by the Council were reviewed in a series of consensus meetings with the Hospital Safety/Quality committee and Human Resources and then referred to the hospital policy approval committees and ultimately, signed by executive leadership. In our case, the upper age limits for inpatient and outpatient admission were determined as follows:

1. Hospitalization of existing patients would be permitted up to age 21 years.
2. New inpatients over 18 years would be accepted coincident with providing a plan to subsequently transition to an adult program.
3. Planned inpatient care for unique patient groups over 21 years would require:
   - A comprehensive plan of care including a review of data that indicates improved outcomes of care within a pediatric center
   - A business plan that takes into account revenue, expense, and patient volume
   - Identification of necessary resources such as physicians, allied health providers, radiology and laboratory services, and equipment
   - Provision of additional training needs
   - Available patient psychosocial support
4. Individual patients >21 could be admitted urgently with consent of the physician-in-chief but would require a plan for subsequent care in an adult hospital.
5. There would be no age limit for outpatient care as long as there is a plan for inpatient care at an adult hospital.

Children's Hospital Log Angeles policies, once approved, are required to be accompanied by a formal communication and education process, provided on an institutional intranet site, and reviewed every 3 years. Discussions around outpatient services concluded that guidelines would allow needed flexibility around the needs of diverse programs, as long as providers were working within the bounds of their certification. It was recommended that subspecialists combine forces with adult primary providers in order to recognize complicating conditions involving other organ systems. Developing a plan for potential hospitalization at an adult facility requires partnership with an adult subspecialist to provide backup for the primary physician or privileging of the pediatric subspecialist, which can be difficult. For that reason, explicit plans should be agreed upon in advance by the patient and primary physician.

The process of policy development that we followed is presented in Fig. 11.1 and Table 11.2. An important aspect of policy development that is expressed in Fig. 11.1 is the requirement for policy review at 3-year intervals. It is feasible for the Policy Development Committee to review the results of the hospital admission policy, as inpatient demographics

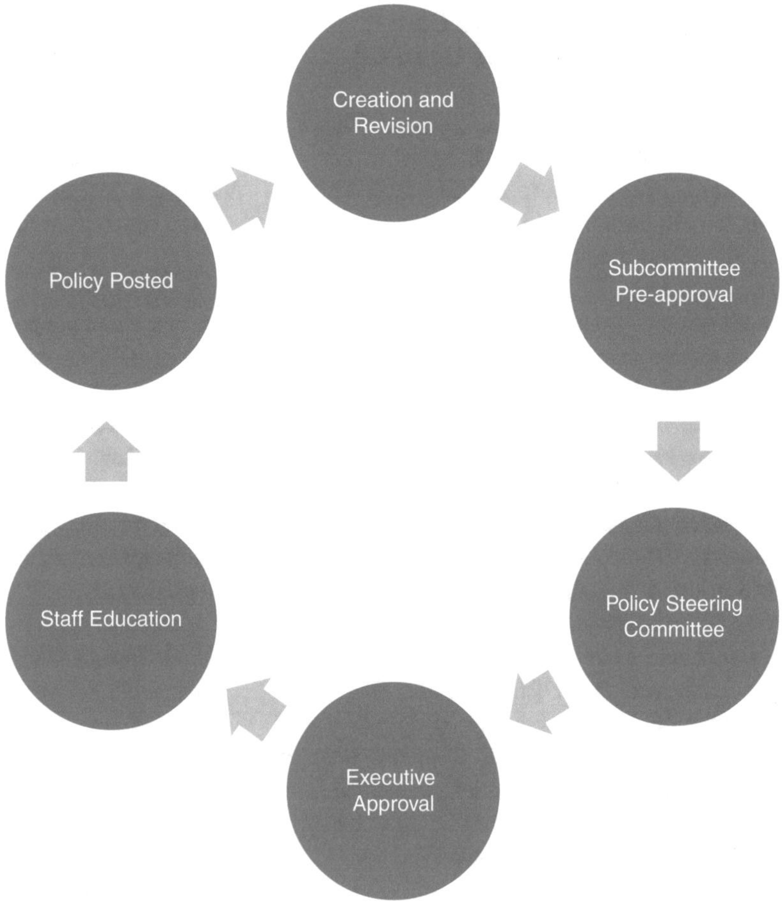

Fig. 11.1 The process of Transition Policy Development at Children's Hospital of Los Angeles

Table 11.2 Policy approval process

1. Policy owner works with subject experts to create and review/revise every 3 years
2. Policy is previewed by appropriate subcommittees as determined by policy coordinator
3. Policy is reviewed by Policy Steering Committee
4. Policy coordinator sends policy for executive approval via one of the following routes: (a) Chief Administrative Officer (CAO), (b) Chief Clinical Officer (CCO), or (c) Quality Improvement Committee (QIC), Medical Executive Committee to Medical Executive Committee, and the Board of Trustee
5. Hospital staff must be educated on the policy through professional conferences and house-wide email notification
6. Coordinator will post policy on internal website

are easily available and satisfaction of program leaders can be surveyed. This requires time and effort for personnel to summarize admitted patients' demographic data and surveying program leaders to present to the Policy Development committee. It is far more difficult to review the success of transfer because of the many different medical destinations of our diverse population. Transition Council leadership meets regularly with physicians and patient navigators at destination programs to review transfer outcomes and problem-solve for the obstructions encountered. Until there is government funding to follow patients in a lifelong registry, however, the assessment of transition and transfer outcomes will be incomplete (see Chap. 12).

Other Policies Related to Care of Adults in a Children's Hospital

For pediatric programs providing care to adults, it is appropriate to deliver an adult model of care. In addition to a policy about age of transfer, it is important to have institutional policies regarding healthcare decisions, communication, and protections that address changes in legal status once adolescents reach adulthood. This includes legal issues related to disclosure, confidentiality, end-of-life decisions, and guardianship as well as financial issues such as insurance coverage and social security requirements for health care and income supplementation (see Chap. 30) [3]. Pediatric teams should be proactive anticipating these changes and actively engage patients and families in discussions about how they will manifest in both inpatient and outpatient services. For example, parents of 18-year-olds or above should be included in a patient interview or exam only with the patient's consent. Well before patients turn 18, teams should also help patients and families navigate benefits and insurance changes, especially supplemental security income (SSI), as this process often requires specific documentation from providers (see Chaps. 8 and 25).

Developing a Transition/Transfer Policy at a General Hospital

There is less need for a formal hospital policy at a general hospital because adult patients are admitted to adult inpatient services with appropriate nursing and other staffing. Medical staff offices generally determine the appropriateness of age limits of hospital privileges for individual practitioners. It is important to have a clear agreement with the internal medicine residency program director about the role of pediatric subspecialists in oversight of internal medicine residents and fellows.

Deploying a Policy on the Upper Age of Care

Hospital policy about the upper age of care should be visible to patients and providers by signage and materials provided to the patient and family at least one year prior to the age of transfer. Ideally, this should be presented years earlier as part of transition planning. Policies should be available on the internet to all providers and reviewed at least every three years since the conditions that govern transition and transfer success will not remain static.

Conclusions

A hospital-wide policy about the age of transfer of patients with childhood diseases must balance difficult issues related to appropriate provider availability and the relative risks of the childhood disease versus the risk of acquired adult morbidities. Although appropriate care may be provided to young adults in the outpatient arena, problems occur when the patient is admitted, and the range of providers involved in their care have differing training experience and comfort levels. Therefore, it is preferable to meet these issues head-on in order to develop a consensus that is enforceable and responsive to local realities. This may be accomplished by informal discussion or a more formal process such as the Nominal Group Technique [4]. Because a rigid policy may not be ideal for all situations, a process for redress should be included. Providing patients and providers with early, accessible information about this policy will facilitate appropriate planning and enhance patient and provider satisfaction.

References

1. American Academy of Pediatrics; American Academy of Family Physicians; American College of Physicians-American Society of Internal Medicine. A consensus statement on health care transitions for young adults with special health care needs. Pediatrics. 2002;110(6 Pt. 2):1304–6.
2. Goodman DM, Halil M, Levin A, Watson RS, Williams RG, Shah SS, Slonim AD. Adults with chronic health conditions originating in childhood: inpatient experience in Children's Hospitals. Pediatrics. 2011;128:5–13.
3. https://www.hhs.gov/hipaa/for-professionals/index.html?language=es
4. Delbecq A, Van de Ven A. A group process model for problem identification and program planning. J Appl Behav Sci. 1971;7:466–92.

12 Establishing a Method to Monitor Transition Planning and Track Patient Outcomes Following Transfer

Gregory Sawicki

Case Vignette

A primary care pediatric practice network is located in the suburbs of a major metropolitan area with multiple academic medical centers, including one freestanding children's hospital. With five locations and 20 providers, the network provides primary care services to approximately 8000 families. Two locations have different EMR systems, and specialty referrals are handled at each location separately. The majority of specialty referrals are sent to the urban freestanding children's hospital, which has developed its own EMR different from any of the community practices. Approximately 15% of the children served by the network have a chronic medical condition for which they periodically receive subspecialty care. Some of these children have higher levels of complex disease requiring multiple specialty care referrals, and others only need intermittent follow-up outside the network. The leadership of the network is interested in developing a transition program for adolescents in their practices with chronic health conditions and has begun discussions with a local adult primary and subspecialty care network. A transition policy is developed stating that pediatric practices will no longer provide services to patients over age 22. A transition coordinator is hired, is asked by the network leadership to determine the expected volume of patients that will need transition and transfer-related services, and is tasked with creating reports for each provider and practice on transition-related needs.

Overview

The American Academy of Pediatrics, the American College of Physicians and the American Academy of Family Physicians joint clinical report on transition outlines an algorithm for a practice-based approach to healthcare transition from pediatric- to adult-focused care [1]. The algorithm includes recommendations for all adolescents and specifies additional steps for youth with chronic medical conditions. Fundamentally, this algorithm relies on a series of specific, coordinated, and proactive care practices starting in early adolescence and ending in young adulthood. A healthcare transition program should empower youth and their caregivers to gain transition skills during adolescence, enable smooth care coordination and communication during transfer of care, and facilitate intake into an adult-focused health-

G. Sawicki, M.D., M.P.H.
Division of Respiratory Diseases, Department of Medicine, Boston Children's Hospital, Harvard Medical School, Boston, MA, USA
e-mail: Gregory.sawicki@childrens.harvard.edu

A. C. Hergenroeder, C. M. Wiemann (eds.), *Health Care Transition*,
https://doi.org/10.1007/978-3-319-72868-1_12

care system. A key component of any healthcare transition program, therefore, is a well-planned and executed mechanism to track youth throughout the process of transition and transfer. The case vignette above illustrates the need for an accessible and up-to-date source for information to manage a complex and varied patient population that requires differing levels of services during the process of healthcare transition. A valuable tool for this type of tracking is a patient registry. At the provider or practice level, developing and maintaining a patient registry serve multiple purposes, including active population management. Recently, advances in health information technology have simplified the processes to create and sustain such registries. This chapter reviews the key components of a transition registry, including the purpose of a registry, why it is important to track healthcare transition preparation processes, the necessary steps in establishing and maintaining a registry, the various uses of a registry, and the value of a registry in tracking population-based measures for practice-based quality improvement.

Patient Registries: A Definition

Broadly defined, a patient registry is an organized data collection tool incorporating clinical, demographic, and other relevant information often from multiple data sources across a healthcare system or systems [2]. Unlike an electronic medical record, a registry is not intended for point-of-care use during clinical encounters. Rather, the primary goals of a registry should be focused on population management. Registries can be good sources of data for clinical research, particularly comparative effectiveness research. In addition, a registry often is the backbone for quality improvement initiatives at the clinician, group practice, or patient population level. Some registries are designed to capture data for diagnosis-specific groups of patients, whereas others include data for tracking multiple different patient populations.

Registry data is usually obtained through an observational study design, mimicking common epidemiologic study methods. Data should be collected using a standard approach, including uniform definitions for all data elements. This standardization also applies to data pulled into registries from EMRs. Data elements should be pre-specified to include information necessary and relevant to clinical, scientific, quality improvement, or policy goals. Although excessive data in any registry leads to challenges with implementation and feasibility, insufficient data can similarly undermine the ability of registries to aid in population management. If data collection becomes too burdensome, the registry can become difficult to sustain. Therefore, careful planning and foresight at the outset of registry development are crucial and require consensus on purpose, data sources, and scope.

Over the past several decades, patient registries have been developed and used to improve health outcomes in many distinct populations. The Cystic Fibrosis (CF) Foundation created a patient registry in 1966 in order to understand the natural history of CF, and over the next 50 years, their patient registry has become a vital tool to healthcare providers, policy makers, and researchers attempting to improve clinical care [3]. In recent years, patient registries have been developed by multiple organizations, and the Center for Medicaid and Medicare Services approves Qualified Clinical Data Registries to support quality improvement-based payment structures to healthcare systems [4]. Such registries have led to improvements in care in multiple areas of clinical medicine, including cardiology, endocrinology, rheumatology, and urology [5–8].

Designing a Registry for Healthcare Transition

A key benefit of a patient registry is the ability to track processes and outcomes over a long period of time using data sources with multiple potential inputs. Since transition from pediatric- to adult-focused healthcare is a process spanning a decade for many youth, a transition registry is a critical component for a well-functioning transition program. Establishing a transition registry is one of the Six Core Elements of transition outlined by Got Transition [9, 10]. In the Six Core Elements, the goals of a transition registry are to establish criteria and a process for identifying transitioning youth within a practice, to develop a mechanism to track the transition progress of the identified youth, and to incorporate transition processes into electronic health records when possible [11].

In order to be successful, a patient registry needs to be more than simply a database derived from a single electronic medical record source. At its core, a transition registry should be developed as a tool based on the following principles:

- Data collection is an active observational process occurring over time.
- Data collection is focused on clinical care elements relevant to healthcare transition processes and outcomes.
- All data elements have specific, easily measurable definitions which are clinically meaningful.
- Data is collected in the same manner regardless of patient or practice setting.
- Data is derived from multiple sources, including patient-reported information.

At the practice level, a transition registry should provide data that can assess variations in clinical practices at the provider level, including provider adherence to transition policies and guidelines set forth by the practice. Registry data can be provided to clinicians in order for them to compare their patient populations with those of their peers. Registry data can also be used to evaluate patient outcomes, for instance, the degree to which patients with a specific diagnosis or cared for in a specific practice have achieved adequate transition readiness skills. Process measures such as the distribution of transition plans or percentage of successful transfers across a population can also be tracked using a registry-based approach.

The logistics of creating a registry are far from trivial and often require dedicated informational technology support and staff, particularly for developing data integration strategies and data reporting tools. Data security and privacy concerns need to be addressed for all registries as well. Registries created with a research component in mind would require patient or caregiver informed consent and may be subject to review by local research ethics boards. Consent should also be considered for registries developed purely for quality improvement purposes, particularly if patient-reported outcomes or measures are planned as data elements.

Although basic spreadsheet or database software (such as Excel or Access) may be most familiar to clinicians, such platforms generally require manual data entry, may not easily link to multiple existing data sources, and could be prone to data entry errors. More often than not, a registry created in such a way is difficult to maintain because it requires extra steps for clinical staff, steps that are quick to fall off when a clinical practice is busy or staff turnover occurs. Some EMRs are able to create population-level dashboards to monitor patient progress within a healthcare system. Leveraging existing technology and tailoring it to transition needs can be a strategy to overcome these limitations [12, 13].

Got Transition has developed an assessment of each of the Six Core Elements, allowing individual practices to self-rate their transition programs on a scale of 1–4 [11]. In the domain of transition tracking and monitoring, the assessment levels are:

- *Level 1*: clinicians in the practice vary in identifying transitioning youth, and many youth are not identified until close to the age of transfer.
- *Level 2*: clinicians in the practice document relevant transition information in an electronic medical record, but not necessarily in an organized registry.
- *Level 3*: the practice develops a transition registry, identifying and tracking transitioning youth starting at age 14.
- *Level 4*: the practice actively uses a transition registry for population management in order to ensure that all youth receive necessary transition planning and transfer-related services.

Data Elements for a Transition Registry

A patient registry needs to include the necessary and relevant data aligned with the goals of the individual practice or program for which it is designed. Data collection needs to be uniform, and data elements need to be pre-specified. The data should address the needs of all relevant stakeholders, including practice leaders, individual clinicians, patients, and families. Maintaining an active patient data registry without regard to these elements leads to significant challenges for maintenance, sustainability, and utility. Finally, once a transition registry is developed and launched, it requires active, ongoing maintenance and evaluation. This requires institutional resources.

At a minimum, a patient registry focused on healthcare transition should include data elements encompassing sociodemographics (including insurance), clinical-medical information, healthcare utilization data, patient-reported data, and transition-specific data (Table 12.1). In general, the level of detail for each of the data categories needs to be tailored to the unique goals of an individual transition program. If the focus of a registry is on a patient population with a single diagnosis (i.e., at a subspecialty practice), the clinical information should be more expansive, but if the registry is intended for use at a primary care or multispecialty level, the detail on specific diagnoses could be left more general. Transition-specific data should incorporate patient-reported outcomes relevant to transition preparation and planning. Examples of such measures include transition readiness assessments and quality of life questionnaires that could be collected at routine clinical visits or as part of structured transition programs [14, 15]. Patient experience measures are often collected after routine healthcare encounters. One example is the Adolescent Assessment of Preparation for Transition (ADAPT) survey, a youth-reported measure capturing information on the degree of transition counseling and preparation received by adolescents during visits with their main healthcare providers [16]. Many patient-reported measures may not be found in standard electronic health records and would need to be collected at routine clinical visits.

Table 12.1 Key data elements for a transition registry

Category	Examples of relevant data elements
Sociodemographic data	Age/date of birth Sex/gender Race/ethnicity Health insurance Family structure Educational level (youth/caregiver) Primary language
Clinical data	Primary diagnosis Secondary diagnoses Active subspecialty referrals
Healthcare utilization data	Dates of prior appointments Dates of upcoming appointments Urgent care (emergency department) visits Hospitalization dates
Patient-reported data	Quality of life Patient experience measures Symptom measures

Transition-specific data	Transition policy shared with family/youth
	Readiness assessments
	  Date administered
	  Scores
	Transition plan developed/updated
	Health insurance after transfer identified
	Adult provider identified
	  Transfer package sent to adult provider
	Transfer completion assessed

Using a Transition Registry for Quality Improvement and Patient Safety

A well-planned transition registry incorporating data elements from multiple clinical and patient-reported sources can fundamentally improve the quality of services and care provided to transitioning youth and their families. As such, a registry needs to be more than simply a list of transitioning youth in a practice. It should be a tool for clinicians or practices to flag individual patients preparing to transfer care and ensure that they have identified an adult-focused doctor or practice, had a transition plan provided, and had medical records/summaries sent to accepting care teams. A transition registry should also identify patients who may have left pediatric care but for whom the outcome of their first appointment in an adult setting has not yet been determined, thus facilitating appropriate outreach and follow-up.

In order to promote high-quality transitional care, registry data needs to be leveraged through structured reports at the patient or population level. Such reports can augment clinical decision support tools targeting guidelines of care. For example, a registry report can flag individual youth that are scheduled for appointments that are due for a transition readiness assessment or can identify populations of youth that have lower readiness scores as a group for more specific intervention. In assessing transfer completion or care coordination, reports can identify gaps in care during transfer, providing opportunities to intervene to reduce such gaps whenever possible. Reports can also highlight differences in practice and outcomes between clinicians, spurring improvement initiatives at the provider or practice level.

Summary

Developing a transition program within a busy primary care or subspecialty care practice can be a daunting endeavor. A fundamental component for any transition program is a system to track and monitor progress of transitioning youth, and thus patient data registries are essential. By using systematic data collection, choosing appropriate data elements, and creating actionable provider or practice-level registry reports, a transition program can leverage a patient registry to improve healthcare services and quality of care, ensuring that all youth benefit from a structured, family-centered approach to transition from pediatric to adult care.

References

1. American Academy of Pediatrics; American Academy of Family Physicians; American College of Physicians; Transitions Clinical Report Authoring Group, Cooley WC, Sagerman PJ. Supporting the health care transition from adolescence to adulthood in the medical home. Pediatrics. 2011;128(1):182–200.
2. Gliklich RE, Dreyer NA, Leavy MB, editors. Registries for evaluating patient outcomes: a user's guide [Internet]. 3rd ed. Rockville, MD: Agency for Healthcare Research and Quality (US); 2014. https://www.ncbi.nlm.nih.gov/books/NBK208616/
3. Schechter MS, Fink AK, Homa K, Goss CH. The Cystic Fibrosis Foundation Patient Registry as a tool for use in quality improvement. BMJ Qual Saf. 2014;23(Suppl 1):i9–14.
4. https://www.cms.gov/Medicare/Quality-Initiatives-Patient-Assessment-Instruments/PQRS/Downloads/2016PQRS_QCDR_MadeSimple.pdf. Accessed 3 Oct 2017.
5. Peterson A, Hanberger L, Akesson K, Bojestig M, Andersson Gäre B, Samuelsson U. Improved results in paediatric diabetes care using a quality registry in an improvement collaborative: a case study in Sweden. PLoS One. 2014;9(5):e97875.
6. Harris JG, Bingham CA, Morgan EM. Improving care delivery and outcomes in pediatric rheumatic diseases. Curr Opin Rheumatol. 2016;28(2):110–6.
7. Tyson MD, Barocas DA. Improving quality through clinical registries in urology. Curr Opin Urol. 2017;27(4):375–9.
8. Clauss SB, Anderson JB, Lannon C, Lihn S, Beekman RH, Kugler JD, Martin GR. Quality improvement through collaboration: the National Pediatric Quality improvement Collaborative initiative. Curr Opin Pediatr. 2015;27(5):555–62.
9. McManus M, White P, Barbour A, Downing B, Hawkins K, Quion N, Tuchman L, Cooley WC, McAllister JW. Pediatric to adult transition: a quality improvement model for primary care. J Adolesc Health. 2015;56(1):73–8.
10. McManus M, White P, Pirtle R, Hancock C, Ablan M, Corona-Parra R. Incorporating the six core elements of health care transition into a Medicaid managed care plan: lessons learned from a pilot project. J Pediatr Nurs. 2015;30(5):700–13.
11. http://www.gottransition.org/resources/index.cfm. Accessed 23 Sept 2017.
12. Wiemann CM, Hergenroeder AC, Bartley KA, Sanchez-Fournier B, Hilliard ME, Warren LJ, Graham SC. Integrating an EMR-based transition planning tool for CYSHCN at a Children's Hospital: a quality improvement project to increase provider use and satisfaction. J Pediatr Nurs. 2015;30(5):776–87.
13. Hergenroeder AC, Wiemann CM, Bowman VF. Lessons learned in building a hospital-wide transition program from pediatric to adult-based health care for youth with

special health care needs (YSHCN). Int J Adolesc Med Health. 2016;28(4):455–8.
14. Zhang LF, Ho JS, Kennedy SE. A systematic review of the psychometric properties of transition readiness assessment tools in adolescents with chronic disease. BMC Pediatr. 2014;14:4.
15. Fair C, Cuttance J, Sharma N, Maslow G, Wiener L, Betz C, Porter J, McLaughlin S, Gilleland-Marchak J, Renwick A, Naranjo D, Jan S, Javalkar K, Ferris M, International and Interdisciplinary Health Care Transition Research Consortium. International and interdisciplinary identification of health care transition outcomes. JAMA Pediatr. 2016;170(3):205–11.
16. Sawicki GS, Garvey KC, Toomey SL, Williams KA, Chen Y, Hargraves JL, Leblanc J, Schuster MA, Finkelstein JA. Development and validation of the adolescent assessment of preparation for transition: a novel patient experience measure. J Adolesc Health. 2015;57(3):282–7.

13

Incorporating Healthcare Transition Readiness Assessment

Lisa A. Schwartz, Alexandra M. Psihogios, and Emily M. Fredericks

Introduction

Advancements in medicine have led to a growing population of adolescents and young adults with special health-care needs (AYASHCN), subsequently resulting in approximately 750,000 AYASHCN transferring from pediatric to adult-centered health-care systems each year [1]. The transition from pediatric to adult health care is considered a purposeful, planned process where an AYASHCN transfers from pediatric-, family-oriented health care to adult-, individual-oriented health care, with the goal of high-quality, developmentally appropriate, uninterrupted health-care services [2]. This medical transition occurs during a complex developmental period when AYASHCN are beginning to form and consolidate critical health behaviors and accept increasing responsibility for their own health [3]. AYA must navigate the transition to adult health care while also traversing other emerging adulthood milestones, such as pursuing academic/career goals, forming intimate relationships, moving away from the family home, and assuming increasing financial impendence [4].

The process of transitioning from pediatric- to adult-based health care poses concurrent risks and opportunities for altering the trajectory of AYASHCN health outcomes. Poor transition readiness results in devastating gaps in health care, morbidity, and mortality [5, 6], while robust transition readiness promotes increased personal responsibility for health and self-management [7]. Across recent decades, research and clinical initiatives increasingly focused on routine assessment and promotion of transition readiness [8]. The American Academy of Pediatrics (AAP), the American Academy of Family Physicians, and the American College of Physicians jointly published a clinical report, transition-planning algorithm, and transition tools for youth with and without special health-care needs [2]. Also in 2011, the National Committee on Quality Assurance Patient-Centered Medical Home standards included a specific requirement to address health-care transitions in primary care [9]. Healthy People 2020 incorporated a new public health goal on transition planning from pediatric- to adult-centered health care [10]. Notably, the research literature has emphasized routine,

L. A. Schwartz, Ph.D. (✉)
Division of Oncology, The Children's Hospital of Philadelphia, Philadelphia, PA, USA

Perelman School of Medicine of the University of Pennsylvania, Philadelphia, PA, USA
e-mail: schwartzl@email.chop.edu

A. M. Psihogios, Ph.D.
Division of Oncology, The Children's Hospital of Philadelphia, Philadelphia, PA, USA

E. M. Fredericks, Ph.D.
C.S. Mott Children's Hospital, Ann Arbor, MI, USA

University of Michigan Medical School, Ann Arbor, MI, USA

A. C. Hergenroeder, C. M. Wiemann (eds.), *Health Care Transition*,
https://doi.org/10.1007/978-3-319-72868-1_13

evidenced-based assessment of AYA transition readiness as one key priority for improving transition outcomes [11–15].

Unfortunately, there is substantial evidence that routine transition readiness assessment and preparation is not in place for many AYA and their families [16, 17]. The 2009–2010 National Survey of Children with Special Health Care Needs found no discernable improvements in transition outcomes since the original 2005–2006 report [18], and it remains to be seen if the subsequent national initiatives and tools will stimulate improvements in transition readiness preparation. A recent systematic review [19] and previous reviews [20–23] identified insufficient transition planning and preparation as central barriers to optimal transition outcomes. While many clinical programs strive to enhance the acquisition of self-management skills in AYASHCN, they do not routinely assess transition readiness [24, 25]. It is recommended that pediatric patients not transfer to adult health services unless they have the skills and supports necessary for functioning effectively in the adult health-care system [26–28].

Preparation for transition to adult medical care includes two dynamic, reciprocal processes: (1) evaluating transition readiness and (2) developing and implementing transition plans [29]. This chapter focuses primarily on the first process, the assessment of transition readiness, and provides a summary of available transition readiness assessment tools and their scientific evidence. Based on emerging research and quality improvement science, we also describe current clinical recommendations for promoting and incorporating transition readiness assessment into health-care settings while overcoming common clinical barriers. We describe a clinical case vignette which depicts how routine transition readiness assessments may be integrated into routine clinical care to ultimately improve transition readiness and adult health outcomes. Finally, we outline future directions for advancing the state of transition readiness assessment science.

Transition Readiness

Construct Definition

In order to appropriately measure transition readiness, it is necessary to define transition readiness and describe the socio-ecological factors that influence it [30]. Transition readiness is a component of disease self-management and refers to indicators that the AYASHCN and those in their support system (family and providers) can successfully begin, continue, and finish the transition process [31, 32]. The specific features of transition readiness may be operationalized differently for different populations. For example, medication adherence, activities of daily living, and keeping track of clinic appointments may represent components of transition readiness for some but not all AYASHCN [19]. Consequently, the definition of a *successful* transition to adult-centered health care may vary across AYASHCN disease populations.

Social-Ecological Conceptualization of Transition Readiness

Emerging research suggests that transition readiness is influenced by patients' social-ecological context [15, 30, 33–35]. The Social-ecological Model of AYA Readiness to Transition (SMART; [30, 36]) is an empirically supported ecological model of transition readiness developed with AYA cancer survivors. SMART proposes that transition readiness is influenced by pre-existing objective indicators that are less amenable to change (e.g., sociodemographics/culture, health status/risk, access/insurance, and neurocognition/IQ), as well as by subjective indicators that are modifiable and represent targets for transition planning interventions (e.g., patient developmental maturity, knowledge, skills/self-efficacy, beliefs/expectations, goals/motivation, relationships, communication, and psychosocial functioning/emotions of patients, parents, and providers). Prior to the development of SMART, research primarily focused on age, skills, and knowledge as components of transition readiness without investigating the patient's broader social-ecological environment, including the influence of multiple stakeholders [14, 37, 38]. To date, researchers have applied and adapted SMART to multiple pediatric populations, including youth with sickle cell disease, inflammatory bowel disease, and diabetes [33–35].

Transition Readiness Assessment

Assessing transition readiness helps to (1) identify intervention targets to increase likelihood of engagement in adult-oriented care and (2) measure changes in transition readiness across time [30, 39]. The Maternal and Child Health Bureau and The National Alliance to Advance Adolescent Health "Got Transition" program established Six Core Elements of Health Care Transition, which define the basic components of the health-care transition process. Among these components, core element 3, "Transition Readiness," directly emphasizes the importance of routine transition readiness assessment beginning at the age of 14. Core element 4, "Transition Planning/Integration into Adult Approach to Care," describes the importance of assessing transition readiness in order to develop self-management goals, determine the optimal timing of transfer to adult-centered care, and identify support needs (e.g., legal changes in decision-making). Taken together, the results of transition readiness assessments should guide transition planning (such as skill-based instruction or obtaining more support) to improve the likelihood of optimal health outcomes during and after the transfer to adult care [27].

Despite calls for evidence-based assessment of AYASHCN transition readiness [11–14] and national initiatives for improving transition from child-centered to adult-centered health care (e.g., the American Academy of Pediatrics transition algorithm and the Maternal and Child Health Bureau and The National Alliance to Advance Adolescent Health "Got Transition" initiative), few validated measures exist that assess and track transition readiness for AYA patients with chronic health conditions [14, 40]. Indeed, one barrier to the routine transition readiness assessment in clinical practice is the lack of validated instruments [14, 24]. There remains a need for transition readiness tools that are feasible in clinic settings, have adequate levels of sensitivity and specificity, and have utility in goal setting and planning transition readiness interventions [27].

Transition Readiness Assessment Measures

In a prior review, the first author of this chapter identified 56 measures of transition readiness [14]. Of the 56 measures, only 10 reported psychometric data in peer-reviewed publications and met the American Psychological Association Division 54 Evidence-Based Assessment (EBA) Task Force criteria for a "promising assessment."

Four generic measures of transition readiness were identified: the (1) California Healthy and Ready to Work (HRTW) Transition assessment tool: health-care self-care [37], (2) Self-Management Skills Assessment Guide (SMSAG; [41]), (3) TRxANSITION Scale ([42]), and (4) Transition Readiness Assessment Questionnaire (TRAQ; [15, 43]). Regarding disease-specific transition readiness, six measures were identified: (1) Cystic Fibrosis Health Care Transition Readiness Scale (CFHCTS; [44]), (2) Readiness Questionnaire (RQ) for patients with cystic fibrosis [38], (3) Readiness for Transition Questionnaire (RTQ) for patients with kidney transplant [45], (4) Transition Readiness Questionnaire (TRQ) for patients with HIV [46], (5) Transition Readiness Survey: Adolescent/Young Adult (TRS: A/YA) for patients with liver transplant [24], and (6) Sickle Cell Transfer Questionnaire (SCTQ; [32, 47]). Since the 2014 review, we identified three additional measures: (1) the Self-management and Transition to Adulthood with Rx = Treatment (STARx) Questionnaire (generic self-reported measure of the TRxANSITION Scale; [48, 49]), (2) TRANSITION-Q (generic measure; [50]), and

(3) Transition Intervention Program-Readiness for Transition (TIP-RFT) assessment for sickle cell disease [51, 52]. Notable strengths of measure development included using mixed-method participatory approaches, testing with racially and ethnically diverse samples (HRTW, RTQ, TRAQ, TRQ, TIP-RFT, STARx), and drawing upon relevant developmental or health psychology theories (TRAQ, HRTW, CFHCTRS).

Despite these identified assessments, there remains a paucity of well-validated transition readiness measures. With the exception of the STARx Questionnaire [48], these measures did not provide data on the predictive validity for actual transition outcomes, which limits our understanding of the long-term impact of transition readiness assessment. The STARx Questionnaire demonstrated initial predictive validity by predicting other self-management constructs (health literacy, self-efficacy, and adherence; [48]), but not health-care utilization. Three measures demonstrated content validity (TRAQ, TRxANSITION, and SCTQ). Most measures demonstrated construct validity, including known-groups validity (HRTW, SMSAG, TRAQ, TRS, SCTQ, TIP-RFT, and STARx) or convergent validity (SMSAG, TRxANSITION, RTQ, and TRQ). Validity findings showed that increased transition readiness was related to older age, lower disease severity, lower anxiety, higher confidence in adult providers, and participation in a transition clinic. The TRAQ, TRS, TIP-RFT, and STARx were factor analyzed, yielding strong subscales with the exception of one subscale of the TRS and one subscale of the TIP-RFT. Most measures also employed convenience samples, assessing patients already coming to clinic. This leads to a biased sample of patients already engaged in care and hinders our understanding of how the measures perform in groups of disengaged patients most at risk for poor transitions. Only a few measures (RTQ, TRS) included parent report, despite the importance of parents in the transition process [53]. Finally, many of the measures were not informed by theory or developed with rigorous methods of measure development (e.g., eliciting stakeholder feedback or assessing multiple indices of validity).

The TRAQ was and still remains the most tested and validated transition readiness measure [15, 43] with good validity and reliability [15, 54, 55]. The initial TRAQ has 29 items and is a patient-reported, generic measure of transition readiness that assesses mastery of disease self-management skills. Responses are based on the Stages of Change model [56]. A briefer, 20-item version of the TRAQ with five factors emerging from exploratory factor analysis demonstrated good internal consistency and criterion validity, though research is needed to determine predictive validity [15]. A potential limitation of the TRAQ is the focus on broad disease management skills (e.g., filling a prescription and calling the doctor's office to make an appointment) that may not apply to all AYASHCN. The narrow focus of the TRAQ is also limiting in that it does not focus on broader social-ecological factors related to transition readiness (e.g., multiple stakeholder perspectives; [23, 30, 35, 36]).

Another new emerging measure is the Transition Readiness Inventory (TRI; [57]). The TRI item pool was developed following guidelines from NIH's Patient-Reported Outcomes Measurement Information System (PROMIS; [58, 59]). PROMIS aims to provide standardized rigorous methods of development of patient-reported outcome measures [58–60]. TRI measures social-ecological components of the SMART model. It was developed for AYA survivors of childhood cancer but is intended to be adapted and modified for other populations. TRI development to date addresses limitations of prior transition readiness measures in that it has incorporated feedback from multiple stakeholders and experts via mixed-method data collection, was theoretically informed, and includes a patient and parent version. The TRI item pool will soon be tested in a larger validation study.

Translation of Transition Readiness Assessment to Clinical Care

Despite consensus statements and policy papers from numerous pediatric and adult organizations supporting the importance of transition preparation [61, 62], many pediatric programs do not systematically address transition readiness. Frequently cited challenges to routinely assessing transition readiness include time, resources, physician training, barriers to care coordination, and lack of validated measures [27, 60, 63–65]. These barriers underscore the importance of translational research and quality improvement initiatives [66, 67] to promote uptake of evidence-based practices in patient care settings [68].

As an example, within our (co-author EF) institution, we identified a gap in services with respect to preparing pediatric liver transplant recipients for the transition to adult transplant care. Specifically, we observed that patient adherence and health status often deteriorated following transfer from pediatric- to adult-centered care. Our program did not have a systematic method of assessing transition readiness or planning for the transfer of care. As part of a quality improvement (QI) initiative, we implemented a clinic-based survey to document the current state of our program, specifically measuring transition readiness skills using the TRS [24] and transition-related attitudes [69] of our AYASHCN and families. The TRS measured health-related knowledge, self-management skills, psychosocial adjustment, and allocation of responsibility for health management tasks. Prior to the implementation of this project, on average, patients transferred care when they reached 18 years of age. Subsequently, as part of ongoing program evaluation, the average transfer age is 21.5 years of age.

The goal of this QI project was to increase documented TRS screening to at least 95% for pediatric liver transplant recipients aged ≥11 years (see [24] for additional details). Results demonstrated that the TRS screening program was successful in assessing 98% of the target pediatric liver transplant recipients. Recipients who completed the TRS prior to transferring care had higher clinic attendance following the transfer to adult care compared to those who did not complete a transition readiness assessment prior to transfer. Unfortunately, adherence declined following the transfer of care for the TRS group and remained suboptimal for the control group, suggesting that merely assessing transition readiness skills in pediatrics may not be sufficient to promote adherence following the transfer of care. Rather, it may be necessary to continue to assess and intervene on self-management skills before and after the transfer to adult care.

Case Vignette

Michael was 2 years old when he underwent liver transplant. As a young teenager, despite adequate knowledge of his health history and regimen, Michael had a pattern of medication nonadherence and experienced graft rejection. His parents increased their monitoring of his medication administration, and his adherence improved. When he was 17 years old, Michael and his parents completed the TRS (see Table 13.1). He evidenced high levels of health-related knowledge and knew the names, doses, and functions of his medications. Because he was not using a reminder system to assist with medication administration, he reported missing several doses per month. While he reported high levels of self-efficacy regarding his ability to manage his medical regimen, he endorsed low levels of confidence in his ability to communicate independently with health-care providers, including the ability to obtain refills and schedule clinic visits. His parents reported that Michael was independent with managing his health-care needs but did not endorse high levels of confidence in his ability to manage these tasks without their support. Because of Michael's history of medication nonadherence and his reliance on his parents for communication with health-care providers, his transfer to an adult provider was deferred.

Over the next several years, Michael set transition-related goals to obtain prescription refills, schedule clinic visits, obtain necessary lab draws, communicate independently with health-care providers at clinic visits, and improve medication

Table 13.1 Case vignette: performance on the Transition Readiness Survey (TRS) over a 4-year transition preparation period

TRS domains	Year 1	Year 2	Year 3	Year 4
Adolescent self-efficacy (1 = low, 3 = high)	2.29	2.5	2.57	2.5
Parent-reported self-efficacy (1 = low, 3 = high)	1.58	2.17	2.42	2.67
AoR communication (1 = parent, 2 = shared, 3 = adolescent)	1.71	1.57	2.14	2.86
AoR self-management (1 = parent, 2 = shared, 3 = adolescent)	2.5	2.67	2.83	3.0
AoR communication—parent (1 = parent, 2 = shared, 3 = adolescent)	1.57	1.88	2.25	2.38
AoR self-management—parent (1 = parent, 2 = shared, 3 = adolescent)	–	2.8	2.8	3.00

Note: *AoR* allocation of responsibility for health management tasks

adherence. He was accepted into college, and despite improvements in his transition-related skills, transferring care to an adult provider was again deferred until he completed his first year of college. Although Michael expressed reluctance to transfer to the adult providers given his comfort level with the pediatrics team, he attended a transfer clinic visit during which time he met representatives from the adult team. His final TRS results demonstrated that Michael and his parents agreed that he had high levels of self-efficacy and competence in his ability to independently manage his health-care needs. Thus, at age 21 years, Michael successfully transferred care to the adult transplant clinic. One year following transfer, Michael continues to demonstrate high levels of adherence, medical stability, and independence with respect to his health-care management.

Conclusions

The last decade has seen advances in transition readiness assessment as evident by many new transition readiness assessment measures and recommendations for the use of readiness assessments from national medical associations and initiatives. However, there remains a paucity of measures that have been rigorously developed, tested, and incorporated into clinical care. While the rigorous development of measures can be a slow process, it is important to move forward with testing the implementation of transition readiness assessment in clinical care. As shown in the case above, such assessment can inform clinical care and outcomes while also helping to refine measures and identify new aspects of transition readiness to assess. Table 13.2 contains recommended strategies

Table 13.2 Recommended strategies to help advance the development of transition readiness assessments

1. **Test for psychometric properties with appropriate sample sizes**. It is important to consider in advance the necessary sample size for testing internal consistency of individual subscales, factor analysis, and multivariate models that identify associates of transition readiness.
2. **Assess predictive validity using longitudinal designs** (see [70]). It is unclear whether transition readiness assessment is related to successful transfer and competence in adult systems and subsequent health outcomes. Therefore, longitudinal studies are needed to establish the predictive validity of existing and future measures.

Table 13.2 (continued)

3. **Test measures with diverse and non-convenience samples**. It is critical that transition readiness measurement development research include diverse samples to enhance the generalizability and validity of measures. A balance of race/ethnicity, income, gender, condition severity, age (early to mid-adolescence through young adulthood), and engagement in care (recruiting those less engaged in care and not solely relying on convenience samples in clinic) is ideal.
4. **Measures should be theoretically informed**. A theoretical model can provide a framework for the measure and the components to be assessed. This helps to inform the constructs assessed and support the validity of the measure.
5. **Consider strengths and weaknesses of generic versus condition-specific measures**. The clinical utility and psychometric attributes of generic versus condition-specific measures need further study. While generic measures can transcend diagnoses and allow for comparisons across samples, factors related to successful transition may vary by diagnosis and require nuanced assessment [2].
6. **Evaluate ability to inform targets of intervention and respond to interventions**. Transition readiness measures should help identify targets of intervention to increase transition readiness and prepare for transfer [30]. Further, transition readiness assessment should allow for longitudinal assessment of change over time.
7. **Distinguish between frequency and competency in self-management behaviors.** Assessing the frequency with which health management tasks are completed does not effectively capture whether AYASHCN are either incorrectly performing or receiving significant assistance to complete tasks. Therefore, transition readiness measures must assess frequency and competency of related self-management tasks.
8. **Involve multiple stakeholder perspectives in measure development and assessment.** Collaboration between medical teams, parents, and patients is key for successful transition [2, 62, 63, 71]. As such, it is important to include various stakeholder perspectives and expertise in the development phase to increase ultimate acceptability and face validity of the measure. Furthermore, there are clinical utility and research-related advantages in assessing transition readiness from multiple perspectives. For one, it can facilitate the ability to promote collaboration between patients, parents, and providers. Additionally, comparison across stakeholders can reveal discrepancies in variables such as knowledge, goals, and expectations, which may influence transition outcomes. Such discrepancies may be important intervention targets [72]. Furthermore, the predominance of existing transition readiness measures is self-report. The accuracy of AYASHCN reports on their own health management and readiness skills remains to be seen. Therefore, multiple informant and objective methods of assessment should be incorporated as much as possible in future research designs.

to help advance the development and refinement of transition readiness assessments, many of which have been previously described [8, 29, 73].

References

1. Scal P, Ireland M. Addressing transition to adult health care for adolescents with special health care needs. Pediatrics. 2005;115(6):1607–12.
2. American Academy of Pediatrics, American Academy of Family Physicians, & American College of Physicians. Clinical report—supporting the health care transition from adolescence to adulthood in the medical home. Pediatrics. 2011;128:182–200.
3. Patterson P, McDonald FE, Zebrack B, Medlow S. Emerging issues among adolescent and young adult cancer survivors. Semin Oncol Nurs. 2014;31(1):53–9.
4. Arnett JJ. Emerging adulthood. A theory of development from the late teens through the twenties. Am Psychol. 2000;55(5):469–80.
5. Pai ALH, Ostendorf HM. Treatment adherence in adolescents and young adults affected by chronic illness during the health care transition from pediatric to adult health care: a literature review. Child Health Care. 2011;40(1):16–33.
6. Van Walleghem N, MacDonald CA, Dean HJ. Evaluation of a systems navigator model for transition from pediatric to adult care for young adults with type 1 diabetes. Diabetes Care. 2008;31(8):1529–30.
7. Betz CL, Lobo ML, Nehring WM, Bui K. Voices not heard: a systematic review of adolescents' and emerging adults' perspectives of health care transition. Nurs Outlook. 2013;61(5):311–36.
8. Devine KA, Monaghan M, Schwartz L. Transition in pediatric psychology: adolescents and young adults. In: Roberts MC, Steele RG, editors. Handbook of pediatric psychology. 5th ed. New York, NY: The Guilford Press; 2017.
9. National Committee on Quality Assurance. Standards for Patient-Centered Medical Home (PCMH). Washington, DC: NCQA; 2011.
10. Healthy People 2020 Summary of Objectives. www.healthypeople.gov/2020/topicsobjectives2020/pdfs/disability.pdf. Accessed 4 June 2012.
11. Crowley R, Wolfe I, Lock K, McKee M. Improving the transition between paediatric and adult healthcare: a systematic review. Arch Dis Child. 2011;96(6):548–53.
12. Freed GL, Hudson AJ. Transitioning children with chronic diseases to adult care: current knowledge, practices, and directions. J Pediatr. 2006;148:824–7.
13. Henderson TO, Friedman DL, Meadows AT. Childhood cancer survivors: transition to adult-focused risk-based care. Pediatrics. 2010;126(1):129–36.
14. Schwartz LA, Daniel LC, Brumley LD, Barakat LP, Wesley KM, Tuchman LK. Measures of readiness to transition to adult health care for youth with chronic

physical health conditions: a systematic review and recommendations for measurement testing and development. J Pediatr Psychol. 2014;39(6):588–601.
15. Wood DL, Sawicki GS, Miller MD, Smotherman C, Lukens-Bull K, Livingood WC, et al. The Transition Readiness Assessment Questionnaire (TRAQ): its factor structure, reliability, and validity. Acad Pediatr. 2014;14(4):415–22.
16. Lotstein DS, Ghandour R, Cash A, McGuire E, Strickland B, Newacheck P. Planning for health care transitions: results from the 2005–2006 National Survey of Children with Special Health Care Needs. Pediatrics. 2009;123(1):e145–52.
17. Quinn CT, Rogers ZR, McCavit TL, Buchanan GR. Improved survival of children and adolescents with sickle cell disease. Blood. 2010;115(17):3447–52.
18. McManus MA, Pollack LR, Cooley WC, McAllister JW, Lotstein D, Strickland B, Mann MY. Current status of transition preparation among youth with special needs in the United States. Pediatrics. 2013;131(6):1090–7.
19. Zhou H, Roberts P, Dhaliwal S, Della P. Transitioning adolescent and young adults with chronic disease and/or disabilities from paediatric to adult care services—an integrative review. J Clin Nurs. 2016;25(21–22):3113–30.
20. Jalkut MK, Allen PJ. Transition from pediatric to adult health care for adolescents with congenital heart disease: a review of the literature and clinical implications. Pediatr Nurs. 2009;35(6):381–8.
21. Lotstein DS, Kuo AA, Strickland B, Tait F. The transition to adult health care for youth with special health care needs: do racial and ethnic disparities exist? Pediatrics. 2010;126(Suppl 3):S129–36.
22. Lugasi T, Achille M, Stevenson M. Patients' perspective on factors that facilitate transition from child-centered to adult-centered health care: a theory integrated metasummary of quantitative and qualitative studies. J Adolesc Health. 2011;48(5):429–40.
23. Wang G, McGrath BB, Watts C. Health care transitions among youth with disabilities or special health care needs: an ecological approach. J Pediatr Nurs. 2010;25(6):505–50.
24. Fredericks E, Dore-Stites D, Well A, Magee J, Freed G, Shieck V, Lopez M. Assessment of transition readiness skills and adherence in pediatric liver transplant recipients. Pediatr Transplant. 2010;14:944–53.
25. McDonagh JE, Southwood TR, Shaw KL. Unmet education and training needs of rheumatology health professionals in adolescent health and transitional care. Rheumatology. 2004;43(6):737–43.
26. de Silva PS, Fishman LN. Transition of the patient with IBD from pediatric to adult care—an assessment of current evidence. Inflamm Bowel Dis. 2014;20(8):1458–64.
27. Fredericks E, Magee J, Eder S, Sevecke J, Dore-Stites D, Shieck V, Lopez M. Quality improvement targeting adherence during the transition from a pediatric to adult liver transplant clinic. J Clin Psychol Med Settings. 2015;22(2–3):150–9.
28. Huang JS, Gottschalk M, Pian M, Dillon L, Barajas D, Bartholomew LK. Transition to adult care: systematic assessment of adolescents with chronic illnesses and their medical teams. J Pediatr. 2011;159(6):994–8.
29. Devine KA, Monaghan M, Schwartz LA. Introduction to the special issue on adolescent and young adult health: why we care, how far we have come, and where we are going. Journal of Pediatric Psychology. 2017b;42(9):903–9.
30. Schwartz LA, Tuchman LK, Hobbie W, Ginsberg JP. A social-ecological model of readiness for transition to adult-oriented care for adolescents and young adults with chronic health conditions. Child Care Health Dev. 2011;37(6):883–95.
31. Betz CL, Nehring WM. Promoting health care transitions for adolescents with special health care needs and disabilities. Baltimore, MD: Paul H. Brookes Pub; 2007.
32. Telfair J, Alexander LR, Loosier PS, Alleman-Velez PL, Simmons J. Providers' perspectives and beliefs regarding transition to adult care for adolescents with sickle cell disease. J Health Care Poor Underserved. 2004;15:443–61.
33. Mulchan SS, Valenzuela JM, Crosby LE, Sang CDP. Applicability of the SMART model of transition readiness for sickle-cell disease. J Pediatr Psychol. 2016;41(5):543–54.
34. Paine CW, Stollon NB, Lucas MS, Brumley LD, Poole ES, Peyton T, et al. Barriers and facilitators to successful transition from pediatric to adult inflammatory bowel disease care from the perspectives of providers. Inflamm Bowel Dis. 2014;20(11):2083.
35. Pierce JS, Wysocki T. Topical review: advancing research on the transition to adult care for Type 1 Diabetes. J Pediatr Psychol. 2015;40(10):1041–7.
36. Schwartz LA, Danzi L, Tuchman LK, Barakat L, Hobbie W, Ginsberg JP, et al. Stakeholder validation of a model of readiness to transition to adult care. JAMA Pediatr. 2013;167(10):939–46.
37. Betz CL. California healthy and ready to work transition health care guide: developmental guidelines for teaching health care self-care skills to children. Issues Compr Pediatr Nurs. 2000;23(4):203–44.
38. Cappelli M, MacDonald NE, McGrath PJ. Assessment of readiness to transfer to adult care for adolescents with cystic fibrosis. Child Health Care. 1989;18:218–24.
39. Miller KA, Wojcik KY, Ramirez CN, Ritt-Olson A, Freyer DR, Hamilton AS, Milam JE. Supporting long-term follow-up of young adult survivors of childhood cancer: correlates of healthcare self-efficacy. Pediatr Blood Cancer. 2017;64(2):358–63.
40. McPheeters M, Davis AM, Taylor JL, Brown RF, Potter SA, Epstein Jr RA. Transition care for children with special health needs. Technical Brief No. 15 (Prepared by the Vanderbilt University Evidence-based Practice Center under Contract No. 290-2012-00009-I) AHRQ Publication No. 14-EHC027. Rockville, MD: Agency for Healthcare Research and Quality; 2014.

41. Williams T, Sherman E, Dunseith C, Mah JK, Blackman M, Latter J, et al. Measurement of medical self-management and transition readiness among Canadian adolescents with special healthcare needs. Int J Child Adolesc Health. 2010;3:527–35.
42. Ferris M, Harward D, Bickford K, Layton J, Ferris M, Hogan S, et al. A clinical tool to measure the components of health-care transition from pediatric care to adult care: the UNC TRxANSITION Scale. Ren Fail. 2012;34:744–53.
43. Sawicki GS, Lukens-Bull K, Yin X, Demars N, Huang I, Livingood W, et al. Measuring the transition readiness of youth with special healthcare needs: validation of the TRAQ—Transition Readiness Assessment Questionnaire. J Pediatr Psychol. 2011;36:160–71.
44. Dudman L, Rapley P, Wilson S. Development of a transition readiness scale for young adults with cystic fibrosis: face and content validity. Neonatal Paediatr Child Health Nurs. 2011;14:9–13.
45. Gilleland J, Amaral S, Mee L, Blount R. Getting ready to leave: transition readiness in adolescent kidney transplant recipients. J Pediatr Psychol. 2012;37:85–96.
46. Wiener LS, Zobel M, Battles H, Ryder C. Transition from a pediatric HIV intramural clinical research program to adolescent and adult community-based care services: assessing transition readiness. Soc Work Health Care. 2007;46:1–19.
47. Telfair J, Myers J, Drezner S. Transfer as a component of the transition of adolescents with sickle cell disease to adult care: adolescent, adult and parent perspectives. J Adolesc Health. 1994;15:558–65.
48. Cohen SE, Hooper SR, Javalkar K, Haberman C, Fenton N, Lai H, et al. Self-management and transition readiness assessment: concurrent, predictive and discriminant validation of the STAR x questionnaire. J Pediatr Nurs. 2015;30(5):668–76.
49. Ferris M, Cohen S, Haberman C, Javalkar K, Massengill S, Mahan JD, et al. Self-management and transition readiness assessment: development, reliability, and factor structure of the STAR x questionnaire. J Pediatr Nurs. 2015;30(5):691–9.
50. Klassen AF, Rosenberg-Yunger ZR, D'agostino NM, Cano SJ, Barr R, Syed I, et al. The development of scales to measure childhood cancer survivors' readiness for transition to long-term follow-up care as adults. Health Expect. 2015;18(6):1941–55.
51. Treadwell M, Johnson S, Bitsko M, Gildengorin G, Medina R, Barreda F, et al. Development of a sickle cell disease readiness for transition assessment. Int J Adolesc Med Health. 2016a;28(2):193–201.
52. Treadwell M, Johnson S, Bitsko M, Gildengorin G, Medina R, Barreda F, et al. Self-efficacy and readiness for transition from pediatric to adult care in sickle cell disease. Int J Adolesc Med Health. 2016b;28(4):381–8.
53. Gutierrez-Colina AM, Reed-Knight B, Eaton C, Lee J, Loiselle Rich K, Mee L, et al. Transition readiness, adolescent responsibility, and executive functioning among pediatric transplant recipients: caregivers' perspectives. Pediatr Transplant. 2017;21(3):1–9.
54. Beal SJ, Riddle IK, Kichler JC, Duncan A, Houchen A, Casnellie L, et al. The associations of chronic condition type and individual characteristics with transition readiness. Acad Pediatr. 2016;16(7):660–7.
55. Eaton CK, Davis MF, Gutierrez-Colina AM, LaMotte J, Blount RL, Suveg C. Different demands, same goal: promoting transition readiness in adolescents and young adults with and without medical conditions. J Adolesc Health. 2017;60(6):727–33.
56. Prochaska JO, DeClemente CC. Toward a comprehensive, transtheoretical model of change: stages of change and addictive behaviors. In: Miller WR, Heather N, editors. Treating addictive behaviors: processes of change. New York: Plenum Press; 1986. p. 3–28.
57. Schwartz LA, Hamilton JL, Brumley LD, Barakat LP, Deatrick JA, Szalda DE. Development and content validation of the transition readiness inventory item pool for adolescent and young adult survivors of childhood cancer. J Pediatr Psychol. 2017;42(9):983–94.
58. Cella D, Yount S, Rothrock N, Gershon R, Cook K, Reeve B, et al. The Patient-Reported Outcomes Measurement Information System (PROMIS): progress of an NIH roadmap cooperative group during its first two years. Med Care. 2007;45(5 Suppl 1):S3–S11.
59. DeWalt DA, Rothrock N, Yount S, Stone AA. Evaluation of item candidates: the PROMIS qualitative item review. Med Care. 2007;45(5 Suppl 1):S12–21.
60. Kenney LB, Melvin P, Fishman LN, O'Sullivan-Oliveira J, Sawicki GS, Ziniel S, et al. Transition and transfer of childhood cancer survivors to adult care: a national survey of pediatric oncologists. Pediatr Blood Cancer. 2017;64(2):346–52.
61. Blum RW, Garell D, Hodgman CH, Jorissen TW, Okinow NA, Orr DP, Slap GB. Transition from child-centered to adult health-care systems for adolescents with chronic conditions. A position paper of the Society for Adolescent Medicine. J Adolesc Health. 1993;14(7):570–6.
62. Rosen DS, Blum RW, Britto M, Sawyer SM, Siegel DM. Transition to adult health care for adolescents and young adults with chronic conditions: position paper of the Society for Adolescent Medicine. J Adolesc Health. 2003;33(4):309–11.
63. Gray WN, Monaghan MC, Marchak JG, Driscoll KA, Hilliard ME. Psychologists and the transition from pediatrics to adult health care. J Adolesc Health. 2015;57(5):468–74.
64. Okumura MJ, McPheeters ML, Davis MM. State and national estimates of insurance coverage and health care utilization for adolescents with chronic conditions from the National Survey of Children's Health, 2003. J Adolesc Health. 2007;41(4):343–9.
65. Zhang LF, Ho JS, Kennedy SE. A systematic review of the psychometric properties of transition readiness assessment tools in adolescents with chronic disease. BMC Pediatr. 2014;14(1):4.
66. Kotagal U, Nolan T. Commentary: the application of quality improvement in pediatric psychology:

observations and applications. J Pediatr Psychol. 2010;35(1):42–4.
67. Stark LJ. Introduction to the special issue: quality improvement in pediatric psychology. J Pediatr Psychol. 2010;35(1):1–5.
68. Gabler NB, Duan N, Vohra S, Kravitz RL. N-of-1 trials in the medical literature: a systematic review. Med Care. 2011;49(8):761–8.
69. Fredericks EM, Dore-Stites D, Lopez MJ, Well A, Shieck V, Freed GL, Eder SJ, Magee JC. Transition of pediatric liver transplant recipients to adult care: Patient and parent perspectives. Pediatr Transplantation 2011:15:414–24.
70. Colver AF, Merrick H, Deverill M, Le Couteur A, Parr J, Pearce MS, et al. Study protocol: longitudinal study of the transition of young people with complex health needs from child to adult health services. BMC Public Health. 2013;13(1):675.
71. Van Staa A, Jedeloo S, van Meeteren J, Latour JM. Crossing the transition chasm: experiences and recommendations for improving transitional care of young adults, parents, and providers. Child Care Health Dev. 2011;37:821–32.
72. De Los Reyes A. Introduction to the special section: more than measurement error: discovering meaning behind informant discrepancies in clinical assessments of children and adolescents. J Clin Child Adolesc Psychol. 2011;40(1):1–9.
73. Pai A, Schwartz LA. Introduction to the special issue: health care transitions of adolescents and young adults with pediatric chronic conditions. J Pediatr Psychol. 2011;36:129–33.

14 Employing Healthcare Transition Planning Tools

Constance M. Wiemann and Albert C. Hergenroeder

Introduction

In the United States, chronic disease and disability in children, adolescents, and young adults up to age 21 affect approximately one in five families [1]. Ninety percent of children and youth with special healthcare needs of a physical nature will enter adulthood, numbering one-half million annually; an estimated additional 600,000 16–17-year-olds in the United States have serious mental illness.

Children's hospitals that serve adolescents and young adults with special healthcare needs (AYASHCN) want to improve the structures and processes to facilitate healthcare transition (HCT) into adult-based care [2–4]. Pediatric providers recognize that their AYASHCN patients are living into adulthood and are concerned about the morbidity/mortality following poorly planned transfer to adult-based care. However, most lack formal training in HCT planning methods (see Chaps. 6 and 10). Providers are looking for evidence-based methods to help prepare their patients for medical self-management.

Potential solutions to improve HCT planning include using electronic medical record (EMR)-based transition planning tools (TPT) designed to facilitate the preparation for HCT in the clinic or hospital setting [5]. The use of EMR-based interventions has demonstrated improved adherence to practice guidelines for Pap smear screening in ob-gyn and primary care physicians [6]. Similarly, pediatricians' use of handheld computers that provided guideline-based decision support was associated with increased physician adherence to asthma treatment guidelines [7].

However, provider uptake and sustained use of these new technologies and tools remain a challenge [8–10]. And, incorporating HCT planning into pediatric practice and letting patients graduate from pediatric service requires a cultural shift [11–13].

In response to the need to develop an HCT planning program, Texas Children's Hospital formed a Transition Committee in 2004 and developed an electronic medical record (EMR)-based transition planning tool (TPT) as one component of a larger institution-wide approach to transition planning. This chapter will describe the authors' experience with promoting TPT use among care providers, highlighting how several services incorporated the TPT into their clinic.

Getting Started

At the first Transition Committee meeting in 2004, representatives from all clinical services were invited to discuss the HCT program initiative.

C. M. Wiemann, Ph.D. (✉) • A. C. Hergenroeder, M.D.
Section of Adolescent Medicine and Sports Medicine, Department of Pediatrics, Baylor College of Medicine, Texas Children's Hospital, Houston, TX, USA
e-mail: cwiemann@bcm.edu; alberth@bcm.edu

A. C. Hergenroeder, C. M. Wiemann (eds.), *Health Care Transition*,
https://doi.org/10.1007/978-3-319-72868-1_14

Many attendees described the AYASHCN on their services with the most pressing medical, psychosocial, and financial needs, along with frustration at being unable to facilitate HCT. They wanted help with those individual patients who were the most problematic to transition. This need underscored the importance of establishing the framework for the Texas Children's Hospital Transition Committee: good clinical outcomes could follow after structures and processes are in place to facilitate those outcomes [14]. The goal was to build a hospital-wide set of core HCT structures and processes to be used by all services, rather than designating one clinic or service as responsible for patient-specific HCT planning. The cornerstone structure would be an EMR-based TPT that the committee would develop and provide technical assistance to implement. The TPT was to serve two purposes: (1) evaluate the patient and family condition-specific knowledge and skills and (2) encourage teachable moments between the provider and patient, which facilitates HCT planning. Rather than developing a paper-based tool, the TPT was integrated into Epic, the hospital's EMR.

The use of the TPT by clinical services was one of the first steps in developing service-specific HCT planning programming. The tool could not be customized—all services would use one tool; however, how they used the tool, what resources they attached to complement the tool, and how they developed a referral network with their adult counterparts were in the control of the services. At the outset, pediatric providers were not routinely assessing for patient and family HCT readiness in part because they had no training on how to prepare AYASHCN and their families for HCT. Preparation for the actual transfer to adult care is discussed in Chaps. 15 and 16.

The remainder of the chapter describes steps taken to introduce the TPT and increase its use across subspecialty services using a quality improvement approach. A description of the Texas Children's Hospital TPT is presented first, followed by quality improvement methods used, summary data on TPT use, and then four vignettes of clinics that piloted the process of implementing the TPT as part of a quality improvement study, before going system-wide.

The Texas Children's Hospital Transition Planning Tool

The TPT is an EMR-based HCT readiness tool designed to identify and help rectify patients' gaps in knowledge and skills about their disease and its management as they approach transition from pediatric- to adult-based healthcare. It encourages teachable moments between the provider and patient, which facilitates HCT planning. The TPT has 13 core questions that can be asked by the provider in any order (see Table 14.1); questions are intended to guide the interaction between the provider and the patient. There is a caregiver version of the core questions, to initiate transition planning for patients not cognitively able to answer the questions. For those with the Epic EMR, the link to the TCH TPT is https://galaxy.epic.com/?#Browse/page=1!68!421!2815780.

A unique feature of the TPT is that questions are asked in the context of what the patient needs to know to advocate for themselves or communicate with a new provider. The TPT asks if the patient had a chance to talk to their doctor alone, a cornerstone of promoting self-management and advocacy. Seen this way, transition planning using the TPT is an extension of regular pediatric care, expanding the provider's role.

When a patient masters a skill, knowledge, or behavior in the TPT, the clinician assigns them a successfully accomplished (SA) score for that question. If a patient does not answer adequately, an explanation of the answer is given, or homework or educational support materials are provided. These resources are linked to each core question to better equip the patient with the knowledge and skills needed to successfully accomplish the question at the next clinic visit. The provider prints these materials in the patient's room.

Table 14.1 Epic transition planning tool core patient questions (and example responses indicating mastery)

Q1.	Tell me about your diagnosis (Patient can communicate basic disease process)
Q2.	Tell me what signs you need to be aware of that indicate you are approaching an emergency situation with your diagnosis? How can you avoid the emergency? When do you call the doctor or go to the emergency room? (Patient can communicate basic signs/symptoms and plan of action in an emergent situation)
Q3.	What number do you call in an emergency? Who are your doctors and how do you contact them? Do you have an in case of emergency (ICE) contact in your cell phone? (Patient can communicate 911 emergency number and appropriate contact information for all of his/her physicians. Patient has an ICE contact in his/her cell phone, if applicable)
Q4.	How do you schedule your doctor's appointments? (Patient can communicate how to schedule an appointment)
Q5.	Did you meet with your doctor without your parent and ask a question today? (Patient met with doctor without a caregiver present and asked an age-appropriate question. A suggested topic could be "what would you like more information about or what are you concerned about?")
Q6.	What are the names of your medications? What are they for? When do you take them? How much do you take? Are there any foods, beverages, or other medications you should avoid when taking your prescriptions? (Patient can communicate name, action, dosing, and contraindications of medications)
Q7.	Do you take your medications and treatments by yourself?
Q8.	What is the danger of mixing your medications with alcohol or drugs not prescribed by your doctor? (Patient can communicate if there is and the danger of mixing current medications with alcohol or other drugs, including over the counter if applicable)
Q9.	How do you fill and refill your prescriptions? (Patient can communicate procedure for getting prescriptions filled and refilled)
Q10.	What questions do you have about sex and birth control? (Implied that clinician has asked about current or future sexual activity)
Q11.	What are the names of your medical/dental/vision insurance companies? Do you know your insurance identification numbers? Do you know the phone numbers for your insurance companies? (Patient can identify name, identification number, and contact information for all insurance carriers)
Q12.	Will your current insurance benefits continue as you transfer to adult-based healthcare? If not, how will you get insurance? (Patient has or can communicate a plan for insurance coverage after leaving TCH)
Q13.	When you transfer to adult-based healthcare, do you know who your doctor is going to be? If not, do you know how to find a doctor? (Patient can identify and knows how to contact the adult care provider for future visits, or patient can communicate how to find a doctor)

The TPT has an extensive library of 81 handouts in English and Spanish, updated annually, including a directory of resources with contact information for over 42 social services ranging from education, employment and vocational training, drug/alcohol rehabilitation programs, dental care, and transportation, and a 41-page handout on adult providers by specialty (e.g., obstetrics and gynecology, psychiatry, dermatology, and internal medicine), who have agreed to take young adults into their practice. The library also includes information sheets with step-by-step instructions on a variety of topics such as how to find private or public insurance and understand insurance coverage. Lastly, the TPT includes a portable medical summary (PMS), which is a letter created within the EMR that when invoked as a smart phrase populates a summary of the patient's medical record, including the active problem list, current prescriptions, immunization history, allergies, insurance information, pharmacy information, emergency contact information, medical insurance information, and recent diagnostic study results, the latter being entered by the provider sending the letter. This letter can be sent directly to the new adult provider by email or electronically through Epic or printed and given to the patient. When generated, the PMS is automatically sent to the EMR patient portal, accessible via the Internet with their name and password.

Improvement Methods to Promote TPT Use

A multidisciplinary team of investigators consisting of an adolescent medicine physician, psychologist, quality improvement specialist, the parent of a young adult with special healthcare needs, transition project manager, and transition research coordinator lead this quality improvement initiative. Seven Plan-Do-Study-Act (PDSA) cycles, used to promote and evaluate the main outcome measure, TPT utilization, were carried out over a 6-year study period and are described in Table 14.2. The PDSA, an improvement science method, is a strategy for "developing, testing and implementing changes that should lead to improvement" [15]. In each PDSA cycle, the objective is identified, and a plan is developed to test the change

Table 14.2 Plan-Do-Study-Act cycles to promote TPT use across the study period

PDSA #	Change strategies/what was learned
1	**Baseline phase**: • TPT available for use in Epic, no formal education provided
2	**Formal training phase—promote TPT use in four pilot clinics**: • Teach providers how to use TPT • Send list of upcoming patient visits each week to encourage TPT use • Provide laminated step-by-step instructional cards on how to access the TPT in the EMR • Host quarterly meetings to review TPT use by all providers and discuss enablers and barriers to HCT planning • Provide additional training and technical assistance on a one-on-one basis, when requested • Administer Provider Survey #1 to measure provider satisfaction with the TPT and identify barriers to use *What was learned*: TPT use increased incrementally; providers cited barriers to TPT use: lack of time, using TPT disrupted the patient flow, could not remember how to use it
3	**Increase intensity of TPT technical assistance in four pilot clinics**: • Troubleshoot barriers to use—contact TPT users (in person, via email, phone, or pager) to remind them to use the TPT • Visit individual clinics to meet with providers to facilitate TPT use • Conduct monthly clinic team meetings to address TPT usage barriers • Continue quarterly provider meetings across all services • Administer Provider Survey #2 to measure provider satisfaction with the TPT and identify barriers to use *What was learned*: TPT use increased; providers reported barriers to TPT use: difficult to locate in the EMR and cumbersome to use; wanted a mechanism to indicate transition planning already completed with each patient
4	**Release of upgraded TPT (TPT 2.0)**: • Streamlined, user-friendly upgrade was developed and made available (see Table 14.3 for list of changes between TPT 1.0 and TPT 2.0) – Addition of a transition button on the EMR navigation pane to facilitate easy access to the tool – A flow sheet reporting the patient's transition planning progress to facilitate continuity between providers and over time – A simplified user interface with fewer clicks needed to access the TPT • Promotion of its use was limited; limited technical assistance *What was learned*: This served as a baseline phase with passive introduction of an upgraded TPT; despite revisions, TPT use did not increase in the absence of active promotion
5	**TPT 2.0 available and promoted across the entire TCH enterprise**: • Distributed user guide to assist with accessing and navigating the TPT • Trained TCH Epic educators to use the TPT and to help others • Presented at Pediatric Grand Rounds on transition, demonstrated TPT use • Provided in-person technical assistance to users who requested it • Administer Provider Survey #3 to measure provider satisfaction with the TPT and identify barriers to use *What was learned*: The numbers of patient encounters with TPT use increased substantially; providers cited insufficient time to integrate the TPT into clinic workflow as a barrier to optimum TPT use

Table 14.2 (continued)

PDSA #	Change strategies/what was learned
6	**TPT 2.0 available and promoted across the entire TCH enterprise**: • Provided in-person technical assistance to users who requested it • Fewer meetings with individual services as efforts to provide technical assistance to outside institutions wanting to adopt the TPT increased *What was learned*: Providers need frequent reminders to use the TPT, and new providers must be trained; regularly scheduled meetings with services during which top users are recognized are important reminders and motivators that HCT is important for optimal patient care
7	**Release of upgraded TPT (TPT 3.0):** • See Table 14.4 for list of changes between TPT 2.0 and TPT 3.0 • Added name of service documenting TPT use – Added dot phrase to copy TPT use to the clinic note – Two questions added to facilitate billing for transition planning – PMS was made accessible to patient via patient's EMR portal • 81 handouts in English and Spanish revised • Meetings with individual services every 6 months; the highest user recognized with prize (candy bar) • In-person technical assistance provided upon request • Best Practice Alert was initiated in a pilot service *What was learned*: Changes to TPT were well received; providers need to be reminded about the importance of EMR documentation of HCT planning for reimbursement; despite an improved TPT, regularly scheduled meetings with services during which top users are recognized are important reminders and motivators and provide structured opportunities for services to review transition planning activities

Table 14.3 TPT improvements from version 1.0 to 2.0

Item improved	TPT 1.0	TPT 2.0
Location in Epic	• Patient education	• Doc (Review) Flowsheets
Ease in accessing	• Three screens to access	• Front screen
Number of clicks per question	• 19 for first question; at least 10 for subsequent questions	• 2–3 clicks per question
Status of HCT planning	• Not available	• Separate HCT status buttons
View progress made	• Four steps to review each question	• Click on flowsheet to see everything completed
Incorporate TPT notes into clinic note	• Not available	• Cut and paste into clinic note

(Plan), and the test is carried out (Do) while collecting data throughout the process. The data from the test is examined and compared to benchmarks (Study). Changes are then planned or implemented for the next cycle of change (Act).

During PDSAs 1–4, the primary focus was on providers in four pilot clinics who expressed interest in developing a HCT program as their patients were at risk for morbidity due to poor HCT (see Wiemann et al. [16]). Serial provider surveys described elsewhere [16] implemented in PDSAs 2, 3, and 5 evaluated provider satisfaction and self-reported transition planning activities. The TPT was actively promoted throughout the Texas Children's Hospital enterprise during PDSAs 5, 6, and 7, including subspecialty services, community pediatric practices, and medical homes. Two sets of upgrades to the TPT were implemented in PDSAs 4 and 7; these changes are summarized in Tables 14.3 and 14.4, respectively. The context of HCT was expanded in PDSA 7 with the addition of the following two questions that are linked to billing codes: "How important is it to you to prepare for/change to an adult doctor before age 22?" and "How confident do you feel about your ability to prepare for/change to an adult doctor?"

Table 14.4 TPT improvements from version 2.0 to 3.0

Items improved	TPT 2.0	TPT 3.0
Review Flowsheet tab	• Don't know the name of the user or section doing HCT planning unless they enter it manually	• Added department name to the Review Flowsheet • Added dot phrases to copy TPT use to the user's clinic note
Department and billing questions	• Not existent	• Added new department button and billing questions
Portable medical summary (PMS)	• No easy way to identify if the PMS has been sent	• PMS accessible by patients via My Chart

Quarterly Epic-generated TPT use reports were reviewed by the team and by the services. The reports included the number of patient encounters with use and the number of providers using the TPT. Qualitative information gathered during provider feedback sessions and from open-ended questions on serial provider surveys assessed barriers to use, and suggestions for improvement were summarized as part of planning for the next PDSA cycle. During PDSA 6 there was a shift in team activity from local TPT promotion to providing technical assistance on TPT implementation to institutions across the nation, resulting in less frequent meetings with individual services.

Resulting TPT Use

Figure 14.1 displays the total number of encounters with TPT use across the TCH enterprise by PDSA cycle. The use during the first four PDSAs was largely confined to the four pilot clinics. Once the TPT became available enterprise-wise, there was a considerable jump in the number of patient encounters with use. The total numbers of encounters with use increased from 1255 in 2015 to more than 1500 in each of 2016 and 2017. Physicians have consistently been the highest users, using more than twice as often as registered nurses and nurse practitioners, the next highest user group (not shown). The third highest user group is social workers or counselors.

Figure 14.2 graphically reports results of provider satisfaction surveys. The percent of providers who reported being "satisfied" or "very satisfied" with certain TPT features significantly increased after introduction of the streamlined, user-friendly upgrade in PDSA 5.

The number of encounters in which each of the 13 TPT core questions was asked in 2017 is presented in Fig. 14.3. The most commonly asked question is also the first question that appears in the TPT: Tell me about your diagnosis. The least commonly asked questions were about insurance, alcohol or illicit drug use, and reproductive health, topics providers noted they were least comfortable discussing with their patients.

Of note, at the start of the study period, TPT use was focused on older adolescent patients as most services were experiencing a backlog of AYASHCN who needed transitioning. As the study progressed, the TPT was used with younger patients, indicating that HCT planning was also occurring at younger ages. See Table 14.2 for a summary of what was learned as a result of each PDSA cycle.

Case Vignettes of Four Individual Clinics

Clinic A was a busy, subspecialty clinic staffed by physicians, nurses, case workers, and social workers. The transition team met with the service chief, faculty, and staff, and the initial plan was that all faculty and staff would use the TPT in clinic. However, through the first four PDSA cycles of the quality improvement project, the physicians reported that they had no time to use the

TPT. Subsequently, the task of using the TPT was given to the social workers and case managers. During the fifth PDSA cycle when TPT version 2.0 was introduced, the service chief went from never using the tool to being one of its main users and advocates. During PDSA 6, the service chief determined that TPT use should become part of the case manager annual evaluation, and the use has been high ever since.

Clinic B was a busy subspecialty service, with a similar composition as Clinic A. The nurse practitioner was an early adopter of the TPT and the highest user. This clinic had the most physicians trained by the transition team to use the TPT, yet only two physicians accounted for the majority of the use in addition to the nurse practitioner. TPT use remained at a high level over PDSAs 6 and 7 with the addition of two more nurse practitioners who became prominent users. TPT use by one of the early physician adopters dropped off as he started seeing more children and fewer transition age youth. Nurse practitioners are now expected to be the drivers of transition planning in this clinic.

Clinic C. Despite the section chief's strong support of the TPT, physicians did not use it. The chief then assigned two research nurses to integrate the TPT into transition planning for every patient participating in a quality improvement study [16]. In this clinic, TPT use did not spread beyond the study patients. Patients in this clinic often transitioned to an adult healthcare clinic that is within the same building. The use on the pediatric side stopped completely at the end of PDSA 5 when the research nurses were no longer available and increased dramatically with the hire of a nurse and social worker dedicated to HCT planning in PDSA 6, who used the TPT in both the pediatric and adult healthcare clinics.

Clinic D. This subspecialty, multiservice clinic sees patients who are medically complex, cognitively delayed, and dependent upon caregivers. Although three physicians and one nurse were trained to use the TPT, TPT use was minimal, with inadequate time in clinic being the limiting condition. Moreover, patients in this clinic are often seen my multiple services, which complicates the timing of transfer to adult care. In this clinic, HCT planning was not designated as part of an individual's job description, and HCT or TPT champion did not emerge.

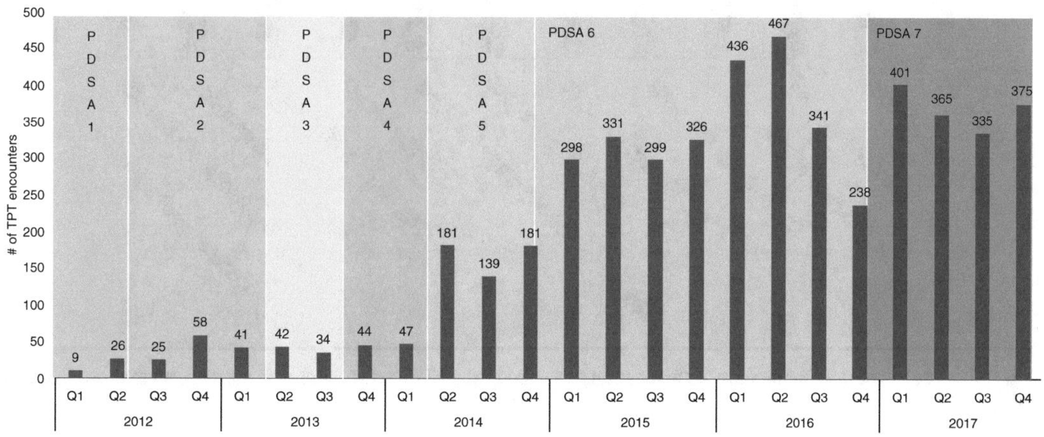

Fig. 14.1 TPT utilization across the TCH enterprise by PDSA cycle (2012–2017)

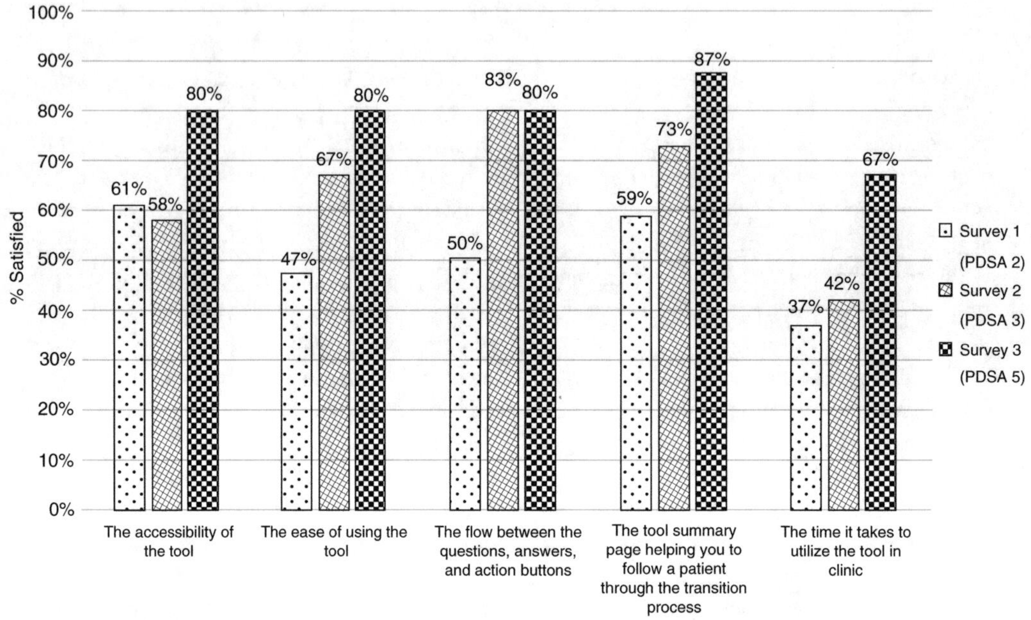

Fig. 14.2 Provider satisfaction with the transition planning tool over three survey periods

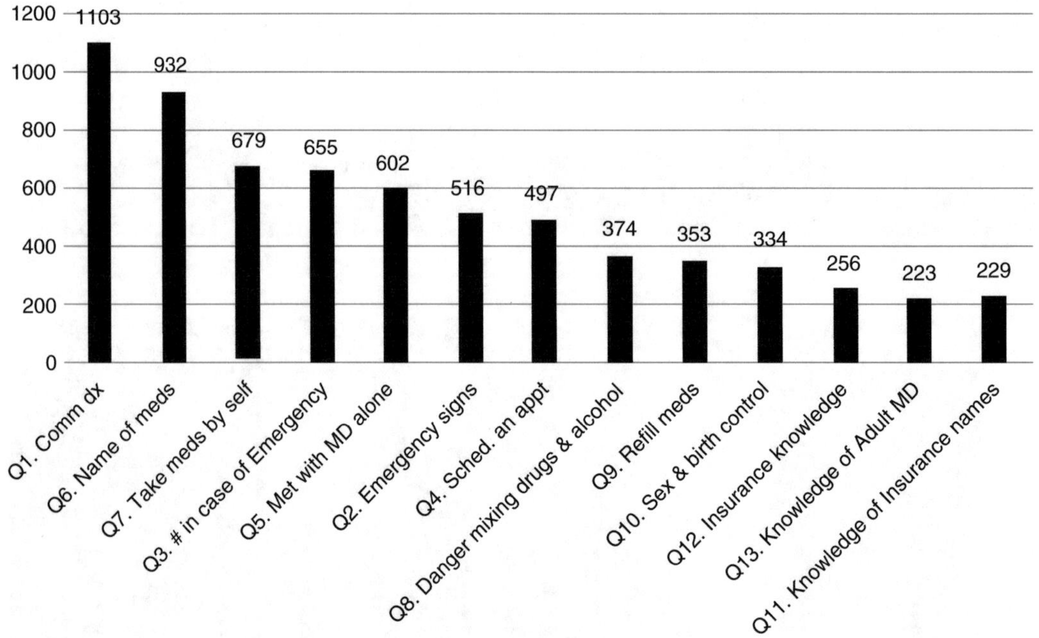

Fig. 14.3 The number of encounters each question was asked in 2017 (question numbers correspond to those listed in Table 14.1)

Conclusions

The use of a HCT TPT sets the expectation that transition planning will occur and that AYASHCN knowledge and skills will increase as a result. The use of the TPT can be increased through regular meetings between a dedicated transition team and the providers and staff of each service. In at least two cases, physicians who initially said they had no time to use the TPT came to see the tool as an asset rather than a burden. They learned to view transition planning as being as important as all other aspects of the care plan and became top TPT users and advocates on their respective services. The TPT by itself is not a transition planning program; rather, it can serve as the key to unlock the door for services to initiate disease self-management conversations with AYASHCN and families, with the expectation that one day they will transition into adult healthcare. It took more than 7 years to develop, implement, and evaluate this Epic-based TPT to the point where it can be used in clinic settings. It is therefore recommended that those wishing to use such tools as part of their HCT programming not create their own, but rather work with this existing structure as a starting point.

References

1. U.S. Department of Health and Human Services, HRSA, Maternal and Child Health Bureau. National Survey of Children with Special Health Care Needs Chart book 2009–2010. Rockville, MD: U.S. Department of Health and Human Services. p. 2013.
2. Cooley WC, Sagerman PJ. Supporting the health care transition from adolescence to adulthood in the medical home. Pediatrics. 2011;128(1):182–200. https://doi.org/10.1542/peds.2011-0969.
3. National Association of Pediatric Nurse Practitioners. NAPNAP position statement on age parameters for pediatric nurse practitioner practice. J Pediatr Health Care. 2014;28(4):A15–6. https://doi.org/10.1016/j.pedhc.2014.03.001
4. Peters A, Laffel L. Diabetes care for emerging adults: recommendations for transition from pediatric to adult diabetes care systems: a position statement of the American Diabetes Association, with representation by the American College of Osteopathic Family Physicians, the American Academy of Pediatrics, the American Association of Clinical Endocrinologists, the American Osteopathic Association, the Centers for Disease Control and Prevention, Children with Diabetes, The Endocrine Society, the International Society for Pediatric and Adolescent Diabetes, Juvenile Diabetes Research Foundation International, the National Diabetes Education Program, and the Pediatric Endocrine Society (formerly Lawson Wilkins Pediatric Endocrine Society). Diabetes Care. 2011;34(11):2477–85. https://doi.org/10.2337/dc11-1723.
5. Sharma N, O'Hare K, Antonelli RC, Sawicki GS. Transition care: future directions in education, health policy, and outcomes research. Acad Pediatr. 2014;14(2):120–7.
6. White P, Kenton K. Use of electronic medical record-based tools to improve compliance with cervical cancer screening guidelines: effect of an educational intervention on physicians' practice patterns. J Low Genit Tract Dis. 2013;17(2):175–81.
7. Shiffman RN, Freudigman KA, Brandt CA, Liaw Y, Navedo DD. A guideline implementation system using handheld computers for office management of asthma: effects on adherence and patient outcomes. Pediatrics. 2000;105(4):767–73.
8. Carlfjord S, Lindberg M, Bendtsen P, Nilsen P, Andersson A. Key factors influencing adoption of an innovation in primary health care: a qualitative study based on implementation theory. BMC Fam Pract. 2010;11:60. https://doi.org/10.1186/1471-2296-11-60.
9. de Veer A, Fleuren M, Bekkema N, Francke A. Successful implementation of new technologies in nursing care: a questionnaire survey of nurse-users. BMC Med Inform Decis Mak. 2011;11(1):1–12. https://doi.org/10.1186/1472-6947-11-67.
10. Doerr M, Edelman E, Gabitzsch E, Eng C, Teng K. Formative evaluation of clinician experience with integrating family history-based clinical decision support into clinical practice. J Pers Med. 2014;4(2):115–36. https://doi.org/10.3390/jpm4020115.
11. Magrab P, Millar H, Jekyll IG. Surgeon General's conference. Growing up and getting medical care: youth with special health care needs. Washington, DC: National Center for Networking Community Based Services, Georgetown University Child Development Center; 1989.
12. Blum RW, Garell D, Hodgman CH, Jorissen TW, Okinow NA, Orr DP, et al. Transition from child-centered to adult health-care systems for adolescents with chronic conditions. A position paper of the

Society for Adolescent Medicine. J Adolesc Health. 1993;14(7):570–6.
13. Reiss J, Gibson R. Health care transition: destinations unknown. Pediatrics. 2002;110(6 Pt 2):1307–14.
14. Donabedian A. Evaluating the quality of medical care. Milbank Mem Fund Q. 1966;44(3 Suppl):166–206.
15. Deming WE. The new economics for industry, education, government. Cambridge, MA: MIT Press; 1994.
16. Wiemann CM, Hergenroeder AC, Bartley KA, Sanchez-Fournier BE, Hilliard ME, Warren LJ, Graham SC. Integrating an EMR-based Transition Planning Tool for CYSHCN at a Children's Hospital: a quality improvement project to increase provider use and satisfaction. J Pediatr Nurs. 2015;30(5):776–87.

Understanding the Pediatric and Adult Healthcare System: Adapting to Change

15

Megumi J. Okumura, Ian S. Harris, and Mary Ellen Kleinhenz

Vignette

Sara is a 20-year-old woman with severe autism and cystic fibrosis. She is limited in her ability to communicate her needs and cooperate with caregivers and providers. She is dependent on her parents for her medical management. Her family has been hesitant about the prospect of transferring her care to adult healthcare providers. She has a primary care pediatrician and pediatric neurologist who cares for her autism and is followed by the pediatric cystic fibrosis team. The pediatric cystic fibrosis team has been discussing the plan to transfer care of the patient to the adult cystic fibrosis center. Due to the patient's developmental needs, it was unclear to the adult cystic fibrosis program how to modify their services to meet Sara's care needs.

Overview

Pediatricians and adult providers often bring up differences between the pediatric and adult healthcare systems during transition. For example, differences in the investment level for management of the childhood-onset chronic diseases are frequently discussed. Lack of resources, lack of expertise, and cultural differences between the two systems are cited as barriers to successful transfer and used as justification as to why patients remain in pediatrics [1–4]. Notions of how to mitigate the handoffs and processes that challenge patient and families and frustrate clinicians to improve health outcomes have been one of the driving forces in the development of transition programs [5, 6]. While there are many exemplars of approaches to this process, consensus on best practices for transition from pediatric to adult healthcare in the setting of childhood-onset chronic illness has not emerged

M. J. Okumura, M.D., M.A.S. (✉)
Departments of Pediatrics and Medicine, Divisions of General Pediatrics and General Internal Medicine, University of California, San Francisco, San Francisco, CA, USA
e-mail: megumi.okumura@ucsf.edu

I. S. Harris, M.D.
Department of Medicine, Division of Cardiology, Adult Congenital Heart Program, University of California—San Francisco, San Francisco, CA, USA
e-mail: Ian.Harris@ucsf.edu

M. E. Kleinhenz, M.D.
Department of Medicine, Division of Pulmonary, Critical Care, Allergy and Sleep, Adult Cystic Fibrosis Program, University of California—San Francisco, San Francisco, CA, USA
e-mail: MaryEllen.Kleinhenz@ucsf.edu

A. C. Hergenroeder, C. M. Wiemann (eds.), *Health Care Transition*,
https://doi.org/10.1007/978-3-319-72868-1_15

Table 15.1 Differences between pediatric and adult care

Domain	Pediatric medicine	Adult medicine
Age related	Growth and development focus Future oriented	Maintenance and disease management "medical" focus. Optimize present
Philosophy	Family-centered: Assumes dependence on family, including decision-making for medical management and social life Focus on child social growth and schooling	Patient-centered: Assumes independence in medical self-management and independence in social and personal life
Insurance	Insurance is an entitlement	Insurance eligibility depending on disability, income, or work
Nonadherence	More assistance	More tolerance
System	Subspecialist often as key coordinator of care Multispecialty centers of care	Primary care as medical home with specialty consultation. Care is spread among various providers

[6–8]. This chapter examines differences seen between pediatrics and adult healthcare systems (see Table 15.1). We consider how to mitigate differing expectations of patients, parents, and pediatric and adult healthcare providers. Finally we explore how to navigate the differences to ensure the highest possible care delivery for patients who are entering the adult healthcare system.

The System

Patient Epidemiology

Significant chronic illness burden in pediatrics is relatively rare as compared to the adult population. While the number of children with special healthcare needs (CSHCN) is increasing, the disease burden is still lower than in the adult population. Technologies have not only benefitted our smallest patients but our older population as well. The trend for chronic disease burden has been increasing for all age sectors and will continue to increase with improvements in medical treatment. There is a monotonic relationship of increasing chronic disease burden with increasing age across all types of patients. In aggregate 45% of the U.S. population has a chronic disease with 21% having multiple chronic diseases. The prevalence of two or more chronic conditions in those under age 17 is 5%, while among persons over 65 years of age, the prevalence of two or more chronic conditions is 62% [9]. The predominant etiology for disease development differs between pediatric and adult diseases (genetic/developmental vs. acquired). Additionally, approaches to disease and management differ, as discussed in the previous chapters. Nonetheless, the developmental concerns focused on in pediatrics related to acquisition of disease management skills during adolescence parallel the adaptations to illness or disability encountered in chronic disease management in the adult system. It is important to think about the trends in chronic disease management to understand the differences and parallels found in both pediatric and adult chronic disease management systems to ensure that transition programs between pediatric and adult systems adequately address patient needs.

Having a life-threatening condition may be relatively rare in pediatrics, and thus these children are considered special or unique in the pediatric system. Having a life-threatening disease in the adult healthcare system, while concerning and life changing for adult patients, is more prevalent. Arguably, ensuring compassionate, high-quality patient-centered care for anyone with a chronic disease is paramount in any healthcare system. In pediatrics, resources for chronic disease management and family supports derive from the health system, schools, and community. In adult medicine, the individual is the focus of disease management, restorative services, and entitlement programs. The historic shortage of adult specialists knowledgeable about management of rare pediatric diseases is a barrier that is slowly being addressed by training programs and medical societies [10]. On the other hand, because the adult healthcare system supports a high burden of chronic illness, chronic illness management for the lifespan is understood by healthcare providers and those who provide ancillary patient services in the adult healthcare setting. Healthcare resources and services try to maintain adults in the work environment, decrease morbidity, and improve quality of life. Because of the large numbers of patients with chronic disease such as diabetes and congestive heart failure, interventions such as disease navigation programs, patient supports, and mental health supports are often robust within individual institutions or within healthcare plans.

Vignette

Sara's pediatric cystic fibrosis care team has reached out to the adult cystic fibrosis care team. The adult team has never had a patient with autism; however they have several patients with developmental delay. The patient would first establish care in adult primary care and then transfer to the adult cystic fibrosis center. The patient's primary pediatrician reached out to an internist who was interested in adults with special healthcare needs to start the transfer process in primary care. The general internist then reached out to the pediatric neurologist to clarify when and to whom the neurologist wanted to transfer the patient. The pediatric neurologist stated that she would follow the patient indefinitely, due to a shortage of autism specialists in the area. Normally for patients on public plans, the general internist otherwise would have referred the patient to an adult psychiatrist within network to manage the mental health and behavioral needs of the patient. The primary care physician also reached out the pediatric and adult cystic fibrosis teams to confirm care management and how to best coordinate the needs for the patient.

Pediatric Healthcare System and Funding in the Pediatric System

The epidemiology of pediatric diseases and need for specialized medical and surgical care have led to the regionalization of services for children with special healthcare needs and, with this pooling of resources, the improvement of child healthcare [11]. Regionalization channels funding to a few institutions within or across states to maximize availability of resources and specialty care access for children with rare chronic diseases. Specifically, Title V funding, State Child Health Insurance Programs, insurance payer funds, and state funds are consolidated into children's hospitals to support the specialized services found in regionalized care. In addition, philanthropy and support by voluntary health agencies (e.g., Cystic Fibrosis Foundation, local disease-specific foundations) augment disease programs that otherwise would not be financially viable. Finally, school systems augment programs, such as with special education programs and school nursing to allow a youth with severe developmental disabilities to function in society within the school setting. Through the consolidation and often augmented funding of child regional healthcare, rare diseases can be addressed. To accommodate patients, regionalized services include multispecialty clinics such as cystic fibrosis, spina bifida, and congenital heart disease programs. This often leads to the expectation of patients and parents that multiple specialty care providers are available within one clinic setting supported by social work, case management, and disease specialty resource creating "one stop shopping" as the norm for chronic disease care. This model system has been subsidized by the children's hospitals through the funding streams mentioned above. Unfortunately, for community hospitals, this multidisciplinary care model may not be fiscally viable. Pooling of resources and adequate philanthropic support are not often found in the adult medicine health system.

Vignette
Sara had comprehensive services (e.g., child life support, social work, and case management) in the pediatric health system. She also had support through comprehensive autism services at the children's hospital. Lacking adult autism services, the pediatric neurologist agreed to manage medication and the behavioral needs of the patient. The pediatric and adult cystic fibrosis teams coordinated services to accommodate the patient's severe autism. The adult primary care physician then worked within her system to find parallel resources to the pediatric program. For example, instead of child life, the primary care physician assisted the family and coordinated with nursing staff on how to meet the patient's needs and make her comfortable in the clinic.

Adult Healthcare System

With the large burden of the aging population and high disease prevalence, the adult healthcare system has focused on detection and modification of risk factors for disease, disease diagnosis, and chronic disease management in local areas. While wellness is increasingly important, the focus has been largely on disease maintenance and ensuring adequate control of diseases such as diabetes, hypertension, and cardiovascular disease. Programs to achieve these goals are based within local hospitals, health maintenance organizations, and physician practices. A focus on the developmental needs of the patient includes the patient's functioning in society with attention to work, financial independence, and self-care needs. Areas of medicine concerned with adult life transitions such as geriatric or hospice provide examples of dependent care and family-based supports built to sustain family members caring for the patient. The resources for and funding to support disabled adults are often less generous than in the pediatric setting [12]. There are notable exceptions to these trends. The Cystic Fibrosis Foundation sponsors a nationwide system of high-quality adult cystic fibrosis care centers to continue lifelong age of its growing adult population [13]. Similarly the American College of Cardiology has made efforts to increase the number of adult congenital heart care centers and specialists to meet the clinical demand of an aging population [14]. Other clinical programs in the adult health system focus on the most prevalent diseases, such as heart disease, diabetes, dementia, and multiple sclerosis. These adult chronic disease programs have the infrastructure to address the medical complexity of more challenging young adults with complex chronic illnesses and, thus, may serve as avenues to ensure that transferring young adults receive the care coordination and case management they need. For example, in complex care programs in adult medicine, support for tracheostomies and G-tubes occurs through different specialties and programs as compared to pediatrics (e.g. geriatrics), but may serve as a resource to manage maintenance. Thus, partnering with adult complex care programs represents potential mechanism to address the needs of transferring young adults.

Vignette
Sara had been on Medicaid and the child health Title V program in California. With her social worker, the family had switched their coverage to the Genetically Handicapped Person's Program that would cover cystic fibrosis and general medical care into adulthood.

Funding in the Adult Healthcare System

For most adults, medical coverage is self-funded, provided through the patient's employer-based insurance or supported through an entitlement program. Because income eligibility varies between those who were less than 19 vs. those 19 years of age and older, many young adults age out of coverage. The Affordable Care Act mitigated this somewhat by extending coverage to young adults until age 26 [15]. While some patients have conditions that are not so disabling that they can be expected to work, other adolescents and young adults with special healthcare needs (AYASHCN) may enter entitlement programs such as condition-specific Title V program extensions [16] (e.g., Genetically Handicapped Persons Program in California) due to their condition and disability without expectation of work. Adults with childhood-onset diseases leave a subsidized pediatric insurance program and transition into the Medicaid system [17]. Being on the Social Security Income and the public health programs offers patients limited financial maneuverability in the healthcare system. This, coupled by a move away from a regionalized pediatric healthcare system to local community-based adult care providers and caregivers, may make finding resources needed to sustain complex disease management a challenge. Many physician practices in the community do not take public insurance as reimbursement rates of public insurance plans make practices less willing to take on the complexity of these patients. Solutions to this problem are dealt with differently depending on access to federally qualified health centers, public safety net programs, and academic medical centers. Working with local clinics and individual providers in these safety net programs or seeing which practices will take a few patients on public plans is often required to find a new medical home for AYASHCN who are transferring to adult care.

Vignette

Sara's adult CF care team had no experience with autism. They were able to get a complete developmental, behavioral, and family situation intake from the pediatric team. They learned that the patient could not sit in a room for long periods and often had her caretaker take her off the clinic's floor. The adult CF providers explored Autism Speak's resource materials to learn how to adapt the clinic visit to a patient with autism and set up a reward for the patient (a book that made noises). The patient was in the room long enough to have the exam and address critical aspects of the visit, at which point the patient was allowed to go outside while one parent remained to discuss the medical needs of the patient. The primary care physician undertook a similar process by ensuring the patient had the first appointment of the day, to minimize noise and traffic in the office waiting room. She initiated the physical exam first before intake so that the patient could go with the family outside and walk around when the physician and caretaker discussed care management.

The Provider

Overview of the Philosophies in Pediatrics and Adult Medicine

Pediatricians and adult care providers have identical goals for their patients—to ensure that patients are well cared for, receive high-quality care, and have the best possible quality of life. In pediatrics, patients are completely dependent on their parents. Families are primarily responsible to execute the care plan in pediatrics. Families, and their pediatric providers, often expect themselves to continue this role even in late adolescence, when autonomy, independence, and self-care are normally supposed to emerge. In the adult healthcare system, autonomy and self-care are assumed. For most pediatric patients, dependence gradually evolves to independence as the working construct of adult healthcare. The approach to disease management in pediatrics is often referred to as "family-centered care," while in the adult care system, the approach is "patient-centered care" [18, 19]. As young adults, their capacity for disease management falls in between family-centered and patient-centered models. AYASHCN need family support, while pediatricians and parents struggle to balance the rigidity of supervised care with the hazards of autonomy. The challenges faced by adolescent patients are multiple: developing an understanding of disease and treatment, learning how to access and sustain treatments, and receiving support when choices have adverse health consequences. The tension between patient- and family-centered care is not unique to pediatrics. In the adult healthcare system, adults who are aging increasingly have relied on children or other family members to care for their needs; thus, family-centered care also occurs. Inclusion of family to accommodate the patient's needs and self-management ability is common practice for adult providers. The apparent well-being and vigor of AYASHCN may mask their need for continued support from family. Hence, explicitly detailing how the family manages the patient's care and whether such responsibility can be assumed by the AYASHCN is essential to a well-executed transfer of care.

A fundamental driver of pediatric care is the principle of beneficence, whereas adult medicine is founded on the principle of autonomy. "Beneficence is defined as an act of charity, mercy, and kindness with a strong connotation of doing good to others including moral obligation. All professionals have the foundational moral imperative of doing right. In the context of the professional–client relationship, the professional is obligated to, always and without exception, favor the well-being and interest of the client" [20]. Beneficence in pediatrics is operationalized in the ability of pediatricians to help ensure that patients are safe and the disease well managed. Pediatricians try to ensure that parents adhere to medication and treatment regimens for their children. If this does not happen and a child's life is threatened, child protective services can be called, and the child can be brought into the hospital without parental consent to receive care. This aspect of beneficence recurs in the care of the elderly where after age 65 years, elderly protective services mirror the function of child protective services [21].

Between patient ages 18 and 65, however, disease management is founded on and limited by the principle of autonomy, which "is usually associated with allowing or enabling patients to make their own decisions about which health care interventions they will or will not receive" [22]. This may not be in line with the treating physician's medical opinion. The ability of the clinician or family member to force medical management on a patient is limited. Thus, trusting, respectful relationships among patient, parents, and pediatric and adult providers are critical to assuring the patient's wellness and optimal disease management. Working on the patient–physician relationship may help mitigate issues parents have with medical-legal constraints as their disabled children achieve their legal majority. Legal issues specific to pediatric and adult health systems are discussed in Chap. 30.

Relative Roles of Primary Care Providers and Specialists in Pediatrics and in Adult Healthcare

Over the last two decades, the medical home has emerged as a dominant model for structuring pediatric and adult medical care. The American Academy of Pediatrics (AAP) and the American College of Physicians (ACP) have published position statements advocating the medical home model and prioritizing access to medical homes for all patients [23]. Within the adult medicine community, the model clearly and consistently envisions the relationship between the patient and the primary care physician as central [24] with the primary care physician and the patient together taking primary responsibility for disease management. Such a view is compatible with the logistical realities of adult primary care where the coordinated management of multiple complex, chronic diseases is common. Adult issues such as childbirth, sexually transmitted diseases, hypertension, and diabetes are all prevalent conditions found in AYASHCN and are within the purview of adult primary care. Adult primary care physicians typically coordinate input from various specialties while maintaining primary responsibility for disease management [25]. Importantly, primary care physicians serve a critical role as a conduit to specialty care as new issues arise. They know the various specialists in their area and can help facilitate the transfer to adult specialty care.

In contrast, primary care pediatrics often focuses on patients' healthy development and overall well-being rather than specific chronic disease management. Children with complex chronic diseases are less likely than adults to have multiple acquired comorbidities, and the management of these chronic diseases tends to be dominated by a single specialty. In light of this, there is ongoing debate within the pediatric community about the optimal relationship between primary care and specialty practices within the family-centered medical home model [26]. This debate has played out on several levels. Institutionally, the increasing prevalence of complex medical conditions among infants and children has prompted the emergence and promotion of multidisciplinary specialty centers designed to provide care related to specific conditions, frequently housed within children's hospitals. In this context, pediatric specialty providers often take the role of both disease-specific and primary care pediatrician. They are willing to take care of acute and chronic care needs. In the early years of a child's life, primary care pediatricians tend to work together closely with their specialty colleagues. However, as CSHCN grow into early adolescence, many have a single, dominant chronic illness, and patients and their families frequently come to view their specialty providers as their primary care providers. Table 15.1 summarizes the differences between the pediatric and adult systems discussed thus far [4].

Aligning Resources

The following section discusses strategic ways to partner with adult providers. This chapter recognizes that the adult program is more likely to parallel then mirror the pediatric program.

Find Strategic Ways to Allow Providers to "Work in Their Scope of Practice"

Adult providers work in the context of primary care with subspecialty consultation. A few adult subspecialists will provide wraparound care for their patients. Dialysis/end-stage renal disease patients may have both their primary care and specialty care needs met by their nephrologists. In general though, the adult chronic illness model can be facilitated by working with the primary care physician and the adult specialty care physician. Most specialists will not want to provide wraparound care, and having clearly laid out the patient's needs, the adult colleagues can assist in assigning the roles of each provider and the additional services that may be needed.

Understand the Processes That Allow Continuity of Services and Care

By understanding the needs of the patient, adult providers can help the pediatric providers plan for needed services. Certain disease management functions found in the pediatric specialty service may not be mirrored in the adult specialty service, but instead found in other specialty or generalist services. For example, a child with a G-tube who is followed by the pediatric gastroenterologist may need to be followed by a G-tube nurse in the adult general medicine practice if adult gastroenterology does not take care of G-tubes. Understanding the parallel services and coordinating between them will help the planning process. Since the pediatric provider does not practice in the adult system, they need to work with their adult colleagues to ensure services are bridged. Service-based, rather than specialty-based, transition planning is critical to ensure that the patient has no interruption in their care.

Vignette

Sara had established with a primary care physician who happens to work with the adult cystic fibrosis center. To encourage interaction with the primary care physician, the CF team would defer general health questions to the primary care doctor. Sara's parents, due to her autistic needs, dreaded hospitalization that required initiation of parenteral antibiotics for management during previous CF pulmonary exacerbations, even with the resources of child life services. The adult CF team was pleased to learn that Sara's parents had successfully supervised home IV therapy once a PICC had been placed. Together, the parents and adult CF team agreed to work with interventional radiology and anesthesiology to place the PICC as a same-day, come-and-go procedure, avoiding the need for hospitalization, as a hospital would likely not be able to accommodate her developmental needs.

Identify the Developmental Needs of the Patient and How to Accommodate for Them

A fundamental difference between pediatrics and adult medicine is the approach to development. In pediatrics, a child is growing and acquiring skills to function and relate to their environment. While a hospital is foreign to children and adults, pediatric systems of care try to normalize the experience through child life services by trying to decrease the anxiety that a child may experience in a medical space. In addition, the structure of a children's environment is meant to be playful and inviting to a child and often includes classrooms and playrooms to allow a child to be comfortable. In the adult healthcare system, there are often few accommodations for these developmental concerns. Unfortunately, for the developmentally delayed, these accommodations are often useful, allowing the patient to be comfortable in the medical environment, and when removed can be anxiety provoking to the patient and families. Accommodations will need to be made to address the patient's developmental needs. This will require coaching by the pediatric team to the adult team to consider how to adapt clinical care delivery to meet the patient's medical needs. Asking pediatric providers what has worked in accommodating the developmental needs of the patient will better prepare adult providers to anticipate potential problems, work with their staff, and make the clinic visit proceed more smoothly.

Vignette

Sara's primary care physician reached out to the adult cystic fibrosis center to ask if they could be the primary site for case management as the adult CF program had a dedicated social worker. While the primary care physician had their own case management services, due to Sara's medication needs, the primary care physician thought that coordination and open communication with the CF program's case manager to coordinate social services and medical needs would be easier for both the patient and providers.

Identify Where to Find the Resources for Case Management and Support

Case management and support can be found at primary care and specialty care levels. Because adult specialty care operates within silos, a patient may require numerous different encounters to address specialty needs. Coordinating between primary care and specialists with technology-based services such as electronic consultations or telehealth may reduce expense and disruption of patient experience. Multidisciplinary clinics, such as adult cystic fibrosis or adult congenital heart disease programs, recognize that certain morbidities are common within their population and embed providers with expertise to address these conditions. Primary and specialty care providers need to agree on the primary coordination site; identify who is responsible for services, equipment, and specialty medications; and educate patients and caregivers about process for requests, authorizations, and assessments. If multiple social workers and case managers are involved, coordination and communication are required to ensure that all issues are taken care of promptly.

Communicate the Components of Care Important to the Individual Needs of the Patient

Education regarding systems of adult care and their differences from pediatric services facilitates a smooth transition from pediatric to adult care. This educational process should occur over a period of years before transfer of care occurs and is a shared responsibility of the pediatric and adult practices. To make such a process work, the two practices must understand each other's approaches and communicate clearly and explicitly so that each practice understands the other's resources and care components. This communication must occur both on a general level (e.g., describing general operations, such as clinic policies) and on a more specific level (specific resources required by a patient), when discussing the needs of individual patients to be transferred.

Communicate the Expectations of Patients and Caregivers Regarding Services, Access, and Outcomes

In the course of managing a significant chronic illness over a child's life, strong emotional bonds form among the physician, patient, and the family. This relationship may create tacit expectations on the part of the patient and his/her caregivers regarding the nature of interactions between family and provider. These expectations may include the availability of providers to deal with different issues (e.g., having the personal cell phone of the provider rather than going through an answering service) and possibly disease-related outcomes (e.g., pediatricians may not discuss long-term outcomes of disease out of fear of frightening families and patients). This dynamic change between family/patient and provider constitutes one of the potential major cultural differences between pediatric and adult care and can pose a major barrier to smooth and effective transition. These expectations of the patient and his/her family are often not clearly recognized by the adult practitioners assuming the patient's care. During transition planning, the pediatric and adult practitioners must discuss these expectations explicitly and frankly and not assume that both sides understand intuitively the differences in approach.

Conclusion

The often referred to cultural differences between pediatrics and adult medicine can be adapted to meet the needs of the patient [27]. Understanding the patient's need to gradually gain self-management skills and foster growing autonomy needs to be recognized as clinicians prepare young adults for the adult system and beyond. Most people understand growth and development in the social environment as young adults graduate from high school and move on to college or the work force. Similar changes are expected in the transfer to adult care. Thus, working closely with adult specialty and primary care providers to ensure that needed medical supports and services are in place is critical for successful transfer to adult care.

References

1. Okumura MJ, Kerr EA, Cabana MD, Davis MM, Demonner S, Heisler M. Physician views on barriers to primary care for young adults with childhood-onset chronic disease. Pediatrics. 2010;125(4):e748–54.
2. Okumura MJ, Heisler M, Davis MM, Cabana MD, Demonner S, Kerr EA. Comfort of general internists and general pediatricians in providing care for young adults with chronic illnesses of childhood. J Gen Intern Med. 2008;23(10):1621–7.
3. Fox A. Physicians as barriers to successful transitional care. Int J Adolesc Med Health. 2002;14(1):3–7.
4. Mulvale GM, Nguyen TD, Miatello AM, Embrett MG, Wakefield PA, Randall GE. Lost in transition or translation? Care philosophies and transitions between child and youth and adult mental health services: a systematic review. J Ment Health (Abingdon, England). 2016;January:1–10.
5. Watson R, Parr JR, Joyce C, May C, Le Couteur AS. Models of transitional care for young people with complex health needs: a scoping review. Child Care Health Dev. 2011;37(6):780–91.
6. Crowley R, Wolfe I, Lock K, McKee M. Improving the transition between paediatric and adult healthcare: a systematic review. Arch Dis Child. 2011;96(6):548–53.
7. Gabriel P, McManus M, Rogers K, White P. Outcome evidence for structured pediatric to adult health care transition interventions: a systematic review. J Pediatr. 2017;88:263–269.e15.
8. McPheeters M, Davis AM, Taylor JL, Brown RF, Potter SA, Epstein RA. Transition care for children with special health needs. Technical Brief No. 15 (Prepared by the Vanderbilt University Evidence-based Practice Center under Contract No. 290-2012-00009- I). AHRQ Publication No. 14-EHC027-EF. Rockville, MD: Agency for Healthcare Research and Quality; 2014.
9. Anderson G, Horvath J. The growing burden of chronic disease in America. Public Health Rep. 2004;119(3):263–70.

10. Child JS, Collins-Nakai RL, Alpert JS, Deanfield JE, Harris L, McLaughlin P, et al. Task force 3: workforce description and educational requirements for the care of adults with congenital heart disease. J Am Coll Cardiol. 2001;37(5):1183–7.
11. Lorch SA, Myers S, Carr B. The regionalization of pediatric health care. Pediatrics. 2010;126(6):1182–90.
12. Lewis V. California Healthcare Foundation Issue Brief: assessing the California Children's Services Program. 2008.
13. Cystic Fibrosis Foundation Patient Registry Annual Data Report 2013. 2013. http://www.cff.org/UploadedFiles/research/ClinicalResearch/PatientRegistryReport/2013_CFF_Annual_Data_Report_to_the_Center_Directors.pdf. Accessed 20 June 2015.
14. Williams RG. Transitioning youth with congenital heart disease from pediatric to adult health care. J Pediatr. 2015;166(1):15–9.
15. Breslau J, Stein BD, Han B, Shelton S, Yu H. Impact of the affordable care act's dependent coverage expansion on the health care and health status of young adults. Med Care Res Rev. https://doi.org/10.1177/1077558716682171.
16. Fishman E. Aging out of coverage: young adults with special health needs. Health Aff. 2001;20(6):254–66.
17. Fishman LN, Barendse RM, Hait E, Burdick C, Arnold J. Self-management of older adolescents with inflammatory bowel disease: a pilot study of behavior and knowledge as prelude to transition. Clin Pediatr (Phila). 2010;49(12):1129–33.
18. Kitson A, Marshall A, Bassett K, Zeitz K. What are the core elements of patient-centred care? A narrative review and synthesis of the literature from health policy, medicine and nursing. J Adv Nurs. 2013;69(1):4–15.
19. Kuo DZ, Houtrow AJ, Arango P, Kuhlthau KA, Simmons JM, Neff JM. Family-centered care: current applications and future directions in pediatric health care. Matern Child Health J. 2012;16(2):297–305.
20. Kinsinger FS. Beneficence and the professional's moral imperative. J Chiropr Humanit. 2009;16(1):44–6.
21. National Adult Protective Services Association. http://www.napsa-now.org. Accessed 27 June 2017.
22. Entwistle VA, Carter SM, Cribb A, McCaffery K. Supporting patient autonomy: the importance of clinician-patient relationships. J Gen Intern Med. 2010;25(7):741–5.
23. American Academy of Family Physicians (AAFP) American Academy of Pediatrics (AAP) American College of Physicians (ACP) American Osteopathic Association (AOA) Joint Principles of the Patient-Centered Medical Home March 2007. http://www.aafp.org/dam/AAFP/documents/practice_management/pcmh/initiatives/PCMHJoint.pdf. Accessed 18 Mar 2016.
24. Policy statement: organizational principles to guide and define the child health care system and/or improve the health of all children. Pediatrics. 2004;113(5 Suppl):1545–7.
25. Starfield B, Shi L, Macinko J. Contribution of primary care to health systems and health. Milbank Q. 2005;83(3):457–502.
26. Van Cleave J, Okumura MJ, Swigonski N, O'Connor KG, Mann M, Lail JL. Medical homes for children with special health care needs: primary care or subspecialty service? Acad Pediatr. 2016;16(4):366–72.
27. Rosen D. Between two worlds: bridging the cultures of child health and adult medicine. J Adolesc Health. 1995;17(1):10–6.

16 Developing the Process for Transferring Care from Pediatric to Adult Providers

Megumi J. Okumura and Erica Lawson

Overview

When pediatric providers and patients discuss the process of transition, the conversation, unfortunately, often focuses only on the transfer procedure, that is, identifying adult providers to whom the patient should transfer and the timing of graduation from the pediatric practice. Transfer of care is only one of the later stages of the process of transition [1, 2]. If the focus of transition is transfer, it is likely that the provider and patient have missed the opportunity to fully prepare a patient for the adult healthcare system. We urge pediatric providers to ensure that the preparation work has been done, as described in the previous chapters, so that the transfer process outlined in this chapter can be productive and proceed as smoothly and seamlessly as possible. The planning for actual transfer to an adult provider should happen at least 1 year prior to when the pediatric provider anticipates transfer of care. *Transfer planning should never be initiated at the last pediatric visit.* The transfer preparation process consists of deciding when is the most appropriate time to transfer care, finding an adult provider who can assume the care of the patient, ensuring that a comprehensive medical summary and care plan is prepared and received, and a follow-up process to ensure that transfer has been completed [3–7].

M. J. Okumura, M.D., M.A.S. (✉)
Departments of Pediatrics and Medicine, Divisions of General Pediatrics and General Internal Medicine, University of California, San Francisco, CA, USA
e-mail: megumi.okumura@ucsf.edu

E. Lawson, M.D.
Department of Pediatrics, Division of Rheumatology, University of California, San Francisco, CA, USA
e-mail: erica.lawson@ucsf.edu

Transfer Preparation

Transfer Timing

Transfer timing is a critical determinant of transition success. Timing may be determined by the practice's transition policy, insurance coverage restrictions, or patient needs (e.g., moving out of the area). Regardless of these circumstances, the alignment of three primary factors is necessary to facilitate a smooth transfer:

1. Control of active medical conditions
2. Patient and family readiness for the adult model of care
3. Access to adult care

Control of active medical conditions. Whenever possible, transfer should occur when (1) chronic medical conditions are under good control, (2) the treatment regimen is stable, and (3) there are no new or urgent healthcare needs. Transfer while disease is active increases the complexity of provider-to-provider handoffs,

A. C. Hergenroeder, C. M. Wiemann (eds.), *Health Care Transition*,
https://doi.org/10.1007/978-3-319-72868-1_16

consequently increasing risk of miscommunication and suboptimal medical management. If transfer is occurring between different healthcare systems (e.g., from an academic center to a community-based practice) and the patient's condition and management plan are in flux, it may be particularly difficult for accepting providers to access the most up-to-date information. Similarly, major medication changes immediately prior to transfer may create confusion for the patient or between providers. Finally, for patients with complex chronic conditions, transfer to an adult provider in the setting of new or urgent healthcare needs necessitating immediate changes to the care plan may make it difficult to carefully integrate past history (e.g., previous medication failure or intolerance) into the current management plan.

Patient and family readiness for the adult model of care. As discussed in Chap. 15, significant differences in resource allocation and style of care delivery exist between pediatric and adult healthcare providers. Even for patients who are cared for by a provider that sees patients across the age spectrum (i.e., with training in family medicine or combined pediatrics and internal medicine), a transition from child-centered to adult-oriented medical care still occurs. In child-centered care, the parent plays a significant role in history-taking and medical decision-making. The child should play an increasingly prominent role in the visit as they age; however, ultimate decision-making responsibility rests with the parents. While the patient becomes the legal decision-maker at age 18, parents often continue to play a prominent role. Parents may wish to be present during the medical visit and, more importantly, may continue to perform critical tasks to manage the patient's health at home. In contrast, in adult-oriented care, the patient is expected to communicate primarily with the physician, although parents may still play an important ancillary role. The patient will be expected to follow through on healthcare tasks as directed by their adult provider, such as lab and radiology testing. Furthermore, ancillary support to coordinate care, such as social workers, is typically less available in adult care systems as compared to pediatrics. Therefore, to achieve a smooth transfer to adult care, the patient must be ready to serve as primary manager of his or her healthcare, as well as the primary point person for communication with the healthcare team. If the patient will not be able to meet these goals due to developmental disability or other cognitive or behavioral challenges, conservatorship, or other legal proxy, must be put in place to allow a parent or other caregiver to continue as primary manager of the patient's care (see Chap. 30).

Providers are encouraged to measure patient readiness for an adult model of care at regular intervals, using a validated self-care or transition readiness assessment (see Chap. 13). While these assessments can provide a useful jumping-off point for self-management discussions and goal setting, multiple studies have been unable to correlate higher transition readiness scores with successful transfer to adult care [8]. This may reflect the complexity of the transition process: while self-care skills are clearly important in the adult model of care, additional factors independent of self-management, such as healthcare provider availability and social supports, may also be critical determinants of transfer success [9, 10].

Access to adult care. Graduating pediatric patients need access to adult providers in order to transfer successfully. Provider availability, provider expertise, and health insurance limitations may all pose barriers to establishing care with adult providers [11, 12]. In some geographic regions, particularly rural areas, the number of adult primary care providers and specialists is often not adequate to meet patient demand [13]. Older adolescents and young adults seeking to transfer care to adult providers may find that local practices are not accepting new patients, or that adult specialists with the necessary expertise to manage rare or complex childhood-onset conditions are not readily available. Finally, even when adult primary care providers and specialists with the necessary expertise are available and accepting new patients, insurance plans may pose barriers to access. For patients with health maintenance organization plans (HMOs), adult providers with the necessary expertise in a patient's condition may be out-of-network. Furthermore, due to poor reimbursement rates, community-based providers often limit the number of patients insured by Medicaid or other public plans in their practice, making it difficult for patients with public insurance plans to establish care [14].

When patients are unable to identify accepting adult providers, there are a few possible options to find appropriate care. (See Table 16.1 for a list of common barriers to transfer and troubleshooting approaches.) If adult specialists are not available or accessible, the patient may transfer to an adult primary care provider while continuing to obtain consultative services from one or more pediatric specialists. Alternately, in rural or remote areas, adult primary care providers may be able to use telemedicine services to obtain subspecialist consultation remotely. When HMO restrictions limit access to specialists, the patient and primary care physician may be able to successfully petition the HMO to access necessary out-of-network care.

While transfer should ideally occur when the above criteria are met (stable medical conditions, readiness for adult model of care, and access to adult providers), healthcare systems may impose restrictions on the timing of transfer. For example, in California, the county-based Title V program, California Children's Services (CCS), reimburses at higher rates than traditional Medicaid and allows patients to be seen at regionalized medical centers. This expanded coverage terminates on patients' 21st birthday. It may be difficult for patients to be seen by adult providers if they are ready to transfer prior to age 21 (as only pediatric providers typically contract with Title V); however after age 21, Medicaid may not cover pediatric care if the patient's existing providers are out-of-network. Therefore, depending on state, young adults may face an abrupt, age-based change in healthcare coverage and provider access, which occurs regardless of readiness for transfer [15, 16].

Table 16.1 Troubleshooting common barriers encountered during transfer to adult care

Barriers	Troubleshooting approaches
Unable to identify local adult provider	• Search subspecialty professional organization's provider directory
	• Contact insurance company or Medicaid office to identify local providers or clinics
	• For inability to find specialty providers, start with local primary care providers for assistance in identifying subspecialty providers
Unable to get appointment with local adult provider	• Schedule first adult visit before terminating care with pediatric practice, as it may take several months to get an initial appointment especially if the practice is oversubscribed and has a waitlist
Adult provider uncomfortable caring for patient with childhood-onset condition	• Pediatric provider may offer to provide ongoing consultation during the post-transfer period
	• Telehealth may be used to conduct reimbursable joint patient visits
	• Provide an expanded transfer summary to address management issues specific to disease such as routine screening/guidelines for condition or providing resources for provider
Unable to find an adult provider who accepts patient's insurance	• Contact insurance company or Medicaid office to identify local providers or clinics
	• For specialty services, work with local primary care to assist in finding specialty services. For those patients in remote areas, consider finding adult providers who provide telehealth to outlying areas and receive insurance waiver for treatment
Patient leaving pediatric practice prior to identifying an adult provider	• Provide patient with an up-to-date medical summary to share with new providers, which should include contact information of current pediatric providers to help facilitate knowledge exchange

Transfer Planning and Logistics

In the immediate pre-transfer period, the following steps should be taken by providers and practices to support a successful transfer to adult care:

1. Systematically identify patients who are approaching the age of transfer.
2. Determine the amount of support each patient is likely to need to transfer successfully.
3. Orient patients and families to the adult approach to care.
4. Help patients identify adult providers.
5. Provide insurance resources, self-management information, and culturally appropriate community supports as needed.
6. Create transfer documentation, including medical summary and plan of care, and ensure that this information is received by adult providers.

Identify patients approaching the age of transfer. In order to ensure that all patients are prepared for a timely transfer, it is helpful to systematically identify patients within the practice who are approaching transfer age. The age at which patients are identified should be guided by the practice's transition policy (see Chap. 11). Standard electronic medical system queries can be developed and run on a scheduled basis, e.g., quarterly, to identify all patients who are within 18 months of transfer. See Chap. 12 for a discussion of transition registries to identify and track pediatric patients preparing to transfer to adult care.

Determine the amount of support each patient will need to transfer successfully. The need for transition support varies greatly among patients and families. While some patients will, without prompting, identify adult providers and ensure continuous insurance coverage, others will require significant support to prevent loss to follow-up after leaving pediatric care. Patients with a history of loss to follow-up and poor adherence to the plan of care are at particular risk for failed transfer to adult providers [17, 18]. There are multiple tools in use to identify patients with the greatest need for support during transfer. One example is the "PREPARE" acronym [19] (Fig. 16.1), developed by Rebecca E. Sadun, M.D., Ph.D. and Richard J. Chung, M.D. (used with permission from authors), which provides a useful structure to help determine which patients will need extra support during transfer.

Orient patients and families to the adult approach to care. Patients should be prepared for their first visit with the new provider by orienting them to the expectations of patients in an adult practice. Specifically:

- The patient is the primary person that the adult provider will try to interact with unless the patient gives permission or asks the adult provider to include other individuals in the conversation.
- Some practices will require a form to indicate that they can share information with the parent. It may be helpful to clarify the practice's requirements on sharing information with other family members while scheduling the first appointment.
- The adult provider serves as a guide for the patient. As outlined in Chap. 15, adult care operates under a shared management model, which may differ from the more paternalistic

- **P**rescription medications (≥2)?
- **R**eferrals and subspecialists (≥2)?
- **E**xacerbations or hospitalizations (w/in the past 2 years)?
- **P**sychiatric, behavioral, or cognitive difficulties?
- **A**dded challenges (autonomous skills like glucose finger sticks or self-injections, allergies, ADL impairments, activity restrictions, etc)?
- **R**oadblocks to care (e.g., socioeconomic, linguistic, cultural, or family structure challenges)?
- **E**ngagement difficulties (e.g., prior no shows, lost to follow - up)?

Fig. 16.1 Adolescent criteria for a successful transfer

model of pediatric practice. The clinician provides guidance and will value autonomy of the patient, even if the patient decides against the clinician's preferred management approach.

- Depending on the practice, the adult provider may not be completely familiar the patient's condition, especially if the condition is rare. The adult provider will likely work with their network of colleagues to ensure that the patient receives appropriate care. While the adult provider will experience a learning curve, if they are willing to work with the patient, they will gain the expertise that is needed to ensure a long-lasting relationship and optimize health outcomes for the patient. The patient should understand that the adult provider does have a wealth of knowledge in adult-onset conditions and adult healthcare needs.
- Preparing a prioritized list of questions for the first visit may help the patient to get accustomed to their more proactive role in the adult practice.

Help patients identify adult providers. As discussed above, several factors influence access to adult providers. While restrictions due to geography and insurance may be in play, patients will appreciate referrals from their pediatric providers to trusted adult providers. Practices should consider compiling a list of local adult providers who are comfortable caring for young adults with childhood-onset chronic conditions and have successfully received former pediatric patients, which can be provided to patients prior to transfer. Patients should also be encouraged to contact their insurance plan to obtain a list of in-network providers. Furthermore, if multiple subspecialists care for the patient, the order of transfer should be considered. It may be practical to first transfer the patient to adult-oriented primary care; the adult primary care provider can then facilitate referral to the appropriate adult specialists in the patient's local insurance network.

Provide insurance resources, self-management information, and culturally appropriate community supports as needed. Particularly for patients who will be aging out of a Title V program or child insurance program, active efforts to ensure insurance continuity are essential (see Chap. 8). These patients and their families should be encouraged to contact their Title V or Medicaid caseworker at least 1 year before coverage expires in order to create a plan to maintain continuous coverage. Patients may also benefit from self-management support as they prepare for adult-oriented care. See Chap. 14 for tools that can be used in the clinic setting to guide discussions about self-management among providers, patients, and caregivers. Self-management resources exist across the spectrum of chronic conditions; foundations and patient advocacy organizations, such as the American Diabetes Association, the Arthritis Foundation, or the National Kidney Foundation, may be excellent sources. For other patients, culturally appropriate community supports may be particularly helpful in developing self-management skills. Local patient advocacy organizations, or local chapters of national organizations, are often able to provide culturally appropriate mentoring and support for patients and families at the time of transfer and beyond.

Create transfer documentation, including medical summary and plan of care, and ensure that this information is received by adult providers. One of the most critical components of a successful transfer is ensuring that the adult provider has access to accurate and concise medical documentation prior to a patient arriving in their practice. This document may consist of a medical summary and emergency care plan, plan of care with transition goals and pending actions, final transition readiness assessment, and, if needed, legal documents, condition fact sheet, and additional provider records. The medical summary and plan of care should allow the adult provider to pick up where the pediatrician left off. Many organizations have provided medical summaries and transfer summaries, which are readily available online and can be adapted for an individual provider or clinic. Most transfer summaries share basic core elements (see Table 16.2 and Fig. 16.2 for contents of a transfer summary) [20, 21]. Often, pediatricians assume it is sufficient to simply identify an adult provider and then consider the transition and transfer work completed. Unfortunately, many patients and parents subsequently complain that the adult provider is unaware of their medical condition or is not prepared for the initial encounter to establish care. This may be due to the fact that the adult provider received little or no information about the patient prior to their first visit, or alternately, that records were not provided in a concise format. It is impossible for an adult provider, in their limited initial visit, to adequately review up to two decades of medical records. Therefore, for a successful transfer to occur, it is critical that the pediatric provider provides a concise transfer summary, including medical history and plan of

Table 16.2 Core elements of a transfer or medical summary

• Past medical history
• Past surgical history
• Current medication list
• Allergies and adverse reactions to medication
• Social summary
• Current pediatric and potential future adult providers and transfer plan
• "Plan" for each condition

Patient Legal Name: **Preferred Name:**
Date of Birth: **Preferred Language:**
Active Problem List: **Preferred Communication Style** (In case patient is non-verbal, or blind or communication is facilitated by family)

Current Medications:
Summary:
Problem-Based Immediate Care Plan: *(a medical plan to help the new provider help prioritize needs and immediate next steps at the first visit)*

Current Provider and Adult Provider Transfer Plan Primary transfer contact: *(designate person who is coordinating the transfer contacts)*			
Specialty	**Pediatric Provider**	**Adult provider**	**Transfer Plan**

Past Medical History:
Past Surgical History:
Adverse reactions to any medications or treatments:
Most Recent Vital Signs:
Immunizations:
Allergies:
Family History:
Social History:
Sexual History:
Cultural considerations:
Developmental History
Social: Cognitive:
Fine Motor: Language:
Gross Motor:
Speech - Assisted communication:
Durable Medical Equipment Needs:
Resources/Services Utilized:
Hospitalizations in past year:
Insurance lapses or financial hardships anticipated by patient within 3 years:
Patient's ability to manage diagnoses and care plan:
□ Fully Independent □ Some Support needed
□ Needs significant support □ Cannot manage without help

Contact Information:
Address: Email:
Mobile phone: Home phone:
Best way to reach: Best time to reach:
Insurance/Plan: Group and ID #:

Emergency Care:
Primary Emergency Contact: Relation
Mobile phone: Primary caregiver/guardianship:
Conservatorship or Advance Care Directive:

Fig. 16.2 Content of sample transfer summary

care. Fortunately, many organizations have developed transfer and medical summaries to help pediatricians generate the key data elements needed by adult providers [1]. Ideally this summary is mailed, e-mailed, or faxed to the new adult provider with confirmation that the information is received. If possible, a verbal communication with the new provider is helpful to prepare for the visit, especially if there are ongoing critical healthcare needs or complex social situations. In addition, the patient should be provided with a copy of their transfer summary.

The Transfer

The initial appointment with the adult provider. Once the new adult provider has been identified, the patient should schedule the appointment and notify the pediatric practice that an appointment had been made. The transfer process should be planned such that the pediatric provider has time to generate the appropriate transfer documentation prior to this first appointment. Patients should be prepared with a copy of the transfer documentation provided by the pediatric practice. Without transfer planning, these young adults will often "fall off" the pediatric provider panel because they are no longer eligible to see the provider due to insurance or age restrictions of the practice.

The adult provider and patient and the patient's caregivers should expect their first appointment to be an introduction to the practice and an opportunity to address immediate needs. Follow-up appointments can be generated either solely with the adult provider or with appointments alternating between adult and pediatric providers until the patient is comfortable with their care in the adult practice.

Considerations Post-transfer

During the transfer process, there is a period of time when the patient is waiting for their new adult appointment or perhaps has not quite established all their care because of missing medical records or incomplete information. It is important to have a clear plan of action for the patient; until the adult provider has all the necessary information to assume full care of the patient, the pediatric provider is obligated to serve as a bridge for acute care needs. The purpose of bridging is not to extend care beyond the time of transfer decided by the provider and patient; rather, this process ensures that continuity of care is maintained and any acute needs are addressed.

To minimize attrition, the pediatric provider should follow up with the patient 6 months after the last pediatric visit to confirm that the patient either has an adult provider visit scheduled or has already been seen by the adult provider [17]. Patients often do not follow through on scheduling an appointment with the adult provider, fail to appear at their first appointment, or cancel their first scheduled visit. It is not routine for an adult provider to seek out a new patient who does not show up or cancels their visit. The responsibility therefore belongs to the pediatric provider to assure that the transfer visit has been completed. This process can be performed by the pediatrician's administrative staff and integrated into routine practice. Another method to ensure transfer is to schedule a final visit with the pediatrician after the patient has met with the adult provider. For patients with complex healthcare needs, this may allow for clarification of treatment plan in case any questions arise from the first visit with the adult provider. Further discussion on developing a system for ensuring transfer completion can be found in Chap. 18.

Summary

Prior to initiation of transfer, the patient and family should be prepared for the move to adult-oriented care through transition processes. Transfer planning must begin early enough to identify appropriate adult providers and mitigate potential barriers to transfer. Transfer should occur while the patient still has the ability to obtain care from the pediatric provider to prevent any lapses in care and maintain access to critical medications or services. Ensuring that the patient has successfully transferred to an adult provider, either by follow-up phone call to the patient or a follow-up visit after the patient has met the adult provider, will help prevent loss to follow-up following exit from pediatric care.

References

1. National Center for Health Care Transition. Six Core Elements of Health Care Transition. http://www.got-transition.org. Accessed 2 July 2017.
2. A consensus statement on health care transitions for young adults with special health care needs. Pediatrics. 2002;110(6 Pt 2):1304–6.
3. Sable C, Foster E, Uzark K, Bjornsen K, Canobbio MM, Connolly HM, et al. Best practices in managing transition to adulthood for adolescents with congenital heart disease: the transition process and medical and psychosocial issues: a scientific statement from the American Heart Association. Circulation. 2011;123(13):1454–85.
4. American Academy of Pediatrics, American Academy of Family Physicians, American College of Physicians, Transitions Clinical Report Authoring Group, Cooley WC, Sagerman PJ. Supporting the health care transition from adolescence to adulthood in the medical home. Pediatrics. 2011;128(1):182–200.
5. Bloom SR, Kuhlthau K, Van Cleave J, Knapp AA, Newacheck P, Perrin JM. Health care transition for youth with special health care needs. J Adolesc Health. 2012;51(3):213–9.
6. Mahan JD, Betz CL, Okumura MJ, Ferris ME. Self-management and transition to adult health care in adolescents and young adults: a team process. Pediatr Rev. 2017;38(7):305–19.
7. McPheeters M, Davis AM, Taylor JL, Brown RF, Potter SA, Epstein RA. Transition care for children with special health needs. Technical Brief No. 15 (Prepared by the Vanderbilt University Evidence-based Practice Center under Contract No. 290-2012-00009-I). AHRQ Publication No. 14-EHC027-EF. Rockville, MD: Agency for Healthcare Research and Quality; 2014.
8. Schwartz LA, Daniel LC, Brumley LD, Barakat LP, Wesley KM, Tuchman LK. Measures of readiness to transition to adult health care for youth with chronic physical health conditions: a systematic review and recommendations for measurement testing and development. J Pediatr Psychol. 2014;39(6):588–601.
9. Javalkar K, Johnson M, Kshirsagar AV, Ocegueda S, Detwiler RK, Ferris M. Ecological factors predict transition readiness/self-management in youth with chronic conditions. J Adolesc Health. 2016;58(1):40–6.
10. Betz CL, Ferris ME, Woodward JF, Okumura MJ, Jan S, Wood DL. The health care transition research consortium health care transition model: a framework for research and practice. J Pediatr Rehabil Med. 2014;7(1):3–15.
11. Okumura MJ, Heisler M, Davis MM, Cabana MD, Demonner S, Kerr EA. Comfort of general internists and general pediatricians in providing care for young adults with chronic illnesses of childhood. J Gen Intern Med. 2008;23(10):1621–7.
12. Okumura MJ, Kerr EA, Cabana MD, Davis MM, Demonner S, Heisler M. Physician views on barriers to primary care for young adults with childhood-onset chronic disease. Pediatrics. 2010;125(4):e748–54.
13. IHS Markit. The complexities of physician supply and demand 2017 update: projections from 2015 to 2030. Association of American Medical Colleges. https://aamc-black.global.ssl.fastly.net/production/media/filer_public/a5/c3/a5c3d565-14ec-48fb-974b-99fafaeecb00/aamc_projections_update_2017.pdf
14. Allen EM, Call KT, Beebe TJ, McAlpine DD, Johnson PJ. Barriers to care and health care utilization among the publicly insured. Med Care. 2017;55(3):207–14.
15. Gulley SP, Rasch EK, Chan L. Ongoing coverage for ongoing care: access, utilization, and out-of-pocket spending among uninsured working-aged adults with chronic health care needs. Am J Public Health. 2011;101(2):368–75.
16. Dahlen HM. "Aging out" of dependent coverage and the effects on us labor market and health insurance choices. Am J Public Health. 2015;105:S640–50.
17. Goossens E, Bovijn L, Gewillig M, Budts W, Moons P. Predictors of care gaps in adolescents with complex chronic condition transitioning to adulthood. Pediatrics. 2016;137(4):1–10. http://pediatrics.aappublications.org/content/pediatrics/137/4/e20152413.full.pdf
18. Mistry B, Van Blyderveen S, Punthakee Z, Grant C. Condition-related predictors of successful transition from paediatric to adult care among adolescents with Type 1 diabetes. Diabet Med. 2015;32(7):881–5.
19. Sadun RE, Chung RJ. Creating a clinical culture that supports the needs of transitioning adolescents. National MedPeds Residency Assoc. Western Regional Meeting: The Underserved, April, 2014; Los Angeles, CA.
20. Got Transition Transfer of Care. 2017. http://www.gottransition.org/providers/leaving-5.cfm. Accessed 13 July 2017.
21. American College of Physicians Pediatric to Adult Care Transitions Initiative: Condition Specific Tools. 2017. https://www.acponline.org/clinical-information/high-value-care/resources-for-clinicians/pediatric-to-adult-care-transitions-initiative/condition-specific-tools. Accessed 13 July 2017.

Preparing the Adult Practice to Accept Adolescents and Young Adults

17

Marybeth R. Jones, Marilyn Augustine, and Brett W. Robbins

Introduction

High-quality health care requires productive interactions between a practice team and patients. Patients need the information, skills, and confidence to make best use of their involvement with their practice team. Practice teams must have the expertise, relevant patient information, time, and resources to ensure effective clinical and behavioral management [1]. When accepting an adolescent and young adult with special healthcare needs (AYASHCN) into a practice, it is essential to prepare the practice team to meet the unique needs of this population. Senior leadership support, transition improvement team champions, and sufficient dedicated time are key resources to implement meaningful practice change [2]. The process of establishing the administrative struc-

ture and support for a healthcare transition program and mobilizing pediatric providers are reviewed in Chaps. 9 and 10. Developing a healthcare policy is covered in Chap. 11. Here we will review the specific steps required to establish a self-sustaining transition structure and process within an adult (receiving) practice.

Preparing the Office Environment

We will use Alexi's case to consider adolescent and young adult (AYA) patients with a single chronic illness who are planning for a first visit to the adult practice. Offering an AYA-friendly ambiance is important to patient satisfaction and to helping the young adult feel welcomed. This might include providing AYA-specific resources in the waiting room or on the office website or access to an office Wi-Fi password during waiting times. AYA may appreciate the opportunity to voice their opinions on how to improve their office experience [3].

M. R. Jones, M.D., M.S.Ed. (✉)
Division of General Pediatrics, University of Rochester Medical Center, Rochester, NY, USA
e-mail: Marybeth_Jones@URMC.Rochester.edu

M. Augustine, M.D.
Division of Endocrinology and Metabolism, University of Rochester Medical Center, Rochester, NY, USA
e-mail: marilyn_augustine@URMC.Rochester.edu

B. W. Robbins, M.D.
Division of Adolescent Medicine, University of Rochester Medical Center, Rochester, NY, USA
e-mail: Brett_Robbins@URMC.Rochester.edu

> **Case**
> *Alexi is coming to see you for her first appointment with an adult primary care provider, after being transferred from her*

© Springer International Publishing AG, part of Springer Nature 2018
A. C. Hergenroeder, C. M. Wiemann (eds.), *Health Care Transition*,
https://doi.org/10.1007/978-3-319-72868-1_17

pediatrician's office where she received her care since birth. She is a 21-year-old female and is living with her family. During the rooming process, her mother stays in the waiting room. Alexi shares that she liked having the Wi-Fi password available, allowing for internet access in the waiting room.

Creating a Process

Before implementing any changes, it is helpful for the adult practice that will be accepting AYA patients to develop materials and guidelines to standardize the transfer of care and to help prepare patients, family members, and clinicians who will be involved in the process. Previous chapters have reviewed the development of the essential components of a transition program (Chaps. 11–14). In brief, input from local youth, family, and pediatric and adult clinician perspectives should guide the revision and adaptation of existing tools into practice. At a minimum, these transition materials should be reviewed during a "get acquainted" visit with an AYA patient. Although data supporting the effectiveness of specific components of a transition program are lacking [4], the six core elements of transition (www.gottransition.org) have been recommended by adult and pediatric national societies [5, 6].

The six core elements' transition policy, practice welcome letter, and FAQ materials describe a practice's approach to accepting and partnering with new AYA-age patients and their families, including privacy and consent information. Materials can highlight information specific to a practice, such as the availability of medical information and access to appointments, special services offered by the practice, or refill requests through online- or app-based resources. Practice staff and clinicians may explicitly review expectations for making and keeping appointments, using answering service or afterhours care, and obtaining refills (see Chap. 11). A key component to success in implementing components of a transition program will be to raise awareness and understanding of transition materials, to assign clear roles and responsibilities to ensure their use, and to identify care team members who can monitor and track success of transition improvement initiatives in your practice [7].

An office staff member reviews the office's transition policy, the welcome letter, and FAQ with Alexi. She is completing a self-care assessment as you enter the room. You ask if Alexi has any questions about the orientation materials. She tells you that she saw the transition policy posted in the waiting room and she understood the staff member's explanation of the materials. She knows that she received these same papers in the mail prior to the visit, and she thinks her mom read them. She and her mother decided together that Alexi would spend most of her visit alone today. Alexi wants to be sure that what she tells you is confidential and tells you that her mother expects to be a part of this visit at some point. You reassure confidentiality and let her know that she can provide consent to have (or not have) any friend or relative as part of any visit.

It is important that all medical staff and clinicians consider unique AYA needs. The prefrontal cortex, the area of the brain responsible for executive functions including planning, decision-making, and moderating complex cognitive behavior, is not fully developed until an average age of 26 (see Chaps. 2 and 3). For this reason, AYA patients will be different from older patients in an adult practice [8]. AYA patients have developed healthy and/or unhealthy lifestyles, and reinforcing preventative care and healthy decision-making is appropriate. While AYA understand health risks, they often overestimate the rewards of unhealthy behaviors. Many will still look to their parents for help with decision-making, even though they do not prefer to do so.

A practice might start by identifying staff and clinicians who have a specific interest in or more experience with caring for AYA. These may include younger, new graduates from training looking to build a practice or clinicians with teenage children at home. Clinicians should have strengths including an interest in developing relationships, patience with overcoming barriers to medical adherence, and dedication to providing an inclusive care environment. Additionally, these clinicians need to be dedicated to providing good continuity of care, including spending time upfront to review previous records and condition fact sheets from pediatric primary care or subspecialty providers.

Implementing Components of the Transition Program

AYA start to disengage from regular preventive health care around age 15. Up to 15% of AYA (ages 19–25) report no identified primary care provider, and up to 40% have not seen a primary care provider in the previous year [9]. As a result, AYAs are the second highest utilizers of emergency room services in the nation, second only to those over age 75 [10, 11]. To keep AYA engaged in preventive and primary care, population health management techniques should be developed to identify and track them. AYA patients should be tracked through their first several appointments, or age 26, to ensure engagement in the adult healthcare system. Aligning this tracking effort with other population health initiatives in a practice (improvements in vaccine administration, cancer screening, or adolescent counseling rates) is likely to increase the success and sustainability of transition improvement initiatives. A champion for this initiative needs to be identified (see Chap. 10) and should set focused goals in order to achieve identified process and clinical outcome measures. A transition improvement team with pediatric, adult, patient, family, nursing, and care management members should plan to lead rapid cycles of practice improvement to measure and improve the success of integrating planned practice initiatives, such as the six core elements, into clinical workflows. In addition to monitoring process measures, which may be assisted with the use of transition planning tools (see Chap. 14), the transition team needs to consider clinical outcomes to provide evidence for meaningful practice improvements. The definition of successful transition from pediatric- to adult-based care has not been established. The "Triple Aim" provides a framework for key outcomes, with goals of improving patient experience, healthcare resource utilization, and clinical outcome measures [12]. Additional key outcomes aim to optimize young adult quality of life and functional status [13, 14].

You have reviewed Alexi's previous records in advance of her appointment. She has a history of mild persistent asthma and has been prescribed inhaled corticosteroids by her pediatrician. She struggled with her school performance during mid-adolescence and was diagnosed with anxiety and depression. These were successfully treated with psychotherapy and medications that were tapered off at the age of 19.

Ideally, prior to the first visit, office staff should ensure receipt of transfer package from a pediatrician, which may include components such as an AYA patient's final transition readiness assessment, plan of care with transition goals and pending actions, medical summary and emergency care plan, and, if needed, legal documents, condition fact sheet (a brief summary of congenital disorders that may be rare among adult patients), and subspecialty provider records. The use of population health management strategies can assist staff members in tracking and collecting this information and providing it to the accepting clinician in advance of the first "get acquainted" visit.

Alexi shares with you that she uses her prescribed inhaled corticosteroid correctly on an average of 6 days each week immediately after an exacerbation. She admits that this consistent use wanes as time goes by when she is feeling well. She has an average of two exacerbations annually, usually around the time of year her seasonal allergies flare and when she has not been using her inhaled corticosteroid routinely. Her triggers are upper respiratory infections, seasonal allergies, and tobacco smoke. In reviewing her self-care assessment, you note that she understands and is fervent about spacer use but has a vague understanding of the role of her inhaled corticosteroid. She prefers e-mail or text messaging for communication and reminders as she rarely answers her phone.

Similar to the transition readiness assessment completed during pediatric years (Chap. 13), a self-care assessment helps a clinician to gather information on a patient's perception of their own health literacy. It can help to provide insight into an AYA's knowledge, beliefs, and motivations to self-manage their health care. It can help guide conversation about chronic care management skills during an encounter and ensure that a patient's questions and needs are met.

Preparing the Patient

After a discussion about the role of inhaled corticosteroids, you realize you will likely have to repeat and reinforce this at future visits, likely just as her pediatrician did. You give her the instructions on accessing her chart through the internet so she can get text message or e-mail reminders, renew medications, ask advice, and make appointments through her chosen route of communication. You also ask questions about her background and social history. She has never smoked cigarettes. She denies substance abuse. You discuss her sexual health and options for contraception. She reports having a good support system and screens negative for mental health concerns today.

It is important to provide the patient with age-appropriate self-management tools. Often teens will prefer web-based tools [3]. Comprehensive AYA care also includes an assessment of risky behaviors and mental health comorbidities, as they are the most common causes of morbidity and mortality in this population.

Establishing the Comprehensive Care Team

After discussing and agreeing on a 3-month follow-up visit, you invite her mother in for further questions. The mother asks what happened at the visit, and you reply that Alexi has a good handle on her health and health issues and that you welcome her to the practice and plan on following her closely for the first year as you both get accustomed to the new relationship and logistics of her care. Her mom is wondering if she'll need to see any subspecialty doctors soon.

The availability of adult clinicians who are trained in and comfortable managing specific childhood-onset chronic conditions will dictate the need for additional subspecialty referrals [15–17]. Often, adult primary care will be the first receiving practice of an AYA patient and can help coordinate additional referrals as needed [6]. Typically, AYA with simple or no chronic illnesses will be transferred directly from the pediatric to the adult primary care clinician. In addition to the pediatrician, adult clinicians should be prepared to discuss a patient's specific needs with any pediatric subspecialty team members in order to determine the optimal adult care team. AYA with more complex chronic illnesses will often need transfers involving both direct primary care pediatric to primary care adult provider communication and pediatric subspecialty to adult subspecialty communication. See Table 17.1 for lessons learned during the process of accepting AYA into an adult practice and Fig. 17.1 for possible relationships between the pediatric and adult primary care and subspecialty providers. The next chapter will address the com-

Table 17.1 Lessons learned for successfully accepting AYA into a practice

• The adult practice needs to collaborate with the pediatric practice and the patients
• The adult practice needs to share the design of a systematic process of accepting an AYA into a practice (i.e., six core elements) with the patients, their families, and their pediatric providers
• Understand that the 18–26-year-old age group is unique in their cognitive development and many continue their reliance on parents for assistance
• Be explicit, concrete, and consistent in your expectations, directions, and teaching
• Be prepared to receive transfers from both pediatric primary care and specialty providers

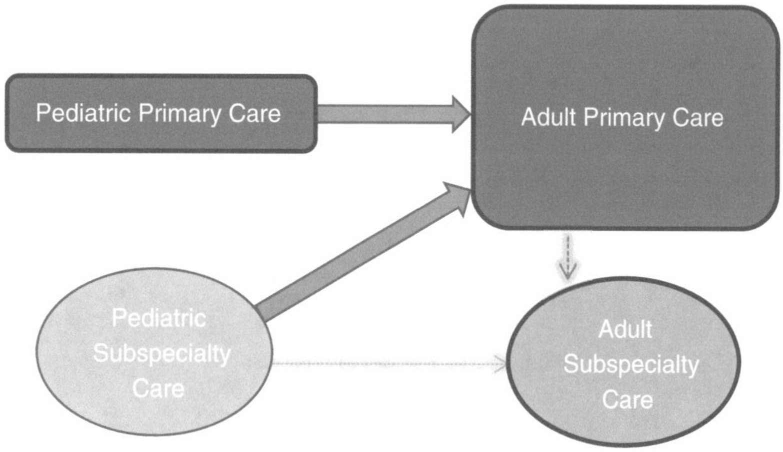

Fig. 17.1 Possible transition relationships among pediatric and adult primary care and subspecialty providers

plexities of establishing a comprehensive care team and ensuring transfer completion in more detail.

References

1. Wagner EH, Austin BT, Davis C, Hindmarsh M, Schaefer J, Bonomi A. Improving chronic illness care: translating evidence into action. Health Aff. 2001;20(6):64–78.
2. White P, Cooley WC, McAllister J. Starting a transition improvement process using the six core elements of health care transition. Got Transition Practice Resource. 2015. http://www.gottransition.org/resourceGet.cfm?id=369. Accessed 18 May 2017.
3. Dovey-Pearce G, Hurrell R, May C, Walker C, Doherty Y. Young adults' (16–25 years) suggestions for providing developmentally appropriate diabetes services: a qualitative study. Health Soc Care Community. 2005;13(5):409–19.
4. Chu P, Maslow G, vonIsenburg M, Chung R. Systematic review of the impact of transition interventions for adolescents with chronic illness on transfer from pediatric to adult healthcare. J Pediatr Nurs. 2015;30:e19–27.
5. Transitions Clinical Report Authoring Group. Supporting the health care transition from adolescence to adulthood in the medical home. Pediatrics. 2011;128(1):182–200.
6. Greenlee MC, D'Angelo L, Harms SR, Kuo AA, Landry M, McManus M, Talente GM, White P, American College of Physicians Council of Subspecialty Societies Pediatric to Adult Care Transitions Initiative Steering Committee. Enhancing the role of internists in the transition from pediatric to adult health care. Ann Intern Med. 2017;166(4):299–300.
7. McManus M, White P, Barbour A, et al. Pediatric to adult transition: a quality improvement model for primary care. J Adolesc Health. 2015;56:73–8.
8. Beresford B, Stuttard L. Young adults as users of adult healthcare: experiences of young adults with complex or life-limiting conditions. Clin Med (Lond). 2014;14(4):404–8.
9. Summary Health Statistics: National Health Interview Survey. 2014. Table 16a. https://ftp.cdc.gov/pub/Health_Statistics/NCHS/NHIS/SHS/2014_SHS_Table_A-16.pdf. Accessed 14 July 2017.
10. Fortuna RJ, Robbins BW, Halterman JS. Ambulatory care among young adults in the United States. Ann Intern Med. 2009;151(6):379–85.
11. Fortuna RJ, Robbins BW, Mani N, Halterman JS. Dependence on emergency care among young adults in the United States. J Gen Intern Med. 2010;25(7):663–9.
12. Prior M, McManus M, White P, Davidson L. Measuring the "triple aim" in transition care: a systematic review. Pediatrics. 2014;134(6):e1648–61.
13. Fair C, Cuttance J, Sharma N, Maslow G, Wiener L, Betz C, Porter J, McLaughlin S, Gilleland-Marchak J, Renwick A, Naranjo D, Jan S, Javalkar K, Ferris M, International and Interdisciplinary Health Care Transition Research Consortium. International and interdisciplinary identification of health care transition outcomes. JAMA Pediatr. 2016;170(3):205–11.
14. Suris JC, Akre C. Key elements for, and indicators of, a successful transition: an international Delphi study. J Adolesc Health. 2015;56(6):612–8.
15. Okumura MJ, Heisler M, Davis MM, Cabana MD, Demonner S, Kerr EA. Comfort of general internists and general pediatricians in providing care for young adults with chronic illnesses of childhood. J Gen Intern Med. 2008;23(10):1621–7.
16. Tuchman LK, Slap GB, Britto MT. Transition to adult care: experiences and expectations of adolescents with a chronic illness. Child Care Health Dev. 2008;34(5):557–63.
17. McLaughlin SE, Machan J, Fournier P, Chang T, Even K, Sadof M. Transition of adolescents with chronic health conditions to adult primary care: factors associated with physician acceptance. J Pediatr Rehabil Med. 2014;7(1):63–70.

18 Establishing a System for Ensuring Transfer Completion

Niraj Sharma, Kitty O'Hare, and Ahmet Uluer

Preparing the transfer of a young adult with a chronic condition from pediatric to adult-centered medical care requires a well-thought-through process to ensure success. This chapter begins with two contrasting patient experiences.

Case Vignette 1

Maria is a 20-year-old female with a history of type 1 diabetes mellitus who presents to the emergency room feeling ill. As part of the initial work-up, it is found that her blood sugars are very high and she is noted to have acidosis. She confides that she has not seen a physician or a specialist for her diabetes since she was 18 years old, when she lost her health insurance. At that time, she was told by her pediatrician that it was time for her to find an adult doctor. She reports that she has lost a lot of weight and has not had her menses in 2 years. She works part-time but has a difficult time maintaining her job because she rarely feels well. She found it challenging to regularly obtain insulin or other supplies due to her lack of insurance and access to a physician.

This vignette highlights several systems issues that could have allowed Maria to stay healthy and productive. The pediatrician has the responsibility to prepare her for the transition to adult care. Maria should have been educated about her disease and the responsibilities associated with managing it, such as scheduling appointments, learning about health insurance and its relationship to transition, and filling prescriptions.

Equally important is identifying and partnering with an adult provider as part of routine practice. This facilitates provider-to-provider communication

N. Sharma, M.D., M.P.H. (✉) • K. O'Hare, M.D.
Division of General Medicine, Department of Medicine, Brigham and Women's Hospital, Harvard Medical School, Boston, MA, USA

Division of General Pediatrics, Department of Medicine, Boston Children's Hospital, Harvard Medical School, Boston, MA, USA
e-mail: nsharma@bwh.harvard.edu; fohare@bwh.harvard.edu

A. Uluer, D.O.
Division of Pulmonary Medicine, Department of Medicine, Brigham and Women's Hospital, Harvard Medical School, Boston, MA, USA

Division of Pulmonary Medicine, Department of Medicine, Boston Children's Hospital, Harvard Medical School, Boston, MA, USA
e-mail: ahmet.uluer@childrens.harvard.edu

A. C. Hergenroeder, C. M. Wiemann (eds.), *Health Care Transition*,
https://doi.org/10.1007/978-3-319-72868-1_18

so that when the transfer takes place, there is a method in place to ensure patients are not be lost to follow-up. This could include following-up after the transfer has occurred and obtaining feedback from Maria to improve the process for future patients.

The care of young adults with chronic conditions was particularly challenging in the era before the Affordable Care Act (ACA). The ACA expanded healthcare access for young adults through several provisions, including an allowance that young adults could stay on their parents health insurance until they are 26 years old [1].

Maria's case can be contrasted with another complex case of transition and transfer with a better outcome.

Case Vignette 2

Josie is a 23-year-old woman referred to the transition program at a freestanding children's hospital due to recent failure in transitioning care to an adult medical home as well as for medical co-management. Her complex medical history includes mast cell activation syndrome, recurrent anaphylaxis with multiple drug and food allergies requiring admission to the intensive care unit, dysfunctional uterine bleeding with concern for endometriosis, chronic chest pain with dyspnea due to obstructive lung disease, seizure disorder, protein-calorie malnutrition with gastrostomy tube placement, history of upper and lower GI bleed, and acute and chronic pain involving multiple joints and back. Previous attempts with transition ended with Josie returning to the pediatric emergency department despite appointments being made at the nearby adult institution.

Team members from the Boston Children's Hospital Transition Program received a consult regarding this patient. Transitional care tools were administered, including the Transition Readiness Questionnaire (TRAQ) [2], screening for depression (PHQ-9 [3] and anxiety (GAD-7 [4]), identification of healthcare proxy, and sexual health, alcohol, and drug use history. In addition, the consult team identified barriers to her transition. This included reaching out to her primary care pediatrician and subspecialists individually to better understand her medical history and barriers to transition from a provider perspective. These discussions led to a personalized and thoughtful approach to identifying providers at adult institutions. Once stakeholders were identified, a combined conference call and in-person meeting were arranged for all providers to attend, and subspecialists were connected electronically. Key adult providers also met with Josie prior to transfer of care.

During the following year, Josie continued to be admitted to the children's hospital where her usual emergency care plan was implemented. A similar care plan, molded by the framework of adult hospital, was also developed, shared with the patient and others in her care team. Josie was kept updated throughout the process and felt empowered by the knowledge of discussions between members of her care team. A second teleconference was arranged and a timeline of final preparations was created, transitional care assessment was reviewed and remediated, and a date of full transfer including emergency care was established. The emergency room at the adult institution also uploaded her emergent care plan easily identified in their electronic health record platform.

Josie had her first successful admission to an adult hospital 14 months after her initial consultation for transitional care support and has not returned to the children's hospital for emergent or ambulatory care since that time. The transitional care team remains in contact with Josie and provides support at the adult institution. A post-transfer interview identified some issues, but the overall experience of the patient was positive, and she feels comfortable with the care she is receiving from her adult medical home. Her providers all expressed gratitude for the completeness of her transitional care work, and previously identified barriers were resolved.

Although Josie's medical care is in many ways more complicated than Maria's, there is a clear difference in the outcome. Josie did not begin learning about transition as an adolescent as is recommended [5], but she did benefit from the existence of a formal transition program at her institution.

In the event that a hospital or department decides to establish a transition consult service, the recommended goals of such a program should include:

1. Inpatient and outpatient transition consultation: the consult service can be called to assist in the transition process, including overcoming barriers, identification of adult providers, care coordination with public agencies external to the healthcare system, and care integration into adult services [6].
2. The flexibility to assist with routine healthy adolescents; patients with chronic medical conditions (e.g., diabetes, cystic fibrosis); patients with developmental disabilities (e.g., autism); patients with mental health conditions, including substance use; and patients with technology dependence or other medical complexity (e.g., tracheostomy, gastrostomy, ventilators).
3. Adult medical co-management for conditions such as management of deep vein thrombosis, hypertension, type 2 diabetes, or perioperative management of adult-age patients.
4. Education of care teams, trainees, patients, and families.
5. Coaching teams in systems redesign and quality improvement strategies to facilitate a smoother transition process.
6. Advocacy for young adult health at the local, regional, state, and federal levels.
7. Development of tools to facilitate care transitions. These tools include, but are not limited to, electronic health records flow sheets, portable medical summaries, resource directories, and how-to guides.

Key team members of a transition consult service and their possible roles can be seen in Table 18.1. There will be overlap in roles. An example of transition care process can be seen in Fig. 18.1. There are seven key elements to this transition process.

Table 18.1 Key team members of a transition consult service and their roles

Team member	Role
Patient/family advisor	Consumer perspective on scope of services
	Community needs assessment
	Available as coach or mentor to other patients/families
Physician	Team leader
	Background in Med-Peds or Adolescent Medicine very helpful
	Establishes and strengthens links between pediatric and adult health systems Advises on routine adolescent/young adult health needs Develops protocols for adult medical condition management (DVT, stroke) Assists with medical condition co-management as needed during the period of transfer
Advanced practice clinician	Assess unmet medical needs at the time of transfer
	With the physician, may provide medical condition co-management as needed during the period of transfer
	Performs inpatient consults
	Providers day-to-day care on the inpatient service
Nursing	Assesses patients' readiness to transition to adult care
	Educates patients around disease self-management and self-care
	Educates patients around medication use
	Assesses patients' home care needs

(continued)

Table 18.1 (continued)

Team member	Role
Social work	Assesses mental health needs
	Provides referrals to community mental health services
	Assists families with guardianship applications
	Counsels families around advanced directives and shared decision-making
	May provide short-term mental health treatment around the time of transfer
Navigator/community health worker	Assesses resource needs and develops resource directories
	Connects patients/families to community-based resources
	Assists patients/families with scheduling their first adult medical appointments. May accompany patients to their first visits
	Advises the team on cultural considerations and community needs
Administration	Manages the day-to-day business affairs of the team
	Manages grants and philanthropic funds
	Coordinates outreach efforts
Technology Consultant	Works with the team to develop EHR-based care plans, questionnaires, and tracking tools
	Serves as a consultant around strategies to share health information electronically
Hospital champion	High-level administrator who advocates for the transition team's activities at hospital level committees Establishes and strengthens links between pediatric and adult healthcare systems
	Provides legislative advocacy
	Alerts the transition team to opportunities for grant funding or philanthropic support
Community partner	Could include the state Title V agency, the state Medicaid plan, Department of Public Health, nonprofits, and/or state medical societies
	Advises the team on new opportunities for collaboration and funding, as well as the latest state/federal regulations
	Provides legislative advocacy

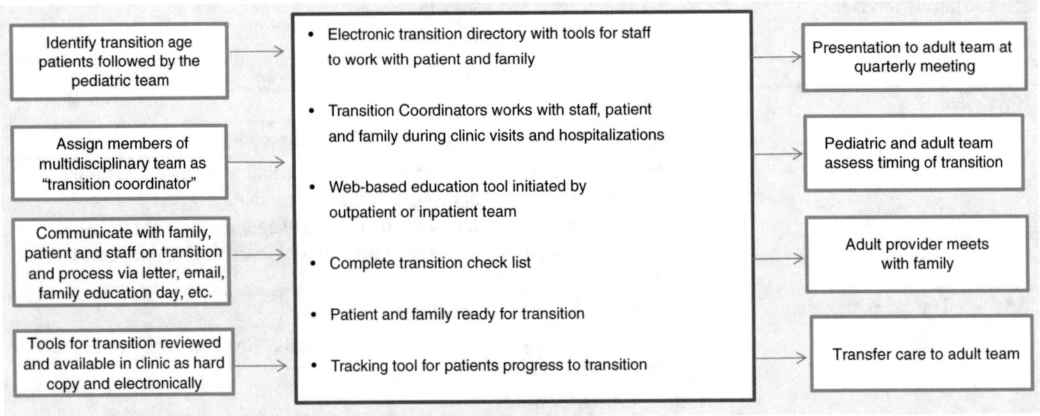

Fig. 18.1 Transition care process. Used with permission from the Boston Children's Hospital and Brigham and Women's Hospital Cystic Fibrosis Center

Build and Maintain Partnerships with Pediatric Primary and Specialty Care Providers

In some respects, this was the most challenging aspect in addressing Josie's case. Many pediatric specialty providers become the de facto primary care provider (PCP) for those with chronic illness as patients become more reluctant to engage with PCPs, particularly as visits to specialists become more frequent. However, with increasing age, a healthcare system requiring referrals and attention to surveillance and preventative care for adults necessitates the transfer to adult providers.

With Josie, when she would fall ill and present to the adult hospital, there were no identified medical providers for her. As a result, she would not receive adequate care as the adult providers did not know how to treat her and she would make her way back to her pediatric providers.

The establishment of the transition consult service allowed the team members to take advantage of existing relationships to coordinate Josie's care. In her case, it was helpful that there was an adult medical system associated with the pediatric hospital. As such, the key leaders at the pediatric and adult facilities could be brought together to develop a plan that could be presented to Josie. Beginning the process with a higher-level discussion, rather than finding individual physicians for each patient, allows for a more efficient transition and transfer process to begin. For Josie, involvement of her newly identified adult PCP early in the process helped preemptively address potential future barriers to transition.

Assist the Young Adult to Connect with Adult Specialists and Other Support Services

One of the decisions that assisted the most in Josie's case was including her in all of the discussions regarding her transition and transfer. A critical part of transition readiness is the achievement of self-advocacy and self-management, but these skills often continue to mature after transfer of care to an adult medical home. It is not enough to simply provide a contact number for an adult specialist to a patient, and it is not optimal for pediatric providers to just send medical records to an adult provider without first discussing the case [7]. In a study from 2011, the researchers interviewed 24 young adults, 24 parents, and 17 providers, all of whom agreed on the need for better organization and communication among pediatric and adult providers.

Josie's case of a successful transition had much to do with the personal correspondence between specialists, whether in person, teleconference, or email, as the conversation led to a more substantive discussion about issues that cannot be shared via medical records alone. Some of these nuances may lead to disruption in care if expectations are not properly calibrated. For example, confrontation may be averted if providers understand how a patient might engage them about particular therapies without the provider feeling undermined.

Communication Between Pediatric and Adult Providers in the Period Between the Last Pediatric and the First Adult Visit

An unplanned transition process often leads to an increase in emergency room utilization, worse health outcomes, and poor adherence to preventative therapies [8]. As can be seen with Josie, the transition program team ensured that there was ongoing and open communication between the adult and pediatric providers. It is critical that as the process is progressing, all the providers are given an opportunity to allow potential problems to arise and solutions identified.

Communication from the Adult Providers to the Pediatric Providers Confirming Transfer into the Adult Practice and Consultation with the Pediatric Providers(s) as Needed

Transfer to adult care does not mean that the relationship between the adult and pediatric providers ends. As noted in the vignette, the transition consult team remained in contact with the medical care teams to ensure the smooth transition process. It is also important to note that although there was a great deal of preplanning, unanticipated issues arose. The pediatric team remained available to address any questions that arose to assist in Josie's ongoing care.

Continue with Ongoing Care Coordination Tailored to Each Young Adult

In Josie's case, the transition consult service continued to provide care management until she had successfully transferred to the adult providers. In reviewing other transition programs, a variety of other models have been attempted. As an example, a study utilizing web based and SMS text messaging to assist adolescents with chronic illness demonstrated improvement in disease management skills, health-related self-efficacy, and patient-initiated communications [9]. This randomized control study tailored an approach that is aimed at the needs of a particular "generation" as opposed to a "disease-specific" model for those with chronic healthcare needs without cognitive delay. Other programs continue to endorse creation of a disease-specific approach and report success [10, 11]. Godbout et al. implemented both universal and endocrine disorder-specific questionnaires to help create a tailored transition program. Most notably, care coordination has been shown to greatly assist achieving transition care process outcomes [12].

Referral Tracking and Loop Closure Between the Last Pediatric and the First Adult Visit

As with any transfer between specialties, it is important to avoid getting lost to follow-up, which is what happened to Maria in the first vignette. Given the success that has occurred with the improvement in pediatric survivorship, ensuring that a patient follows through to engage in adult care is critical. Patients must first learn responsibility and adherence. Beyond that, there are opportunities for processes to be developed that can reduce any lapses.

Josie's case illustrates key steps for the successful transfer from pediatric to adult care (Table 18.2). First, Josie was involved from the beginning in developing a transfer plan, which gave her ownership in her success. Second, there was direct communication between the adult and pediatric providers. This opened a line of communication to answer questions or address problems that could arise, such as missing appointments. Third, a summary of her medical records was given to the adult providers, and appropriate care plans were uploaded to the adult healthcare providers' electronic health records in advance. All of this required forethought and action on the part of the patient and the pediatric and adult providers but results in an overall successful transfer to adult care.

Table 18.2 Steps for successful transfer from pediatric to adult care

1. Achieve understanding with patient and/or family to proceed with transition process
2. Identify adult PCP as key team member to coordinate transition
3. Communicate with all providers, if possible, together in person or via teleconference to identify barriers and adult specialists
4. Patient and/or care coordinators make appointments with adult specialists
5. Connect pediatric and adult specialists individually or as group to communicate medical and transition management
6. Alternate visits during a specified period and provide other support as needed
7. Transfer care while pediatric specialists remain available for consultation
8. Transition team to monitor patient following transfer for feedback and support

Elicit Feedback from Young Adults to Assess Experience with Adult Health Care

Obtaining feedback from all of the participants when transitioning a patient to adult care is critical not only for improving the care of the individual patient but also for improving the process for future patients. The feedback should be obtained from the patient, family, and pediatric and adult medical providers. As with Josie, she experienced a positive transition and transfer. The lessons learned from her case inform the quality improvement efforts for future transition and transfer. Every transfer is different, but it is incumbent on the leaders of these transition programs to learn from each experience to improve the process to ensure positive outcomes.

Conclusion

The transfer to adult care can be successfully achieved even in the most complex cases. It is beneficial to have case management to assist in coordinating the efforts. Developing relationships at a higher level between institutions creates opportunities and assists in aligning interests in transfer. Furthermore, establishing open and ongoing relationships between pediatric and adult providers can help anticipate and prevent problems with transfer. Most importantly, involving the patient and caregivers in the process and obtaining their feedback throughout allows them to play an active role and invest in the effort to ensure a successful transition and transfer outcome.

References

1. The Patient Protection and Affordable Care Act (PPACA), Pub. L. 2010. Mar 23, No. 111-148, 124 Stat. 119.
2. Wood DL, Sawicki GS, Miller MD, Smotherman C, Lukens-Bull K, Livingood WC, et al. The Transition Readiness Assessment Questionnaire (TRAQ): its factor structure, reliability, and validity. Acad Pediatr. 2014;14(4):415–22.
3. Kroenke K, Spitzer RL, Williams JB. The PHQ-9: validity of a brief depression severity measure. J Gen Intern Med. 2001;16(9):606–13.
4. Spitzer RL, Kroenke K, Williams JB, Löwe B. A brief measure for assessing generalized anxiety disorder: the GAD-7. Arch Intern Med. 2006;166(10):1092–7.
5. American Academy of Pediatrics; American Academy of Family Physicians; American College of Physicians; Transitions Clinical Report Authoring Group, Cooley WC, Sagerman PJ. Supporting the health care transition from adolescence to adulthood in the medical home. Pediatrics. 2011;128(1):182–200.
6. Sharma N, O'Hare K, Antonelli RC, Sawicki GS. Transition care: future directions in education, health policy, and outcomes research. Acad Pediatr. 2014;14(2):120–7.
7. Van Staa AL, Jedeloo S, van Meeteren J, Latour JM. Crossing the transition chasm: experiences and recommendations for improving transitional care of young adults, parents and providers. Child Care Health Dev. 2011;37(6):821–32.
8. Chua KP, Schuster MA, McWilliams JM. Differences in health care access and utilization between adolescents and young adults with asthma. Pediatrics. 2013;131(5):892–901.
9. Huang JS, Terrones L, Tompane T, Dillon L, Pian M, Gottschalk M, et al. Preparing adolescents with chronic disease for transition to adult care: a technology program. Pediatrics. 2014;133(6):e1639–46.
10. Herbert LJ, Sweenie R, Kelly KP, Holmes C, Streisand R. Using qualitative methods to evaluate a family behavioral intervention for type 1 diabetes. J Pediatr Health Care. 2014;28(5):376–85.
11. Godbout A, Tejedor I, Malivoir S, Polak M, Touraine P. Transition from pediatric to adult healthcare: assessment of specific needs of patients with chronic endocrine conditions. Horm Res Paediatr. 2012;78(4):247–55.
12. Sharma N, O'Hare K, O'Connor KG, Nehal U, Okumura MJ. Care coordination and comprehensive electronic health records are associated with increased transition planning activities. Acad Pediatr. 2017. pii: S1876-2859(17)30161-4. https://doi.org/10.1016/j.acap.2017.04.005. [Epub ahead of print].

Part V

Defining Successful Transition

19 Defining Successful Transition: Young Adult Perspective

Teresa Nguyen and Mallory Cyr

Successful Transition

In the previous chapters, you have learned about the different aspects, processes, and stakeholder perspectives of specifically health-care transition. However, what constitutes a well-rounded, successful transition from the perspective of an adolescent or young adult with special health-care needs (AYASHCN)? The two authors have made the transition to adulthood and will share their perspectives.

Case
Katie is a 20-year-old woman who is starting to navigate the adult health-care system. Katie was born with cerebral palsy and uses a power wheelchair for mobility. She often wonders why she must make such large changes to her health care as an adult, such as switching from a pediatric provider to an adult provider or keeping track of all of her medications while she goes to college. She understands she must be healthy in order to achieve her goals for adulthood, but what does it take for success? As Katie thinks about her future, she must consider all of the important components and skills that contribute to a successful transition (see Fig. 19.1).

T. Nguyen, M.P.H. (✉)
Got Transition, Washington, DC, USA
e-mail: teresa.nguyen@ucdenver.edu

M. Cyr, M.P.H.
Mallory Cyr, LLC, Denver, CO, USA
e-mail: MhCyr@bu.edu

A. C. Hergenroeder, C. M. Wiemann (eds.), *Health Care Transition*,
https://doi.org/10.1007/978-3-319-72868-1_19

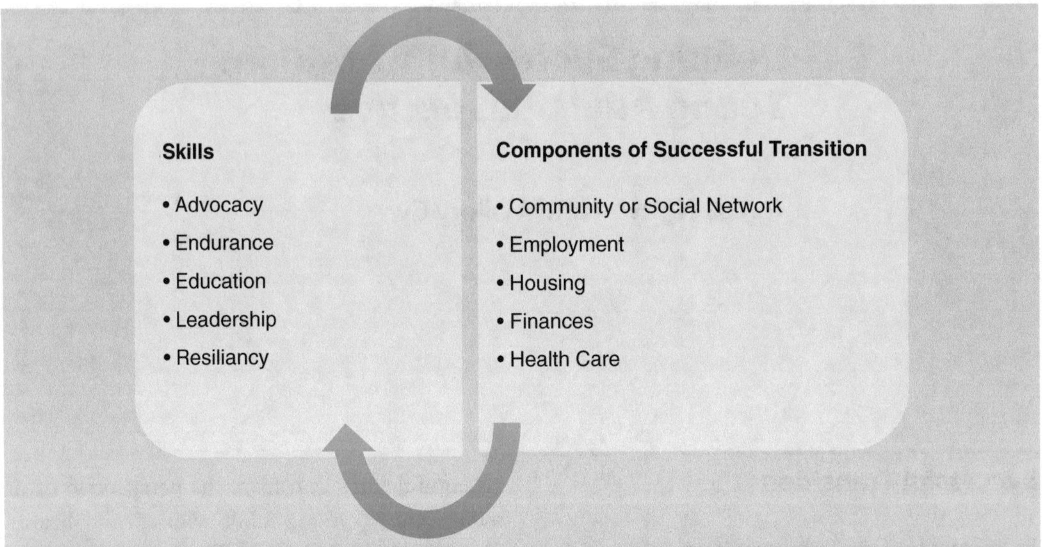

Fig. 19.1 It is important to keep in mind that the components of a successful transition are accompanied by skills that allow for the success of a transition into adulthood

Community and Social Network

Katie learned at a young age that inclusion and integration are crucial to her success. Katie's parents encouraged her to join extracurricular activities that fit her passions, goals, and needs during high school, and it was in those activities that Katie starting building her own support system. For Katie's parents, it was always a challenge to be in-between letting her take risks while allowing her to be integrated into adolescence experiences. Katie was persistent with her parents about her wishes to participate in the *same* activities as her friends and not partaking in anything that separated her from her peers. She built a support network of her peers at school and had good relationships with her medical providers, high school staff, and public transportation staff as she started to navigate independent living. Katie found the network of support she built was helpful when it was time to transition her life into college and employment. The smallest connection to the local pharmacist in her college town helped her have a successful transition because the pharmacist became familiar with Katie's medication. Even with a typical busy college schedule, Katie found a way to always keep in touch with the pharmacist for her medication needs.

Katie carried her communication and charismatic skills to college. She knew when to advocate for her needs and when to just have fun with her college peers. These skills enabled Katie to build a strong bond with her friends and explore romantic relationships.

Things for the AYASHCN to think about:

- Who can you rely on in a new town or setting?
- Does your participation in activities require accommodations? If so, know who to talk to.
- How to communicate with family members or parents about risk taking and being a normal young adult. What is important for them to know?

Financial

As Katie is thinking about moving out on her own, there are a few critical decisions she needs to make to set the foundation: Where will she live? Will she live by herself or with someone (and who)? And, what will her budget be?

In today's pop culture and media scene, it is difficult to find something targeted toward young adults that accurately portray the idea of living independently for the first time. Often depicted with large, glamorous city apartments, drinks with friends, and ordering takeout, while the reality is that all those things cost money, and rarely do we see the characters doing anything to earn income. Going from living at home with her family to living on her own, Katie will have to think about her monthly expenses and how she will afford them. Will she have her own cell phone or remain on her family's plan? Will she want cable? How much will she pay for food and groceries? What will her electricity/gas/water bill be? Will she need money for transportation?

These decisions will influence where she chooses to live and if she decides to have a roommate to share these expenses. Since Katie has complex medical needs, she will need to think about how her financial life will impact her health care and about insurance coverage. Because of the Affordable Care Act, or ACA, Katie can stay on her parents' insurance until she turns 26 whether she lives in their home or on her own [1].

Katie is enrolled in her state Medicaid program which covers the things her parents' private insurance does not cover. Katie will need to be thinking about insurance coverage, beyond her current status. If she works, will her employer provide adequate insurance coverage? If it is not adequate, what will she need to do to maintain her secondary coverage with Medicaid? As part of the ACA, 31 states expanded Medicaid to provide coverage to adults with disabilities who earn over the income limit for standard Medicaid [2]. This option (often referred to as "Medicaid Buy-In") allows participants to pay a monthly premium based on their income to access services and supports provided by Medicaid. Katie will need to factor this into her monthly budget if she needs to buy into Medicaid to keep her community supports and additional health-care coverage that help her to be independent (see Chap. 8).

If she does not buy into Medicaid, she will need to calculate her deductible and out-of-pocket costs under her private insurance coverage. Since Katie was in school and not working, she has been receiving Social Security Income (SSI). Once she moves out and begins working, she will need to report her change in income and make sure that her income is sufficient to meet all her monthly expenses. She can do this through the Social Security website or over the phone, but legally, it is Katie's responsibility to notify them that she has begun working. Depending on how much she will be making at her new job, this may reduce her benefits. Katie may also have the option to not receive a payment but remain eligible for SSI in order to receive services through Medicaid. Katie must report her changes within 10–12 days of when the changes occur, or she risks losing her benefits.

Things for the AYASHCN to think about (see also Table 19.1, below):

- Understand income and monthly expenses, including bills and recreation. An Excel spreadsheet can be used to track bills, income, and savings.
- Include expenses like cell phone, cable, or other things that may have been paid by someone else before.
- Will expenses will be paid independently or split between people who are living together?

Table 19.1 Useful resources for understanding finances and benefits

Finance and budget information	Resource website
Social Security Administration and SSI/SSDI information	https://www.ssa.gov/
Information about health-care coverage	https://www.healthcare.gov/
Simple budget worksheet	https://www.moneyunder30.com/really-simple-budget-worksheet

- How will health insurance or out-of-pocket costs impact being able to pay bills or save money?
- Income limits for any essential program or services that are needed to live independently.

Housing

Katie has a conversation with her family about housing options since she is ready to move out! She decides it would be best for her to live with a friend who wants a roommate and wants to live in the same area. If Katie did not want a roommate, she would have to hire someone to help her around the house, for example, reaching things, cooking meals, doing laundry, buying groceries, and running other errands.

Now that she knows who she will live with, Katie and her friend need to find an affordable place to live. This means thinking about things that her peers might not have to think about: If they choose to live in an apartment building, she will need a wheelchair accessible unit or will need to discuss reasonable accommodations and learn the building policies to request them. Katie and her friend make a list of what they will want in an apartment and anything that Katie may need specifically. The list includes:

- Within budget for rent (both will pay $500, can look for units up to $1000)
- Level entry (no stairs to get in building)
- Washer and dryer in unit
- Close to public transportation
- Accessible health care (specifically Katie's providers and hospital)
- ADA compliant doorways
- Bathroom large enough to enter, turn around, and close door
- Spacious kitchen
- Oven with controls on front vs. behind burners (request as reasonable accommodations)
- Elevator or first floor apartment (in case elevator is out of use during fire)

After touring a few apartments, they agreed to fill out applications. If a person is interested in the apartment, they must be approved, to show that they will be a responsible tenant who will follow the rules and pay their bills and rent on time. During this process, a fee and deposit are usually required. The cost of these varies, just like the cost of rent, and all buildings have different application processes. Potential tenants must prove that they can pay for the apartment and that they can afford rent each month. This is done either through showing paystubs to prove how much money is made (which must be more than three times the rent each month) or by showing that there is enough money saved in an account to equal 3 months' rent.

When applying for an apartment, the property management might run the potential tenant's credit score. A credit score is the result of financial actions a person has taken and the results, such as, the amount of debt, lines of credit, and whether credit card payments were late or on time. Table 19.2 lists resources to help with housing decisions.

It is important for young adults to learn about credit, debt management, and how the financial decisions they make can impact their long-term financial goals. Young adults are often the target of credit card and loan offers, as well as debt repayment scams with high interest rates. Many schools do not teach these life skills, so as Katie

Table 19.2 Useful resources for navigating housing options

Housing information	Resource website
Money Smart financial curriculum	https://www.fdic.gov/consumers/consumer/moneysmart/adult.html
Fair housing and accessibility	https://www.ada.gov/doj_hud_statement.pdf
Americans with Disabilities Act Checklist for Readily Achievable Barrier Removal	https://www.ada.gov/racheck.pdf

is thinking about her financial future and how she will be managing her expenses, she may want to have this conversation with her family or with a mentor who has a healthy relationship with finances. Just like some health topics, money can be uncomfortable to talk about, but to achieve success, it is necessary to have these conversations! Our suggestion is to start these conversations early. For example, when the first credit card is obtained, plan on paying the principal monthly, not just the interest payment.

Things for the AYASHCN to think about re: Housing

- Paying Rent. Who will pay how much? What is the highest that everyone can afford monthly?
- Location. Urban or rural? What type of transportation is available?
- What accommodations will be needed? Make a list. Don't forget little things like where the mailbox will be and how you turn your key!
- Prepare all documentation before applying. Get copies of all sources of income and identification
- Applications cost money. Be clear on all upfront costs and what is required to move in!

Employment

Katie has always wanted to become a lawyer. Her passion is to defend those who are vulnerable and underrepresented, like herself. She was accepted to a university in a town that is 1 hour away from where she was born and raised and plans to obtain her bachelor's degree prior to moving on to graduate school to pursue her career in law. Her university receives federal financial assistance; therefore, Katie is entitled to disability accommodations in school, under Section 504 of the Rehabilitation Act of 1973 [3]. She connects with her Office of Disability Services at the University and begins the process to receive accommodations.

Educational accommodations for Katie could include:

- Exams in digital formatting (versus paper)—due to fine motor skill limitations
- Extended time on exams
- Flexible attendance—due to winter weather and wheelchair mobility difficulties and/or spontaneous medical incidents due to disability

Educational accommodations for someone with a learning disability could include:

- Extended time on exams
- Digital format for textbooks or exams
- Word processing and dictation software
- Access to notetakers in classes and tutors

While in school, Katie wants a part-time job. One difference between this job experience and a full-time job is access to employee benefits and health insurance. She knows that in the future, benefits and health insurance will be a priority when she is deciding on where she wants to work. As a low-income student with a disability, Katie is currently on her state Medicaid plan, so a part-time job without benefits is suitable for this phase of her life. When the time comes for a full-time position complete with benefits and health insurance, Katie must assess her health needs and choose the health insurance plan that best fits her needs. If she chooses to utilize Medicaid, Katie knows that there are programs for working individuals who need Medicaid [4].

She wonders if the accommodation process at work is the same as the process she utilizes in college. Through her experience in obtaining a part-time position at the local bookstore, she learns that communication is the key to a successful employment experience. Through several job interviews, Katie found that disclosing her disability was hard. She found it helpful to not disclose her disability until the first interview with each employer, as opposed to before the interview. Sometimes disclosing prior to the first interview causes the employer to focus the job interview on the needs of the interviewee, instead of focusing on the job responsibilities and expectations of the prospective employee. During the first interview, Katie discusses only what she deems is necessary for the employer to know, in order for the organization or company to successfully accommodate her. She talks about how the accommodations would enable her to perform at her best and be successful in her work for the company. Katie, the company's human resources department, and her employer agree to an open communication plan—allowing her to communicate about how things can change or be modified as they see fit.

Skills that are a catalyst to success in obtaining and keeping employment include education, resilience, and endurance. In preparation for any job, there needs to be education or training around the skills that are needed to succeed in a vocational environment. If a young adult chooses an alternate route to education, the young adult and/or their family should have the awareness of available resources, such as partnering with their local Division of Vocational Rehabilitation, to adequately prepare the young adult for employment. Katie does not become discouraged through the process of communicating with her employer and understands that sometimes reframing the same question or concept is necessary for people to understand her perspective. She utilizes the skills she learned from school and her social life to strengthen her communication with employers and faculty. This is an example of resilience, taking what she learned in past experiences and applying the same skills to current experiences. Lastly, endurance is needed when navigating a new aspect of adulthood. Katie needs to make sure she is in her best health to continue working and going to school.

Things for the AYASHCN to think about:

- How to prepare for employment? Is education the best route? If not, what other resources are available for preparation?
- What are the necessary accommodations for an individual to succeed in their workplace?
- What are the top things to look for in an employer?

Medical

Perhaps the most important component of a successful transition is the medical component. Health is the foundation for the outcomes of transition into adulthood, and transitioning into the adult health-care system is a necessary conversation that needs to happen between the pediatric provider and the AYASHCN, ideally beginning at the age of 14 years [6].

As Katie is heading to her last visit with her pediatrician, she remembers some essential things that have prepared her for the switch to an adult health-care provider: the importance of a medical home, an emergency plan, and finding an adult provider that would respect her lifestyle. Katie knows that to be able to thrive in her new environment(s), work, and college, she must continue to be healthy with the right team of health-care providers.

Katie has many specialists that she sees for her health care: a primary care provider, a neurologist, a physical therapist, and a psychologist. Although she is capable of managing her care and appointments with each department, she finds it helpful that her specialists are able to communicate with each other, when needed. For example, to manage her anxiety Katie sees a psychologist for therapy. Although Katie's primary care provider manages her anxiety medication, communication between her psychologist and primary care provider helps Katie understand and maximize her treatment for anxiety. There have been other times when communication and collaboration between her health-care providers proved to be helpful, such as coordination for Katie's surgeries and medical procedures. The team-based, coordinated, patient-centered care approach is also known as the medical home health-care model [5]. Recognizing the importance of her pediatric medical home team, Katie chose adult providers and specialists that have a focus on being patient-centered and collaborative with the individuals that Katie deems necessary in her medical care.

Along with the medical home approach, it was important to Katie to have providers who under-

Table 19.3 Useful resources for navigating health-care transition

Health-care transition tool	Resource website
Medical summary template	http://gottransition.org/resourceGet.cfm?id=227
Sample Transition Readiness Assessment for Youth	http://gottransition.org/resourceGet.cfm?id=224

stand her lifestyle and transition into adulthood. As is true for many young adults, Katie prefers electronic communication (text message, email, etc.) to telephone calls, when it comes to scheduling appointments and/or communicating with her providers. She plans to communicate to her new medical team that as a college student who also works part-time, it is important that there was more than one way for her to conveniently and efficiently connect with her providers. In addition, it was critical to Katie that her adult health-care team provided her with a safe environment to be able to share her goals with them, for the purpose of developing a health plan that would support those goals. Some of her goals focused on sensitive topics such as: reproductive health, family planning, mental health, and drug and alcohol safety. The new adult team respects Katie's lifestyle and empowers her to continue being an advocate for her own health care and health plan.

Katie was beginning a new chapter of her life that involved many changes at once: going to college, moving out on her own, and managing her own health care with new providers. An emergency plan was developed with her family, pediatric providers, and new adult providers so that Katie would have a strategy when an emergency arose. She made a list of medical concerns and/or medical emergencies, who to contact during which scenario, and the most up-to-date contact information for each individual involved. The emergency plan was stored electronically on her keychain USB drive with all of the information regarding: medications she was taking, recent health procedures and their dates, and any other important notes that medical providers need to consider when working with her in an emergency. In addition to storing the plan on her USB drive, she gave a copy to her providers for reference, if needed.

With a new medical team behind her as she enters a new chapter of her life, Katie is confident that she will be able to maintain her health in order to achieve her new adulthood goals!

Things for the AYASHCN to think about: medical issues and transition (see Table 19.3, above)

- When is it appropriate to have a conversation with your current doctor about transitioning into the adult health-care system?
- What are some goals that you want to achieve in adulthood? How does your health fit into those goals?
- What are some key qualities of a health-care provider that you would like to have in a new provider?

Conclusion

As demonstrated, a successful transition consists of many pieces and components that interplay together for AYASHCN. One example, in Katie's case, is financial planning which affects her housing plans and health insurance decisions. While many of the independent components have an effect on transition and its success, the most important takeaway for AYASHCN is how health and health care are a critical foundation for a successful transition. It is essential that all of the individuals involved in transition planning, i.e. families, school faculty, medical providers, friends, care coordinators, social workers, etc., understand and respect the goals and aspirations of the young adult. These aspirations and goals help mold the conversations that center around the topic of transition from pediatric care to adult care for AYASHCN. Medical providers can have a key role in the success of an individual moving into adulthood by starting the transition conversation early, by guiding the young adult to develop or strengthen their advocacy and leadership skills within the health-care system, and by empowering the AYASHCN to make their own choices in managing their health. All of the transition components discussed in this chapter would not be a consideration without a healthy AYASHCN to carry out the necessary steps to obtain an education, secure housing, and become an employed individual.

References

1. HealthCare.gov. Health insurance coverage for children and young adults under 26. U.S. Centers for Medicare and Medicaid Services. https://www.healthcare.gov/young-adults/children-under-26/. Accessed 3 July 2017.
2. Families USA. A 50-state look at Medicaid expansion. Families USA, 1 Apr 2017. http://familiesusa.org/product/50-state-look-medicaid-expansion. Accessed 3 July 2017.
3. United States. US Department of Education. Frequently asked questions about Section 504 and the education of children with disabilities. Office of Civil Rights, 16 Oct 2015. https://www2.ed.gov/about/offices/list/ocr/504faq.html#protected. Accessed 30 June 2017.
4. Medicaid.gov. Medicaid Employment Initiatives. Centers for Medicare and Medicaid Services. https://www.medicaid.gov/medicaid/ltss/employmment/index.html. Accessed 3 July 2017.
5. PCPCC. Defining the Medical Home. Medical Home. Patient-Centered Primary Care Collaborative. 2017. https://www.pcpcc.org/about/medical-home. Accessed 30 June 2017.
6. Gottransition.org. What is health care transition? Youth and families. Got Transition. 2014. http://gottransition.org/youthfamilies/index.cfm#preparing. Accessed 30 June 2017.

Defining Successful Transition: Parent Perspective

20

Rosemary Alexander and Laura J. Warren

Set the Stage

The transition from childhood to adulthood for AYASHCNs occurs between ages 14 and 22 but can play out for years before and after this age span. Often transition never really ends, for as new issues arise, families and AYASHCNs find themselves renegotiating health-care systems. Also, medical transition is only one of the many transitions. Others include post-secondary education, employment, housing, funding, appropriate supports, and social connections.

As families and AYASHCNs face these issues, they may feel overwhelmed by the decisions that need to be made, anxious about the future, hopeless about the availability of resources and opportunities, and burned out by the struggles up to that point. For all of these reasons, families and their AYASHCN may ignore health-care transition planning and simply wait to act until practitioners eject them from their practice at age 18 or they face a health crisis, an interaction with the Emergency Department (ED) or police, or some other cataclysmic events.

Ideally, AYASHCN and their families arrive at adulthood enrolled with adult general practitioners, specialists, and other staff who understand their unique health-care needs and are prepared to treat families and young adults with respect, patience, and effective care. AYASHCN and families must learn that adult health care looks different from pediatric care and that they must move to the next stage of care with knowledge and forethought.

In this chapter we will explore factors that influence the ability to make a smooth health-care transition and how this process can be positive for families and their youth while providing examples of both barriers families have encountered and positive steps they have taken in the transition process. We hope that sharing the parent perspective will provide health-care providers with models for how to support families and youth as they move from pediatric to adult health care.

The authors of this chapter are parents of young adults with disabilities. We have worked for 25+ years in the arena of supporting families of children with disabilities, at both nonprofits and the local school district. We count in the thousands the number of families we have gotten to know. We have known families who successfully connected with vital resources and those who struggled; we have known families who lost their beautiful children and many who have watched their children grow into robust adults; we have watched funding and services ebb and flow, seeing a program that we thought would

R. Alexander, Ph.D. • L. J. Warren (✉)
Texas Parent to Parent, Austin, TX, USA
e-mail: Rosemary.Alexander@txp2p.org; Laura@txp2p.org

A. C. Hergenroeder, C. M. Wiemann (eds.), *Health Care Transition*,
https://doi.org/10.1007/978-3-319-72868-1_20

last forever abruptly vanish; and we believe we have earned the right to hopeful skepticism. We learn so much more from our children about ourselves—resiliency, determination, and unconditional love—and see the beauty of our children's lives, while others just get uncomfortable around them. We hope that these experiences will be helpful to our readers as we explore successful health-care transition.

Family Story

William is a young man who does not read, write, or talk and needs help with all daily living activities. And yet, he has the ability to influence all those in his sphere. When we are with him, we slow down and enjoy the moment. We laugh more and get more hugs. We are reminded not to take for granted the ease with which most of us carry out life's ordinary functions. He surprises us with how knowing he is as he perceives mood changes in others and responds to them. He is comforting to be with. We work for him and with him so that he has a full life, happy and safe, engaged in the community, so that his gifts will be received by more people.

Define the Issues

We have defined six issues that factor into how smoothly health-care transition proceeds. These issues are interwoven, but we will describe them separately.

- How parent culture influences the health-care transition process
- How the AYASHCN's medical needs and ability level influence the health-care transition process
- How families find and interact with adult care providers
- How families find and interact with specialists
- How legal issues affect the transition process after age 18
- What constitutes smooth health-care transition and how we can facilitate it

How Parent Culture Influences the Health-Care Transition Process

Each family has an established method of accessing health care—some have a history of being proactive, actively seeking out what is needed, while others do not have the means or the background to effectively access health care. They may have a belief system that discourages using health care and are not accustomed to using health-care experts.

Families also have a broader culture that influences transition. For example, they may come from a culture that values searching for options or a culture that accepts the first option proposed. How then do families come to have the knowledge to interview a new doctor, rather than using the first referral? Some families may have had negative experiences that they bring to interactions with health-care providers; it may take effort to overcome these experiences and view new health-care professionals as welcoming and available. Other families may be able to set their own boundaries and expectations and seek out and evaluate resources. Knowing the family culture will help the physician better understand which family they are encountering.

What families expect after public school graduation also affects transition. A family and an AYASHCN may imagine a future that is close to home or out in the world, where the youth works full-time, part-time, or not at all and where the youth lives with the family or moves out and goes on to post-secondary education or not. These pictures of adulthood influence the kind of medical services a family seeks. A student going to college needs to learn independence earlier, perhaps, than a student who stays home after graduation. Family expectations are based on how they perceive their child's needs and strengths, whether they expect their child to become independent or if their child will always need assistance.

Family financial and emotional stability and ability level influence transition. Some families have financial resources to supplement what is available through public funding for their young adults. Family emotional stability is impacted by their coping skills, emotional support from family and friends, and how stressful their child's disabilities are. Parents may become discouraged by hearing horror stories about adult services and become anxious or reluctant to access adult care. For example, they may hear statements from other parents, such as "Medicaid funding is terrible!" "Doctors who accept Medicaid aren't accepting new patients!" Such statements paint a gloomy picture and could cause parents to avoid trying to get Medicaid assistance altogether. As a result, parents may be less able to hear the counseling of health-care staff about transition or use their advice to plan for the future.

Families must be educated on transition best practices. Most of us have no prior experience teaching children to take control of their own health issues; most parents have no idea it is even necessary. Health-care providers can teach the parent and youth that he or she is expected to take over their own care as they grow up. Most parents do not know that this planning should take place.

We surveyed 23 families, whom we know well and whom we respect for their ability to care and advocate for their children, about their progress on transition; their responses are contained in Table 20.1.

Even among the most able families, few (25%) have had assistance with transition. There is a wide range of ages when families have made progress on medical transition (most were around 18), and few have been able to assist their child to be truly independent in medical settings (only two thought that their youth could make their own decisions). We believe that the education of families about transition, preferably by the youth's providers, would change this outcome radically. See Table 20.2 for provider tips for tuning into a family's culture.

Table 20.1 Responses to parent survey about transition ($N = 23^a$)

Question	Yes
Has your youth transitioned to adult primary care?	19 (90.5%)
Has your youth transitioned to adult specialist care?	13 (68.5%)
How old was your youth when you started planning for medical transition? mean (range)	17 (9–30 years)
Did you consider any of the following when starting your transition planning:	
How to handle decisions once your youth turned 18	20 (90.9%)
How your youth is learning and developing	16 (72.7%)
How puberty affects your youth's health, behavior, or well-being	10 (45.5%)
How the independence of your youth affects transition	16 (72.7%)
Your youth's ability to navigate the medical system alone	12 (54.5%)
If your youth cannot navigate the medical system alone, do you know who will help them?	16 (72.7%)
How your culture or your family circumstances affect transition	9 (40.9%)
How does your youth's disability affect transition?	16 (72.7%)
Have you worked with your youth to be more independent in making their own health decisions?	12 (60%)
Did you receive any assistance in preparing your youth for medical transition?	6 (30%)
Can your youth help with medical decisions?	5 (71.4%)
Can your youth order their prescriptions?	5 (71.4%)
Does your youth attend their doctor's appointments on their own?	3 (42.9%)
Does your youth make their own medical decisions on their own?	2 (28.6%)
Can your youth give informed consent for a procedure on their own?	5 (71.4%)

[a]Not all parents responded to every question

How the AYASHCN's Medical Needs and Ability Level Influence the Health-Care Transition Process

AYASHCN's medical complexity and cognitive/behavioral level affect the health-care transition process.

A healthy teen who uses the health-care system minimally may hardly notice the shift from pediatric to adult health services. Perhaps all that is needed for a healthy teen is a yearly doctor visit, permission forms signed, and a general checkup. At the other end of the spectrum are children who are medically fragile or have chronic illness; they see many specialists and

Table 20.2 Provider tips for tuning into a family's culture

• We all have a perspective, based on background, culture, and personality. Become aware of your biases and how they influence your interactions with families. Strive to be as free of bias as possible as you work with families
• Find ways to accommodate families who speak a language besides English, both by having a qualified interpreter present and by being aware of cultural norms
• Remember that parents are the experts on their own children; honor their knowledge and expertise. Respect family choices without judgment
• Note that the family and AYASHCN are the ones who will ultimately decide whether they will carry out your directives; find ways to get their buy-in so that they will carry out the plan that you develop together
• Work to establish rapport with a family by calling each person by name and by knowing the relevant facts of their AYASHCN's medical history before you enter the treatment room. Families get tired of repeating their AYASHCN's medical history
• Praise positive steps the family and youth have taken toward transition to adulthood

spend much time in doctors' offices, as well as accessing occupational, speech and physical therapists, nutritionists, dietitians, and other services. For these children and their families, how well transition flows may have life-or-death significance. Many teens reside somewhere in the middle, with some health-care needs but less complexity. Where they fall along this spectrum greatly influences the transition process.

Cognitive and behavioral abilities can greatly influence the transition process. A teen who can speak for himself may be able to take over health-care decisions and actions with ease, while teens with cognitive and/or behavioral issues will face more barriers to a smooth transition.

AYASHCNs with cognitive or communication disabilities often are not able to articulate "where it hurts" or may misrepresent their symptoms; they may not understand the changes caused by puberty and will be anxious or easily upset with medical staff; they may not understand why a treatment is important and will resist what is in their best interest; and they may not be able to undertake the adult role in health care and are dependent on others who may or may not be available for reliable assistance. While pediatric providers may have more experience with child-like communication skills, adult providers may not have the experience to interpret the signs and signals of those who have limited speech. It takes a special kind of listening and learning to treat an AYASHCN who cannot always or effectively speak for himself.

Adult providers may have less knowledge of how to interact with AYASHCN with cognitive disabilities or are who are uncooperative, noncompliant, or disruptive in the waiting room, resistant to assistance, or unable to understand medical advice and decisions. AYASHCNs with behavioral issues may lack the motivation to follow medical recommendations or are subject to pressure from peers to ignore medical issues and daily self-care. Practitioners must avoid personalizing these behaviors and be open to creative solutions to providing health care.

Family Story

Cindy is a young woman who has severe autism and visual impairment, along with self-injurious behaviors and phobias. At an early age, she developed a fear of doctors' offices, and as she grew larger and stronger, her family found it almost impossible to get her into a medical office. Fortunately, they found a pediatric provider who was willing to meet Cindy in the lobby or her mother's car. When Cindy aged out of this practice, the family struggled to find another doctor who would literally meet their daughter "where she was." They are now using a service that provides in-home care, but this remedy restricts their access to health care. Table 20.3 contains tips for providers in providing medical care to patients with special needs.

Table 20.3 Provider tips for being creative in providing medical care

• Schedule youth with disruptive behaviors or medical complexity as the first patient in the morning before the waiting room has filled up or at other times when your waiting room is relatively quiet and empty
• Ask the parent ahead of the first appointment how their AYASHCN works best with a physician
• Ask the parent how the AYASHCN likes to be approached—Does a quiet voice help? Does touching upset them? How do they communicate? Do they use a communication device?
• Provide a contact within the physician's office for parents to call when they have follow-up questions or problems

How Families Find and Interact with Adult Care Providers

The more proactive and organized the family is at transition time, the smoother the transition process will be, as the family is more likely to find and use medical resources. For families who are less organized, the process may be more difficult.

For families living in rural settings, there may be a lack of care providers locally, and the family may have to drive much further to access care. Having to seek care far from home makes it more expensive in travel cost and time off from work. More specialized care also requires families to cast a wider net for adult care, perhaps driving hours to an urban medical center.

Families who are isolated and not linked into parent or disability groups may be cut off from valuable information about how to find providers and who the most receptive adult providers are in their area. The shared wisdom of local groups can be invaluable.

The family's and AYASHCN's access to insurance for medical care is a significant factor in transition. The age and disability level of an AYASHCN may determine what kind of funding is available to pay for medical care, as is a family's access to private medical insurance resources. Insurance provided by an employer changes as a youth becomes an adult; families must be aware of how their employment-based plan treats this change and be proactive in applying for extended care at age 26 (see Chap. 8).

Often families and their AYASHCNs struggle to find providers who will accept their funding source and must be prepared to change providers as funding changes, to appeal insurance decisions that deny coverage for important medications and services, and to become active advocates in the insurance arena.

Families often learn about adult providers who will accept their children from other parents. We hear the question, "Does anyone know of a doctor who works well with youth with Autism?" Answers may be hard to find. Many families are referred to adult providers, only to have the provider reject them, many times for less than credible reasons. Not only does that waste the parent's time but also is terribly frustrating and hurtful for the family.

Family Story

Thomas is a 25-year-old with osteogenesis imperfecta, type II. He has had multiple fractures, extreme spinal curvature, and severe respiratory problems and has had 24-h nursing since birth. Thomas has graduated from high school. His parents started his medical transition early, including how they received insurance coverage. Thomas gave up his Medicaid Waiver Program and moved to managed care Medicaid at age 21, in order to maintain his nursing care. There were multiple meetings between his family and the managed care organizations, with a contract signed, before making this move. Medicaid waivers are precious and families rarely give them up.

Thomas and his mother visited several adult care providers before settling on a new team. They called several offices before settling on a pulmonologist who said they could handle a tracheostomy. However, the provider took one look at Thomas, said he could not treat him, and left the room. That was a hurtful moment for Thomas, and his mother was furious. They found a team, but it took several years and many panicked moments with the fear of having to go to the Emergency Department for treatment. See Table 20.4 tips for providers to engage parents and family members.

Table 20.4 Provider tips for engaging parents and family members

• At the first office visit, ask the parent what has worked well and not so well with previous doctors
• When the child is old enough, start explaining issues to him or her as well as to the parents
• When the teen does not understand a concept or how to take over a medical task, provide written information, if appropriate, for them that they can take home and study. Translate technical language into simple language that is clear to someone with limited understanding
• As the child becomes a teenager, direct information to him or her, and assess their ability to make medical decisions. Work with the parents to develop the teen's decision-making skills
• Introduce the family to a Care Notebook and encourage them to create one together. A Care Notebook is a useful organizing tool for parents who have children with special health-care needs or disabilities. The Care Notebook at the Texas Parent to Parent website is a compilation of PDF fillable documents. Parents can download all or any part of the Care Notebook. These forms allow you to enter your specific information and save it on your computer. You can find an example at https://www.txp2p.org/services/family-to-family-health-info/care-notebook or www.txp2p.org under services and under Family-to-Family Health Information Center. You can also conduct a search for Care Notebooks to find other examples
• Make sure families and AYASHCNs feel that they are part of the medical team by acknowledging their input and using it to make decisions
• Always ask what else you can do to help the family. Parents may need help but may not know how to ask for it. Broaden your concern to include issues that are not strictly medical but involve overall well-being

How Families Find and Interact with Specialists

Families of teens and young adults with more complex medical needs are likely to interact with one or more specialists. Families must sort out which specialists are still required, how to find them, how to pay for their services, and how to deal with the differing medical opinions. Families need to know who is in charge and to whom to turn in different situations. Care coordination is essential and a medical home is the ideal. However, medical home is another concept that families may not be familiar with, and they may require education to learn how to find one.

The transition from pediatric to adult specialists involves the transfer of trust. Families have been with a certain specialist for many years, perhaps their child's whole life, and may find it difficult to move to adult care, both logistically and emotionally. Adult specialists can make this transition easier by working closely with their pediatric counterpart to learn all they can about the AYASHCN's medical history and by helping to transfer records. They can work to establish trust at the adult level by reassuring families that they will get to know the AYASHCN over time and will gradually learn how best to meet the needs of the AYASHCN. It might also help for the adult provider to explain what is different in their practice. For example, will the provider be talking more to the AYASHCN than the parents? Will the adult provider have a different protocol for communicating with parents? Will he or she have a different focus, perhaps more on maintaining health than exploring new treatments? Will the AYASHCN be seen with the same frequency?

Family Story
Larry had a serious seizure disorder through childhood, often requiring trips to the ED. At age 20, his disorder was brought under control. The family remained with the pediatric neurologist, and he approved the same meds annually. When Larry was 30, he experienced a severe seizure. The family met their new adult neurologist in the ED at midnight! They realized belatedly that they should have established a relationship with an adult neurologist years earlier and since then have worked hard to establish a close working relationship with the adult neurologist. See Table 20.5 for tips adults specialists can use when working with AYASHCN.

Table 20.5 Tips for adult specialists working with AYASHCN

• Help the family and AYASHCN have clear expectations for the adult specialty practice
• Ask the family and AYASHCN how the adult specialist can best help to make the move from pediatric services
• Find out who will be the central medical provider for the AYASHCN and what records should routinely be shared with the central provider. Find out how to provide test results with all concerned
• Be sure parents understand the changes in how the medical community shares information after an AYASHCN becomes 18 years old and know what options are available for staying involved

Table 20.6 Tips for helping a family through the legal changes at age 18

• Don't assume that you know best what choice a family should make about guardianship versus other legal tools; make sure families are aware of and able to explore different options
• Remember that getting guardianship is a costly, time-consuming enterprise and a big responsibility, and it strips the AYASHCN of all legal rights
• Find a way to give advice about the parent role in an AYASHCN's decision-making that is nonjudgmental. For example, describe situations where an AYASHCN will be called upon to make decisions and ask if the parent has witnessed the youth making such decisions
• Note that often parents don't know what skills an 18-year-old will be able to develop. Assure parents that everyone is eager for their AYASHCN to learn and grow, and explain what can be done to help in the short term

How Legal Issues Affect the Transition Process After Age 18

Before an AYASHCN reaches age 18, a parent may manage all aspects of medical care. It can be a shock when parents realize that their role changes dramatically when their child is 18: suddenly they cannot take any of these actions without some provision. The big question is, to what extent—if at all—can my child learn to manage his or her own care? (see Chap. 30.)

If a child can learn these skills, the family and professionals should start by age 14 or younger to guide the teen in the transition process. Parents may need to let the teen start trying to do things the parents have traditionally done, like making appointments or calling in medication renewals. Small steps lead toward a higher level of responsibility, and teens begin to feel more competent. Parents must redefine their role as supporter rather than primary decision-maker.

For families whose teens will not be able to take over their own care, parents and physicians must explore how to provide the least restrictive yet supportive path for the future, that is, how to leave as much power as possible in the hands of the AYASHCN while safely and responsibly navigating the health-care arena with them or for them.

Supportive decision-making, medical power of attorney, and guardianship are among the legal tools parents can use to help their youth to make informed decisions or make decisions for them, access health-care information, and continue to have an active role (see Table 20.6 and Chap. 30).

Care Notebooks and similar tools, such as a Portable Medical Summary (a one-to-two page "quick facts" of relevant information) or an Emergency Care Plan, are ways to record medical history, provide important facts, and pass along vital information. (For more information on Portable Medical Summary, go to www.txp2p.org and search for this term.)

What Constitutes Smooth Health-Care Transition and How We Can Facilitate It

Strong collaborations among parents, AYASHCNs, and the medical community increase the chances that youth will move from pediatric to adult services with ease. Each of the participants in this process needs the information essential for planning.

Sharing information among families, AYASHCNs, and medical providers is the first step toward positive transitioning. Emotional support for families gives them hope in the future and the motivation to plan; it can come from other parents and parent organizations, other nonprofits, and encouraging professionals. Medical professionals need financial and logistical support to enable them to have relevant information for families, time to sit down and plan with families, and staff available to assist in the process. Faith is built over time, engendered by success stories and rewarding partnerships; everyone needs positive feedback to keep going!

Here are some of the elements that will facilitate smooth health-care transitions for parents and for AYASHCNs:

- Parents should have the crucial information about what is coming well before the crisis point:
  - Age 18 is a turning point for parent involvement, and parents must be prepared with the legal means to stay involved or know that their AYSHCN is prepared to go it alone or with less assistance.
  - The specific age at which the pediatric practice will require their AYASHCN to move to an adult practice.
  - The changes in funding as their AYASHCN becomes an adult.
- Parents need emotional support during transition. By the time their AYASHCN is nearing 18–21, parents are often burned out, fearful about the future, and discouraged. They need to feel hopeful that their youth will have the resources they need as adults to live as independently as possible. This hope can come from hearing how other parents have created a good life for their adult children, what models are available, and how to link into funding and resources. They should participate in a parent community where they can gain support and work with other families to create great lives for their AYASHCN. Emotional support empowers parents to be strong advocates and gain the skills needed to facilitate medical care transition.
- Parents need to learn the meta-skills of advocacy, such as when to speak up and when to listen and how to take notes, store and access their child's history, and articulate their goals and needs. If possible, the AYASHCN will gain these skills and knowledge for themselves as they mature.
- Families and AYASHCN need the know-how to build a medical team and to discuss creating a medical home with the primary physician, specialists, and other medical professionals who can work together to keep the AYASHCN healthy. This coordination eases the way for families and AYASHCNs so that they know whom to call under what circumstances and what to expect from each team member.
- Families and AYASHCNs need the means to communicate a vision for their future and a sense that their future is important.
- For AYASHCNs with the potential to manage their own care, families and health-care providers must start at age 14 or younger to provide opportunities for the AYASHCN to gain the skills to manage their own care and advocate for themselves.
- For AYASHCNs who will not arrive at this level, families and health-care providers must engage with the youth to learn what level of participation they can attain and find adequate supports to take care of the areas where they cannot make decisions.
- AYASHCNs who are nonverbal need health-care professionals who understand that behavior is communication. Professionals must learn to read the actions and reactions of their patients as language; they must ask parents and others in their patients' lives to describe behaviors that reveal health concerns (see Chap. 32).
- AYASHCNs must have access to adult health professionals who are ready to learn about their medical needs, how the AYASHCN communicates, and how to engage the youth in the transition process.
- AYASHCNs must have access to adequate supports and funding as adults and a safety net for times of change and crisis.

Here are some statements about what families and AYASHCNs value in health-care providers for smooth health-care transitions:

- Families need highly informed and motivated pediatric providers, who will take the lead in medical transition; highly informed and motivated adult providers open to serving AYASHCN; and highly informed and motivated pediatric and adult professionals who are willing to work together for a smooth transition.

- Families need health-care professionals with the information required to help their patients develop the skills to manage their own care.
- There needs to be a mechanism—the time, place, and attention—for parents, AYASHCN, and providers to talk about the future and participate in meaningful transition planning.
- Planning is a process. Families and AYASHCNs learn as they go and need to ask follow-up questions and receive advice that is appropriate at different stages. Information should be provided verbally and in written format.
- We need medical homes for AYASHCNs who have complex needs.

A successful transition for AYASHCN would look like this:

- Between ages 12 and 14 years, the pediatrician would begin teaching the AYASHCN to take control of his medical needs and make medical decisions.
- By age 17, the AYASHCN would already have been introduced by his pediatrician to the adult health-care team.
- By age 18, the AYASHCN would have a primary care physician to work with specialists and help the AYASHCN make health-care decisions.
- By age 21, parents would no longer be a necessary partner in their AYASHCNs health care, except when legally established. For AYASHCN with limited ability to advocate for themselves, legal documents guiding access to information and methods to support AYASHCN health-care decision-making would be in place by age 18.

This would be perfect but we know that nothing is perfect, especially in the disability world. However, we hope that our insights into the parent perspective on health-care transition will enable care providers to strive for this ideal and find numerous ways to be flexible, accommodating, patient, and compassionate in assisting an AYASHCN transition to adulthood and receive the care they need as adults!

21 Defining Successful Transition: Pediatric Provider Perspective

Cynthia Fair, Sophie Rupp, Laura C. Hart, Ana Catalina Alvarez-Elias, Martha Perry, and Maria Ferris

Case Example

TL is an 18-year-old female with asthma that was well-controlled on an inhaled corticosteroid, though when she stopped her controller medication a year ago, she had an exacerbation that required a visit to the emergency department and admission. She doesn't see her pediatrician often but has come in today to have some forms filled out for college. She plans to see the student health clinic for her care while in school. What does successful transition look like for TL?

Current Definitions of Successful Transition

Given that adolescents and young adults with special health-care needs (AYASHCN) are now living beyond childhood, it is imperative that this population successfully moves from a pediatric to adult health-care setting [1]. The main goal of health-care transition (HCT) preparation is to secure the maximum lifelong functioning and well-being for all youth with chronic conditions, requiring a variety of services and strategies to achieve that goal. While this broad definition is from the health-care provider's perspective, what is the meaning of "successful" HCT for AYASHCN [2]?

C. Fair, L.C.S.W., M.P.H., Dr.P.H. (✉)
Department of Public Health Studies, Elon University, Elon, NC, USA
e-mail: cfair@elon.edu

S. Rupp, B.A.
Department of Public Health Studies, Elon University, Elon, NC, USA
e-mail: srupp2@elon.edu

L. C. Hart, M.D., M.P.H.
Cecil G. Sheps Center for Health Services Research, University of North Carolina at Chapel Hill, Chapel Hill, NC, USA
e-mail: laura_hart@med.unc.edu

A. C. Alvarez-Elias, M.D., M.Sc.
Hospital Infantil de Mexico Federico Gomez, Universidad Nacional Autonoma de Mexico, Mexico City, Mexico

Sick Kids, The Hospital for Sick Children, University of Toronto, Toronto, ON, Canada

M. Perry, M.D.
General Pediatrics and Adolescent Medicine, University of North Carolina at Chapel Hill, Chapel Hill, NC, USA
e-mail: mfperry@med.unc.edu

M. Ferris, M.D., M.P.H., Ph.D.
Healthcare Transition Program, University of North Carolina at Chapel Hill, Chapel Hill, NC, USA
e-mail: maria_ferris@med.unc.edu

A. C. Hergenroeder, C. M. Wiemann (eds.), *Health Care Transition*,
https://doi.org/10.1007/978-3-319-72868-1_21

Scholars who have studied the HCT process overwhelmingly agree that the goal of a formal HCT program is to prepare AYASHCN for transfer of care [3]. However, research on the definition of HCT reveals significant variability in what constitutes or defines a successful completion of the process. Pediatric providers have tended to create definitions of successful HCT that are narrow and process-focused. For example, one study defined successful HCT for patients with congenital heart disease as continuing in care with adult congenital heart disease team [4]. Others have suggested that successful HCT should include identifying and addressing any unmet health-care needs [5]. In the transplant literature, the focus of success has tended to be on medication adherence [6, 7].

Other literature discusses more general descriptions that can be applied to a range of chronic illnesses but often retains a focus on procedural success. Out of the ten criteria for successful transition identified by experts, four related to procedures for success, including self-management of illness, one was having a medical home, and quality of life was the highest ranked HCT outcome [8]. Another study identified not being lost to follow-up and attending all scheduled visits as the two most essential pieces of successful transitional care [9]. While there can be no doubt that these process-oriented and procedural elements are critical starting points for successful transition, a focus only on process and procedure may result in missed opportunities to adequately describe successful HCT. Successful HCT is more comprehensive than just staying in contact with providers and should be defined to reflect the comprehensive nature of transitional care.

A Broader Interpretation of Successful Health-Care Transition

Defining successful HCT is complicated, as the process involves not just the medical aspects of their lives but also the developmental, psychosocial, environmental, and cultural aspects that impact the way AYASHCN manage their chronic condition. The psychosocial aspects that affect behavior in AYASHCN include five main areas: control, emotional reactions, acceptance, coping strategies, and search of meaning [3]. Formal investigation made by Olsson et al. reports that resilient AYASHCN adjust better to their diseases, so endorsing resilience builds self-esteem and the acceptance of their condition [10].

The elements that go into a broader definition of successful HCT can be challenging to identify for several reasons. First, pediatric primary care providers care for patients with a wide variety of conditions. Consequently, they must consider the responsibilities an individual must take on to manage their own care, which will depend upon the demands of treatment regimen and a patient's physical and cognitive ability for independence. This means that as providers create individual HCT programs, they must adjust their expectations as patients will each contend with a variety of tasks that can vary in scope and difficulty [11]. Second, subspecialists who lead interdisciplinary teams in the care of their patients need to educate their patients about their condition with interventions that account for level of development and cognition to overcome deficits. Providers, youth, and families have to envision the process in three main areas: envisioning the future, the moment or age to learn responsibility, and the stage of transition [12].

Additionally, many providers confront the challenge of determining when AYASHCN should begin to transition and how to pace a patient's progression toward independence. For example, despite recommendations stating that HCT preparation should start around the age of 12, a majority of pediatricians feel that HCT should start around the age of 18 or near the time of transfer [13, 14]. Although several other scholars have outlined general age ranges associated with stages of the HCT process (e.g., [3, 15]), these can only be taken as broad guidelines. In reality, a patient's ability to enter an adult care setting and take on self-management tasks depends upon their maturity, cognitive functionality, abstract reasoning ability, and personal development, traits that may not be uniformly associated with chronologic age [16]. In addition, patients' experiences moving between medical settings can be greatly influenced by environmental factors including their cultural background, language fluency, literacy, health literacy, socioeconomic status, familial stability, and parental education levels [17].

Overall, providers must view their patients as multifaceted, taking into account the characteristics of their illness as well as the unique traits that define their personality, and yet understand the indicators that are ubiquitous across all successful transitions. What are those generic indicators, and how should providers attend to them? Within the definitions of effective HCT processes, several consistent ones have emerged: behavioral indicators, level of knowledge and skills, psychosocial indicators, and measures of disease control (e.g., [8, 9, 18, 19]). See Table 21.1 for examples of each indicator.

Behavioral Indicators

There are multiple self-management tasks that AYASHCN must learn to complete in order to successfully transition to adult care. At the basic level, attending adult clinic appointments is a first step in determining whether a transition was successful [20]. Other aspects of self-management include the ability to refill and pick up prescriptions and communicate with medical professionals. Securing a medical home is another important aspect of HCT, which may be made more complex by the lack of available adult care providers and changes in insurance status as AYA mature. While the importance of these has been described, providers must think beyond this level to other indicators.

Table 21.1 Pediatric provider perceptions of indicators of successful health-care transition

Behavioral	Measuring level of knowledge and skill for HCT and self-management	Psychosocial	Measures of disease control
AYASCHN can: – Refill prescriptions – Manage appointment schedule and shows up on time – Adhere to medications and diet restrictions – Attend appointments without parents – Live independently – Secure a medical (health) home – Prepare questions for doctors, nurses, and therapists – Communicate with clinicians – Take responsibilities for self-management tasks	AYASCHN have: – Awareness of medical records – Understanding of names and purposes of medications and when to take them – Understanding of access and use of insurance – Understanding of reproductive health – Knowledge of diagnosis/prognosis complications – Understanding of characteristics of conditions and complications – Understanding of how disease will affect their future (see Chap. 13 for description of transition readiness assessment instruments)	AYASCHN: – Establish key aspects of identity – Create social network of friends and peer relationships – Develop complex thinking skills – Pursue educational and vocational endeavors – Achieve optimal quality of life – Satisfaction with transition process	Clinical biomarkers: – FEV1 – HbA1c – Viral load – Mortality – Comorbidities – Graft failure – Immunosuppressant levels Patient-reported measures: – PHQ-9 (measure of depression) – RCADS (measure of depression, anxiety and phobias) – Crohn's disease activity index – Juvenile arthritis activity score – SLEDAI score

Level of Knowledge and Skills

AYASHCN must have a solid understanding of their disease and medications as well as possible limitations their illness may place on future educational/vocational options and effects on sexual and reproductive health [6, 21]. Further, as they mature into adulthood, AYASHCN must know when symptoms require the attention of a medical provider and how to access care.

Level of knowledge and skills can be formally monitored by using structured HCT surveys such as the TR_xANSITION Index™ (formerly known as the TR_xANSITION Score), a provider administered tool to verify HCT skill mastery (English and Spanish version, youth and parent versions) [22, 23], the self-administered STARx Questionnaire English and Spanish version, youth and parent versions [24, 25], or the TRAQ [26]. These tools can be administered annually to track progress. See Chap. 13 for additional readiness assessment tools described in greater detail.

Behavioral indicators of a successful HCT and level of disease-related knowledge require increasing levels of patient autonomy. However, there are several barriers to such independence: parental over-involvement and the physical transition from adult to pediatric care settings [27].

For many AYASHCN and their families, a significant challenge to transition is the transfer of responsibilities from parents to adolescents themselves. When patients are young, parents or primary caregivers are responsible for completing health-related tasks such as managing medications, bringing patients to appointments, communicating with providers, and handling matters related to insurance. However, as AYASHCN near adulthood, many parents worry that their adolescent will be unable to handle these responsibilities resulting in the decline of their health and lapses in treatment [27]. Some parents, who never expected to transfer responsibilities to their child, may struggle to adjust their expectations in order to accommodate the developmental maturation of their adolescent [28]. Other parents recognize the importance of promoting independence yet find it difficult to "let go," as managing their children's health needs defines them as parents [16].

Meanwhile, as adolescents mature and experience more autonomy in other areas of their life, they expect the same within health-care settings. Some may prefer to be spoken to in an adult manner by providers and other health-care professionals, while others look for greater participation in decision-making and an overall greater role in their own care [16, 29]. Providers can look for signs that patients may be willing to take on self-management tasks. However, willingness to become independent may not correspond with an adolescent's ability to do so. Some youth may become overwhelmed as they attempt to maintain their health and navigate the health-care system by themselves for the first time [30]. For this reason, some providers may recommend parents stay involved as they worry that a young patient will be unable to manage their care alone [31].

Psychosocial

Aspects of functioning that occur outside the medical setting such as employment, education, and quality of life fall under the category of psychosocial indicators. Satisfaction with the overall transition experience is another metric. Satisfaction is a necessary but insufficient component of successful HCT. AYASCHN and their families may be satisfied with the transition process yet still fail to engage in adult-oriented care. There appears to be a reciprocal relationship between psychosocial well-being and other features of an effective HCT process. Those who feel successful in other aspects of their lives are likely to have the motivation to continue to self-manage their illness [16].

AYASCHN may struggle with anxiety and depression as they strive to integrate their illness with their search for identity. Some youth may fail to prioritize their health in light of these challenges and refuse to manage their illness independently, while others simply forego care. Paine et al. [16] draw connections between self-management and psychosocial well-being stating: "This lack of motivation and goal-setting was often times attributed to underlying psychosocial difficulties or missed opportunities by the parents or providers to encourage independent ownership of disease management" (p. 6).

Some psychosocial indicators such as the assessment of and intervention to improve quality of life may be outside the purview of traditional medicine. However, integrating quality of life questions into existing medical assessment tools such as the HEADSS assessment [32] is manageable and necessary in order to provide comprehensive care to AYASHCN [33]. As medical providers ask questions about quality of life, this does not imply they will have the resources to address all concerns raised by asking such questions. Yet, it does increase the likelihood that an adolescent patient will feel heard and understood which, in turn, can improve patient-provider relationship. Consequently, high-quality patient-provider relationships are associated with positive outcomes such as improved adherence and retention in care [34].

Measures of Disease Control

Some chronic illnesses have specific biomarkers that reveal whether a patient is adhering to medication, diet, or other medical advice and can serve as an indicator of a successful HCT. For example, an undetectable viral load among HIV-infected AYA may indicate successful transition to adult care [20]. Similarly, HbA1c measurements in adolescents with type 1 diabetes can be an outcome variable to assess the success of transition to adult services [35]. In such a context, "each specialist team needs to operationalize generic [transition] principles and create condition-specific risk assessment measures of readiness for transition-sensitive outcomes" [11, p. 320].

When biomarkers are available, they can assist providers in determining whether patients are ready for transfer to adult-oriented care. Guidelines have recommended that transfer occur at a time of stability [2]. Biomarkers that are within target ranges can serve as indicators that the patient is in a time of stability when transfer is most ideally timed. The most recent biomarker levels can be sent to accepting providers as well, allowing the accepting provider to know how the patient was doing as of the last pediatric visit.

Unfortunately, not all AYASHCN illnesses are easily monitored by biomarkers. In these cases, providers will have to use other indicators to assess clinical stability. For some patients, there may be patient-reported measures of disease activity, such as the PHQ-9 for depression [36], the short Crohn's disease activity index [37], or the juvenile arthritis disease activity score [38]. When these specific scores are not available, providers can assess how the patient and family feel things are going. Providing a sense of how stable a patient is can be helpful to accepting adult providers.

Strategies to Maximize the Likelihood of a Successful HCT

Pediatric providers can use a variety of strategies which target the adolescent, their parents, and the broader environment of adult care settings to increase the likelihood of a successful HCT.

Adolescent

There is general consensus that AYASHCN should begin to take on transition tasks slowly so that HCT is a "lengthy process rather than an abrupt event" [19, p. 217] [16, 29, 31]. Principally, a gradual transfer of responsibilities can allow both young adults and their parents to comfortably adapt to the patient's independence [16]. Pediatric providers should increase direct communication with the adolescent, conduct appointments without a parent present, and allow patients to make more choices about their care. Doing so indicates to AYASHCN that they are "in charge" and allows a safe way for them to practice managing their care. This assumes that patients understand their condition and how to care for themselves [19]. Some clinicians suggest the transition to adult care should be framed as a rite of passage [39] but should not take place during other significant life transitions in order to avoid overwhelming both the patient and their parents [3].

Parents

Providers should initiate early discussions with parents about the transition process and continually explain its importance in the maturation of their young adult. Doing so will not only allow providers to set expectations regarding when patients will begin to practice specific transition tasks but will also allow parents to become accustomed to the idea of transferring care responsibilities [39]. Providers need not completely exclude parents and families from taking part in their child's health care but rather must emphasize limited participation [31]. It can be difficult to navigate patient-parent relationships to ensure that both parents and their children are comfortable, as research suggests that parents and teens have different expectations and views on the transition to adult health care [40]. By engaging in conversations with patients and parents, providers can gain a greater understanding of how the family interprets the illness and what expectations they hold for the HCT process [3].

Broader Environment

Several differences between the pediatric and adult care settings may contribute to a difficult transition (see Chaps. 15, 16, and 17). Pediatric providers are perceived to "coddle" their patients and "everything is arranged" [29, p. 826]. However, AYASHCN perceive a change in the culture of empathy within the adult setting so that a perceived lack of sensitivity and feeling unable to ask questions leads to anxiety and feelings of abandonment [11, 39, 41]. In order to promote a smooth transition, pediatric providers can coordinate with adult providers through in-person visits. Such visits will allow the adolescent to meet new providers, assess their compatibility [19], and help establish the basis for a new relationship [16, 39]. Pediatric providers can also continue to be available to patients and adult providers after the first visit in an adult-oriented care setting.

In addition, it is crucial that pediatric providers ensure that medical records are adequately transferred and that the patient has a copy [16]. Along with the transfer of medical records, pediatric providers can write a transfer-of-care letter with relevant medical and psychosocial information [3]. Ideally, the pediatric provider transmits information to an adult provider through the use of electronic medical records [16]. However, differences in electronic medical record platforms can cause delays in information transfer.

Interface Between Primary Care Provider and Specialist

Pediatric primary care providers and specialists will each have their unique considerations in defining successful HCT. As the provider who does well-child checks, primary care pediatricians are positioned to consider the big picture for patients beyond their chronic health condition, including educational, social, and vocational success. The Bright Futures guidelines [42] recommend a global assessment of health with consideration to these other domains, and tools like the HEADSS exam [43] build that assessment into an adolescent well-child check. By bringing these tools to at least one visit a year for adolescents with chronic illness, the primary care pediatrician can help ensure that the needs an adolescent has beyond their illness get addressed. While specialists will certainly incorporate family concerns and needs into the treatment plan, they may not be as well versed in the general needs of all adolescents. For this reason, a specialist may be more focused on and better suited to addressing disease management.

How these two approaches interact to ensure transition gets addressed will depend on the needs of the adolescent, particularly on whether they see their primary care doctor or specialist more often. For patients who are seen primarily by their primary care provider, addressing transition becomes a function of annual checkups and periodic disease management visits, where pediatricians can work with patients and families on various needs that arise over time. The major coordination required around the time of transfer consists of knowing family practice and internal medicine primary care physicians in the area and communicating with those providers before and after transferring patients to ensure all questions and needs have been addressed.

For patients who primarily see only their specialists, such as patients with a transplant who see a transplant team frequently, the coordination of transition becomes more complicated. For example, pediatric transplant teams tend to be more involved in intervisit care and will provide more frequent reminders to patients and families about health-care tasks that need to be completed than will the adult-oriented transplant teams. Since adult-oriented transplant teams are less involved, a patient leaving a pediatric team and moving to an adult-oriented one may benefit from having a primary care doctor on the adult side who is more involved than the pediatric PCP had been. However, this scenario raises the question: Who's in charge? If a patient is only going to transplant appointments, then it is difficult for the pediatric PCP to take the lead, and in fact, pediatric transplant teams may have already incorporated processes to address transitional care needs into the transplant appointments for adolescents and young adults. However, the pediatric transplant team is unlikely to be familiar with the options for adult-oriented primary care. In these scenarios, pediatric specialists may need to take the lead but may also want to reach out to the pediatric PCPs as a way to ensure that all aspects of a patient's care are transferred, not just those that the specialist tends to focus on.

Most complicated are those patients who see multiple pediatric specialists, such that no specialist is really the "main" doctor. For patients like this in a well-resourced patient-centered medical home, the medical home can serve not only as the central hub for care in the present but also for assisting with transition and moving to adult-oriented care. The care coordination and provider communication involved in this scenario can be extensive, and pediatric providers may feel overwhelmed by the prospect of establishing a network of trusted providers in adult-oriented care. However, this may not be necessary if there are adult-oriented patient-centered medical homes in the vicinity. While the services in an adult-oriented patient-centered medical home are not always as extensive as those in the pediatric world, these types of clinics are more comfortable with providing care coordination and may also manage some chronic problems on their own. For patients like this who are not in a patient-centered medical home, the patient or family may have identified a doctor who they feel is in charge. Pediatric primary care and specialist providers may want to ask patients and families who they feel is in charge. Ideally, this person would then provide the main assistance to families as they transition. Other providers on the care team may need to offer more support than would be required for patients who are being seen in patient-centered medical homes.

Pediatric primary care providers and specialists are also likely to approach addressing the psychosocial aspects of successful transition differently. Because many patients have educational needs, pediatricians tend to be more familiar with the educational resources available than specialists. On the other hand, specialists may be more familiar with the resources available to patients with specific illnesses. For example, a primary care pediatrician may have a better understanding of the accommodations that can be made in a 504 plan for a teenager with arthritis, but a rheumatologist will be more familiar with the support groups that have been organized by the Juvenile Arthritis Association. In this case both providers have contributions to make to maximize the teenager's psychosocial functioning.

In summary, primary care pediatricians and specialists bring different and important skills to addressing transition and ensuring successful transition for patients. The exact role for each provider will depend on the needs of the patient, and we encourage providers to understand and address those needs to ensure successful transition for the patients that they see.

Returning to the Case Example

As a refresher, TL is an 18-year-old with asthma well-controlled on an inhaled corticosteroid, who plans to go to the student health clinic for care once she starts college. She came to what was likely her last visit with her pediatrician to have medical forms filled out for college.

If one focused merely on a procedural definition of successful transition for TL, her forms would get completed as she has requested, the last visit note would be sent to the student health clinic, and TL would be encouraged to make an appointment as soon as she could after starting school. However, what if TL doesn't know how to refill her medications? What if the student clinic won't send a refill to the pharmacy before she is seen there and she runs out? Does TL have her insurance card with her? Is her insurance card accepted at the student health clinic? What if she goes to the first appointment at the student health clinic but doesn't like the providers there and never goes back?

With a broader definition of transition success, many of these questions would be addressed well in advance of TL leaving for school. Her provider would see her for periodic visits to assess her asthma control and would use those visits to address other needs, like ensuring she understands the difference between her controller and rescue inhalers, knows how to order refills, and can navigate a visit with a doctor on her own.

In addition, at the last visit, the pediatrician would have a transfer letter ready, and the patient would be given a copy in addition to the letter being sent to the new provider. This way, she has the tools and information to seek a different adult provider if need be. Finally, the pediatrician would follow-up with the patient and/or the accepting provider to ensure no new issues have come up during the transfer. This can serve not only as an additional means of ensuring patients are staying in care but also an opportunity to address any learning or psychosocial issues that were incompletely addressed previously. Thus, with a broader definition of transition success in mind, the pediatrician takes a more comprehensive approach to transitional care of the patient and helps to address potential pitfalls for patients before they occur.

References

1. Oswald DP, Gilles DL, Cannady MS, Wenzel DB, Willis JH, Bodurtha JN. Youth with special health care needs: transition to adult health care services. Matern Child Health J. 2013;17(10):1744–52. https://doi.org/10.1007/s10995-012-1192-7.
2. Cooley WC, Sagerman PJ, American College of Physicians, Transitions Clinical Report Authoring Group. Supporting the health care transition from adolescence to adulthood in the medical home. Pediatrics. 2011;128(1):182–200. https://doi.org/10.1542/peds.2011-0969.
3. Sable C, Foster E, Uzark K, Bjornsen K, Canobbio MM, Connolly HM, et al. Best practices in managing transition to adulthood for adolescents with congenital heart disease: the transition process and medical and psychosocial issues. Circulation. 2011;123(13):1454–85. https://doi.org/10.1161/CIR.0b013e3182107c56.
4. Jalkut MK, Allen PJ. Transition from pediatric to adult health care for adolescents with congenital heart disease: a review of the literature and clinical implications. Pediatr Nurs. 2009;35(6):381–7.
5. Sawyer SM, Macnee S. Transition to adult health care for adolescents with spina bifida: research issues. Dev Disabil Res Rev. 2010;16(1):60–5. https://doi.org/10.1002/ddrr.98/.
6. Fredericks EM, Dore-Stites D, Well A, Magee JC, Freed GL, Shieck V, et al. Assessment of transition readiness skills and adherence in pediatric liver transplant recipients. Pediatr Transplant. 2010;14(8):944–53. https://doi.org/10.1111/j.1399-3046.2010.01349.x.
7. Pai A, Ingerski L, Perazzo L, Ramey C, Bonner M, Goebel J. Preparing for transition? The allocation of oral medication regimen tasks in adolescents with renal transplants. Pediatr Transplant. 2011;15(1):9–16. https://doi.org/10.1111/j.1399-3046.2010.01369.x.
8. Fair C, Cuttance J, Sharma N, Maslow G, Wiener L, Betz C, et al. International and interdisciplinary identification of health care transition outcomes. JAMA Pediatr. 2016;170(3):205–11. https://doi.org/10.1001/jamapediatrics.2015.3168.
9. Suris JC, Akre C. Key elements for, and indicators of, a successful transition: an international Delphi study. J Adolesc Health. 2015;56(6):612–8. https://doi.org/10.1016/j.jadohealth.2015.02.007.
10. Olsson CA, Bond L, Johnson MW, Forer DL, Boyce MF, Sawyer SM. Adolescent chronic illness: a qualitative study of psychosocial adjustment. Ann Acad Med Singap. 2003;32(1):43–50.
11. Rapley P, Davidson P. Enough of the problem: a review of time for health care transition solutions for young adults with a chronic

illness. J Clin Nurs. 2010;19(3–4):313–23. https://doi.org/10.1111/j.1365-2702.2009.03027.x.
12. Reiss JG, Gibson RW, Walker LR. Health care transition: youth, family, and provider perspectives. Pediatrics. 2005;115(1):112–20. https://doi.org/10.1542/peds.2004-1321.
13. American Academy of Pediatrics, Clinical Report. Supporting the health care transition from adolescence to adulthood in the medical home. Pediatrics. 2011;128(1):182–200.
14. Burke R, Spoerri M, Price A, Cardosi A, Flanagan P. Survey of primary care pediatricians on the transition and transfer of adolescents to adult health care. Clin Pediatr (Phila). 2008;47(4):347–54.
15. Fair CD, Sullivan K, Gatto A. Best practices in transitioning youth with HIV: perspectives of pediatric and adult infectious disease care providers. Psychol Health Med. 2010;15(5):515–27. https://doi.org/10.1080/13548506.2010.493944.
16. Paine CW, Stollon NB, Lucas MS, Brumley LD, Poole ES, Peyton T, et al. Barriers and facilitators to successful transition from pediatric to adult inflammatory bowel disease care from the perspectives of providers. Inflamm Bowel Dis. 2014;20(11):2083. https://doi.org/10.1097/MIB.0000000000000136.
17. Lotstein DS, McPherson M, Strickland B, Newacheck PW. Transition planning for youth with special health care needs: results from the National Survey of Children with Special Health Care Needs. Pediatrics. 2005;115(6):1562–8. https://doi.org/10.1542/peds.2004-1262.
18. Betz CL, Ferris ME, Woodward JF, Okumura MJ, Jan S, Wood DL. The health care transition research consortium health care transition model: a framework for research and practice. J Pediatr Rehabil Med. 2014;7(1):3–15. https://doi.org/10.3233/PRM-140277.
19. Bloom SR, Kuhlthau K, Van Cleave J, Knapp AA, Newacheck P, Perrin JM. Health care transition for youth with special health care needs. J Adolesc Health. 2012;51(3):213–9. https://doi.org/10.1016/j.jadohealth.2012.01.007.
20. Fair CD, Sullivan K, Gatto A. Indicators of transition success for youth living with HIV: perspectives of pediatric and adult infectious disease care providers. AIDS Care. 2011;23(8):965–70. https://doi.org/10.1080/09540121.2010.542449.
21. Sawicki GS, Lukens-Bull K, Yin X, Demars N, Huang IC, Livingood W, et al. Measuring the transition readiness of youth with special healthcare needs: validation of the TRAQ—Transition Readiness Assessment Questionnaire. J Pediatr Psychol. 2009;36(2):160–71. https://doi.org/10.1093/jpepsy/jsp128.
22. Cantú-Quintanilla G, Ferris M, Otero A, Gutiérrez-Almaraz A, Valverde-Rosas S, Velázquez-Jones L, et al. Validation of the UNC TR x ANSITION scale™ version 3 among Mexican adolescents with chronic kidney disease. J Pediatr Nurs. 2015;30(5):e71–81. https://doi.org/10.1016/j.pedn.2015.06.011.
23. Ferris ME, Harward DH, Bickford K, Layton JB, Ferris MT, Hogan SL, et al. A clinical tool to measure the components of health-care transition from pediatric care to adult care: the UNC TRxANSITION scale. Ren Fail. 2012;34(6):744–53.
24. Ferris M, Cohen S, Haberman C, Javalkar K, Massengill S, Mahan JD, Bickford K, Cantu G, Medeiros M, Phillips A, Ferris MT, Hooper SR. Self-management and transition-readiness assessment: development, reliability, and factor structure of the STARx questionnaire. J Pediatr Nurs. 2015;30(5):691–699. pii: S0882-5963(15)00153-0. https://doi.org/10.1016/j.pedn.2015.05.009.
25. Cohen SE, Hooper SR, Javalkar K, Haberman C, Fenton N, Lai H, Mahan JD, Massengill S, Kelly M, Cantú G, Medeiros M. Self-management and transition readiness assessment: concurrent, predictive and discriminant validation of the STAR x questionnaire. J Pediatr Nurs. 2015;30(5):668–76. https://doi.org/10.1016/j.pedn.2015.05.006.
26. Wood DL, Sawicki GS, Miller MD, Smotherman C, Lukens-Bull K, Livingood WC, et al. The Transition Readiness Assessment Questionnaire (TRAQ): its factor structure, reliability, and validity. Acad Pediatr. 2014;14(4):415–22. https://doi.org/10.1016/j.acap.2014.03.008.
27. Rehm RS, Fuentes-Afflick E, Fisher LT, Chesla CA. Parent and youth priorities during the transition to adulthood for youth with special health care needs and developmental disability. ANS Adv Nurs Sci. 2012;35(3):E57. https://doi.org/10.1097/ANS.0b013e3182626180.
28. Cheak-Zamora NC, Farmer JE, Mayfield WA, Clark MJ, Marvin AR, Law JK, et al. Health care transition services for youth with autism spectrum disorders. Rehabil Psychol. 2014;59(3):340. https://doi.org/10.1037/a0036725.
29. van Staa A, van der Stege HA, Jedeloo S, Moll HA, Hilberink SR. Readiness to transfer to adult care of adolescents with chronic conditions: exploration of associated factors. J Adolesc Health. 2011;48(3):295–302. https://doi.org/10.1016/j.jadohealth.2010.07.009.
30. Soanes C, Timmons S. Improving transition: a qualitative study examining the attitudes of young people with chronic illness transferring to adult care. J Child Health Care. 2004;8(2):102–12. https://doi.org/10.1177/1367493504041868.
31. Peter NG, Forke CM, Ginsburg KR, Schwarz DF. Transition from pediatric to adult care: internists' perspectives. Pediatrics. 2009;123(2):417–23. https://doi.org/10.1542/peds.2008-0740.
32. Goldenring JM, Cohen E. Getting into adolescents' heads. Contemp Pediatr. 1988;5:75–90.
33. Scal P. Improving health care transition services: just grow up, will you please. JAMA Pediatr. 2016;170(3):197–9. https://doi.org/10.1001/jamapediatrics.2015.3268.
34. Taddeo D, Egedy M, Frappier JY. Adherence to treatment in adolescents. Paediatr Child

Health. 2008;13(1):19–24. https://doi.org/10.1093/pch/13.1.19.
35. Kipps S, Bahu T, Ong K, Ackland FM, Brown RS, Fox CT, et al. Current methods of transfer of young people with type 1 diabetes to adult services. Diabet Med. 2002;19(8):649–54. https://doi.org/10.1046/j.1464-5491.2002.00757.x.
36. Richardson LP, McCauley E, Grossman DC, McCarty CA, Richards J, Russo JE, Rockhill C, Katon W. Evaluation of the patient health Questionnaire-9 item for detecting major depression among adolescents. Pediatrics. 2010;126(6):1117–23. https://doi.org/10.1542/peds.2010-0852.
37. Hyams JS, Ferry GD, Mandel FS, Gryboski JD, Kibort PM, Kirschner BS, et al. Development and validation of a pediatric Crohn's disease activity index. J Pediatr Gastroenterol Nutr. 1991;12(4):449.
38. Consolaro A, Ruperto N, Bazso A, Pistorio A, Magni-Manzoni S, Filocamo G, Malattia C, Viola S, Martini A, Ravelli A, Paediatric Rheumatology International Trials Organisation. Development and validation of a composite disease activity score for juvenile idiopathic arthritis. Arthritis Rheum. 2009;61(5):658–66. https://doi.org/10.1002/art.24516.
39. Lugasi T, Achille M, Stevenson M. Patients' perspective on factors that facilitate transition from child-centered to adult-centered health care: a theory integrated metasummary of quantitative and qualitative studies. J Adolesc Health. 2011;48(5):429–40. https://doi.org/10.1016/j.jadohealth.2010.10.016.
40. Fair CD, Goldstein B, Dizney R. Congruence of transition perspectives between adolescents with perinatally-acquired HIV and their guardians: an exploratory qualitative study. J Pediatr Nurs. 2015;30(5):684–90. https://doi.org/10.1016/j.pedn.2015.06.001.
41. Schwartz LA, Daniel LC, Brumley LD, Barakat LP, Wesley KM, Tuchman LK. Measures of readiness to transition to adult health care for youth with chronic physical health conditions: a systematic review and recommendations for measurement testing and development. J Pediatr Psychol. 2014;39(6):588–601. https://doi.org/10.1093/jpepsy/jsu028.
42. Hagan JF, Shaw JS, Duncan PM. Bright futures: guidelines. 3rd ed. Elk Grove Village: American Academy of Pediatrics; 2007.
43. Katzenellenbogen R. HEADSS: the 'Review of Systems' for adolescents. Virtual Mentor. 2005; 7(3):1–2.

22 Defining Successful Transition: Adult Provider Perspective

Gregg Talente

Vignette

MR is a 23-year-old Hispanic female. She was diagnosed with lupus at the age of 12. She is coming today for an appointment with her primary care physician to discuss reproductive health issues. She married a year ago and has decided to have a child. She had previously discussed this with her primary care provider on a couple of occasions but had not decided what she wanted to do, and those discussions focused on the medical risks of pregnancy and the financial costs since she has limited insurance coverage. She has seen the same primary care provider at the internal medicine clinic for the last 3 years since transitioning from her pediatric clinic along with the clinic pharmacist who manages the clinic's Anticoagulation Clinic. In childhood her lupus was complicated by nephritis and problems with clotting in addition to skin and joint symptoms. She was hospitalized numerous times, and early on her disease was difficult to control. For the last 5 years, her lupus has been under control. She takes Plaquenil and low-dose prednisone. She has been maintained on warfarin due to her history of clotting and antiphospholipid antibody syndrome. Her doctor and the clinic pharmacist who she has good relationships with have been objective with her about the gravity of this decision. She appreciates the open discussions with them even though they have recommended against this decision. She knows that she may not be able to sustain a pregnancy due to her illness and that even if she can, there are other risks. Because of these discussions, she has taken birth control regularly since she became sexually active. The one thing that everyone agreed on was if she was to consider pregnancy, it needed to be planned and prepared for. At the suggestion of her primary care provider, she has also discussed this with the adult rheumatologist who she has been seeing since she transitioned to the internal medicine clinic. Feeling that she understands the risks and costs, today, she wants to discuss coming off of her birth control and transitioning from warfarin to low molecular weight heparin for management of her clotting. The latter step had been a barrier to this decision. She was told that the switch to the low molecular weight heparin was necessary, but unfortunately she doesn't have insurance coverage to pay for this. She pays for her medications in cash. Her regular medications aren't too expensive. She and her husband have had to save to be able to afford to pay for the injectable heparin. Having worked that out, she has made up her mind.

G. Talente, M.D., M.S.
Department of Medicine and Pediatrics, University of South Carolina School of Medicine,
Columbia, SC, USA
e-mail: Gregg.Talente@uscmed.sc.edu

A. C. Hergenroeder, C. M. Wiemann (eds.), *Health Care Transition*,
https://doi.org/10.1007/978-3-319-72868-1_22

When thinking about a completed and successful transition, the above vignette has many of the characteristics one would hope for, a mature young woman who has transitioned not only from a pediatric to an adult health-care setting but in life as well. She is working, married, and making decisions about her life, her finances, and her health. In the 2002 AAP, ACP, and AAFP consensus statement, the goal of transition was to "maximize lifelong functioning and potential through the provision of high quality, developmentally appropriate health care services that continue uninterrupted as the individual moves from adolescence to adulthood" [1]. MR seems to have achieved this. She has a trusting, continuous relationship with a primary care medical home and a primary care team. She has adult subspecialty care that is working well with her medical home and her to manage her health and meet her goals, she has an understanding of her illness that allows her to make autonomous decisions about her care goals, and not only is her lupus, the condition she has had since childhood, being well managed, she is also getting care for all of her adult health needs. This contrasts greatly with the status of MR at the time of her first visit with her adult primary care provider.

At age 19, MR presented for the first time to establish care with a new internal medicine clinic. MR had been followed for the past 6 years in an academic general pediatric clinic by a single pediatrician. She had received specialty care from a pediatric nephrologist and had intermittently seen a pediatric rheumatologist who had clinic in the community once a week but resided in a nearby city. Her lupus was under good control. She was taking prednisone, Plaquenil, and warfarin as she would be a few years later. The transition had been necessary because her primary care pediatrician moved out of the state. When she knew she was leaving, she had arranged for MR to meet once with a med/peds trained colleague to talk about the internal medicine clinic. Prior to this there had been little discussion about transition. Over the first few months at the internal medicine clinic, her new primary care provider and the pharmacist who ran the Anticoagulation Clinic that would manage her warfarin noted that MR was only intermittently adherent mostly due to lack of understanding about her condition and medications. The pediatric office had always reminded her when she needed to come get her INR checks or had appointments or if she forgot to refill her medications. It was also noted that she was getting her medications through a charitable program affiliated with the children's hospital that was supposed to stop at age 18 but had been allowed to continue for her at least temporarily. MR was quiet and reserved and rarely questioned the recommendations of her new care team at the adult clinic.

The difference between MR when she first transitioned to her new adult primary care provider and the MR who presented 3 years later makes it clear that for adult providers, as it is for patients and their families, a successful transition for AYASHCN has not occurred just because a patient kept several appointments with an adult provider. To view transition as successful, adult providers have greater expectations. This is not surprising. The guidelines for transition make it clear that the work of transition is not finished after a patient establishes with a general internist, family practitioner, or adult subspecialist [2]. As outlined in more detail in Chaps. 7 and 18, there are a series of steps required of adult providers and patients and families after the initial appointment. In general, adult providers should assess and further help develop patient self-management skills and maintain communication with pediatric providers to ensure transition of records and seamless care and to close the loop on the transition, and, finally, adult providers need to facilitate any other transition tasks including vocational and social transitions [2].

So what makes for a successful transition for an AYASHCN from the perspective of an adult provider? The simplest way to understand this is to look at the factors that increase adult provider satisfaction with any patient-physician relationship. Because while AYASHCN present a unique challenge for adult providers at the time of transition, adult providers' goals for these relationships are not different from their goals for relationships with other patients. There may be additional goals surrounding the unique needs and challenges of AYASHCN, but overall what an adult provider would want in a successful transition would be a continuous relationship built on good rapport and trust [3].

Trust and rapport are probably the most important factors in both a good patient-physician relationship and a successful transition. Patients and providers have better care experiences when trust and rapport are strong [4–6]. Moreover, patients have less anxiety and greater involvement in decisions when they have trust in their providers [4–6].

Table 22.1 lists factors that increase or are barriers to physician satisfaction with patient relationships and encounters and the factors that decrease physician satisfaction as well. Continuity of care has been consistently cited as important to providers [7, 8]. Access to health records and the information needed to care for patients has also been shown to be important [7, 9]. Team-based care and the ability to delegate tasks or share responsibility with ancillary staff in the care of complex patients have also been shown to improve physician satisfaction [8, 9]. Having adequate time with patients is valued by providers [8]. Many of these factors are not just important to providers. Patients share similar views of what makes for a good patient-physician encounter and relationship [8].

Just as having more time with patients is seen by providers as desirable, not having enough time with their patients and time pressures in general are barriers to provider satisfaction with their patient relationships [10–16]. Similarly, just as continuity of care is valued, an inability to maintain an ongoing relationship is seen as a barrier to a satisfying relationship [13–16]. Along with time pressures, increased administrative burdens in providing care increase provider frustration [17]. Physicians find patient encounters and relationships less satisfying when they feel that they lack control and the ability to make decisions [7, 17]. This can be due to patient factors such as a disagreement with the provider or nonadherence, system factors such as insurance barriers, or poor interactions with other providers such as specialists that the patient is seeing. Providers are more dissatisfied when they cannot obtain the services that they feel are needed for their patients [13–16]. Providers find certain types of patients more difficult. Patients with somatic complaints and no identified organic etiology, increased symptom severity, and lower levels of function due to either physical, emotional, or social factors are rated as more difficult or challenging [18]. Patients with complex psychosocial problems and patients with mental health issues are associated with greater physician dissatisfaction [17].

Table 22.1 Provider perspectives on factors impacting patient-physician relationships and provider satisfaction

Factors in a good patient-physician relationship	Barriers to a good patient-physician relationship
Trust and rapport	Time pressures
Continuity of care	Lack of continuity
Access to medical records and patient information	Administrative burdens
Patient adherence	Lack of control
Team-based care	Inability to obtain needed services for the patient
More time spent with patients	Patients with somatic complaints
	Patients with complex psychosocial needs
	Patients with decreased function and capacity

Research into the internists' role in the transition of AYASHCN reported that they lack time to provide ideal care, lack needed support staff, and lack institutional and health system support for resources and reimbursement [19]. In other words, they do not always have what they need to move a newly transitioned young adult from where they are when they first present to where they should be to consider the transition successful. The issues that adult providers identify as barriers to successful transition are listed in Table 22.2. Many of these issues are the same as the factors that impact all of their patient-physician relationships. A few are different. Concern that they lack the training to manage young adult patients is an issue specific to transitioning patients. Too much or too little family involvement and patient immaturity during this unique adolescent to young adult transition

Table 22.2 Factors impeding transitions from the adult provider perspective [20]

Physician competency and availability
Lack of training in the care of adolescents
Lack of training in the conditions of transitioning young adults
Lack of access to needed subspecialists
Patient psychosocial needs
Family issues
High expectations
Too little support for patients who need help from their families
Too much involvement for patients that do not need it
Patient immaturity
Patients are not prepared to take responsibility for their health needs
Dependency on past relationships
Patients are closed-minded to new approaches
System issues
Lack of insurance
Lack of time to meet the patient's needs
Transition coordination issues
Inadequate transfer of records
Issues with transitioning specialist care

period are two issues that have been discussed as impacting the patient-physician relationship.

So in the eyes of an adult provider, a successful transition for an AYASHCN would be one that has addressed or minimized the factors that inhibit a good patient-physician relationship and has achieved the factors that are valued by the adult provider in all of their patient interactions. Not surprisingly, when one considers the barriers to successful transition as outlined in detail in Chap. 7 and more briefly in Table 22.2 and the process for achieving a successful transition as outlined in Chap. 18, all of the factors listed above, both good and bad, are what a good transition process is designed to address. Trust and report are more likley to develop when AYASHCN receive transition preparation from an early age, have an organized agreed upon transition plan, and have been oriented to the adult health-care practice, trust and rapport with the new adult provider are more likely to occur. Achieving the steps in the previous sentence is helpful in increasing the young adult's or their caregiver's ability to function within the adult health-care environment which is associated with better patient and physician satisfaction [18]. Portable medical summaries and good communication between pediatric and adult providers are intended to insure the adult provider has access to the information he/she needs. Care coordination before and after transition [2] is helpful in addressing administrative issues, eliminating barriers to care and barriers to obtaining services for newly transitioned young adults, and fostering the team-based approach to care that adult providers find useful in caring for all of their patients, especially those that are most complex.

A successful transition process is one that, using whatever tools and resources are available, not only moves the AYASHCN into an adult practice but moves that patient into a relationship with an adult health-care team that is satisfying to both the patient and the care team. Looking back at our vignettes, this is the difference between MR at her first visit and MR at the visit 3 years later. She still has complex care needs, issues with access to care and insurance, and significant health issues. The biggest difference is that she was a mature active participant in her care and decision-making and she has a trusting relationship with the adult care team.

One issue that is critical to a successful transition for AYASHCN is the subspecialty needs of AYASHCN and a strong, highly functioning interface between the patient, their adult primary care team, and the subspecialty practices. One factor that adult providers find to be a barrier to good patient-physician relationships is a lack of control. This does not mean control over the patient. Rather it refers to interference in the patient-physician relationship by external factors. Systems-based interference such as insurance limitations to shared decision-making and care is one example. Fractured care among the primary care team and specialists is another way the patient-physician relationship can be disrupted [21]. Lack of partnering with subspecialists was identified by adult providers as a barrier to successful transition for AYASHCN [20].

So how is the correct relationship between the patient, the primary care team, and all of the subspecialists involved in the care of AYASHCN achieved during and after transition? Depending on the patient's condition, AYASHCN often have multiple specialists, frequently require care from specialists that the adult primary provider does not typically work with, or may receive some of their ongoing care from a pediatric subspecialist. Understanding how to achieve a successful transition requires a look at the accepted principles for primary care/subspecialty partnership that apply to all patients in the adult health-care world.

As the concept of the patient-centered medical home has come to encompass the goals and tasks that primary care providers are charged with fulfilling in the care of all patients, especially patients with chronic conditions, and transitioning young adults [2], it became necessary to define the role of the subspecialist in relation to the evolving primary care paradigm. The American College of Physicians as part of their high-value care initiative attempted to do that. They outlined the ideal components of the primary care-subspecialty partnership in a 2011 position paper [22]. The main principles that should guide subspecialists in providing services and working with medical homes are listed in Table 22.3. In addition, the position statement defined types of primary care-subspecialty interactions [22]. These different interactions included informal exchange of information, formal consultation for a specific question, comanagement, and transfer of care. An overriding principle was the need for the scope and type of interaction to be clear to all involved.

Table 22.3 Characteristics of ideal subspecialty practice in partnering with a primary care medical home (PCMH) [22]

Effective communication and coordination with the PCMH
Timely consults and delivery of requested services
Efficient and effective flow of information between all of the patient's providers
Effective determination of each specialty and primary care practice's responsibilities toward the patient
Patient-centered, high-quality care
Support for the PCMH practice as the provider having overall responsibility for care coordination and care integration along with the patients primary care needs

In the 2011 position statement of the AAP, AAFP, and ACP regarding best practices for the care of AYASHCN as they transition from pediatric to adult health-care settings, similar goals for the interaction between the medical home and subspecialty practices were recommended [2]. Good communication between providers and clearly defined roles in the care of the patient were the two most important factors [2]. Application of the principles outlined by the ACP for ideal partnership between a patient's medical home and their subspecialists would ensure better, more coordinated, and more satisfactory care for patients and providers. Adherence to these principles also reduces the need for subspecialists and adult primary care providers to have a pre-existing relationship which, as noted earlier, is sometimes a barrier for transitioning young adults who are seeing specialists with expertise different than the specialists to which most adult patients are referred. Application of these principles to ensure high-functioning collaboration between the medical home and subspecialty practices would represent an adult provider's ideal successful transition.

In summary, to an adult provider, a successful transition would be one where the patient not only is being seen and cared for by an adult primary care team but one where the care team and the patient have a trusting relationship. From this follows all the other factors that are needed to successfully care for the patient after transition, continuity, shared decision-making, and a setting where barriers to transition, to quality care, and to satisfaction for the patient, their caregivers, and the health-care team can be addressed and overcome. In a successful transition, all of the teams helping the patient with their health-care and life goals work in partnership with clearly defined roles and responsibilities. Achieving this is hard. Pathways to successful transition have been discussed earlier in this book.

There is no one pathway for successful health-care transition that applies to all AYASHCN, and this is illustrated in MR's case presented in this chapter. The desire to achieve successful health-care transition, however, is shared by all patients and adult providers.

References

1. American Academy of Pediatrics, et al. A consensus statement on health care transitions for young adults with special health care needs. Pediatrics. 2002;110:1304–6.
2. AAP, AAFP, ACP Transition Clinical Report Authoring Group. Supporting the health care transition from adolescence to adulthood in the medical home. Pediatrics. 2011;128:182.
3. Dang BN, Westbrook RA, Mjue SM, Giordano TP. Building patient trust and rapport early in the new doctor-patient relationship: a longitudinal qualitative study. BMC Med Educ. 2017;17:32.
4. Dean M, Street RL. A 3-stage model of patient-centered communication for addressing cancer patients' emotional distress. Patient Educ Couns. 2014;94(2):143–8.
5. Thorne SE, Kuo M, Armstrong E, McPherson G, Harris SR, Hislop TG. 'Being known': patients' perspectives of the dynamics of human connection in cancer care. Psychooncology. 2005;14(10):887–98.
6. Shepherd HL, Tattersall MHN, Butow PN. Physician-identified factors affecting patient participation in reaching treatment decisions. J Clin Oncol. 2008;26(10):1724–31.
7. DeVoe J, Fryer GE, Straub A, McCann J, Fairbrother G. Congruent satisfaction: is there geographic correlation between patient and physician satisfaction? Med Care. 2007;45(1):88–94.
8. Linn LS, Brook RH, Clark VA, Ross Davies A, Fink A, Kosecoff J. Physician and patient satisfaction as factors related to the organization of internal medicine group practices. Med Care. 1985;23(10):1171–8.
9. Lictenstein R. Measuring the job satisfaction of physicians in organized settings. Med Care. 1984;22(1):56–68.
10. Lipsitt DR. The challenge of the "difficult patient" (deja vu all over again--only more so). Gen Hosp Psychiatry. 1997;19:313–4.
11. Barsky AJ, Borus JF. Somatization and medicalization in the era of managed care. JAMA. 1995;274:1931–4.
12. Freidson E. Prepaid group practice and the new "demanding patient". Milbank Mem Fund Q Health Soc. 1973;51:473–88.
13. Landon BE, Reschovsky J, Blumenthal D. Changes in career satisfaction among primary care and specialist physicians, 1997–2001. JAMA. 2003;289:442–9.
14. Stoddard JJ, Hargraves JL, Reed M, et al. Managed care, professional autonomy, and income – effects on physician career satisfaction. J Gen Intern Med. 2001;16:675–84.
15. Devoe J, Fryer GE, Hargraves JL, et al. Does career dissatisfaction affect the ability of family physicians to deliver high-quality patient care? J Fam Pract. 2002;51:223–8.
16. Haas JS. Physician discontent—a barometer of change and need for intervention. J Gen Intern Med. 2001;16:496–7.
17. Krebs EE, Garrett JM, Konrad TR. The difficult doctor? Characteristics of physicians who report frustration with patients: an analysis of survey data. BMC Health Serv Res. 2006;6:128.
18. Jackson JL, Kroenke K. Difficult patient encounters in the ambulatory clinic. Arch Intern Med. 1999;159:1069–75.
19. Scal P. Transition for youth with chronic conditions: primary care physicians' approaches. Pediatrics. 2002;110:1315–21.
20. Peter NG, Forke CM, Ginsburg KR, Schwarz DF. Transition from pediatric to adult care: internists perspectives. Pediatrics. 2009;123:417–23.
21. Greer RC, Ameling JM, Cavenaugh KL, et al. Specialist and primary care physicians' views on barriers to adequate preparation of patients for renal replacement therapy: a qualitative study. BMC Nephrol. 2015;16:37.
22. The patient centered medical home neighbor, the interface of the patient centered medical home with specialty/subspecialty practices. American College of Physicians Position Paper. 2010. http://www.acponline.org/advocacy/where_we_stand/policy/pcmh_neighbors.pdf.

Defining Successful Transition: Payer Perspective

23

Angelo P. Giardino

Introduction: Payer Perspective Is Transactional

The payer perspective is fundamentally transactional in nature and rooted in the management of an insurance benefit provided to the adolescents and young adults with special health-care needs (AYASHCN). Essential to understanding this perspective are the interactions between the payer and other entities, including (1) the purchaser of the AYASHCN's benefit, (2) the health-care providers and institutions who deliver the care and services within the benefit, (3) the AYASHCN and their families, and (4) the payer's regulators (see Fig. 23.1). A key point to understanding the payer perspective is that managing a benefit to an AYASHCN means managing the dollars available to support the care and services. Over time, the transactions around benefits and cost have broadened to include a balance with the measured quality of the care and services provided. This balance of cost and quality leads to the notion of value (i.e., quality divided by cost), and discussions around value are now routinely part of the benefit management discussion.

A. P. Giardino, M.D., Ph.D.
Texas Children's Hospital, Houston, TX, USA

Academic General Pediatrics, Department of Pediatrics, Baylor College of Medicine, Houston, TX, USA
e-mail: apgiardi@texaschildrens.org

Applying the payer's transaction-based perspective to defining a successful health-care transition (HCT), the fundamental question asked by the payer organization is "How does AYASHCN transitioning from a pediatric to an adult setting make sense from either a fiscal, operational, programmatic, or fiscal standpoint?" Additionally, if AYASHCN HCT does not tangibly save money or have a significant fiscal return on investment (ROI), then what other intangible benefits can be measured that might be used to define success, for example, enhanced reputation, compliance with a government mandate, or meeting a stated expectation from the purchaser? Chapter 8 speaks about insurance options for AYASHCN. This chapter will focus more on broader, general aspects of benefit management for the population of AYASHCN at the level of the payer organization.

Understanding the payer perspective on HCT is important for AYASHCN, their health-care providers, and the advocacy community since these stakeholder groups will interact with payer organizations as they seek to influence the approach to the services and supports necessary for effective HCT. While Chap. 24 deals more specifically with financing and cost issues at a population level related to providing HCT services to AYASHCN, this chapter will focus on structural and programmatic aspects of how payers address HCT. In order to understand the payer perspective, basic issues related to how

A. C. Hergenroeder, C. M. Wiemann (eds.), *Health Care Transition*,
https://doi.org/10.1007/978-3-319-72868-1_23

Fig. 23.1 Transactional nature of the payer's role

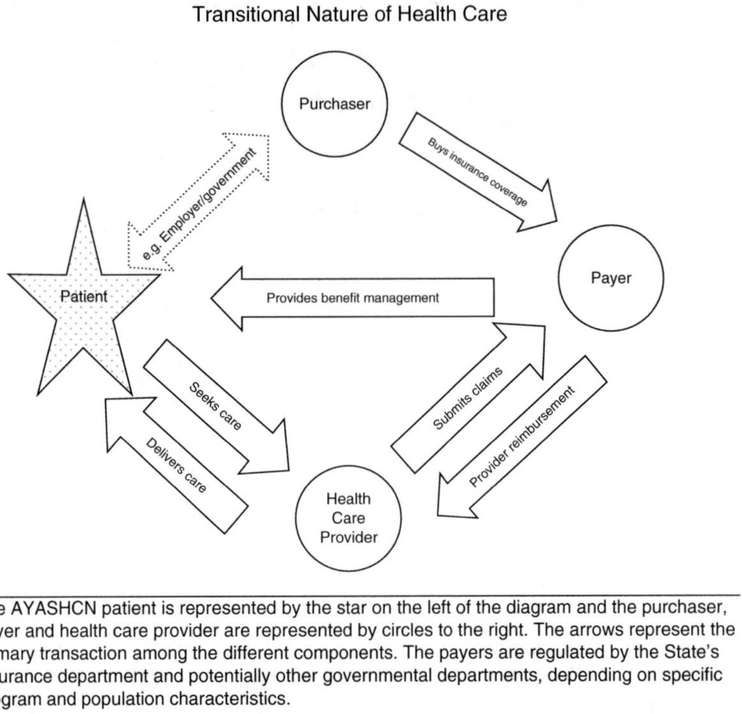
Transitional Nature of Health Care
Purchaser
Buys insurance coverage
e.g. Employer/government
Payer
Patient
Provides benefit management
Seeks care
Submits claims
Provider reimbursement
Delivers care
Health
Care
Provider
The AYASHCN patient is represented by the star on the left of the diagram and the purchaser, payer and health care provider are represented by circles to the right. The arrows represent the primary transaction among the different components. The payers are regulated by the State's insurance department and potentially other governmental departments, depending on specific program and population characteristics.

payer organizations are structured and how they operate are described next.

Payer Basics: Governance

Payer is a generic term that typically describes an organization, namely, an insurance company that manages a benefit and pays health-care provider claims for services rendered to patients. It is important to discuss several high-level distinctions among payers as, at a practical level, they impact how payer priorities are established. Additionally, these distinctions have a tremendous influence on what would be considered successful, either fiscally, operationally, or programmatically, by a payer in terms of a benefit package offered to the AYASHCN, such as HCT planning.

For-Profit Versus Not-for-Profit

The first defining characteristic is the distinction between for-profit and not-for-profit payers. All business entities should generate more revenue than expense if they are to be viable. However, what happens with excess revenue, the profit or margin, at the for-profit versus the not-for-profit level, is important to understand. In a for-profit entity, at times called an investor-owned entity, the excess profit is typically distributed back to the owners or stockholders. In contrast, at the not-for-profit entity, which is not "owned" by investors but is instead incorporated by a board of directors drawn from another not-for-profit organization or from the community itself, the profit is reinvested into the mission of the organization. Other than salaries and performance-related bonuses paid to employees, the not-for-profit entity is not permitted by law to provide excess revenue to any individuals for personal gain. It is too simplistic to think that for-profits will only pursue a benefit element if it makes money and contributes to the profit. There are other aspects that factor into a payer's business decision including intangible benefits related to enhanced reputation, meeting a regulatory mandate in the State in which the payer operates, or, possibly, satisfying an expectation from the purchaser of the insurance coverage. These intangible benefits must be balanced with the fiscal reality of generating a profit. The not-for-profit payer may have a lower fiscal target for the profit or margin that it generates from its operations, but it is not immune from financial considerations. A frequent refrain in not-for-profit organization boardrooms is "if no margin, then no mission," which reflects the fiscal reality of being financially viable regardless of governance.

One emerging concept that goes beyond profit calculation is value. A key goal for any payer is to increase the quality of the care being delivered divided by the lowest cost to deliver that care or benefit, representing the highest value: value = quality/cost [1].

> Payers, physicians, patients, … each use a different lexicon when defining and discussing value. Each stakeholder group also comes to the table with perceptions on how the other groups are defining value. As stakeholders engage to assign value to therapies, these gaps become glaringly obvious and make it clear that while we are all talking about the same thing, we are not always speaking the same language [1, p. 1].

Hence, with regard to HCT of AYASHCN, sharing perspectives will help all stakeholders to understand how each defines value.

Private Versus Public

The second defining characteristic describing payers relates to the benefit being managed as either being a private or commercial benefit as opposed to being a government or public-type benefit such as Medicaid. This distinction has become less clear in recent years with the privatization of government services whereby government agencies contract with nongovernmental businesses to deliver services traditionally delivered by that government agency. However, the basic private/public distinction remains. Private or commercial insurance typically is provided by an employer to their employees and dependents. Small business owners or individuals may purchase private or commercial insurance policies. The main point is that the entity purchasing the insurance is the primary customer setting expectations for the payer. The entity who pays the bill gets to define what is included in the benefit that is managed by the payer (within regulatory corridors). Thus, for private or commercial insurance, the payer interacts with the purchaser to design and deliver an insurance benefit consistent with what the purchaser wants, constrained by applicable regulations. The receivers of the insurance, typically the purchaser's employees and their dependent family members, have some say in the benefit design, but they are one step removed from the transaction between the payer and the purchaser.

Public insurance is defined by the government program of which it is a part. The program is defined by laws or regulations in terms of eligibility for the benefit, the range of services that are covered, and how much of the cost is shared with the patient and family. The type of public insurance that most often is discussed when considering AYASHCN and HCT is the Medicaid program. This chapter will focus on Medicaid as an exemplar of public insurance for HCT. As stated previously, a State government may offer the Medicaid program's benefits directly, via a State agency, or the State agency may contract with either for-profit or not-for-profit insurance companies to offer this public benefit. The main point is that the government is the purchaser of the insurance, and it therefore, via the program's design, defines what is included in the benefit and what is not.

For government programs, such as Medicaid, there are laws and regulations that form the basis of what is and what is not part of the benefit. For example, in the Medicaid program (defined in Title XIX of the Social Security Act), there is a specific section, 1905(r), which defines the Early and Periodic Screening, Diagnostic, and Treatment (EPSDT) services that provide a comprehensive array of health-care services for children and adolescents under the age of 21 years. According to the Center for Medicare and Medicaid Services (CMS) [2], "EPSDT's goal is to assure children get the health care they need when they need it—the right care to the right child at the right time in the right setting." Thus, for AYASHCN under 21 years of age, the EPSDT services mandate provides for a broad range of covered health-care services. Paradoxically, AYASHCN under 21 years old, with only commercial or private health-care insurance coverage, have less comprehensive benefit plans than do those covered under the Medicaid program and the EPSDT mandate. Prior to age 21 years, AYASHCN have access to a broad range of health-care services and supports, and, then, they "fall off the cliff" of coverage as they celebrate their 21st birthday [3]. They no longer have the federally mandated EPSDT services, so coverage for care and supports commonly used to maintain function and health such as physical therapy, occupational therapy, and speech-language pathology services are often discontinued. This cliff is visually demonstrated in Fig. 23.2 [3].

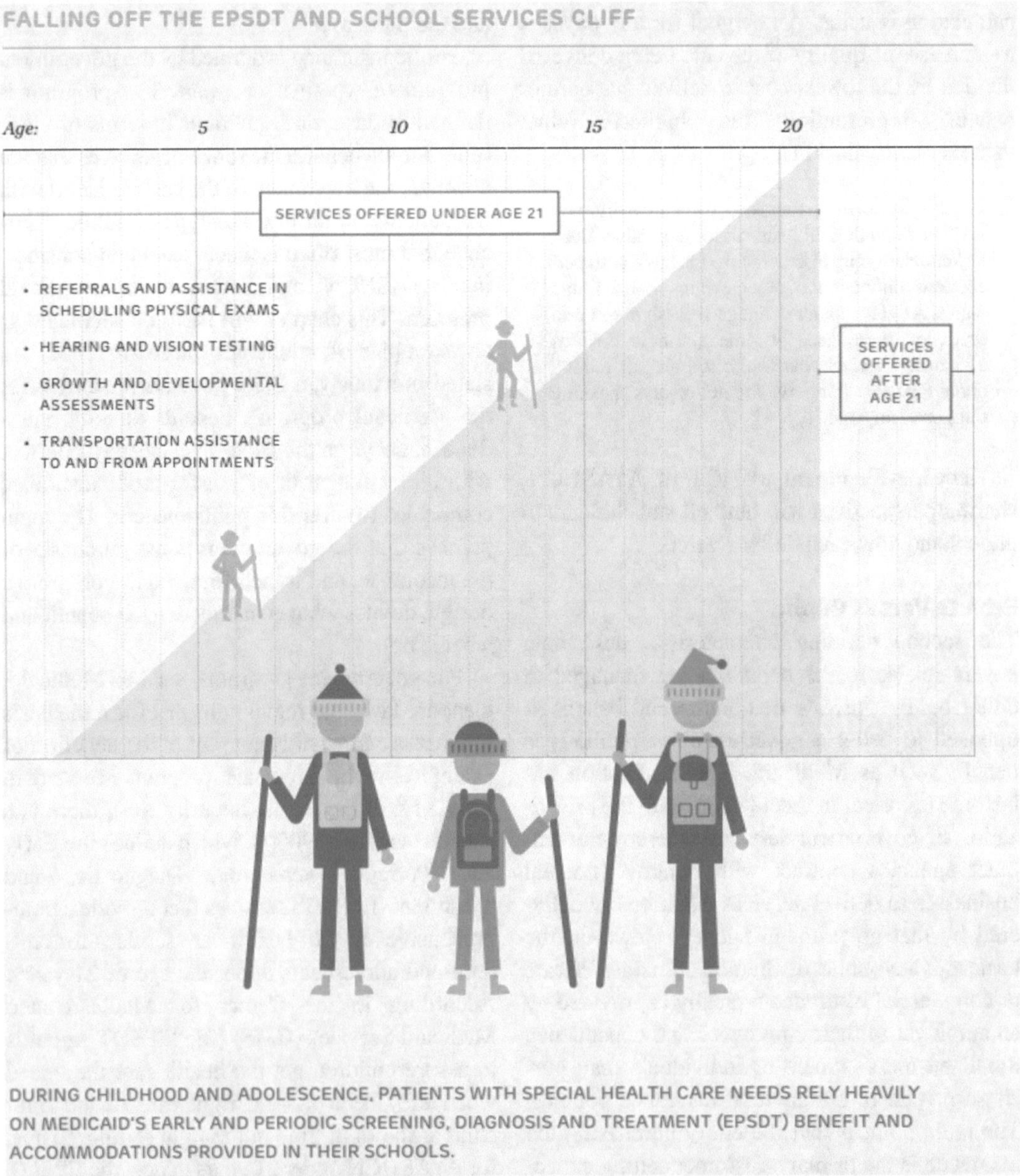

Fig. 23.2 The EPSDT cliff for AYASHCN older than 21 years of age (Used with Permission. Steinway C. Gable JL, Jan S., and MINT. *Transitioning to Adult Care: Supporting Youth with Special Health Care Needs.* PolicyLab at Children's Hospital of Philadelphia; 2017. Retrieved from http://bit.ly/E2A_TransitionsOfCare). Used with permission

According to the Agency for Healthcare Research and Quality (AHRQ) (2014), this concern for AYASHCN falling off the cliff around the time of transition to the adult care setting is very real, and the insurance coverage issues are significant. AHRQ [4] notes that approximately "one-third of youth experience gaps greater than 6 months in health care coverage when moving from a pediatric to adult provider and between 15 and 30% of young adults with special health care needs have no insurance coverage…[and] many have difficulty maintaining employment, which can pose additional challenges to paying for health care." [4, p. 23]

Payer Basics: Payment Models: Fee-for-Service Versus Value-Based Reimbursement

A fundamental transaction to understand when considering the payer perspective is how money is exchanged between the payer and the health-care provider for the care delivered to the AYASHCN. Over the past decade, owing to massive health-care reform efforts, a great deal of attention has been directed toward payment models in health care with a focus on how financing and reimbursement may impact the delivery of care. Reforms have been proposed which seek to ensure that financial incentives are aligned in ways to promote ideal care. The traditional payment model that pervades the current U.S. health-care system is referred to as fee-for-service (FFS) reimbursement. In a FFS payment model, the provider is compensated for the volume of covered services delivered and not necessarily for the quality and measured outcome of those services. To manage a FFS model, a great deal of effort is expended in developing complex coding systems that identify specific diagnoses being treated and which help identify and count the specific procedures and services provided during the encounter. A detailed explanation of these coding systems is beyond the scope of this chapter, but the result is a highly technical process that requires training and expertise to use. The coding systems result in large reference documents, long lists of approved codes specific to each type of insurance benefit, a billing system at the provider's office, and a claims management system at the payer's office that occupies a significant amount of time and effort to accurately count and pay for what was done during the encounter.

Reformers have proposed alternative payment models (APM) that seek to shift from this volume of service, or counting, approach to reimbursement to a model that reimburses for the quality of the care delivered and, ultimately, toward a model that pays for achieving actual positive outcomes for the patient. Value in APM is defined as value = quality/cost. The concept of paying for value in health care rather than volume or counting of services is generally seen as ideal, but the practical aspects to implementing this newer, operational approach are challenging. Chapter 25 discusses several APMs. In brief, the Centers for Medicare and Medicaid (CMS) has developed a four-category framework to describe the shift toward value-based reforms from the traditional fee-for-service system, described in Fig. 23.3 [5]. The CMS four-category framework for value-based reforms includes:

1. Fee-for-service with no link to quality
2. Fee-for-service linked to quality
3. Alternative payment models built on a fee-for-service architecture
4. Population-based payment

Figure 23.3 [5] describes the framework and time frame over which CMS envisions the U.S. health-care system adopting alternative payment models. CMS is focused initially on the Medicare system, but the expectation is that Medicaid as well as much of the commercial insurance system would likely embrace this effort as well.

In considering the potential benefit of these APMs as they apply to children and adolescents, Dr. Sandra Hassink [6], then president of the American Academy of Pediatrics (AAP), highlights the longitudinal value of pediatric quality and preventive measures noting specifically that the return on investment should not be limited to a benefit plan year since much of the potential benefit may extend beyond that period as would be seen with immunizations and obesity prevention.

Fig. 23.3 CMS framework for value-based reimbursement evolution

Aim: When it comes to improving the way providers are paid, we want to reward value and care coordination - rather than volume and care duplication. In partnership with the private sector, the Department of Health and Human Services (HHS) is testing and expanding new health care payment models that can improve health care quality and reduce its cost.

Framework:

Payment Taxonomy Framework

	Category 1: *Fee for Service–No Link to Quality*	Category 2: *Fee for Service– Link to Quality*	Category 3: *Alternative Payment Models Built on Fee-for-Service Architecture*	Category 4: *Population-Based payment*
Description	*Payments are based on volume of services and not linked to quality or efficiency*	*At least a portion of payments vary based on the quality or efficiency of health care delivery*	*Some payment is linked to the effective management of a population or an episode of care. Payments still triggered by delivery of services, but opportunities for shared savings or 2-sided risk*	*Payments is not directly triggered by service delivery so volume is not linked to payment. Clinicians and organizations are paid and responsible for the care of a beneficiary for a long period (e.g ≥1 yr)*
Medicare FFS	• Limited in Medicare fee-for-service • Majority of Medicare payments now are linked to quality	• Hospital value-based purchasing • Physician Value-Based Modifier • Readmissions/Hospital Acquired Condition Reduction Program	• Accountable care organizations • Medical homes • Bundled payments • Comprehensive primary care initiative • Comprehensive ESRD • Medicare-Medicaid Financial Alignment Initiative Fee-For-Service Model	• Eligible Pioneer accountable care organizations in years 3-5

Value-based purchasing includes payments made in categories 2 through 4. Moving from category 1 to category 4 involves two shifts: (1) increasing accountability for both quality and total cost of care and (2) a greater focus on population health management as opposed to payment for specific services.

Timeline:

Target percentage of Medicare FFS payments linked to quality and alternative payment models in 2016 and 2018

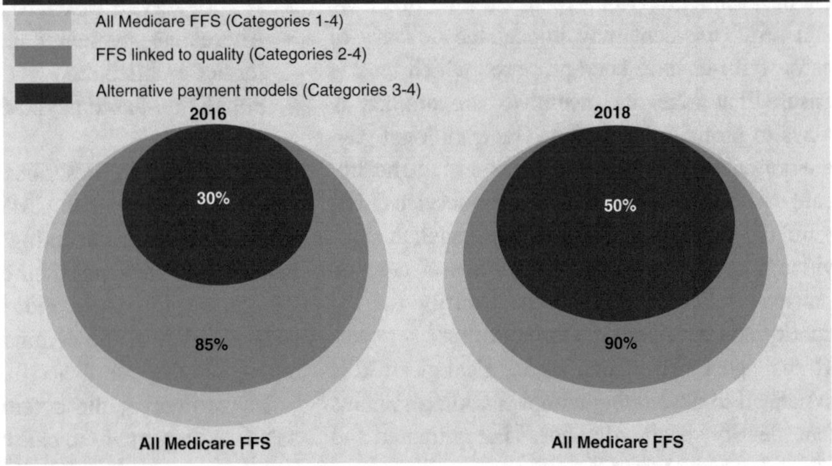

All alternative payment models and payment reforms that seek to deliver better care at lower cost share a common pathway for success: providers must make fundamental changes in their day-to-day operations that improve the quality and reduce the cost of health care. Making operational changes will be attractive only if the new alternative payment models and payment reforms are broadly adopted by a critical mass of payers. When providers encounter new payment strategies for one payer, but not others, the incentives to fundamentally change are weak. In fact, a provider that alters its system to prevent admissions and succeed in an alternative payment environment may lose revenue from payers that continue fee-for-service payments.

A focus on value of care delivered rather than on the delivery of a volume of services has the potential to be useful in promoting HCT for AYASHCN in that a value-based approach would likely avoid the challenges of counting and billing of specific services and would instead provide a pathway for the patient education and case management necessary for effective transition. Specifically, AHRQ [4], in its technical brief, addresses the financial challenges that a fee-for-service reimbursement model causes for health-care providers who must balance the transition planning needs for AYASHCN with other practice responsibilities as well:

> Health care providers are often held to benchmarked standards for volume of patients seen and levels of reimbursement within their practice. Transition care requires a significant amount of provider time, which results in a decrease in the number of patients seen by an individual provider. However, this care does not result in a substantial increase in per visit reimbursement and can therefore translate into a financial loss to clinics that provide this type of service [4, pp. 23–24].

Payer Basics: Medical Necessity and Standard of Care

In order to provide health-care insurance coverage and conduct benefit management activities, the payer must have a framework from which to determine if a specific health-care service or support is covered. A fundamental element to this determination is deciding if a service or support is "medically necessary." Typically, both private/commercial and public payers work toward covering those services that are recognized as a standard of care based on a review of current evidence and best practice. Publicly funded programs such as Medicaid must by law and regulation only cover medically necessary care and services. Establishing medical necessity is rooted in the scientific study of health-care interventions. The AAP [7] defines medical necessity as:

> ...health care interventions that are evidence based, evidence informed, or based on consensus advisory opinion and that are recommended by recognized health care professionals, such as the AAP, to promote optimal growth and development in a child and to prevent, detect, diagnose, treat, ameliorate, or palliate the effects of physical, genetic, congenital, developmental, behavioral, or mental conditions, injuries, or disabilities [7, p. 400].

Ideally, there will be robust scientific literature to support the establishment of the evidence base for a standard of care that justifies a medical necessity determination. However, while that evidence base is being developed, e.g., during the approximately 17 years described by Green below, payers must rely on professional consensus and best practices as promulgated by authoritative organizations such as professional organizations like the AAP or governmental authorities such as the Centers for Disease Control and Prevention (CDC) and AHRQ [4] (see Fig. 23.4 [8]).

Looking specifically at the evidence generation process related to HCT for AYASHCN transitioning from pediatric settings, a number of influential position statements and best practices have been developed and disseminated which provide a platform for scientific study, the emergence of scientific evidence, and for a medical necessity determination.

In 2014, Got Transition, a federally funded national center initiative focused on HCT, issued the Six Core Elements of Health Care Transition, which describe the process of HCT. Despite these processes being widely available in professional publications and on the Internet, they have not been uniformly adopted. Payers are aware of the evolutionary and incremental adoption of process for best practices and use medical advisory committees to stay informed of emerging best practices. Specifically, the AHRQ (2014) in its technical brief on transition care for children with special health needs reports that fewer than half of children with special health-care needs receive adequate support and HCT services, less so for those children living in poverty. One-third of pediatricians indicate referrals to adult-serving physicians, and less than 15% of pediatricians reported providing transition educational material to adolescents and their parents [4].

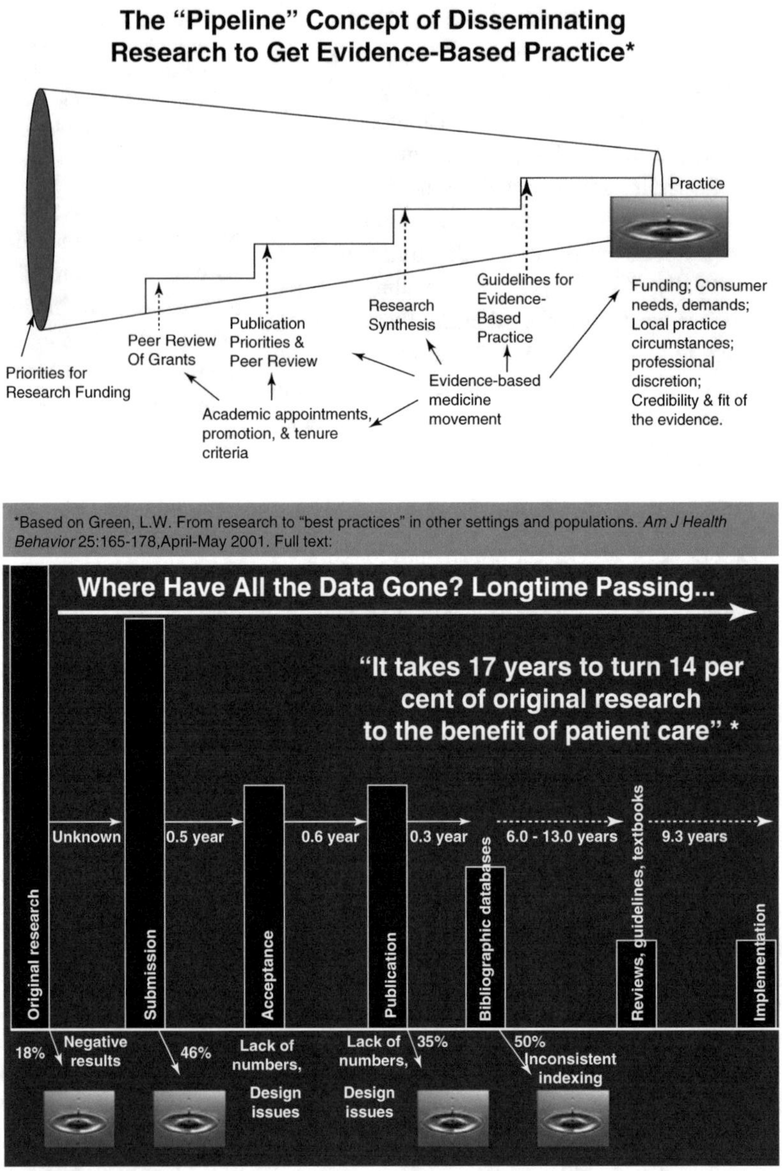

Fig. 23.4 The extended time period for evidence generation and adoption in practice. Used with permission

In addition, every 10 years, the CDC issues national, aspirational goals meant to guide improvement efforts in the U.S. health-care system in the ensuing 10-year period. In 2010, the CDC issued Healthy People 2020, which included a goal around increasing the proportion of AYASHCN whose health-care provider discusses HCT planning. Based on baseline data from 2005 to 2006, a modest goal of a 10% improvement from 41.2% having that conversation to 45.3% by 2020 was set. Based on data collected in 2010 and reported in 2016 in the Healthy People 2020 mid-course review, little to no improvement has been observed in this indicator. There is minimal agreement among pediatricians with the best practice of beginning HCT planning at or before age 14 noting that 62% of pediatricians think transition planning should start between 18 and 20 years of age for adolescents with special needs followed by 25% who think 15–17 is the time to begin [9, 10].

Application to AYASHCN HCT

From the transactional nature of the payer perspective, the purchaser of the health-care benefit can demand transition for AYASHCN to be part of the benefit and then pay for adequate resources to be made available to support a HCT initiative. More likely, however, the payer incorporates a focus on transition in its transaction with the health-care provider from either a financial, operational, programmatic, or regulatory point of view.

The financial return on investment in a HCT program would likely be long term in nature. From a payer's perspective, the measurement of an ideal financial return on investment is often short term and somewhat linear. For example, an initiative that assists the patient in following an optimal medical management plan for their asthma, typically, would result in less exacerbations, less emergency department visits, and fewer inpatient admissions. The investment in the relatively inexpensive initiative leads to less expenditures on the expensive emergency department and inpatient stays which make for a favorable return on investment. Transition is likely not going to have that relatively short-term measured financial benefit owing to the years-long, longitudinal nature of transitioning for AYASCHN. As a result, operational, programmatic, and regulatory returns on investment are more likely to be associated with HCT programs. As a starting point, however, the payer would need to establish the medical necessity for AYASHCN transition services and supports as a standard of care. At this point, with professional organizations like the AAP along with others calling for HCT services, with authoritative governmental agencies such as AHRQ and CDC defining transition as part of the national agenda, and with a federally funded national center initiative catalyzing research and practice innovation regarding transition, medical advisory committees working with payers who seek to be well informed would have ample emerging evidence to determine that HCT for AYASHCN is a standard of care and would meet criteria for a medically necessary service. In the transactional nature of the payer perspective, how might transition become part of an intangible return on investment for a payer?

First, many payers embrace a public commitment to quality improvement that goes beyond just a financial calculation around a short-term monetary return on investment and maintain instead a focus on their reputation as defined by high-quality and responsive service delivery. Numerous national quality initiatives that are supported by payers across the board have defined a vision for performance improvement in the nation's health-care system. Among the most prominent models adopted by a large number of health-care organizations, including both private and public payers, is the Institute for Healthcare Improvement's (IHI) Triple Aim model. Essentially, the health-care system is envisioned as working to improve the health of the population by delivering appropriate care and services while enhancing the experience of the patient and family for a reasonable cost. Value then would be delivery of high-quality care and services for low cost in a manner that is experienced as acceptable by the patient and family. Arguably, transition services for AYASHCN would be a component of the optimal care envisioned via a system that aspires to the IHI's Triple Aim (see Fig. 23.5 [11]).

Second, Group Health of Puget Sound in Washington State (a well-recognized not-for-profit organization) has popularized a model for optimal care for those with chronic conditions that is applicable to HCT. Wagner's Chronic Care Model is generally accepted as sound and is frequently cited as a goal which health care should move toward (see Fig. 23.6 [12]). The key to the

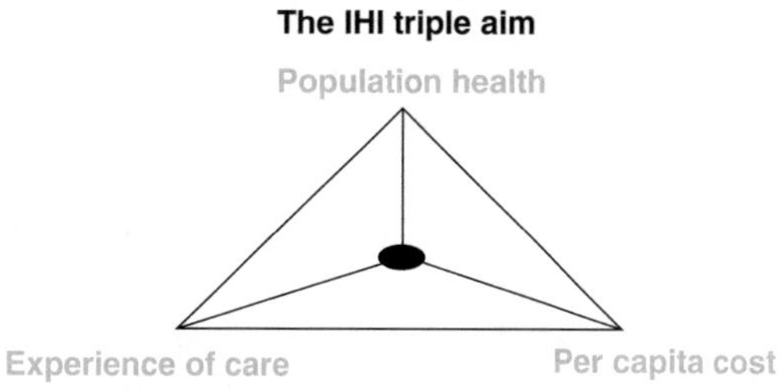

Fig. 23.5 IHI's Triple Aim (Used with permission)

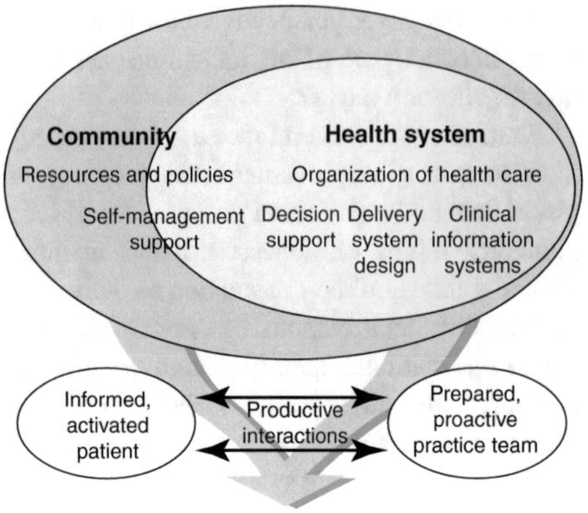

Fig. 23.6 Chronic Care Model (Used with permission). Edward H. Wagner, MD, MPH, Chronic Disease Management: What Will It Take To Improve Care for Chronic Illness? Effective Clinical Practice, Aug/Sept 1998, Vol 1

Chronic Care Model's success is the productive interactions that are envisioned between a "prepared, proactive practice team" and the "informed activated patient" that lead to desired functional and clinical outcomes. Clearly, the payer, in its transactional processes, can do much to facilitate these productive interactions by promoting attention on the part of the practice team and by removing barriers that may be in the way of HCT. The productive interactions can be of value from operational, programmatic, or regulatory efforts, and the ideal functional and clinical outcomes likely will enhance the payer's reputation as an organization interested in being innovative and delivering high-quality care and support to its patients.

Third, the AAP has for decades promoted the need for ideal primary care to occur via a patient family-centered medical home characterized as accessible, family-centered, continuous, comprehensive, coordinated, compassionate, and culturally effective. Payers have recognized the potential value for this ideal primary care model and will provide financial incentives to practices that implement this type of care in a measurable way (see Chap. 26). A medical home would be ideally suited to support and encourage HCT.

Case Study #1: Managed Care Organization Pilot—Transition as Part of Quality Improvement [13]

In 2013, a pilot project to further understand the process of HCT for AYASHCN using the six core elements model was undertaken with 35 participants enrolled in the Health Services for Children with Special Needs (HSCSN), a not-for-profit payer in Washington DC. The pilot project demonstrated the feasibility for a payer to support the health-care system in customizing and delivering recommended transition services [13]. From the payer's perspective, HCT made sense as part of the quality improvement process within the payer organization's operational structure. The return of investment was not monetary but quality.

Case Study #2: Texas Children's Health Plan (TCHP) and STARKids Program—Transition as a Regulatory Requirement

Transition services, such as ongoing case management to implement a care plan that includes a transition process beginning at age 14, are not typically called out explicitly in many benefit packages, either private or public. However, beginning on November 1, 2016, the State of Texas explicitly included, as a requirement, the development and ongoing maintenance of transition care plan for enrollees in a newly created benefit program (i.e., STARKids) for children and adolescents receiving Medicaid as part of their qualification for being in the Supplemental Security Income (SSI) program. This explicit requirement is written into the State's uniform managed care contract (UMCC) and as such requires compliance as a condition of participation. Thus, as the STARKids program is fully implemented, this contractual requirement can be expected to drive the development and maintenance of transition processes.

Challenge for the Future

At present, from a transaction perspective, there is a mismatch between the effort expended to achieve effective HCT for AYASHCN and the financial benefit that is likely to result from the more coordinated care results. The healthcare providers, AYASHCN, and their families continue to expend a great deal of effort to navigate through the transition process. Thus, while in the Chronic Care Model all stakeholders can be expected to experience the benefit of the activated patient and the well-informed team producing ideal HCT, the potential financial savings in a fee-for-service-based model that would come from avoiding fragmented care only go now to

the payer and ultimately to the purchaser (see Fig. 23.7).

Clearly, a more equitable approach would be if the up-front costs required for a well-functioning AYASHCN HCT process could be defrayed by the later savings. Value-based purchasing models hold great promise toward achieving both the Triple Aim and the Chronic Care Model's ideal goals. The value-based reimbursement approach trusts the clinicians to do what needs to be done to generate, in partnership with the AYASHCN and their family, the functional and clinical outcomes desired. In Steinway, Gable, and Jan's (2017) policy brief, there are sets of recommendations for various stakeholders in the transition to adult care realm and the

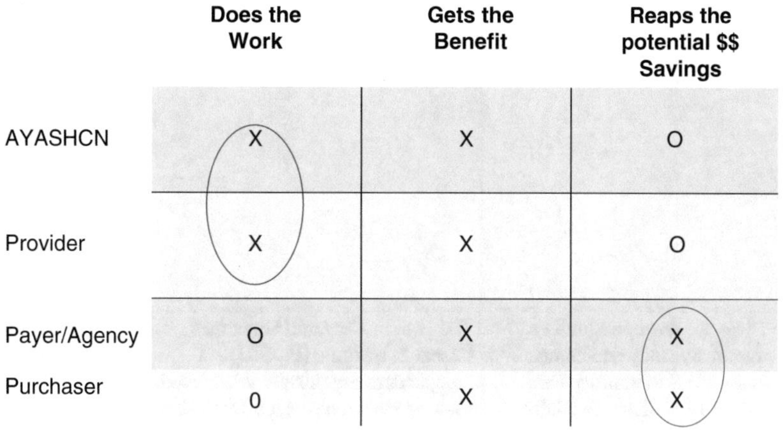

Fig. 23.7 Effort versus benefit for transition among the stakeholders

	Does the Work	Gets the Benefit	Reaps the potential $$ Savings
AYASHCN	X	X	O
Provider	X	X	O
Payer/Agency	O	X	X
Purchaser	0	X	X

Table 23.1 Recommendations for policymakers

Problem	Recommendation	Recommendation details
Young adults aging out of the pediatric health system face challenges accessing adequate health insurance coverage or referral networks to meet all of their special health-care needs	State Medicaid directors should help to prevent the often predictable gaps in health-care coverage and access by	• Employ methods to avert the specific "falloff" from Medicaid coverage as youth age out of children's coverage • Extend habilitative services
Pediatric and adult providers, practices, and hospital systems have few incentives to interact with one another or to provide transition services	The Centers for Medicare and Medicaid Services (CMS) should utilize innovative, consistent, and thorough transition payment models that would allow compensation for transition-related services, thus incentivizing their use Shift care coordination and care management to payers	• Enhanced fee-for-service (FFS) payments • Pay-for-performance (P4P) • Administrative or infrastructure payments • Capitation • Bundled payments and shared savings

(continued)

Table 23.1 (continued)

Problem	Recommendation	Recommendation details
Youth with complex medical conditions on capitated Medicaid managed care plans are unable to gradually transition care from pediatric to adult primary care providers. Typically, if multiple providers of the same specialty see a patient in the same visit, only one of these providers can bill for services, which creates disincentives for joint visits	CMS, State Medicaid programs, and private insurers should create more flexible billing policies to allow both pediatricians and adult primary care providers to bill for the same patient during the transition and transfer process	Adult providers should have the opportunity to meet and assess pediatric patients in a familiar setting before the transfer process and then have the opportunity to work alongside pediatric providers if patients are ready for transfer
There is an insufficient number of dually trained internal medicine and pediatrics (Med–Peds) clinicians who are ideally suited to provide continuity of care across the life span of individuals with pediatric complex chronic conditions	Medicare—which covers the majority of the cost teaching hospitals spend on training medical residents—should increase training opportunities and residency slots for physicians working with medically complex adolescents and young adults	In the 2015 residency match cycle, there were 380 Med–Peds resident slots at 78 institutions across the United States. Med–Peds residents comprised less than 2% of all residents in all specialties through the National Residency Matching Program. An increase in the number of residents who specialize in Med–Peds would create a pipeline of providers that have the expertise to care for patients with pediatric-onset chronic illness across the life span Family medicine residencies should also add core competencies in providing primary care for persons with pediatric chronic conditions, which would increase provider knowledge and comfort in managing complex young adult patients
There are few opportunities to rigorously study and compare innovations to improve the quality of pediatric to adult care transitions	The Patient-Centered Outcomes Research Institute (PCORI), an independent organization dedicated to funding research projects that enhance patient, provider, and policymaker clarity around informed health-care decision-making, and the U.S. Department of Health and Humans Services' Agency for Healthcare Research and Quality (AHRQ) should continue to fund research around the transition process from pediatric to adult health care	For example, PCORI recently announced a funding opportunity entitled, "Management of Care Transitions for Emerging Adults with Sickle Cell Disease." Although national guidelines from Got Transition outline ideal transition goals, little has been done to explore best practices and concrete processes that achieve these goals

Used with permission

Steinway C. Gable JL, Jan S., and MINT. *Transitioning to Adult Care: Supporting Youth with Special Health Care Needs*. PolicyLab at Children's Hospital of Philadelphia; 2017. Retrieved from http://bit.ly/E2A_TransitionsOfCare

recommendations for policymakers that are most applicable to the transactional nature of the payer perspective (see Table 23.1 [3]).

In summary, as the nation moves toward the adoption of alternative payment models that are value-based, there is a great reason for optimism that the medically necessary transition services for AYASHCN will find paths forward that satisfy the transactional needs of the payers who are tasked with the benefit management process.

References

1. Abedi S. Defining value: the payer perspective. PharmExec.com. 2016;35(12). http://www.pharmexec.com/print/304915. Accessed 20 June 2017.
2. Centers for Medicare and Medicaid Spending (CMS). EPSDT – a guide for states: coverage in the medicaid benefit for children and adolescents. 2014. https://www.medicaid.gov/medicaid/benefits/downloads/epsdt_coverage_guide.pdf.
3. Steinway C, Gable JL, Jan S, MINT. Transitioning to adult care: supporting youth with special health care needs. PolicyLab at Children's Hospital of Philadelphia. 2017. p. 11. http://bit.ly/E2A_TransitionsOfCare.
4. Agency for Healthcare Research and Quality (AHRQ), McPheeters M, Davis AM, Taylor JL, Brown RF, Potter SA, Epstein RA. Transition care for children with special health needs. Technical Brief No. 15 (Prepared by the Vanderbilt University Evidence-based Practice Center under Contract No. 290-2012-00009-I). AHRQ Publication No.14-EHC027-EF. Rockville, MD: Agency for Healthcare Research and Quality. June 2014. www.effectivehealthcare.ahrq.gov/reports/final.cfm.
5. Centers for Medicare and Medicaid Spending (CMS). Better Care. Smarter Spending. Healthier people: paying providers for value, not volume. 2015. https://www.cms.gov/Newsroom/MediaReleaseDatabase/Fact-sheets/2015-Fact-sheets-items/2015-01-26-3.html.
6. Hassink, SK. Letter to Sam Nussbaum, MD. Alternative Payment Model Framework and Progress Tracking (APM FPT) Work Group. American Academy of Pediatrics. November, 18, 2015.
7. American Academy of Pediatrics Committee on Child Health Financing. Essential contractual language for medical necessity in children. Pediatrics. 2013;132(2):396–401. http://pediatrics.aappublications.org/content/pediatrics/132/2/398.full.pdf
8. Balas EA, Boren SA. Managing clinical knowledge for health care improvement. Yearbook of Medical Informatics 2000: Patient-centered Systems. Stuttgart, Germany: Schattauer; 2000. p. 65–70.
9. Healthy People 2020. Washington, DC: U.S. Department of Health and Human Services, Office of Disease Prevention and Health Promotion. DH-5. https://www.healthypeople.gov/node/4153/data_details
10. Healthy People 2020 Objective (DH-5). Midcourse review. 2016. https://www.cdc.gov/nchs/data/hpdata2020/HP2020MCR-C09-DH.pdf
11. Institute for Healthcare Improvement (IHI) The IHI Triple Aim. http://www.ihi.org/Engage/Initiatives/TripleAim/Pages/default.aspx.
12. Wagner EH. Chronic disease management: what will it take to improve care for chronic illness? Eff Clin Pract. 1998;1:2–4.
13. McManus M, White P, Pirtle R, et al. Incorporating the six core elements of health care transition into a Medicaid managed care plan: lessons learned from a pilot project. J Pediatr Nurs. 2015;30:700–13.

Part VI

Financing Healthcare Transition

Financial Cost of Healthcare Transition

24

Angelo P. Giardino

"…, everything we discuss in reference to medicine, health care delivery or policy will merely be symptomatic of the overarching tension between our aspirations for health care and our resources to pay for them." (Surgeon General C. Everett Koop, [1, p. 5]

Introduction

Clearly, there is an aspiration in the health-care field for a transition process for adolescents and young adults with special health care needs (AYASHCN) that is "uninterrupted, coordinated, developmentally appropriate, psychosocially sound, and comprehensive," but the resources to pay for those services are in question [2, p. 570]. This book explores many facets of the health care transition (HCT) process, and this chapter addresses financing transition services at the system level to promote effective HCT. The finances for HCT have long been recognized as a cornerstone of the process [3]. As early as 1989, the Surgeon General of the U.S.A., Dr. Koop [1], commented about the need for financing to support effective HCT. In specific, at the 1989 Surgeon General's Conference entitled "Growing Up and Getting Medical Care: youth with Special Health Care Needs," Dr. Koop highlighted the following:

> "The financing of care must be regarded as an immediate priority. We are talking about labor-intensive care, increasingly expensive, and the reimbursement systems which have not caught up with these facts. Children with special needs entering the adult system are not overly welcomed because:

- They should many times overstay their DRG [diagnosis related group] norm.
- They may not be covered—any longer—by their parents' insurance
- If employed—even part time—they may be part of the working poor—uninsured but not destitute enough … for [M]edicaid." (p. 5)

Since HCT is a process rather than a discrete event, the discussion of costs and financing is complex. The process is longitudinal and occurs within many encounters over an extended period and requires a broader view of how to support teams as they build relationships that result in a successful HCT. Despite a clear need for, and the well-recognized value of, measuring costs for a variety of services and supports delivered in support of HCT, this cost remains elusive:

> "Measuring per capita costs is still a big challenge; it requires that we capture all relevant expenditures, include them appropriately to local market

A. P. Giardino, M.D., Ph.D.
Texas Children's Hospital, Houston, TX, USA

Academic General Pediatrics, Department of Pediatrics, Baylor College of Medicine, Houston, TX, USA
e-mail: apgiardi@texaschildrens.org

A. C. Hergenroeder, C. M. Wiemann (eds.), *Health Care Transition*,
https://doi.org/10.1007/978-3-319-72868-1_24

> circumstances, and be able to measure actual costs in a care system whose current methods of pricing and discounting obscure them. Population measures would require some form of registration or sampling for defined populations and would be speeded by widespread implementation of electronic health record systems. Citing one serious gap, the IOM [Institute of Medicine] recently concluded that measures of both cost and care across the continuum, impeded by the fragmentation of delivery itself, still need much more developmental work." [4, p. 762]

The emerging literature is replete with efforts to improve transition for specific clinical populations. A recent PubMed search on cost for HCT from pediatric to adult settings yielded 87 citations, none of which had generalizable financial data; the majority of these papers focused upon developing models for condition-specific groups or proposing best practices to guide clinicians. Thus, with a paucity of peer-reviewed literature regarding cost and financing, this chapter will focus on the health-care system and its approach to funding HCT. No specific dollar amount will be prescribed for a transition event nor for the transition process; instead, there will be a discussion of the ideal health-care delivery system that likely could support processes that facilitate effective HCT over time. The patient family-centered medical home [5], when joined with value-based reimbursement models, is described as having the potential to be the optimal care delivery system for transitioning AYASHCN from pediatric to adult health.

The chapter begins with a general discussion of health-care costs in the U.S.A. The cost and utilization of services for children with special health-care needs (CSHCN) and adults with special health-care needs (ASHCN) are discussed next. The chapter concludes with a discussion of the financial aspects of an ideal patient- and family-centered medical home. The opportunity presented by the move toward value-based reimbursement combined with the medical home delivery system is described as opening up the door for aspirations around HCT and AYASHCN as described by Dr. Koop to be aligned with the resources available to pay for this process.

U.S. Health-Care System

Overall

In 2014, U.S. health-care spending from all sources was 3.031 trillion dollars, representing 17.5% of the gross domestic product (GDP) at an average cost of $9523 per person [6]. Health-care spending as a percentage of GDP and per capita spending has risen over the past several decades. In 1970, U.S. health-care spending was 75 billion dollars, accounting for 7.2% of the GDP and representing an average of $356 per person [7]. The per capita expense of $9523 per person on health-care spending is the highest for any developed nation [6].

On January 1, 2014, a significant expansion of enrollment in the health-care insurance programs supported by the Affordable Care Act (ACA) of 2010 caused shifts in insurance coverage and a 19.5% reduction in the number of uninsured Americans. In 2014, there were 35.5 million uninsured Americans having fallen from 44.2 million in 2013 as a result of the massive expansion of insurance coverage ushered in by the implementation of the ACA. In 2014, private (or commercial) insurance accounted for the largest source of health-care spending at $991 billion, followed by Medicare at $618.7 billion, and Medicaid at $495.8 billion. Individuals and families contribute personal funds toward the payment for some or all of their insurance premiums and frequently also incur out-of-pocket expenses for health care. Out-of-pocket expenses alone (not counting the contribution toward the insurance premiums) accounted for $329.8 billion during 2014 as well. Table 24.1 [6, 8] presents data related to source of insurance and related health-care spending comparing 2013 and 2014.

In the aggregate, in 2014, 28% of the dollars for the health-care spending in the U.S.A. came from individuals (a combination of personal outlays to cover insurance premiums and their own out-of-pocket expenses), and 28% came from the federal government, 27% from businesses, and another 17% from state and local governments [6]. Thus, 55% of U.S. health-care spending comes

Table 24.1 Source of insurance and related health care spending calendar years 2013 and 2014

Source of funds	2013	2014
Private health insurance		
Expenditure (billions)	$949.2	$991.0
Per enrollee expenditure	$5.056	$5.218
Enrollment (millions)	187.7	189.9
Medicare		
Expenditure (billions)	$586.3	$618.7
Per enrollee expenditure	$11,434	$11,707
Enrollment (millions)	51.3	52.8
Medicaid		
Expenditure (billions)	$446.7	$495.8
Per enrollee expenditure	$7676	$7253
Enrollment (millions)	58.2	65.9
Uninsured		
Uninsured (millions)	44.2	35.5
Uninsured (growth)	−1.3% (from 2012)	−19.5%

2013 U.S. population (millions) = 315.9
2014 U.S. population (millions) = 318.3

from private sources, and 45% is covered by a combination of federal, state, and local governments [6]. At a national level, the dollars are spent on a variety of services and supports and large categories of expense that include (1) purchasing private insurance, (2) funding the Medicaid and Medicare programs, (3) buying prescription drugs, (4) paying for hospital care and other institutional care, (5) reimbursing physician, and (6) the costs associated other clinical service providers.

Children

Turning specifically to the portion of health-care spending directed toward health care for children (i.e., those under 19 years of age), Bui and colleagues [9] examined data from 1996 to 2013 and found that health-care spending on children increased from $149.6 billion to $233.5 billion during that period. Clearly, children account for a relatively small but important and growing component of the total U.S. health-care expenditure. The $233.5 billion spent on health care for children was 8.4% of the total U.S. health-care expenditure in 2013, accounting for 1.42% of the GDP at a cost of $2788 per child. The top 10 condition categories and their associated costs were:

1. Well newborn care in the hospital setting ($27.9 billion)
2. Attention-deficit/hyperactivity disorder (ADHD) ($20.6 billion)
3. Well dental care including dental checkups and orthodontia ($18.2 billion)
4. Asthma ($9 billion)
5. Oral disorders including caries, extractions, and oral surgery ($8.7 billion)
6. Well child care in the ambulatory setting ($8.5 billion)
7. Upper respiratory infections (URI) ($8.4 billion)
8. Long-term respiratory conditions such as sleep apnea, allergic rhinitis, and chronic sinusitis ($8.1 billion)
9. Dermatologic conditions such as cellulitis, cysts, acne, and eczema ($8 billion)
10. Mechanical forces such as striking an object and cuts ($7.8 billion) [9]

Other behavioral health-related conditions joined ADHD among the top 20 conditions with depressive disorders accounting for $5 billion and anxiety accounting for $3.4 billion in expense. This data reflects a population based view of health-care spending on all children and highlights the investment in well care that is made in pediatrics, as well as the dollars that get spent on specific conditions and disorders affecting children and adolescents. Equipped now with this general health-care spending context, the costs and utilization associated with children and adults with special health-care needs will be discussed next.

Children with Special Health-Care Needs (CHSCN)

According to the national representative of National Survey of Children with Special Health Care Needs (NS-CSHCN) conducted in 2005–2006, 14% of U.S. children and youth (birth through 17 years of age) have special health-care needs, and 22% of U.S. households with children include at least one child or youth with a special health-care need [10]. The federal Maternal and Child Health Bureau (MCHB) defines children and youth with special health-care needs (CYSHCN) as "those who have or are at increased risk for a chronic physical, developmental, behavioral or emotional condition and who also require health and related services of a type or amount beyond that required by children generally" [11, p. 138]. Using this definition, Kogan, Strickland, and Newacheck [12] estimated that one in seven children or about 10.2 million children in the U.S.A. had an existing special health-care need and had expenditures about three times higher than routinely developing children, accounting for 42% of the health-care costs spent on child health care. Newacheck and Kim [13] estimate that, on average, out-of-pocket expenses for CSHCN are about twice what they are for routinely developing children. The share of health-care bills paid out of pocket varies by type of service: 12% of non-physician services such as physical and occupational therapy; 14% of physician services; 30% of prescription costs; 40% of related services including vision aids, medical supplies, and other equipment; and 67% of dental services. A quarter of families with a CSHCN spend at least $1000 out of pocket. For lower-income families, expenditures of $250 or more are associated with family perception of a financial burden [14]. Table 24.2 [13, 15, 16] compares the cost data for children with and without special health-care needs.

Where CSHCN get their insurance is an important aspect of the financing for their care. According to the Kaiser Family Foundation [17], Medicaid and other public health insurance programs cover 44% of CSHCN. Publicly funded insurance is the sole source of funding for 36% of CSHCN, and an additional 8% have public insurance as a supplement for their private coverage. Figure 24.1 [17] arrays the types of health insurance among CSHCN.

The costs described above are expected to increase as a function of increased prevalence of CHYCN. There was a 15.6% increase in children with neurodevelopmental and mental health conditions between 2001 and 2011, accounting for the largest increases in chronic conditions [18].

Adults with Special Health-Care Needs (ASHCN)

In the adult health services literature, costs for ASHCN attributed as a result of the onset or worsening of a chronic or disabling condition are referred to as "disability-associated health-care expenditures (DAHE)" [19, p. 45]. In 2006, 18.2% of the U.S. adult population had a disability; the DAHE accounted for 26.7% of overall health-care expenses, or $397.8 billion. The average DAHE per capita cost was $11,637. Considering this from a population level and spreading the additional costs related to disability across the population of the nation, the per capita cost for DAHE is $2190 per U.S. resident. Turning to the insurance coverage for ASHCN and examining the funding sources for the nearly $400 billion spent on DAHE in 2006, Medicaid provided for the largest portion of spending, accounting for nearly $161 billion, followed by Medicare

Table 24.2 Costs and utilization for CSHCN (adapted)

Category	Children and youth with special health care needs	Children without disabilities	Comparison
Hospital days	552 days/1,000	90 days/1,000	7 times higher
Physician visits	4.6 visits/year	1.9 visits/year	2 times more visits
Nonphysician professional visits	3 visits/year	0.6 visits/year	5 times more visits
Prescriptions	6.94 medications/year	1.22 medications/year	5 times the number of prescriptions
Home health provider days	1.73 days/year	0.002 days/year	865 times more days
Health care expenditures	$2335/year	$652/year	3 times the cost
Out-of-pocket expenditures	$352/year	$175/year	2.0 times the cost

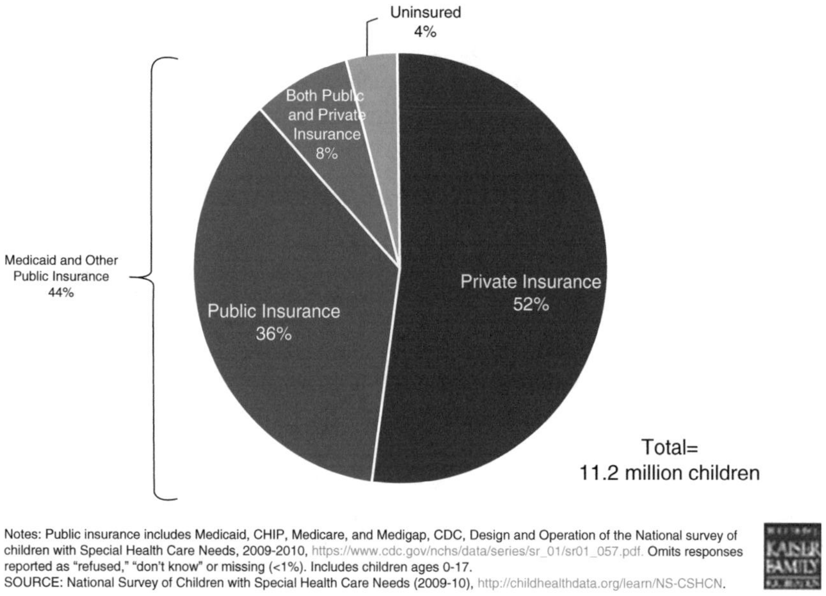

Fig. 24.1 Type of health insurance among children with special health-care needs. Muscemi, MaryBeth, Poindexter, Danielle. Medicaid Restructuring and Children with Special Health. Care Needs, The Henry J. Kaiser Family Foundation, Issue Brief January 2017. (http://files.kff.org/attachment/Issue-Brief-Medicaid-Restructuring-and-Children-with-Special-Health-Care-Needs). Used with permission

spending at $119 billion, and private insurance costs at $117 billion [19]. Medicaid's high proportion of the expense is due to its coverage for long-term care services, which are typically not part of Medicare and private insurance.

As with CSHCN, ASHCN also incur out-of-pocket costs. Adults between 21 and 61 years of age with a disability, on average, incur $1102 of out-of-pocket costs for health-care-related expenses which is 65% greater than the same age group without disabilities [20]. Looking specifically at those adults with disabilities that are covered by Medicaid, 80% of their out-of-pocket costs are for prescription medications followed by costs for ambulatory services [21].

Paying for the Costs of Transition: Embedding the Process in the Medical Home

The Six Core Elements of HCT promulgated by Got Transition, the Center for Health Care Transition Improvement, presents a best practice process for delivering effective HCT for AYASHCN from pediatric to adult settings. The payment models for financing the costs of this process remain a work in progress. White and McManus [22], co-directors of Got Transition, note that current payment models do not reimburse for the additional time, training, and infrastructure needed to establish transition programs and processes. Nor do they adequately reimburse care coordination activities such as identifying adult providers, transferring medical records, and verifying successful transfer [22].

Without successful HCT, the AYASHCN's health is diminished, the quality of care delivered is compromised and health-care costs are increased owing to duplication, fragmentation, and providing treatment later rather than earlier [23, 24]. Thus, a mandate exists for the development and implementation of a financing strategy that will support the HCT process.

Despite this urgency and mandate, the mismatch between our aspirations for effective HCT and the resources to pay for them remains. An Institute of Medicine [25] report 15 years ago suggested that the fragmentation of health care for everyone, including those with disabilities and special needs in the U.S.A., jeopardized quality of care and led to costly duplication of services and missed opportunities to deliver care in lower-cost settings. As early as 1992, the American Academy of Pediatrics (AAP) [26] called for all children to have "a medical home that provides accessible, continuous, comprehensive, family-centered, coordinated, and compassionate health care in an atmosphere of mutual responsibility and trust among clinician, child, and caregiver(s)" [27]. The AAP [5] expanded the statement with a more comprehensive interpretation of the concept and defined the patient- and family-centered medical home as the ideal way to deliver primary care to children and adolescents with or without special health-care needs. This family-centered medical home also includes personalized care that demonstrates the clinician's knowledge of the patient and family environment, including work, personal, emotional, and, at times, financial concerns [27]. For the child and adolescent with special health-care needs, the team at the medical home also assists with the coordination of care with the patient's subspecialist(s), the school system, and community providers to ensure comprehensive care (see Chap. 26). The AAP along with three other prominent medical organizations have issued a joint statement calling for the medical home principles to be extended to all primary care for children, youth, and adults throughout the U.S.A. referred to as the Patient-Centered Medical Home (Joint Principles, 2007). In 2011, the AAP along with the American Academy of Family Practice and the American College of Physicians issued a report on HCT that defined an algorithmic approach to care planning with a specific branch for those patients with special health-care needs which is applicable to primary and specialty-based practices [28].

Despite the value of addressing the fragmentation in care and toward reducing health-care costs promised by the medical home and effective HCT, in a fee-for-service health-care system focused on counting events, more than half of the time that a health-care provider spends with AYASHCN may involve activities such as care coordination that are not reimbursed by insurance [29, 30]. Berry and colleagues [27] summarize the financing dilemma of a process such as delivering primary care according to a medical home model as well as services and supports for HCT as follows:

> "In general, outpatient structured clinical programs providing high quality of care for children with medical complexity have not been profitable in a traditional fee for service payment arrangement. Reasons to explain the lack of profitability include (1) lengthy outpatient visits (e.g., a 1 hour visit) are routinely needed to address health issues and care needs of [children with medical complexity], and (2) a large percentage of the time spent on care coordination does not occur during face-to-face health care encounters; the extensive non-face-to-face time required to effectively coordinate care (e.g., with phone conversations, email, home visits, and health information review) is poorly reimbursed or not reimbursed at all." (p. 9)

According to the National Survey of CSHCN (NS-CSHCN) in 2005–2006, 46% of parents of CYSCHN received care in a medical home type format that helped them coordinate their child's care, 32% lacked one or more elements of adequately coordinated care, and 22% felt they did not need coordinated care. In response to a question about their ability to get help in coordinating their child's care, 55% of parents reported they did not need any help with care coordination, 30% reported that they needed help and usually got it, and 15% reported they needed help and did not get it [10]. Care coordination and patient education can favorably impact the patient's and the family's experience. An analysis of the NS-CSHCN in 2005–2006 found that children who received adequate care coordination had an increased chance of receiving family-centered care, experiencing partnerships with professionals and reporting satisfaction with services [31]. Paradoxically, the more severely affected CSHCN, among the most in need of coordinated care, were the least likely to have a medical home and were also less likely to receive HCT services [32].

What is needed to promote medical homes and effective HCT for AYASHCN are alternative payment models that focus more on the value of the care delivered and less on volume of patients seen and on billing of discrete services delivered. Several promising alternative payment models summarized by Steinway and colleagues that could promote effective HCT as listed next [33]:

- "Enhanced Fee-for-Service (FFS) Payments
  - In a FFS setting, providers are compensated based on the reporting of medical billing codes. Insurers could enhance current medical billing codes by providing additional compensation (for example, at 150 percent) around the time of transition, recognizing that ensuring successful transfer to adult care requires additional time and work. While billing codes exist for transition services, these are usually not reimbursed by most public and private insurers.
- Pay-for-Performance (P4P)
  - The P4P mechanism pays providers based on a set of previously agreed upon metrics. In this model, insurers could incentivize pediatric providers to transfer patients before they reach age 22, for instance, and incentivize adult providers to accept complex young adult patients.
- Capitation
  - Capitation is the monthly payment for a service. Monthly payments for care coordination services needed for the transition from pediatric to adult health care could ensure that providers are properly compensated for their time preparing the documents for transfer, educating patients and families and communicating with adult providers.
- Bundled Payments and Shared Savings
  - Bundled payments are a group of services that receive one amount of money per episode of care and help align incentives for different providers. Bundled payments currently exist for transitions from hospital to home, but not for transitions from pediatric to adult health care. Alternatively, savings that the health system incurs through successful transfer could be equally shared with pediatric and adult providers. Payments could be linked to completion of services by both the sending pediatric and receiving adult providers.
- Administrative or Infrastructure Payments
  - These types of payments have been utilized by both Medicare and Medicaid. Instead of compensating for direct clinical activities, administrative or infrastructure payments are compensation for systems change. In the case of transition, these payments could be used for EMR adaptations that include, for example, Got Transition's Six Core Elements of Health Care Transition." (p. 21)

A value-based approach will likely generate cost savings that can then be redirected toward the care processes and care coordination so essential to delivering effective HCT [33]. A number of examples offer support for the value of clinical programs designed to coordinate care and optimize health [27]. Table 24.3 [27] summarizes these promising examples. In addition, the Center for Health Care Transition Improvement is working with six large integrated care systems on value-based initiatives to design and deliver care models that incorporate the Six Core Elements in a clinically relevant and cost-effective manner [23].

In summary, while a specific cost figure cannot be stated at the time of this writing, the path forward for how best to finance HCT for AYASHCN moving from the pediatric to adult settings of care calls for multiple strategies to overcome the payment barriers encountered when seeking to fund a process rather than a discrete procedure or event [22]. Health-care advocates interested in promoting HCT are increasingly focused on delivering value and utilizing one of the alternative payment models that gives health-care providers and institutions more flexibility in directing dollars toward activities that coordinate care but which have traditionally not been covered in fee-for-service volume-based reimbursement [34]. The literature supporting the value and financial benefit for the patient- and family-centered medical home cited above provides reason for a sense of optimism that supports for the process of care underlying HCT will also emerge [27]. However, overcoming payment barriers to HCT

Table 24.3 Examples of clinical programs designed to coordinate care and deliver value [adapted]

Location	Description	Citation
Outpatient consultative program at the Children's Hospital of Wisconsin	Provides intensive care coordination for ~230 CMC reported a $400,000 annual loss to operate the program while contributing to a 3-year reduction in hospital resource utilization of more than $10 million for its patients	Gordon JB, Colby HH, Bartelt T, Jablonski D, Krauthoefer ML, Havens P. A tertiary care-primary care partnership model for medically complex and fragile children and youth with special health-care needs. *Arch Pediatr Adolesc Med.* Oct 2007;161(10):937–944
Outpatient primary care program for children with medical complexity at Arkansas Children's Hospital	Reported a one-year decrease in the mean annual cost per patient per month (PPPM) of $1800 for inpatient care and $6 for emergency department care. Although PPPM cost for outpatient claims and prescriptions increased, the overall cost to Medicaid PPPM decreased by ~$1200	Casey PH, Lyle RE, Bird TM, et al. Effect of hospital-based comprehensive care clinic on health costs for Medicaid-insured medically complex children. *Arch Pediatr Adolesc Med.* May 2011;165(5):392–398
Two community-based pediatric clinics in Canada staffed with tertiary care nurse practitioners to coordinate care	Eighty-one patients with medical complexity reported a mean [standard deviation (SD)] decrease in per-member-per-month total health system cost from $244 (SD 981) to $131 (SD 335) without an increase in out-of-pocket costs to families. Fewer inpatient days was the primary reason for the decrease in per-member-per-month child quality of life improved after enrollment in the clinic intervention	Cohen E, Lacombe-Duncan A, Spalding K, et al. integrated complex care coordination for children with medical complexity: a mixed-methods evaluation of tertiary care community collaboration. *BMC Health Serv Res.* 2012;12:366
Six primary care pediatric practices in Massachusetts	A care coordination intervention for ~150 CMC/ CSHCN that included a case manager, parent consultant, and an individualized plan of care within was associated with a decrease in hospitalization rate (58–43%) and a decrease in the rate of parents missing 3 or more weeks of work (26–14%). The intervention cost $400 per patient	Palfrey JS, Sofis LA, Davidson EJ, Liu J, freeman L, Ganz ML. The Pediatric alliance for coordinated care: Evaluation of a medical home model. *Pediatrics.* May 2004;113(5 Suppl):1507–1516
A medical home for ~ at University of California Los Angeles	30 CMC were offered an hour-long intake appointment, 30 min. follow-up visits, access to a family liaison, and a family notebook, reported a decrease in the average number of emergency department visits from 1.1 (SD 1.7) to 0.5 (SD 0.9) after enrollment	Klitzner TS, Rabbitt LA, Chang RK. Benefits of care coordination for children with complex disease: a pilot medical home project in a resident teaching clinic. *J Pediatr.* Jun 2010;156(6):1006–1010

Adapted from: Berry J., Agrawal RK, Cohen E., Kuo DZ. The Landscape of Medical Care for Children with Medical Complexity. Children's Hospital Association. June 2013

will not be easy. Despite optimism that alternate payment models will be a useful development along the path toward sustainable HCT funding for AYASHCN, families and professionals must continue to advocate that HCT is part of ideal care. While the alternative payment models provide clinicians and administrators with flexibility to support the care coordination efforts fundamental to HCT, adequate tracking and data analysis are essential so that the value of HCT for AYASHCN as well as to the overall health-care system can be measured and used to justify additional efforts and investment.

References

1. Koop CE. Introductory remarks. In: Magrab PR, Millar HEC, editors. Surgeon General's conference. Growing up and getting medical care: youth with special health care needs, Summary of conference proceedings. Washington, DC: Georgetown University, Child Development Center; 1989. p. 3–5.
2. Blum RW, Garell D, Hodgman CH, Jorissen TW, Okinow NA, Orr DP, Slap BB. Transition from child-centered to adult health-care systems for adolescents with chronic conditions. J Adolesc Health. 1993;14:570–6.
3. Scal P. Transition to youth with chronic conditions: primary care physicians' approaches. Pediatrics. 2002;110(6):1315–21.
4. Berwick DM, Nolan TW, Whittington J. The triple aim: care, health, and cost: the remaining barriers to integrated care are not technical; they are political. Health Aff. 2008;27(3):759–69.
5. American Academy of Pediatrics. Medical home initiatives for children with special needs project advisory committee: the medical home. Pediatrics. 2002;110:184–6.
6. Martin AB, Hartman M, Benson B, Catlin A, the National Health Expenditure Account Team. National Health Spending in 2014: faster growth driven by coverage expansion and prescription drug spending. Health Aff. 2016;35(1):150–60.
7. Kaiser Family Foundation (KFF). Trends in health care costs. 2009. http://kff.org/health-costs/fact-sheet/trends-in-health-care-costs-and-spending.
8. Centers for Medicare and Medicaid Services (CMS). Office of the Actuary. National Health Expenditure. 2017. https://www.cms.gov/Research-Statistics-Data-and-Systems/Statistics-Trends-and Reports/National-HealthExpendData/NationalHealthAccountsProjected.html. Accessed 21 Mar 2017.
9. Bui AL, Dieleman JL, Hamavid H, Birger M, Chapin A, Duber HC, Horst C, Reynolds A, Squires E, Chung PH, Murray CJL. Spending on children's personal health care in the United States. JAMA Pediatr. 2017;171(2):183–9.
10. U.S. Department of Health and Human Services (UHD-HHS), Health Resources and Services Administration, Maternal and Child Health Bureau. The National Survey of children with special health care needs chartbook 2005–2006. Rockville, MA: U.S. Department of Health and Human Services; 2007. http://mchb.hrsa.gov/cshcn05/MI/NSCSHCN.pdf
11. McPherson M, Arango P, Fox H, Lauver C, McManus M, Newacheck PW, Strickland B. A new definition of children with special needs. Pediatrics. 1998;102:137–40.
12. Kogan MD, Strickland BB, Newacheck PW. Building systems of care: findings from the National Survey of children with special health care needs. Pediatrics. 2009;124:S333–6.
13. Newacheck PW, Kim SE. A National profile of health care utilization and expenditures for children with special health care needs. [published correction appears in Arch Pediatr Adolesc Med. 2005 Apr;159:318]. Arch Pediatr Adolesc Med. 2005;159(1):10–7.
14. Lindley LC, Mark BA. Children with special health care needs: impact of health care expenditures on family burden. J Child Fam Stud. 2010;19(1):79–89.
15. Newacheck PW, Inkelas M, Kim SE. Health services use and health care expenditures for children with disabilities. Pediatrics. 2004;114:79–85.
16. Medical Expenditure Panel Survey (MEPS) HC-050 documentation, 2000; main data results. Rockville, MD: Agency for Healthcare Research and Quality; 2003. http://www.meps.ahrq.gov/mepsweb/data_stats/download_data/pufs/h50/h50doc.pdf.
17. Musumeci M. Medicaid and children with special health care needs. The Henry J. Kaiser Family Foundation issue brief. 2017. http://files.kff.org/attachment/Issue-Brief-Medicaid-and-Children-with-Special-Health-Care-Needs.
18. Houtrow AJ, Larson K, Olson LM, Newacheck PW, Halfon N. Changing trends of childhood disability, 2001–2011. Pediatrics. 2014;134(3):530–8.
19. Anderson WL, Armour BS, Finkelstein EA, Wiener JM. Estimates of state-level health-care expenditures associated with disability. Public Health Rep. 2010;125:44–51.
20. Mitra S, Palmer M, Kim H, Mont D, Groce N. Extra costs of living with a disability: a review and agenda for research. Disabil Health J. 2017;10:475–84.
21. Burns MD, Shah ND, Smith MA. Living at the thin margin of health: out-of-pocket health care spending by Medicaid beneficiaries with disabilities. Health Aff. 2010;29(8):1517–22.
22. White PH, McManus M. Facilitating the transitions from pediatric-oriented to adult-oriented primary care. In: Pilapil M, Delaet DE, Kuo AA, Peacock C, Sharma N, editors. Care of adults with chronic childhood conditions. New York: Springer; 2016. p. 3–14.
23. White P. Transition models from pediatric to adult health care: innovative strategies. Center for Health Care Transition Improvement. Nd. https://www.hrsa.gov/advisorycommittees/mchbadvisory/heritabledisorders/meetings/2015/ninth/innovativestrategies.pdf.
24. Prior M, McManus M, White P, Davidson L. Measuring the "Triple Aim" in transition care: a systematic review. Pediatrics. 2014;134:e1648–161.
25. Institute of Medicine. Crossing the quality chasm: a new health system for the 21st century. Washington, DC: National Academies Press; 2001.
26. American Academy of Pediatrics. American Academy of Pediatrics ad hoc task force on definition of the medical home: the medical home (RE9262). Pediatrics. 1992;90:774.
27. Berry J, Agrawal RK, Cohen E, Kuo DZ. The landscape of medical care for children with medical complexity.

Alexandria, VA: Children's Hospital Association; 2013. https://www.childrenshospitals.org/-/media/Files/CHA/Main/Issues_and_Advocacy/Key_Issues/Children_With_Medical_Complexity/Issue-Briefs-and-Reports/LandscapeOfMedicalCare_06252013.pdf
28. American Academy of Pediatrics (AAP), American Academy of Family Physicians, American College of Physicians, Transitions Clinical Report Authoring Group. Clinical report – supporting the health care transition from adolescence to adulthood in the medical home. Pediatrics. 2011;128:182–200.
29. Antonelli RC, Antonelli DM. Providing a medical home: the cost of care coordination services in a community-based general pediatric practice. Pediatrics. 2004;113(5):1522–8.
30. Antonelli RC, Stille CJ, Antonelli DM. Care coordination for children and youth with special health care needs: a descriptive, multisite study of activities, personnel costs, and outcomes. Pediatrics. 2008;122:e209–16.
31. Turchi R, Berhane Z, Bethell C, Pomonio A, Antonelli R, Minkovitz CS. Care coordination for CSHCN: associations with family-provider relations and family/child outcomes. Pediatrics. 2009;124(Suppl 4):S428–35.
32. Singh GK, Strickland BB, Shandour RM, van Dyck PC. Geographic disparities in access to the medical home among US CSHCN. Pediatrics. 2009;124(Suppl 4):S352–60.
33. Steinway C, Gable JL, Jan S, MINT. Transitioning to adult care: supporting youth with special health care needs. PolicyLab at Children's Hospital of Philadelphia; 2017. p. 11. http://bit.ly/E2A_TransitionsOfCare.
34. Agency for Healthcare Research and Quality (AHRQ). Theory and reality of value-based purchasing: lessons from the pioneer. 1997. https://www.ahrq.gov/professionals/quality-patient-safety/quality-resources/tools/meyer/index.html.

Payment for Healthcare Transition Services

25

Margaret A. McManus, Patience H. White, and David Kanter

Introduction

Aligning payment with recommended healthcare transition (HCT) delivery system improvements is a critical need identified by pediatric and adult clinicians. Although the Centers for Medicare and Medicaid Services (CMS) prioritized hospital-to-home transitions for Medicare populations, there have not yet been comparable efforts by CMS or private payers to establish value-based payment arrangements for pediatric-to-adult care transitions.

In 2012, CMS recognized the value of effective hospital-to-home transitions for Medicare populations when it introduced the Medicare Hospital Readmissions Reduction Program. This program established a set of measures to calculate excess readmissions and to make adjusted hospital payments [1]. Further, in 2013, CMS lent its support for new Medicare codes for transitional care management services. These hospital-to-home CPT codes can be used to report an office visit within a specified time frame and a set of non-face-to-face care coordination, communication, and health education services provided by physicians and other health team members [2]. Research has documented the benefits of combining hospital-to-home delivery and payment reforms in terms of cost savings and improvements in population health and consumer experience [3, 4].

While pediatric-to-adult transition encompasses many of the same services as hospital-to-home transitions, there are several important distinctions. First, the time period surrounding pediatric-to-adult transitions extends from early in adolescence through young adulthood—compared to the brief hospital-to-home intervention period. Second, transition to adult care involves a broader set of interventions, including transition preparation to develop patient self-care skills and health literacy, identification of adult care providers, preparation of current medical information, communication and coordination between pediatric and adult providers, and facilitated access, integration, and retention into adult care. In

M. A. McManus, M.H.S. (✉)
The National Alliance to Advance Adolescent Health, Washington, DC, USA

Got Transition, Washington, DC, USA
e-mail: mmcmanus@thenationalalliance.org

P. H. White, M.D., M.A.
Departments of Medicine and Pediatrics, George Washington School of Medicine and Health Science, Washington, DC, USA

Got Transition, Washington, DC, USA
e-mail: pwhite@thenationalalliance.org

D. Kanter, M.D., M.B.A., C.P.C.
Medical Coding, MEDNAX Services, Inc, Fort Lauderdale, FL, USA

CPT Editorial Panel, American Academy of Pediatrics, Fort Lauderdale, FL, USA

A. C. Hergenroeder, C. M. Wiemann (eds.), *Health Care Transition*,
https://doi.org/10.1007/978-3-319-72868-1_25

contrast, hospital-to-home interventions primarily address transfer. Third, transition to adult care is more complex because it involves changing from family-centered pediatric care to patient-centered adult care with a vulnerable age group.

Recognizing the distinctive services that are part of pediatric-to-adult transitions, this chapter attempts to identify payment gaps and options for shared accountability between pediatric and adult care. These payment options align with transition interventions called for in the AAP/AAFP/ACP Clinical Report on Health Care Transition [5] and the clinical approach, called the "Six Core Elements of Health Care Transition" [6]. The chapter begins with a summary of common payment barriers followed by a listing of specific transition-related codes. It also offers suggested guidance to avoid common billing and coding missteps along with suggested advocacy strategies for negotiating coverage with practices, health plans, and payers. Finally, the chapter describes innovative payment approaches related to enhanced fee-for-service arrangements, capitation, pay-for-performance, and bundled payments.

Table 25.1 Specific pediatric-to-adult transition payment barriers

• Codes for care plan oversight, health risk assessment (including transition readiness/self-care assessment), care management services, consultation, and self-care management often not recognized by payers
• Transition readiness assessments and health risk assessments cannot be coded during the same adolescent or young adult preventive visit
• Office visits for transferring patients seeing both pediatric and adult providers on the same day not covered
• No comparable ambulatory care transition code—like the hospital-to-home transition code
• No CPT code for outreach and facilitated access to care
• Relative value units (RVUs) for selected transition-related codes (e.g., health risk assessment) are low or not published in the Medicare physician fee schedule
• If transferring pediatric patient's last visit is a preventive office visit, insurance will not pay for initial adult preventive visit until a year later
• Electronic health record (EHR) adaptations to incorporate transition-related clinic procedures not reimbursed
• Quality improvement (QI) processes to implement recommended transition interventions not reimbursed
• Young adults disproportionally likely to be uninsured
• Young adults have high no-show rates

Payment Barriers Impeding Transition to Adult Care

Numerous studies have examined transition barriers affecting pediatric and adult providers [7–11]. Unfortunately, most of these studies fail to describe specific coding and reimbursement issues; rather, studies simply cite "payment or reimbursement problems." Table 25.1 provides a listing of specific payment issues identified by the authors as part of transition quality improvement efforts that Got Transition, the national resource center on healthcare transition, is involved in.

Transition-Related Codes

Transition is intended to be part of routine preventive, primary, and chronic care for all adolescents and young adults. As such, outpatient office visit and preventive medicine codes—codes that all payers recognize—can be used to provide transition anticipatory guidance, counseling, and coordination. Table 25.2 includes a listing of transition-related codes. Further information about corresponding Medicare fees and RVUs and detailed CPT coding descriptions and clinical vignettes can be found in Got Transition's *2017 Coding and Reimbursement Tip Sheet* [12].

Billing and Coding Documentation Guidance and Advocacy Strategies for Transition Payment

The American Medical Association (AMA) maintains the Current Procedural Terminology (CPT) code set which describes services

Table 25.2 Transition-related codes

• Office or other outpatient services, new/established patient (CPT 99201–99205, 99211–99215)
• Office or other outpatient consultations, new/established patient (CPT 99241–99245)
• Care plan oversight services (CPT 99374–99380)
• Prolonged services (99354, 99355, 99358, 99359)
• Medical team conference (99366–99368)
• Preventive medicine services (99384, 99485, 99394, 99395)
• Health risk assessment (96160, 96161)
• Care management services (99487, 99489, 99490)
• Transitional care management services (99495, 99496)
• Telephone services (99441–99443)
• Online medical evaluation (99444)
• Interprofessional telephone/Internet consultation (99446–99449)
• Education and training for patient self-management (98960–98962)
• Miscellaneous educational services (99078)

performed by physicians and other healthcare professionals[1]. The annual publication of this AMA-maintained code set may include year-to-year additions, deletions, and modifications, and, therefore, it behooves the reporting clinician and other billing staff to be aware of current CPT guidance that pertains to the codes relevant to one's practice. CPT addresses services that are both procedural and surgical in nature as opposed to cognitive and non-procedural. Non-procedural, cognitive services are most aligned with the elements of transitional care, and these cognitive services are represented by both face-to-face codes (such as evaluation and management visits) and non-face-to-face services (such as care management codes). While historically a higher likelihood of payer coverage existed when services were rendered face to face, more recently, payers have provided broader coverage of non-face-to-face services based on the role that such services play in managing complex clinical scenarios in achieving improved patient outcomes [13].

With such a large inventory of coded services relevant to transitional care scenarios (Table 25.2), clinicians can pursue alternatives strategies to maximize potential for payment for service. Clinicians should be aware that with the scope and complexity of the CPT code set, payers may not cover some of the services relevant to transitional care. With regard to assessing likelihood of payer coverage, the Medicare Physician Fee Schedule (MPFS) provides valuable insight into payment policy. Although pediatricians may have limited Medicare exposure among their patients, the MPFS establishes a coverage template that many state Medicaid programs as well as commercial payers follow. Each year CMS publishes the MPFS, which includes CMS-accepted RVUs based on AMA Relative Value Update Committee (RUC) recommendations, as well as Medicare's coverage policy for a particular code. For example, Medicare assignment of provider status A to a particular CPT code represents active coverage by Medicare and increases the likelihood that Medicaid programs as well as commercial payers will also cover the service (as opposed to status B, bundled, or status N, non-covered, which do not support Medicare payment and minimize the likelihood of Medicaid coverage for the service). CMS provides an online look-up tool that allows clinicians to enter any CPT code to determine Medicare RVU valuation along with Medicare coverage status [14]. Such information can be helpful not only in assessing Medicare and other payer coverage but also in negotiating service payment rates with nongovernment payers.

In addition to the MPFS, many state Medicaid programs publish their own physician fee schedules on their online websites. These fee schedules not only provide the Medicaid payment rate for a particular service but also provide insight into Medicaid coverage policy (whereby absence of a service on the fee schedule generally indicates non-coverage). Since Medicaid plays such a central role in pediatric care, clinicians and administrative staff should be familiar with their state's Medicaid fee schedule policies as pertains to the

[1]Qualified healthcare professionals are non-physician clinical personnel who utilize their national provider identifier (NPI) number to report to payers those CPT services rendered within their scope of practice.

types of services relevant to a given adolescent and young adult population. In making coverage and payment determinations, Medicaid programs base their fee schedules on state budget parameters and allowances. Clinicians can play an important role in advocating for Medicaid payment in their respective states. Medicaid programs may not be as quick in assuming coverage for newly created CPT codes even though such services may already be actively covered by Medicare. Absence of a particular service in the Medicaid fee schedule provides an opportunity for the clinician to contact Medicaid representatives to relay the importance of the service to pediatric patients and to encourage coverage as state budget discussions progress. Especially for coordinated services such as those related to transition to adult care, Medicaid programs will be receptive to payment in the context of clinical strategies that offer the possibility of reduced use of downstream acute care services while improving outcome [15].

Although Medicare and Medicaid coverage increases the likelihood of commercial payment for a particular service, clinicians can include any CPT code when establishing contracts with their commercial payers. While commercial payers may have established coverage policies regarding particular types of services, some services may play an instrumental role in healthcare delivery for particular clinicians and patients, and these scenarios provide an opportunity for expansion of commercial payer coverage for those types of services that may have special relevance for a unique patient population. For example, payer coverage of care management services (99487, 99489, 99490) and care plan oversight (99374–99380) is typically inconsistent, yet such services can be instrumental in managing complex patients as they progress through various transitions in care. If claims for such services are denied by the payer based on non-coverage, physicians can use those denials to educate and advocate with the payer when negotiating contractual carve-outs for such services based on the value they provide to beneficiaries. Payers are increasingly attuned to the impact that care management services have on healthcare quality and patient outcome. If certain services are integral to a structured, longitudinal approach to healthcare, and if such services may not be currently covered by the commercial payer, opportunities exist to establish quality measure process and outcome requirements that can support mutual payment agreements between provider and payer that validate effectiveness of service payment.

The evolution of healthcare toward alternative models of payment nicely accentuates the strengths that transitional care services provide to overall patient care. Alternative payment models are typically structured on creation of value by achieving quality at a given cost. Some of the non-face-to-face care coordination services inherent in effective transition have not historically received payment in a fee-for-service environment but contribute value through their impact on a broad scope of patient care. Even though isolated segments of transition services may be represented by individual fee-for-service CPT codes, some of which may not be covered by the payer, the integration of these codes into models of care (e.g., Six Core Elements of Health Care Transition) that encompass multiple providers and environments in pediatric and adult healthcare settings has relevance in assessing the financial value of payment bundles or alternative payment models. By becoming familiar with and reporting the codes that encompass these broad scope services, clinicians have a better opportunity to understand the value of the care being rendered and can thus more effectively engage in discussions regarding modeling of these various services into an integrated approach to care and payment [16]. Therefore, even if a clinician has not received payment for the transition-related codes listed in Table 25.2, it is essential to continue to document provision of these services in order to make the case for expanded coverage.

Alternative Payment Options to Promote Shared Accountability

A range of alternative payment methods can be considered by CMS and other payers as options for strengthening the delivery of healthcare transition services in pediatric and adult settings consistent with the AAP/AAFP/ACP Clinical Report on Transition and the Six Core Elements of Health Care Transition.

Enhanced Fee-for-Service Payments

Fee-for-service (FFS) payments will continue to be important in supporting the delivery of recommended transition services. Reporting the appropriate CPT codes and ensuring that private and public payers are using the current associated values for each code form the foundation for payment in FFS arrangements. Payers could enhance FFS payments—for example, paying pediatric and adult office visit fees at 150% of Medicare rates for the year surrounding the transfer of a new patient, recognizing the added work involved in transferring and accepting patients. They could also increase fees for care plan oversight services to ensure the development and updating of the medical summary as well as of the plan of care.

Pay-for-Performance

Under pay-for-performance (P4P), physicians are paid based on agreed-upon performance metrics for a defined population. Payers could, for example, offer pediatric practices a bonus payment for successfully transferring their patients before age 22 with complete medical records and evidence of communication with adult providers. Similarly, adult providers could receive a bonus for accepting a certain volume of new young adult patients, communicating with the referring pediatric provider, and ensuring a primary care visit is made within 6 months of transfer from the pediatric provider. P4P could also be structured based on improvements made or scores received on either the Current Assessment of Health Care Transition Activities or the Health Care Transition Process Measurement Tool (available at www.gottransition.org).

Capitation

Monthly care coordination payments or capitation can provide a mechanism for reimbursing the added time involved by pediatric and adult practices in preparing youth and their families/caregivers for transfer to adult care, preparing the necessary transfer documents, ensuring coordination and communication between pediatric and adult care systems, and implementing outreach and follow-up strategies for new young adult patients. These monthly capitation payments could also be adjusted for patient complexity.

Bundled Payments

Bundled payments, by definition, include multiple services typically associated with an episode of care. The CPT codes for transitional care management services (99495, 99496) are examples of a combination of services provided by a physician or qualified healthcare professional for a patient with moderate to high complexity transitioning from hospital- to community-based setting. These include a face-to-face visit, communication, education to support self-care, assessment of treatment and medication management, identification of community resources, referrals, and scheduling follow-up. This code, however, does not extend to transition from pediatric to adult ambulatory health care, only from hospital to home. Still, it would be possible to structure a bundled payment arrangement for a package of transfer services from pediatric to adult care, including an updated medical summary and emergency care plan, transition readiness assessment, plan of care, and other services listed under the CPT Transitional Care Management Services. Templates for each of these transition services are available in the Six Core Elements packages (www.gottransition.org).

Shared Savings

By ensuring a successful transfer from pediatric care to adult care at a cost below budgeted amounts, the resultant savings associated with reduced emergency room visits and hospitalizations could be shared with pediatric and adult providers. This payment arrangement generally follows a defined set of structural and quality standards. In the case of transition from pediatric to adult healthcare, a potential option would be to use the measurement tools described above under pay-for-performance.

Administrative or Infrastructure Payments

This payment mechanism has been used by Medicare to support adoption and meaningful use of electronic health record technology and by Medicaid to conduct administrative activities (e.g., outreach, planning, training) to implement a state's Medicaid plan. Demonstration grants and other infrastructure investment grants have been awarded to support system changes. In the case of pediatric-to-adult transition, this payment strategy could be considered for covering costs of customizing electronic health records to align with the recommended core elements of transition and for transition training of pediatric and adult providers, but not for direct services.

Conclusion

Progress in advancing pediatric-to-adult transition improvements will be slow to achieve without payer recognition of transition-related codes and investment in new alternative financial incentives. Much can be accomplished by clinicians effectively coding for transition-related services and working with their state professional chapters and Medicaid and commercial insurance carriers to encourage not only the recognition of existing codes but also consideration of the value-based alternative payment options described in this chapter.

References

1. Centers for Medicare & Medicaid Services. Readmissions reduction program (HRRP). 2017. https://www.cms.gov/medicare/medicare-fee-for-service-payment/acuteinpatientpps/readmissions-reduction-program.html. Accessed 29 June 2017.
2. Medicare Learning Network. Transitional care management services. 2017. https://www.cms.gov/Outreach-and-Education/Medicare-Learning-Network-MLN/MLNProducts/downloads/Transitional-Care-Management-Services-Fact-Sheet-ICN908628.pdf. Accessed 29 June 2017.
3. National Transitions of Care Coalition. Improved transitions of patient care yield tangible savings. 2017. www.ntocc.org/Portals/0/PDF/Resources/TangibleSavings.pdf. Accessed 29 June 2017.
4. Wasfy JH, Zigler CM, Choirat C, Wang Y, Dominici F, Yeh RW. Readmission rates after passage of the hospital readmissions reduction program: a pre-post analysis. Ann Intern Med. 2017;166:324–31.
5. American Academy of Pediatrics, American Academy of Family Physicians, American College of Physicians, Transitions Clinical Report Authoring Group, Cooley WC, Sagerman PJ. Supporting the health care transition from adolescence to adulthood in the medical home. Pediatrics. 2011;128:182–200.
6. McManus M, White P, Barbour A, Downing B, Hawkins K, Quion N, et al. Pediatric to adult transition: a quality improvement model for primary care. J Adolesc Health. 2015;56:73–8.
7. Gray WN, Resmini AR, Baker KD, Holbrook E, Morgan PJ, Ryan J, et al. Concerns, barriers, and recommendations to improve transition from pediatric to adult IBD care: perspectives of patients, parents, and health professionals. Inflamm Bowel Dis. 2015;21:1641–51.
8. Nehring WM, Betz CL, Lobo ML. Uncharted territory: systematic review of providers' roles, understanding, and views pertaining to health care transition. J Pediatr Nurs. 2015;30:732–47.
9. Okumura MJ, Kerr EA, Cabana MD, Davis MM, Demonner S, Heisler M. Physician views on barriers to primary care for young adults with childhood-onset chronic disease. Pediatrics. 2010;125:e748–54.
10. Peter NG, Forke CM, Ginsburg KR, Schwarz DF. Transition from pediatric to adult care: internists' perspectives. Pediatrics. 2009;123:417–23.
11. Sebastian S, Jenkins H, McCartney S, Ahmad T, Arnott I, Croft N, et al. The requirements and barriers to successful transition of adolescents with inflammatory bowel disease: differing perceptions from a survey of adult and paediatric gastroenterologists. J Crohns Colitis. 2012;6:830–44.
12. McManus M, White P, Harwood C, Molteni R, Kanter D, Salus T. Coding and reimbursement tip sheet for transition from pediatric to adult health care. 2017. www.gottransition.org/resourceGet.cfm?id=352. Accessed 29 June 2017.
13. Burton R. Health policy brief: improving care transitions. Health Aff. 2012. https://doi.org/10.1377/hpb20120913.327236.
14. Centers for Medicare & Medicaid Services. Physician fee schedule overview. 2017. https://www.cms.gov/apps/physician-fee-schedule/overview.aspx. Accessed 29 June 2017.
15. Sawicki GS, Garvey KC, Toomey SL, Williams KA, Hargraves JL, James T, et al. Preparation for transition to adult care among medicaid-insured adolescents. Pediatrics. 2017;140(1):e20162768.
16. Porter ME, Kaplan RS. How to pay for health care. Harv Bus Rev. 2016;94:88–100.

Part VII

Special Issues in Healthcare Transition

Healthcare Transition and the Medical Home

26

Jennifer Lail

Case

Pam is a 17-year-old female with repaired complex cyanotic congenital heart disease, a history of learning disabilities, and mild cognitive delays. You have been her pediatrician since birth, initially following her closely in her medical home, Pine Forest Pediatrics. You saw her for checkups and co-management of her heart disease with the Pediatric Cardiology from the nearby medical center before, during, and after her cardiac repair. Pam was entered at birth in your practice's clinical registry of children with special healthcare needs, which is curated by your care coordination staff. Regular preventive care visits at Pine Forest, though, declined after her heart repair and her Kindergarten physical examination was completed. The birth of her brother reconnected the family to the medical home for his well-baby care, but thereafter Pam was seen primarily for sick visits with well-child care requiring outreach by practice care coordinators. When Pam was 12, the emergency department called about her admission to the intensive care unit for accidental head trauma. You discover that the family had suffered a contentious divorce and moved twice, missing contact attempts by Pine Forest. The mother is now the custodial parent and father's involvement is sporadic. Needed follow-up from her intensive care unit stay was done at Pine Forest, with a complete physical examination, including adolescent vaccines and screenings, cardiology appointment facilitated by your staff, and a discussion that Pam would need lifelong preventive care and cardiac follow-up. Pam's 12-year-old understanding of her condition was "I was a really sick baby and had surgery to fix my heart." For a short time after her head injury, Pam and her family remained connected to Pine Forest, as they dealt with her menarche and her emerging learning differences, and you worked with Pam to coach, monitor, and track her self-efficacy in managing her conditions. Your team interfaced with her school around her medical absences and her individualized education program in school and connected the family to financial assistance resources. Your staff made a future chronic care management appointment for Pam and her family, but they did not show up. Your team made several follow-up calls and, when unable to reach an individual, sent a follow-up letter to the latest known address.

The medical home is a model of care that provides a reliable and familiar entry into a comprehensive care system and fosters communication and collaboration between and among patients,

J. Lail, M.D.
Chronic Care, James M. Anderson Center for Health Systems Excellence, Cincinnati Children's Hospital Medical Center, Cincinnati, OH, USA

Complex Care Center, Division of General Pediatrics, Cincinnati, OH, USA
e-mail: Jennifer.Lail@cchmc.org

A. C. Hergenroeder, C. M. Wiemann (eds.), *Health Care Transition*,
https://doi.org/10.1007/978-3-319-72868-1_26

families, clinicians, support staff, and the larger community. The medical home model [1] has been endorsed by pediatricians, internists, family medicine physicians, osteopathic providers, and emergency physicians [2]. The Joint Principles for the Patient-Centered Medical Home—care that is accessible, compassionate, comprehensive, continuous, coordinated, culturally appropriate, and family-centered—are important to adolescents and young adults with special healthcare needs (AYASHCN), since trusted and informed relationships and ready access to such care affects their clinical and functional outcomes [3]. However, data from the 2011 National Survey of Children's Health demonstrates that only about half the children from ages 1 to 17 years in the United States had a medical home, with notable racial/ethnic, socioeconomic, and health-related disparities [4]. The medical home, when established as a reliable touchpoint for preventive, acute, and chronic care, represents system-level support for transition and transfer to both an adult model and adult site of care. While adherence to condition-specific medical and lifestyle regimens [5] is a critical piece of a youth's care, the medical home model offers enhanced opportunities to provide a holistic approach to the adolescent and young adult (AYA). Data from a Minnesota program showed higher receipt of vaccines, preventive care, and screenings in AYA who were enrolled in a patient-centered medical home model of care [6]. An AYASHCN also requires support for preventive health practices, school and work performance, self-esteem, peer relationships, and evolving sexuality, with the goal of care integration across all the domains where the youth functions. A growing body of evidence supports the value and benefits of the medical home, including impacts on healthcare costs, quality of care, health outcomes, and family satisfaction [7]. The Chronic Care Model from Dr. Edward Wagner and the MacColl Institute informs the necessary medical home structures and processes that optimally support improved outcomes for youth with chronic illness [8, 9], highlighting both the prepared, proactive practice team and the informed, empowered patient and family as foundational elements. The National Center for Medical Home Implementation, a technical assistance collaboration between the American Academy of Pediatrics and the United States Health Resources and Services Administration, offers guidance in implementation of such structures, processes, and practices to optimize a youth's medical home [10].

The Medical Home Model: Relationships, Access, Population Management, Communication, and Care Coordination

When a multidisciplinary practice team implements the elements of the medical home model, systems and processes are built to promote trusted healthcare relationships, dependable access to care, proactive population management outside of face-to-face encounters, clinical information systems for continuity and accuracy of health information, supportive links to specialists and the community, and way-finding with care coordination for adult care providers, funding, insurance, privacy, and, when necessary, guardianship. Policies, procedures, and roles and responsibilities across the care team members must be explicit, with the care team's names and contact information available to youth and families. Families may identify more strongly and interact more openly with team members other than physicians. Both licensed and unlicensed staff are valuable to identify clinical gaps in care, assist with refills and pre-authorizations, do condition-specific self-management education, remove barriers to care, help with transportation, maintain a registry, develop a care plan, and address financial and psychosocial needs through links to the local community. Such processes can culminate in the co-creation of a gradual and cumulative plan with each youth and family for a safe and effective transfer from a pediatric to an adult model of care [11]. Even so, as demonstrated in the opening vignette, realizing such a transfer is complicated and labor intensive.

Relationships/Team-Based Care in the Medical Home

When Pam was 16, her mother told your staff that Pam had been tired for several months and wanted papers signed about her heart disease so she could get her driver's license. Your care team, using population management strategies for clinical outreach, had made multiple calls for Pam and her brother, who were overdue for well-adolescent care, and arranged for them to see you in a week. The registry prompted staff that pre-visit planning should be done for Pam because of her known chronic conditions. Your staff accessed specialty records and noted missed cardiology and neurology visits and the absence of recommended lipid screening and vaccines and pended orders for those services in Pam's chart. You saw each young adult separately and alone after a shared interview with mother and each youth. In your psychosocial history, obtained using a validated tool (HEEADSSS 3.0 [12]), Pam told you everything was "just fine," but the brother told the nurse giving his vaccine that Pam and their mother "fight all the time," and Pam was "sneaking out" with her boyfriend. A conversation with Pam revealed that she was having unprotected sex, had no understanding of her cardiovascular risk if she became pregnant, and felt her mother was too focused on her failing grades, since Pam's goal was to become a cosmetologist.

Just as youth and parents mark the earliest signs of puberty as a milestone, so can the medical home care team acknowledge early adolescence as a time to apply their screening processes to meet the needs of children in this vulnerable developmental zone. In their Transitions Clinical Report [11], Cooley, Sagerman et al. suggest the age of 12–13 years to begin the explicit preparations for the transition of care to an adult-oriented healthcare model around the ages of 18–21 years. Such evolving preparation, incorporating models such as the Six Core Elements of Health Care Transition [13], can be accomplished within the medical home, usually in a primary care setting and in collaboration with the youth's specialty providers. The Academic Pediatric Association noted a youth's developmental trajectory and their dependence on family as unique relationship challenges in caring for adolescents [14]. The continuity of care afforded by empanelment, or the patient/family guided assignment of a patient to a provider-led care team, has shown evidence for improved access and care coordination and reduced hospitalizations and healthcare costs in chronic conditions in adults [15, 16]. Trusted relationships developed in the medical home with young people who have chronic illness or disability can be powerful and forged at the tumultuous, and sometimes life-threatening, time of the new diagnosis of the chronic condition. Likewise, a family may be given the diagnosis of a chronic condition in a crisis setting, such as an emergency department or inpatient setting with unfamiliar providers. The American College of Emergency Physicians includes communication with the child's medical home as a guideline for pediatric emergency care [17]. Involvement by providers and staff in the medical home at diagnosis gives opportunities for shared decision-making, goal-setting, and understanding of the larger family structure as the diagnostic and therapeutic care plan evolves [17]. When the care team is familiar, families report relief at not having to repeat their child's medical history at each encounter. Coping with chronic conditions stresses family function and adherence to medical regimens, as well as sibling mental health and interpersonal function [18, 19]. The medical home can address such stressors. For example, medical home team personnel assist with appointments for medical and surgical specialists, school and community supports, and mental/behavioral/financial assistance.

Relationships in the medical home with a child and family necessarily change in adolescence and young adulthood, requiring practice policies around adolescent confidentiality. The medical home practices also must establish legally sound processes and policies for caring for youth who present for care without a parent or guardian (care by proxy) [20]. When clinicians establish, from early adolescence, that the parent(s) may be asked to step out of the exam room for the exam/conversation, both the youth and the parent know they can express their concerns and perceptions, providing qualified confidentiality. Laws around adolescent confidentiality vary by country and state, and it is critical that the medical home provider understands their laws around confidentiality, particularly in multistate care areas [21]. The American Academy of Pediatrics policy statement on chaperones during the physical exam [22] provides for shared decision-making about who should be present for physically or psychologically uncomfortable interactions with a youth. Setting confidentiality rules in early adolescence and reiterating them with the youth and family increases the likelihood of disclosure of important information that may prevent adverse health consequences [23]. Time alone with the clinician also permits discussion of the youth's understanding of their conditions, gives opportunity for information exchange, and validates the youth's concerns as important.

Strong relationships with a medical home team over time prompt the discussion of the practice's policies and procedures for transition to adult care services and the expectations that the family, specialists, and practice will collaborate to establish readiness and a plan for transfer to an adult model of care. By creating actual transition policies and procedures, the medical home care team establishes group consensus on the age at which a youth must leave their practice, so parents and providers begin the necessary planning for a gradual and informed transition to an adult medical home. Such policies and procedures should include processes to identify and contact adult providers willing to care for AYASHCN, a timeline for transitions and tools to track readiness, and any exclusionary criteria that would support delay of transition beyond the age stated in the policy (e.g., AYASCHN is clinically unstable or in palliative care). The transition policy can establish standards around appointments necessary to complete guardianship documentation and essential content of a transition summary and identify provider/staff roles for each step of the transition process.

Access to Care in the Medical Home and Beyond

At this 16-year-old well visit, Pam's mother pulled you aside and said she also wanted contraception prescribed for Pam. She reported that staff layoffs are occurring at her work and she feared losing her job in the next wave of cuts, so she wanted "everything checked out" while Pam and her brother are insured. She could only come to appointments on Saturday or Tuesday, her days off. You signed the pended lab and vaccine orders and added a pregnancy test and sexually transmitted disease screening after taking a sexual history and discussing with Pam. Your staff arranged for Pam to return on Saturday morning to complete her visit. You secure emails to update Pam's cardiologist, and a local gynecologist who sees teens facilitated an urgent appointment and reviewed Pam's cognitive delays and need for contraception. Pine Forest's business manager and care coordinator discussed other funding options for the family, who would meet Medicaid financial eligibility if the mother was laid off. You coded the visit for well-adolescent care and used a 25 modifier to code for your separate evaluation of multiple chronic condition issues.

For an AYASHCN gaining access to care can be fraught with barriers. Lack of insurance, physical barriers/transportation obstacles, time missed from school/work, distance from appropriate specialists, and health literacy/language barriers create disincentives for AYASHCN to get the care they need. Lack of funding for care is a proximal barrier to care. Medical homes can help by accepting public insurance and working with their state's Title V program for direction around eligibility for services. The Catalyst Center: National Center for Health Insurance and Financing for Children and Youth with Special Health Care Needs [24] offers support and technical assistance for financing healthcare delivery. Evolving standards for a youth's continued coverage on the parent's health insurance have expanded coverage options for AYA, but only to age 26 in the United States [25].

Titles II and III and Section 504 of the Americans with Disabilities Act, updated in 2010, require adapted physical access to medical facilities and the services they provide for all people with disabilities. These include parking, doorway and exam room clearance for wheelchairs, and unobstructed paths of travel to restrooms, telephones, and water fountains, as well as adjustable examination tables, lifts, and weighing apparatus. For AYA, privacy for vital signs and the exam and appropriately sized (and decorated) exam rooms and examination gowns are other ways to diminish barriers to care in the medical home. Medical homes may benefit from an active evaluation of their physical access to care for the adolescent and young adult patient. A walk-through with a young adult/family with technological dependence, limited mobility, or sensory sensitivities will help the practice identify barriers to care. Training for staff for safe lifting and transfers protects both patients and healthcare providers.

Access in the medical home also includes communication—with youth and family—so language translation services, use of augmented communication devices, and even visit-sequencing with picture schedules can help remove communication barriers [26]. For youth with intellectual or developmental disabilities, access to care involves dependency on parents, family members, or other care providers for physical transport, communication, and decision-making. Training for staff and providers in the medical home on interaction with people with any sort of disability helps with patient and family experience, legal compliance, and service provision [27, 28].

National standards for certification as a patient-centered medical home endorse expanded office hours on evenings and weekends for routine or urgent care and alternate access points, such as secure electronic patient portals, telephone consultations, and after-hours advice [29]. For youth with work, sports, and school commitments, expanded care hours on evenings and weekends and same-day access to care increases the opportunities for continuity and avoid emergency department utilizations. Acute care encounters offer an opportunity to identify and close care gaps in needed vaccines and screenings and to reenter the youth into regular well-youth and chronic condition care visits. While all needs may not be met in an acute care visit (such as Pam's), acute care is an opportunity to reengage and schedule the youth for preventive and chronic care management, including planning for transition and evaluating readiness skills. Medical homes can adapt time slots for such visits to accomplish many services in one visit (called max-packing [30]) and adjust medical coding to cover the extra time allotted for such care [31]. "No-shows" for appointments can be averted by population prediction based on prior missed appointment rates [32], acknowledging that transportation instability or public transit use may affect both attendance and timeliness for appointments. Medical home providers should establish expectations about visit attendance and timeliness with the youth; details of follow-up care for which the AYASHCN is responsible should be included and reviewed in the after-visit summary.

With the focus on management of their disease, young people with chronic conditions often do not receive preventive care [33]. Preventive care and chronic care visits in the medical home are a good way for AYASHCN to practice accessing care, refilling medications, and obtaining phone advice. Pre-visit contacts and planning (see below) with the youth or family can remind them of an upcoming appointment and identify the issues that matter to them, as well as updating the provider on the interim health history. In the known environment of the medical home, gradual testing of the youth's ability to make their own appointments, call for their medication refills, and identify their own concerns at medical encounters can occur. Such practice could create a phased independence with more responsibility and confidence-building while still within the pediatric model of care. For AYASHCN, the completion of sports, school, and camp forms can serve as a prompt for healthcare maintenance visits, as well as chronic condition management and transition readiness assessments. Access to online patient portals with connections to electronic health records may require adaptation for youth with disabilities, based on state privacy and consent laws for teens [34]. Securing accurate contact data for the youth is critical, as they may have limited data access on cellular devices and resist having their minutes spent on medical interactions. Reminders about upcoming appointments, with some flexibility about late arrivals, may help adolescents continue their connection with a childhood medical home. Gaps in needed care are common in adolescence [35]; the medical home's population management task is to identify those who have unmet needs and provide timely access to care to meet them. Identifying all the places a youth receives care provides a more comprehensive picture of their needs, since care may also be delivered by specialists or at emergency departments, school-based health centers, urgent care centers, or community health options such as Planned Parenthood. Same-day access to care is optimal for adolescents who are still developing their planning and time management capabilities and encourages the youth to align their care within the medical home.

Population Management Infrastructure

Before Pam's Saturday visit, your clinical assistant accessed and unified online records from her cardiologist at one medical center and the discharge summary from her intensive care unit stay for head trauma at a different hospital. She noted a recent fax from an urgent care center with diagnosis of bronchitis (with a reported history of smoking a pack a day of cigarettes). Your assistant contacted the mother for more information, who reported she saw oral contraceptive pills in Pam's bookbag, prescribed at a local family planning center. Your assistant noted that Pam has missed a neurology appointment as part of her head trauma follow-up. Using an electronic template, she copied and pasted this collated information for your review.

In the context of the medical home, population management refers to efforts to optimize health outcomes of the practice's patients by identifying and providing needed preventive care and by addressing gaps in care in chronic condition management. In both pediatric and adult models of care, AYASHCN benefit from elements of population management, such as care coordination, health education, and self-management support delivered in a highly functioning, patient-centered medical home [36]. Practice infrastructures, such as patient registries, proactive outreach for needed services, care-planning processes, and personnel to help navigate health services, all support a medical home's ability to improve care quality and patient experience. Providers' panel sizes vary by practice size and patient complexity, and knowing who your patients are (empanelment) is as important as the patient knowing their provider [16, 37]. Both research- and disease-specific registries have been in use for years, but more primary care practices are using patient registries to identify a provider panel and manage a specific set of metrics at both the population and patient level. Medical homes that use paper or electronic registries to identify patients with higher needs can stratify those needs and apply interventions and appropriate staff to address them. Applying the medical complexity algorithm developed by Simon et al. [38] can be a first step to stratifying the medical complexity of those in a population registry. Such needs may be condition-specific (e.g., HbA1c in diabetes or thyroid-stimulating hormone in Down syndrome), psychosocial (transportation, handicapped parking placards, energy assistance needs), or based on utilization (readmissions, emergency department use). Registries serve as a foundation for population management, with the ability to predict and plan for needed care, visits, or procedures [39].

At a population level, a registry can begin as a list of patients having received services in the practice within a time frame, often the prior 3 years, following the Centers for Medicare & Medicaid Services definition of a new patient [40]. The medical home must define their active subpopulation for measurement and may choose to exclude patients they do not expect to follow over time, such as one-time visits and patients who are outside their service area or are second-opinion consults [41, 42]. Practices can develop the registry to track preventive and condition-specific services for reliable delivery to their population, such as adolescent well care, influenza vaccines, or sexually transmitted disease screening, and to identify which providers have openings in their patient panels. High-functioning registries can be used to measure patient outcomes and utilization and direct a practice's quality improvement initiatives by identifying where care is being missed or inappropriately accessed. Registries provide the data needed to drive and document quality improvement efforts required by insurers or certifying bodies such as HEDIS [43] or the National Committee on Quality Assurance.

At an individual patient level, when a patient is due for or missing care, the youth's identified care team can reach out to the youth to remove barriers to completion. Evidence-based standards of care for more common chronic conditions, such as Down syndrome, attention deficit/hyperactivity disorder, asthma, obesity, and epilepsy, can be applied reliably via a registry with retrievable data to identify all patients coded with that condition. For high-severity, low-frequency conditions such as cerebral palsy, cystic fibrosis, or genetic/metabolic disorders, a registry can be used to assure patients are receiving health maintenance services, such as body mass index, lipid screening, vaccines, and wellness exams. Registry use permits a care team in a medical home to anticipate and plan for a youth with a chronic condition prior to their encounter. Pre-visit planning templates and processes tap the skills of a variety of support staff to gather records and results from interim encounters at other healthcare sites, review vaccine status, and identify needed screenings [44] and to follow up after the visit to close gaps in care. Practices who collaborate within an integrated health system may share electronic records with specialists, easing access to their consults, labs, and imaging. Those without electronic interoperability or access to specialists' medical records may need to facilitate electronic access for staff members, permitting access to records that clarify the patient's clinical picture and do not put the burden of communication on the youth/family [45, 46]. Such preparation [39], which may include a phone or electronic staff contact with the family before the visit, focuses and streamlines the interactions to assure that care needs are met and family concerns addressed before, during, and after a completed appointment. Pre-visit planning with the family can accomplish medication reconciliation and completion of online screenings through a health portal and identify medication and equipment needs even before the encounter. By having a patient's care gaps identified, orders may be placed for labs or vaccines, and needed action included in the after-visit summary for the AYASHCN [47]. For a youth with medical complexity, this medical "to-do" list reminds them/their family of needed follow-up and identifies contact numbers and links to community resources. For efficiency with an electronic health record, smart phrases or autotexts can be created to include condition-specific guidance in the after-visit summary. Such follow-up is especially effective when supported by care coordination staff, who may be licensed or unlicensed but are responsible as a care team member to facilitate needed services. Planned care has been associated with improved clinical and functional outcomes, as well as enhanced joy in work for providers [48, 49].

For youth with multiple or severe conditions, chronic care management visits accomplished between preventive care visits permit closer medication management and offer opportunities for condition education, transition readiness assessments, and co-managed care with specialists. These encounters can be coded as health maintenance visits to address issues outside of preventive care. McManus et al. provide detailed coding guidance for these face-to-face encounters [50]. Such co-management in the medical home may be particularly helpful when a youth's specialty provider is at distance or when the needed surveillance includes laboratory or imaging results. Telephone consults, electronic communications, or alternating visits with specialists after chronic care management visits may prevent the family lost time from school or work and costs of travel and complete missed specialty follow-up.

Personnel and processes within the medical home are needed to perform these critical functions of planning care, co-managing with other health providers, and outreach with the youth and family. Practices who choose to care for AYASHCN will benefit from team-based care design [51], standardizing their roles, responsibilities, and processes to have staff operating at the top of their licensure, communicating efficiently, and coordinating care for their panel of patients. Size of patient panels and time spent in visits and care coordination will vary by patient complexity. Staff support frees up physicians to see patients, helping promote ready access to care. Development of both licensed and non-licensed staff for registry curation and care gap closure closes the loop on outstanding healthcare needs. Such interaction reinforces self-management education with a young adult and encourages a gradual and informed transition to handling their healthcare services.

Communication/Monitoring/Measuring with Clinical Information Systems

Having reviewed the completed pre-visit planning template for Pam's Saturday visit and noted the negative sexually transmitted disease screen and pregnancy tests, you met with her and her mother, together and separately. You explained that you have a bigger picture of Pam's history from reviewing records from multiple sources and heard more about her fatigue, declining school performance, family conflict, and desire to get her driving permit. Pam's adolescent depression screening tool showed evidence of mild depressive symptoms. You completed your online transition readiness assessment tool, noting multiple areas needing attention, and offered your team's collaboration with the local school system to clarify Pam's learning challenges. You elicited no history or symptoms of cardiac deterioration, but explained the risks of smoking and substance use privately to Pam, and used your online directory of resources to provide teen smoking cessation resources in her after-visit summary. With Pam and her mother, you reiterated the need for cardiology and neurology follow-up, placed new electronic referrals, and included your clinical assistant, who helped with appointment scheduling and tracked completion. You received consult notes from cardiology and neurology, both of whom requested annual follow-up with Pam, but note that they transition youth to adult specialists at age 18.

Pam came to see you 13 months later, having turned 17, after multiple outreach efforts by your staff. She reported that her mother was laid off, she is now insured by Medicaid, and she intended to quit high school since she has a job at a fast-food restaurant and is happily living with her boyfriend. She reported that she has quit smoking, gets her own prescriptions filled, and still wants to go to cosmetology school. You again explained the Pine Forest policy that you will continue to see her until the end of her 21st year and would need several chronic care management visits to prepare her and locate an appropriate adult medical home and adult specialty care for her. Your care team linked her to local vocational rehabilitation resources and assured she is receiving reliable family planning services. Pam agreed to another visit in 3 months. She asked if you will still be her doctor if she has a family of her own.

By having and documenting a holistic view of a youth's healthcare, the medical home is one key to a safe transition and transfer of care for AYASHCN. Serving as a communication hub in the youth's healthcare, the medical home multidisciplinary team, in partnership with the youth and family, requires efficient clinical information systems. Information tools and reliable processes for their use promote communication, monitoring, and measurement, particularly when multiple providers are contributing to the youth's care plan.

Optimally, such systems are entirely electronic and interoperable, but more likely include multiple inputs, such as fax and postal communications, paper forms, and phone messages from many sources. Sharing current and accurate clinical information is critical when the youth's specialty care occurs at a distance from their residence and medical home [52]. For youth with medical complexity, communication with home care nursing, durable medical equipment suppliers, and state-mandated plans of care is often external to the patient's electronic health record. Letters of medical necessity and pre-authorizations for medications are common for AYASHCN whose conditions involve progressive decline, technological dependence, or off-label medication prescription. Accordingly, a medical record that accurately reflects the plan of care for a youth with a chronic condition is foundational in the medical home.

O'Malley and Reschovsky reported low reliability in bidirectional communication between specialists and primary care providers in both referral information and consultation reports [53]. Features of practices that supported reliable communication were "adequate" visit time with patients, receipt of quality reports regarding patients with chronic conditions, and nurse support for monitoring patients with chronic conditions. Because the medical home synthesizes input from many sources, electronic access or bridges to permit staff communication across non-interoperable electronic health systems may be necessary to locate consultations and emergency and inpatient reports, labs, and imaging, particularly for pre-visit planning [54]. Human processes, such as reliable medication, nutrition, and vaccination reconciliation in the medical home, are important for safety for AYASHCN, whose care involves multiple providers, therapists, pharmacies, and suppliers and who may elect to add over-the-counter or homeopathic medications or supplements to their regimens. Reliability can be increased by mapping and standardizing processes to maintain problem and medication lists and by using electronic templates for encounters and pre-visit planning. Adolescent well-care standards can be templated within an electronic encounter to give decision support around needed screenings and preventive care. Electronic templates for letters of medical necessity [55], standardized academic testing accommodations, and collegiate housing adaptation can save time for providers. The National Alliance to Advance Adolescent Health provides templates for transition summaries and emergency care plans for completion in the medical home.

Electronic scheduling may require visit types with extended time slots based on clinical complexity and needs noted in pre-visit planning; a patient in the practice registry with medical complexity who needs a college physical examination will need a longer appointment to meet needs, complete necessary documentation, and avoid delays.

Data collection within a clinical information system permits longitudinal monitoring of metrics affecting the youth's clinical and functional outcomes. Flow sheets for data collection or lab results permit data retrieval from discrete fields, averting lengthy chart review and permitting both youth and provider to see condition metrics over time and implement needed changes. By sharing and interpreting such results with the youth, the medical home can enhance the youth's understanding of their condition, empowering them for a safer transition to adult care. Monitoring of chronic conditions, particularly when co-managing with specialists, is aided by condition-specific standards of care (such as acceptable ranges for lab results) and the ability to retrieve and integrate data from multiple sources. Youth may incorporate medical mobile phone apps for condition tracking, risk alerts, and education [56, 57]; personal medical monitoring device integration with the electronic health record is underway. The clinical information system can be used to delineate the youth's care team members inside and outside the practice, including dieticians, specialty providers, and therapists for easier access to collaborative thinking about a youth's care plan and to inform their transition summary on transfer to adult care. Medical homes may create explicit co-management agreements [58] with consulting specialists to define who is monitoring and addressing a specific problem, such as hypothyroidism, or glycemic monitoring for atypical antipsychotic use. The youth's role in a co-management arrangement with a specialist involves knowing who and how to contact the proper individual for concerns. Both the medical home and specialty provider support a youth with a chronic condition in accepting more self-management of their condition over time. Tracking the youth's readiness for transition can be done electronically using validated tools that identify both strengths and areas needing attention [59].

A clinical information system permitting data collection within the medical home also can drive quality improvement in processes of care, outcomes, and utilization. The medical home may, for example, evaluate their performance on HEDIS measures, such as their population's meningococcal and influenza vaccination rates and numbers of youth receiving recommended chlamydia screenings [60] or the National Quality Forum's measurement of Adolescent Assessment of Preparation for Transition (ADAPT) to adult-focused healthcare [61, 62].

Care Coordination, Resources, and Way-Finding

Pam now returns for her 3-month follow-up visit with you and proudly announces that she is pregnant and saving money for cosmetology school while working at her restaurant job. Her mother did not come with her to your visit, and Pam reports her mother and she don't talk since she moved in with her boyfriend. Pam went to her cardiology and neurology appointments, but she does not recall any discussion of how long she would be followed in their practices. While your practice's transition policy indicates transition at age 21, your group included a clause that pregnancy required transfer to obstetrical and adult care practices. Concerned, you call the medical center where Pam receives cardiac care, grateful to find a teen pregnancy support program to which you make a referral. You write for prenatal vitamins for Pam and promise to follow up by phone (confirming her contact number) to assure she attends her obstetrical visit. You explain that her heart, while repaired, may be stressed by the pregnancy and follow-up with her cardiologist is critical. Later that day, you call the pediatric cardiologist, who assures you she can be followed by the adult cardiologist who specializes in congenital heart disease. Your staff works with Pam around her Medicaid coverage and the possibility of Social Security benefits, and they give her contact data for the local Women, Infants, and Children (WIC) program [63], explaining the importance of Pam's nutrition. Your care coordinator collaborates with the nurse practitioner running the teen pregnancy program, in an attempt to assure that Pam attends her scheduled appointment. You and your care coordinator work to create a transition summary for Pam, acknowledging that she needs more preparation for her transition and that you and your staff are available for questions or information.

Medical homes are an integral part of the medical neighborhood [64], an alliance of clinical and community supports that contribute to the health and well-being of a community, as well as that of an individual youth. Schools, faith-based groups, condition-specific nonprofit organizations, camps, specialists, therapists, mental health services, addiction/abuse services, and residential care settings and vocational rehabilitation groups are examples of other members of the medical neighborhood. Anecdotal or personal knowledge of one's medical neighborhood is helpful, but not sufficient, for meeting the needs of AYASHCN and their families. Medical homes may create paper and/or electronic databases of available supports for AYASHCN in their community and include lesser-known resources for AYASHCN such as contact data for compounding pharmacies, legal aid, reproductive health, respite care resources, and supports for individualized education programs. Those teams who care for AYASHCN need awareness of and resource connections to links for family supports around the assignment of full or partial guardianship [65], application for Social Security benefits, and direction to legal assistance for special needs trust funding. Limitations based on geographical location and accepted insurers must be noted. Medical homes will benefit from a database of such supports, which can be drawn from prior completed referrals, patient and family reports, and connections from specialty colleagues. Medical centers have print and online referral directories; medical homes can develop relationships with the referral teams at specialty centers, inviting specialists for information sharing opportunities in their practices. Such connections are facilitated when a particularly productive referral has been completed with a specialty group or when a new specialist joins the medical center and is making new services known. The Internet and social media provide opportunities for family-to-family support, which may or may not be curated for accuracy. Collaborative efforts among families, specialists, community services, schools, camps, respite care services, staff and providers in the medical home, and community leaders foster the development of a database. The National Institute for Children's Health Quality and the American Academy of Pediatrics offer resources and toolkits to develop family advisory councils that may contribute knowledge of community resources to the database [66].

An updated database of available adult primary care and specialty providers who will accept care for AYASHCN is vital to a successful transition program. Strategies used by practices to identify adult providers include surveys to surrounding family medicine and internal medicine practices to identify who is accepting new patients, AYASHCN, and patients with public insurance. Contacts through local medical societies may be useful, and certainly location of and connection with transition medicine or combined medicine-pediatrics training programs at medical centers are opportunities for transition/transfer of care of AYASHCN. Primary and specialty providers may differ on the age at which they expect a youth to move to adult care sites. Both the family and provider benefit from a history of successful transfers of other AYASHCN into a selected practice. Adult practices that have undergone medical home transformation efforts may have systems for care coordination, population management, and referral tracking (see Chapters 12, 16, 17, 18, 22).

Pam calls you several weeks later to report that the baby's fetal echocardiogram looks normal. You explain that you will be delighted to be the pediatrician for her child, but you will also help her find an adult practice for her own health-care, ideally in the same health system with her cardiologist. A call to the medicine-pediatrics training program indicates that Pam would meet criteria to join their practice; your transition summary is sent with your contact data if questions exist.

Summary

The medical home model of care is a highly supportive element in the care of AYASHCN. It is built on relationships, ready access, and practice infrastructure such as electronic records, registries stratified to identify highest need, team-based care coordination, and self-management support. The primary care medical home, covering large age ranges and a diverse array of conditions, must have knowledge of, and contacts for, services they cannot provide directly. Time, staffing, and unbillable services around care coordination [67] and care transitions are being recognized as critical elements to good outcomes and patient experience in health, with opportunities to generate a billing code for such services. Payment for them is not universal; this needs to improve. To promote fiscal viability in the current U.S. healthcare funding environment, medical homes who choose to include AYASHCN must build processes and roles that permit maximal efficiency by all staff members, with all personnel optimizing their talents and working to the top of their license [68]. Electronic record systems should be optimized to template encounters with electronic retrieval of often-used data, such as lab results, imaging reports, and recent consults. Providers and business staff must be educated on coding practices, with regular audits to assure documentation and coding are aligned [50]. Providers and staff must be dedicated to working as a team, using all available contacts and talent to meet the needs of the AYASHCN. The ultimate goal, as in parenting AYASHCN, is to support their optimal outcomes and personal goals, promoting independence and self-sufficiency for a gradual, informed, and successful transition to an adult care model.

References

1. American Academy of Family Physicians, American Academy of Pediatrics, American College of Physicians, American Osteopathic Association. Joint principles of the patient-centered medical home. 2007. http://www.aafp.org/dam/AAFP/documents/practice_management/pcmh/initiatives/PCMHJoint.pdf. Accessed 18 Apr 2017.
2. American College of Emergency Physicians. Clinical & Practice Management. The patient-centered medical model. 2015. https://www.acep.org/Clinical---Practice-Management/The-Patient-Centered-Medical-Home-Model/. Accessed 18 Apr 2017.
3. Rosen DS, Blum RW, Britto MT, Sawyer SM, Siegel DM, Society for Adolescent Medicine. Transition to adult health care for adolescents and young adults with chronic conditions: position paper of the Society for Adolescent Medicine. J Adolesc Health. 2003;33(4):309–11.
4. Strickland BB, Jones JR, Ghandour RM, Kogan MD, Newacheck PW. The medical home: health care access and impact for children and youth in the United States. Pediatrics. 2011;127(4):604–11. https://doi.org/10.1542/peds.2009-3555.
5. Rapoff MA. Adherence to pediatric medical regimens. In: Issues in clinical child psychology. 2nd ed. New York, NY: Springer Science + Business Media; 2010.
6. Garcia-Huidobro D, Shippee N, Joseph-DiCaprio J, O'Brien JM, Svetaz MV. Effect of patient-centered medical home on preventive services for adolescents and young adults. Pediatrics. 2016;137(6):e20153813.
7. American Academy of Pediatrics, National Center for Medical Home Implementation. Why is medical home important? 2016. https://medicalhomeinfo.aap.org/overview/Pages/Evidence.aspx. Accessed 18 Apr 2017.
8. Coleman K, Austin BT, Brach C, Wagner EH. Evidence on the chronic care model in the new millennium. Health Aff (Millwood). 2009;28(1):75–85. https://doi.org/10.1377/hlthaff.28.1.75.
9. Group Health Research Institute. Improving chronic illness care. The Chronic Care Model. http://www.improvingchroniccare.org/index.php?p=The_Chronic_Care_Model&s=2. Accessed 18 Apr 2017.
10. American Academy of Pediatrics, National Center for Medical Home Implementation. About us. https://medicalhomeinfo.aap.org/about/Pages/default.aspx. Accessed 18 Apr 2017.
11. American Academy of Pediatrics, American Academy of Family Physicians, American College of Physicians, Transitions Clinical Report Authoring Group, Cooley WC, Sagerman PJ. Supporting the health care transition from adolescence to adulthood in the medical home. Pediatrics. 2011;128(1):182–200. https://doi.org/10.1542/peds.2011-0969.
12. Klein DA, Goldenring JM, Adelman WP. HEEADSSS 3.0: the psychosocial interview for adolescents updated for a new century fueled by media. Contemp Pediatr. 2014. http://contemporarypediatrics.modernmedicine.com/contemporary-pediatrics/content/tags/adolescent-medicine/heeadsss-30-psychosocial-interview-adolesce?page=full. Accessed 18 Apr 2017.
13. National Alliance to Advance Adolescent Health, Center for Health Care Transition Improvement. Side-by-side version. Six Core Elements of Health Care Transition 2.0. 2014. http://www.gottransition.org/resourceGet.cfm?id=206. Accessed 18 Apr 2017.
14. Stille C, Turchi RM, Antonelli R, Cabana MD, Cheng TL, Laraque D, et al. The family-centered medical home: specific considerations for child health research and policy. Acad Pediatr. 2010;10(4):211–7.
15. Ladapo J, Chokshi D. Continuity of care for chronic conditions: threats, opportunities, and policy. Health Aff Blog. 2014. http://healthaffairs.org/blog/2014/11/18/continuity-of-care-for-chronic-conditions-threats-opportunities-and-policy-3/. Accessed 19 Apr 2017.
16. Brownlee B, Van Borkulo N. Empanelment: establishing patient-provider relationships. Seattle, WA: Qualis Health and the MacColl Center for Health Care Innovation at the Group Health Research Institute; 2013.
17. American Academy of Pediatrics, Committee on Pediatric Emergency Medicine, American College of Emergency Physicians, Pediatric Committee, Emergency Nurses Association Pediatric Committee. Joint policy statement – guidelines for care of children in the emergency department. Pediatrics. 2009;123(4):1233–43. https://doi.org/10.1542/peds.2009-1807.
18. Goudie A, Havercamp S, Jamieson B, Sahr T. Assessing functional impairment in siblings living with children with disability. Pediatrics. 2013;132(2):e476–e83. https://doi.org/10.1542/peds.2013-0644.
19. Herzer M, Godiwala N, Hommel KA, Driscoll K, Mitchell M, Crosby LE, et al. Family functioning in the context of pediatric chronic conditions. J Dev Behav Pediatr. 2010;31(1):26–34. https://doi.org/10.1097/DBP.0b013e3181c7226b.
20. Fanaroff JM, Committee on Medical Liability and Risk Management. Consent by proxy for non-urgent pediatric care. Pediatrics. 2017;139(2):e20163911.
21. Middleman AB, Olson KA. Confidentiality in adolescent health care. In: English A, Blake D, Torchia MM, editors. UpToDate. 2017. https://www.uptodate.com/contents/confidentiality-in-adolescent-health-care#H5. Accessed 2 May 2017.
22. Committee on Practice and Ambulatory Medicine. Use of chaperones during the physical examination of the pediatric patient. Pediatrics. 2011;127(5):991–3.
23. Ford CA, Millstein SG, Halpern-Felsher BL, Irwin CE Jr. Influence of physician confidentiality assurance on adolescents' willingness to disclose information and seek future health care. JAMA. 1997;278(12):1029–34.
24. Center for Advancing Health Policy and Practice, Boston University School of Public Health. The Catalyst Center: National Center for Health Insurance

and Financing for Children and Youth with Special Health Care Needs (CYSHCN). http://cahpp.org/project/the-catalyst-center/. Accessed 2 May 2017.
25. HealthCare.gov. Individuals & families. People under 30. How to get or stay on a parent's plan. https://www.healthcare.gov/young-adults/children-under-26/. Accessed 9 May 2017.
26. Autism Speaks. Family services. visual tools. https://www.autismspeaks.org/family-services/resource-library/visual-tools. Accessed 2 May 2017.
27. American Psychological Association. Enhancing your interactions with people with disabilities. http://www.apa.org/pi/disability/resources/publications/enhancing.aspx. Accessed 2 May 2017.
28. Cooley WC, Cheetham T. Integrating young adults with intellectual and developmental disabilities into your practice: tips for adult health care providers. National Alliance to Advance Adolescent Health. Practice Resource – No. 3. 2015. http://www.gottransition.org/resourceGet.cfm?id=367. Accessed 2 May 2017.
29. National Committee for Quality Assurance (NCQA). Patient Centered Medical Home (PCMH). PCMH 2017 Standards. http://www.ncqa.org/programs/recognition/practices/patient-centered-medical-home-pcmh/pcmh-2017. Accessed 2 May 2017.
30. Institute for Healthcare Improvement. Changes. Decrease demand for appointments. http://www.ihi.org/resources/Pages/Changes/DecreaseDemandforAppointments.aspx. Accessed 2 May 2017.
31. Chariatte V, Berchtold A, Akre C, Michaud PA, Suris JC. Missed appointments in an outpatient clinic for adolescents, an approach to predict the risk of missing. J Adolesc Health. 2008;43(1):38–45.
32. Topuz K, Uner H, Oztekin A, Yildirim MB. Predicting pediatric clinic no-shows: a decision analytic framework using elastic net and Bayesian belief network. Ann Oper Res. 2017. https://doi.org/10.1007/s10479-017-2489-0.
33. Carroll G, Massarelli E, Opzoomer A, Pekeles G, Pedneault M, Frappier JY, et al. Adolescents with chronic disease. Are they receiving comprehensive health care? J Adolesc Health Care. 1983;4(4):261–5.
34. Center for Adolescent Health & the Law. State minor consent laws: a summary. 3rd ed. Chapel Hill, NC; 2010. http://www.cahl.org/state-minor-consent-laws-a-summary-third-edition/. Accessed 2 May 2017.
35. Hargreaves DS, Elliott MN, Viner RM, Richmond TK, Schuster MA. Unmet health care needs in US adolescents and adult health outcomes. Pediatrics. 2015;136(3):513–20.
36. Safety Net Medical Home Initiative. About the initiative. http://www.safetynetmedicalhome.org/about-initiative. Accessed 2 May 2017.
37. Shah AK, Stadtlander M. Building better care "Empanelment". 1st ed. Portland, OR: Multnomah County Health Department; 2009. http://www.safetynetmedicalhome.org/sites/default/files/Clinical-Standards-Empanelment.pdf. Accessed 22 May 2017
38. Simon TD, Cawthon ML, Stanford S, Popalisky J, Lyons D, Woodcox P, et al. Pediatric medical complexity algorithm: a new method to stratify children by medical complexity. Pediatrics. 2014;133(6):e1647–54.
39. American Medical Association Steps Forward, Sinsky S. Pre-visit planning online module. https://www.stepsforward.org/modules/pre-visit-planning. Accessed 18 Apr 2017.
40. Centers for Medicare & Medicaid Services. Frequently asked questions. What is the definition of "new patient" for billing evaluation and management (E/M) services? https://questions.cms.gov/faq.php?id=5005&faqId=1969. Accessed 2 May 2017.
41. Gliklich RE, Dreyer NA, Leary MB. Registries for evaluating patient outcomes: a user's guide. 3rd ed. Rockville, MD: Agency for Healthcare Research and Quality; 2014. Report No. 13(14)-EHC111; https://effectivehealthcare.ahrq.gov/ehc/products/420/1897/registries-guide-3rd-edition-vol-1-140430.pdf. Accessed 2 May 2017
42. National Center for Medical Home Implementation. Building your medical home. An introduction to pediatric primary care transformation. Managing your patient population. https://medicalhomes.aap.org/Pages/Managing-Your-Patient-Population.aspx. Accessed 2 May 2017.
43. National Committee for Quality Assurance. HEDIS 2017 technical specifications for physician measurement (epub). http://store.ncqa.org/index.php/catalog/product/view/id/2507/s/hedis-2018-technical-specifications-for-physician-measurement-epub/. Accessed 2 May 2017.
44. American Academy of Pediatrics, Materials & Tools. Bright futures: guidelines for health supervision of infants, children, and adolescents. 4th ed. https://brightfutures.aap.org/materials-and-tools/Pages/default.aspx. Accessed 19 Apr 2017.
45. Montori VM. NEJM catalyst care redesign talk: the invisible work of the patient. http://catalyst.nejm.org/videos/invisible-work-patient-disruption/. Accessed 2 May 2017.
46. Romley JA, Shah AK, Chung PJ, Elliott MN, Vestal KD, Schuster MA. Family-provided health care for children with special health care needs. Pediatrics. 2017;139(1):e20161287.
47. Hummel J, Evans P. Providing clinical summaries to patients after each office visit: a technical guide. 2012. https://www.healthit.gov/sites/default/files/measure-tools/avs-tech-guide.pdf. Accessed 8 May 2017.
48. Lail J, Schoettker PJ, White DL, Mehta B, Kotagal UR. Applying the chronic care model to improve care outcomes at a pediatric medical center. Jt Comm J Qual Patient Saf. 2017;43(3):101–12.
49. Sinsky CA, Willard-Grace R, Schutzbank AM, Sinsky TA, Margolius D, Bodenheimer T. In search of joy in practice: a report of 23 high-functioning primary care practices. Ann Fam Med. 2013;11(3):272–8.
50. McManus M, White P, Harwood C, Molteni R, Kanter D, Salus T. 2017 Coding and reimbursement tip sheet

for transition from pediatric to adult health care. National Alliance to Advance Adolescent Health. Practice Resource No. 2. 2017. http://www.gottransition.org/resourceGet.cfm?id=352. Accessed 8 May 2017.

51. Bodenheimer T. Building teams in primary care: lessons from 15 case studies. California Health Care Foundation; 2007. http://www.chcf.org/publications/2007/07/building-teams-in-primary-care-lessons-from-15-case-studies. Accessed 22 May 2017.
52. American Academy of Pediatrics, National Center for Medical Home Implementation. Co-management between primary and specialty care. 2017. https://medicalhomeinfo.aap.org/about/Pages/January-2017.aspx. Accessed 8 May 2017.
53. O'Malley AS, Reschovsky JD. Referral and consultation communication between primary care and specialist physicians: finding common ground. Arch Intern Med. 2011;171(1):56–65.
54. HealthIT.gov. What is EHR Interoperability and why is it important? 2013. https://www.healthit.gov/providers-professionals/faqs/what-ehr-interoperability-and-why-it-important. Accessed 8 May 2017.
55. Kerr LM. Writing letters of medical necessity. Medical Home Portal, Department of Pediatrics, University of Utah. 2011. https://www.medicalhomeportal.org/issue/writing-letters-of-medical-necessity. Accessed 8 May 2017.
56. Con D, De Cruz P. Mobile phone apps for inflammatory bowel disease self-management: a systematic assessment of content and tools. JMIR Mhealth UHealth. 2016;4(1):e13.
57. U.S. Department of Health and Human Services, U.S. Food & Drug Administration. Examples of mobile apps for which the FDA will exercise enforcement discretion. 2016. https://www.fda.gov/MedicalDevices/DigitalHealth/MobileMedicalApplications/ucm368744.htm. Accessed 8 May 2017.
58. McAllister J. National center for medical home implementation. Co-management letter and agreement. https://medicalhomes.aap.org/Documents/CoManagementAgreement.pdf. Accessed 8 May 2017.
59. National Alliance to Advance Adolescent Health. Transition readiness. http://www.gottransition.org/providers/leaving-3.cfm. Accessed 8 May 2017.
60. National Committee for Quality Assurance. HEDIS 2017 Standards, Volume 2. Summary table of measures, product lines and changes. http://www.ncqa.org/Portals/0/HEDISQM/HEDIS2017/HEDIS%202017%20Volume%202%20List%20of%20Measures.pdf?ver=2016-06-27-135433-350. Accessed 8 May 2017.
61. Center of Excellence for Pediatric Quality Measurement, Division of General Pediatrics, Boston Children's Hospital. Measuring the preparation for transition from pediatric-focused to adult-focused health care: the adolescent assessment for preparation for transition (ADAPT) survey. 2014. https://www.rmhpcommunity.org/sites/default/files/resource/ADAPT-survey-materials.pdf. Accessed 8 May 2017.
62. National Quality Forum. Pediatric measures. Final Report. Measure 2789. Adolescent assessment of preparation for transition (ADAPT) to adult-focused health care. Washington, DC; 2016.
63. United States Department of Agriculture, Food and Nutrition Service. Women, infants, and children (WIC). 2017. https://www.fns.usda.gov/wic/women-infants-and-children-wic. Accessed 8 May 2017.
64. Fisher ES. Building a medical neighborhood for the medical home. N Engl J Med. 2008;359(12):1202–5.
65. Center for Health Care Transition Improvement, Got Transition. Guardianship and alternatives for decision-making support. 2012. http://www.gottransition.org/resourceGet.cfm?id=17. Accessed 8 May 2017.
66. National Center for Medical Home Implementation. For Practices. Family-centered care. 2016. https://medicalhomeinfo.aap.org/tools-resources/Pages/For-Practices.aspx. Accessed 8 May 2017.
67. U.S. Department of Health & Human Services, Agency for Healthcare Research and Quality. Chapter 2: What is care coordination? In: Care coordination measures atlas update. 2014. https://www.ahrq.gov/professionals/prevention-chronic-care/improve/coordination/atlas2014/chapter2.html. Accessed 8 May 2017.
68. The Advisory Board, Nursing Executive Center. Achieving Top-of-License Nursing Practice. Best practices for elevating the impact of the frontline nurse. 2013. https://www.advisory.com/-/media/Advisory-com/Research/NEC/Research-Study/2013/Achieving-Top-of-License-Nursing-Practice/Achieving-Top-of-License-Nursing-Practice.pdf. Accessed 8 May 2017.

The Hospitalist's Perspective on Healthcare Transition

27

Ryan J. Coller, Sarah Ahrens, and Debra Lotstein

Background

A 19-year-old patient with severe cerebral palsy presents to the emergency department of a busy tertiary academic center in respiratory distress. The emergency department (ED) providers prepare to admit the patient for suspected aspiration pneumonia. After the admitting pediatric hospitalist tells the ED that they don't accept patients over 18, the admitting internal medicine hospitalist is called and accepts the patient. During transfer, the patient's mother realizes that instead of heading to the familiar children's hospital units, they are heading for a bed on an adult unit. This is their first time being admitted outside of the children's hospital; and while they are technically in the same organization, a flood of panic overwhelms her. "Will they know his routines?"; "How will the providers talk with us?"; "Can his sister stay with him?"; "Do they know what Lennox-Gastaut means?"; "What are rounds like?"; "Where do I park?"; "Will we still have child life, social workers, the subspecialists who know him?"….

For children with chronic health conditions and their families, acute hospitalizations are often times of crisis. The fragile and exhausting realities of an acute hospitalization expose medical, financial, and psychosocial vulnerabilities distinct from other healthcare encounters. Abrupt and poorly executed transition to a new adult setting can only exacerbate this stress for families and risk worsening the young adult's health and healthcare through gaps in information transfer. Moreover, poor transitions can also lead to provider frustration in both pediatric and adult inpatient healthcare teams.

The transition from pediatric to adult inpatient medical care also has tremendous ramifications for healthcare policy. At the national level, spending on adult patients admitted to children's hospitals has grown to $1 billion annually [1], as adult-aged patients with childhood-onset, chronic conditions are increasingly admitted to children's hospitals [1]. This suggests that both this patient population

R. J. Coller, M.D., M.P.H. (✉)
Department of Pediatrics, University of Wisconsin School of Medicine and Public Health, Madison, WI, USA

Division of Hospital Medicine, Pediatric Complex Care Program, Madison, WI, USA
e-mail: rcoller@pediatrics.wisc.edu

S. Ahrens, M.D.
Department of Medicine, University of Wisconsin School of Medicine and Public Health, Madison, WI, USA
e-mail: sahrens@medicine.wisc.edu

D. Lotstein, M.D., M.P.H.
Departments of Anesthesia and Pediatrics, Keck School of Medicine, University of Southern California, Los Angeles, CA, USA

Comfort and Palliative Care Division, Los Angeles, CA, USA
e-mail: dlotstein@chla.usc.edu

A. C. Hergenroeder, C. M. Wiemann (eds.), *Health Care Transition*,
https://doi.org/10.1007/978-3-319-72868-1_27

is growing in size and there are important barriers to transitioning adult patients out of children's hospitals.

Inpatient transitions have elements that make them different from other ambulatory transitions of care. For example, because hospitalizations are typically unplanned events, it can be difficult to adequately anticipate all of the issues that can arise with the change to a new location of care. Orchestrating inpatient transitions in the ambulatory setting can be difficult for outpatient providers who may lack relevant knowledge or influence over inpatient systems. As a result, despite its substantial influence on health and healthcare experience, the hospital transition may be neglected altogether.

Although many informative youth-adult transition guidelines and frameworks have been created to help families and providers navigate this major milestone [2–8], far less attention has been paid to how the element of hospital care fits within existing transition models. Practical strategies to anticipate, identify, and address the issues specific to transitioning inpatient care from pediatrics to adult hospital settings are largely missing. As a result, pediatric and adult hospital-based providers (aka physician "hospitalists") have been mostly left out of these planning activities. This is a major gap in improving the transition to adult care process generally, as these providers now carry out the majority of inpatient medical care and are therefore an important part of the medical care plans for adolescents and young adults with special healthcare needs (AYASHCN). The hospitalists' role in the transition process is further complicated by the fact that they usually have less continuity with the family and may not have relationships with the youth's primary medical specialists.

Some of the challenges of *inpatient* youth-adult transitions are tightly connected to other health system challenges, such as difficulties in outpatient transition processes, inpatient-outpatient transitions, and primary care-subspecialty communication. In an ideal health system, many of these failures would be proactively addressed (and people are working on this, as described elsewhere in this book). However in the meantime, it is important to consider specific strategies that can mitigate the confusion and distress caused by poor inpatient transitions.

Throughout the chapter we distinguish "pediatric" and "adult" providers, meaning those providers trained in caring for children vs. those trained in caring for adults. We recognize that many providers are dually training (e.g., joint internal medicine-pediatrics or family medicine) and may span both settings. For consistency and simplicity throughout this chapter, we will describe inpatient providers as either "pediatric" or "adult" hospitalists, referring to their role in the pediatric or adult setting.

Current State

To date, most of what is known about the inpatient transition process relates to experiences of adult-aged patients admitted to children's hospitals. Not surprisingly, adults admitted to children's hospitals tend to be the "sickest of the sick" [1]. Adult patients in pediatric intensive care units (PICUs) are nearly twice as likely to die in the PICU compared to adolescents [9]. Hospital charges and lengths of stay appear to be greater when adults with childhood-onset chronic conditions are admitted to pediatric versus adult inpatient care settings [9–11]. Although severity of illness likely explains why adult-aged patients may both remain in children's hospitals at older ages and have worse outcomes than their younger peers, further research would help to understand what may be specific risks of staying in pediatric settings in adulthood, as well as the preventable risks of moving to a more age-appropriate setting. The mix of risks and benefits is likely to vary with local resources and also with the inpatient pediatric organizational structure, i.e., a free-standing children's hospital, a children's hospital-within-a-hospital, a pediatric unit within a community hospital, and other variations. Policy and practical issues may also influence where a young adult patient may be hospitalized. For example, bed and provider licensure issues, as well as the size of beds and equipment, might prevent a children's hospital from meeting the needs of a young adult.

Assuming an individual's inpatient care will transition out of the children's hospital at some point, pediatric and adult providers need guidance on (1) the important unique aspects of the inpatient transition and (2) how to improve the hospital-based transition process. We will highlight both of these elements of inpatient transitions in the clinical cases that follow.

Clinical Cases in Inpatient Transition

Case #1

A 19-year-old male presents to the emergency department at a large urban hospital following 3 days of severe vomiting and diarrhea. He was born with VACTERL association (*v*ertebral defects, *a*nal atresia, *c*ardiac defects, *t*rachea-*e*sophageal fistula, *r*enal anomalies, and *l*imb abnormalities) and has a history of tracheoesophageal fistula status post repair, tetralogy of Fallot status post repair, and a solitary cystic kidney with chronic kidney disease. He is presumed to have acute gastroenteritis but also has an acute-on-chronic kidney injury, with a creatinine increase to 4.6 from his baseline of 1.9, as well as concerning electrolytes (sodium of 153 and potassium of 6.1).

Plans are made to admit him for monitoring, rehydration, and additional workup. There are no beds on any of the children's units, so the decision is made to admit him to an internal medicine hospitalist service on an adult unit. The internal medicine hospitalist has the nephrologist on call see the patient that evening. Recommendations are made regarding fluid management, antihypertensives, and diuretics. The primary service follows the recommendations.

This is the patient's first stay on a non-pediatric unit. His family is distraught—in part they are confused because the available bed is on a cardiac unit and they are concerned the team believes something is wrong with his heart based on his congenital heart disease. His mother misses having a pullout bed to sleep on like the one in the children's hospital room, and the patient misses seeing the art therapist who knows him well and is an important support for him during his frequent admissions.

The next morning, the patient's pediatric nephrologist receives an email from the patient's mother that he was admitted. The pediatric nephrologist visits them at the bedside and comments that he would have handled the medications differently. He also shares alternative ideas on the fluid choices that were made.

The patient's mother is worried that the overnight decisions might have been wrong and could have harmed her son. When the internal medicine hospitalist arrives for rounds, the family is angry and afraid and has many questions.

Discussion

The scenario in this case is common and more appropriately labeled an abrupt "transfer" than a thoughtful transition of care. The decision to admit a patient to an adult hospitalist service and involve internal medicine subspecialists can be triggered by patient age or availability of beds. The experience is reactive rather than proactive, and there are no actual "processes" to manage information transfer, family or provider expectations, preparation, readiness, or handling potential ambiguities (e.g., call adult or pediatric nephrology?). For patients with chronic or complex medical or social backgrounds, this can lead to many problems including poor experiences for patients, families and providers, as well as worse patient health outcomes.

There are currently no agreed upon standards for when the inpatient location should switch from pediatric to internal medicine care, although the patient's chronological age is a common driver. Some hospitals may draw the line at early adolescence, while others may wait until early adulthood, e.g., 21 or 25 years old. Specific disorders or reasons for admission can also determine whether a young adult is hospitalized on a pediatric vs. adult unit, and some pediatric facilities may use developmental rather than chronological age, e.g., providing ongoing care for adults of all ages when they have severe intellectual disabilities that began in childhood. Nonage triggers to transition inpatient care can also be milestone-based, such as transition of primary care from pediatrics to internal medicine and transition of subspecialty care, employment, graduation from college, or a certain level of chronic disease control.

The most common experience across children's hospitals is inconsistency—either hospitals have no policies on age limits for admission or have policies that are applied haphazardly, requiring flexibility when census is high on either the adult or pediatric side. Young adults may therefore bounce back and forth between units and services during different admissions. Hospitalists and families can be confused about who is really the primary service, and subspecialists on either side can feel uncomfortable making decisions.

There may be differences in policies and supports between pediatric and adult hospital settings. Hospital room sizes and visitor rules may differ outside the children's hospital. Supportive resources in inpatient pediatrics may not exist in internal medicine (e.g., child life), and services available in the internal medicine setting may be unknown or not accessed due to lack of familiarity.

Additionally, differences in the model of healthcare team communication, often rooted in differences in family-centered care and the legal implications of adulthood, can create striking differences for patients and families. For example, inpatient pediatrics is typically anchored in patient- and family-centered care, including daily bedside rounds with members of an interprofessional team and the patient and their family members. Although this model is becoming more common in adult inpatient settings, the practice is not currently widespread. It is often the first major difference that patients and families experience.

Additional important changes experienced after transitioning into adult hospital care can include differences in medical treatment approaches. For example, there may be differences in routine treatments, such as intravenous fluids, enteral feeding, pain control, first-line antibiotics for common infections, and more. Furthermore, patients and families may (rightfully) perceive differences in physician or nurse knowledge of childhood-onset chronic conditions. The lack of understanding may lead to well-intentioned but less well-informed medical recommendations.

Unfortunately, the parents' surprise and fear seen in this case are common initial reactions. Parents often reach out directly to longtime and trusted providers, whether the inpatient provider team is aware of these communications or not. Similarly, providers can be put in challenging-to-navigate situations, potentially feeling undermined. The internal medicine hospitalist in this case is faced with negotiating different treatment recommendations while trying to regain patient and family confidence. He or she also must maintain professional relationships with the subspecialty services involved on both the adult and pediatric sides of the case. The voice of the patient is also lost in this scenario, and the internist will need to work with this adult-aged individual to establish the level of involvement they desire from their family before they can even continue discussing his clinical care with the family.

Potential Inpatient Transitional Care Approaches

First and foremost, inpatient providers should cultivate an appreciation that this transition period can be extremely challenging for patients and families. Many of the issues highlighted in this case are not unlike issues faced every day by inpatient providers regardless of patient age—complex medical care, negotiating treatment plans, determining a care plan with conflicting consultant recommendations, and reassuring families. A key distinction is that many of the negative sides of these issues can be avoided through proactive, deliberate planning. When challenges occur, they have a feeling of "preventability" which can frustrate providers, patients, and families, i.e., "if only it had been done *this* way, we wouldn't be dealing with this…." Furthermore, hospitalizations are times of crisis; they are not effective times to conduct most transitional care processes. When possible, transitional care activities should happen before an acute hospitalization.

Opportunities for communication breakdowns (and therefore opportunities to build bridges) are created from four potential silos: pediatric primary care, internal medicine primary care, pediatric subspecialty care, and internal medicine subspecialty care [12]. Traditionally, communication channels exist between internal medicine primary care and subspecialty care providers. Current best practices for communication during the transition would also occur between pediatric subspecialty and internal medicine subspecialty providers. To provide lifelong care for youth with chronic illness after transitioning primary care to adult-oriented providers, the creation of a set of bidirectional communication links between pediatric subspecialists, internal medicine subspecialty counterparts, and internal medicine primary care providers has been proposed. This approach is easily adaptable to the issues introduced by inpatient care.

The following are approaches which may be undertaken by hospital providers to create a gradual or planned transition rather than a sudden transfer and avoid some of the challenges described in the case above.

- Work with hospital administrators to create a policy or guideline clarifying when youth or young adults are admitted to pediatric vs. adult units. Attempt to address ambiguities and contingency plans in order to clarify the situations and deviations from these guidelines that are allowed.
- Communicate the hospital policy or guideline with patients and outpatient providers so that patients and families can be aware. Managing expectations, even if the inconsistencies cannot be avoided, can be helpful in minimizing distress.
- Providers caring for pediatric patients in the hospital should attempt to identify patient populations in their health system who are likely to be hospitalized throughout adolescence and early adulthood. Proactive planning can begin with these patients.
- When communicating with outpatient providers about patients likely to have ongoing hospitalizations, inpatient pediatric providers should remind them to include hospital transition issues in their transition planning. This can also create an opportunity for inpatient providers to educate outpatient providers on the policies and related issues that could create future challenges for the patient or family (and vice versa).
- Inpatient providers caring for transition-aged patients could ask the patient/family whom they prefer be called prior to placing an inpatient consult, i.e., pediatric or adult subspecialists. It is important to let the patient know that their preference may not be able to be followed if an adult subspecialist is uncomfortable with their condition or if the pediatric subspecialist will not take care of a young adult or is not credentialed in the adult hospital.
- Inpatient providers should become familiar with comprehensive transitional care models such as the Six Core Elements framework [3], whose activities mainly focus on outpatient settings. For example, knowing where to find a transition care plan and information about who/when primary and specialty care providers will transition can be informative for managing inpatient care. This can also shed light on insurance, case management, financial/housing/school plans, guardianship, competence, and other legal issues.
- Inpatient providers should consider developing an "inpatient transition plan" for patients anticipated to need ongoing hospitalization through early adulthood. The content for this plan would serve as a transition summary to describe the key inpatient care issues for future providers. Ideally, these plans would integrate into more comprehensive transition plan documentation and be put together in late adolescence, before the need to be hospitalized on an internal medicine unit. The template for these plans should be developed with input from patients, families, and pediatric and internal medicine providers. An example plan is shown in Appendix.
- When possible, families appreciate an opportunity to become familiar with the new location in advance of an acute hospitalization. Arranging a tour of the anticipated adult unit during adolescence can make the first nonpediatric stay feel more comfortable and answer logistical questions (e.g., where to park, etc.) that can create added stress at times of hospitalization.

As noted above, the issues highlighted by this case can differ markedly based on the hospital's physical and administrative structure, i.e., free-standing children's hospital, children's hospital within a general hospital, etc. This topic is discussed in more detail in a later case.

Case #2

A 22-year-old female with Batten disease, a progressive neurodegenerative disorder, is admitted because of acute hypoxic respiratory failure secondary to pneumonia. Although she is managed with bi-level ventilation and improves with antibiotics, her appetite remains diminished and she becomes increasingly short of breath with the effort of eating. As a result, she often needs bi-level ventilation even after eating small amounts of food. A gastrostomy tube is recommended for safe delivery of adequate nutrition and to promote respiratory recovery. The primary team attempts to discuss this with the patient several times to obtain her consent for the procedure; however, she only shrugs when responding to their questions. Eventually, this becomes the main obstacle to her discharge.

The patient's parents want her to have the gastrostomy tube placed, but they are frustrated they cannot consent for her at this point. After multiple discussions with the patient and family, the primary team asks psychiatry to evaluate the patient for capacity to make this medical decision. The consulting psychiatrist determines that the patient does not have capacity to make this decision and recommends activation of the patient's power of attorney (her parents in this case).

Discussion

This case highlights unique legal and developmental issues introduced when patients with intellectual disability become 18 years old. The age of 18 is a relatively arbitrary legal cutoff that influences many actions in the hospital. Among others, it defines when providers must seek a patient's consent to discuss the care with their family. It is also the age when a patient is expected to make medical decisions and must, if able, provide consent for procedures. Acute illness and hospitalization amplify these issues because providers often ask patients and families to make decisions about potentially life-altering or life-sustaining treatments at this time.

Pediatric providers learn to communicate healthcare decision-making through families, with the intent to increasingly integrate the child into the decision-making process as they gain independence during adolescence. Adult providers learn to communicate directly with adult patients, and they cannot speak with families about the adult patient's care until they have the patient's permission (see Chap. 30). Parent access to health system tools to communicate with healthcare teams or receive results through electronic patient portals in the medical record is typically turned off at age 18, if not sooner.

These legal, cultural, and stylistic communication differences can feel drastic, and parents may feel "shut out" because of the abrupt change in their level of involvement. For patients with severe intellectual disability and/or previously established guardianship, this is less of an issue. However, the cultural differences introduced by this approach to care can still be felt by patients and families.

Patients with severe developmental delays often arrive in the hospital with previously established guardianship. In this relatively straightforward situation, the hospitalist talks to and obtains consent from the guardian in a manner similar to when the patient was younger than 18 years old. The opposite end of the spectrum is the medically complex patient with typical intellectual and social development. The hospitalist can discuss medical decisions and obtain consent from these patients directly, even though these patients may independently choose to discuss their care and decisions with their family members who have been involved for most if not all the patient's life.

The third and more challenging category highlighted in the case involves uncertainty about the patient's capacity to make a specific medical decision. Such patients may have chronic, progressive diseases that require continued and often more intense medical care as they reach the legal age of adulthood. These patients can be mildly intellectually delayed and therefore may not have appointed guardians or activated power of attorneys. However, like the patient presented in the case, these patients may struggle to make major medical decisions. This can be, in part, because they might not have been raised with a goal of achieving independence. Legally, the hospitalist must treat them as independent adults, but they may not be ready or able to take on that level of decision-making. This can lead to delays in care and considerable friction between patients, families, and providers.

Potential Inpatient Transitional Care Approaches

- Providers, both pediatric and adult, need to recognize that there is a spectrum of capacity to make a medical decision. The same patient who can make simple medical decisions may not be able to make complex decisions.
- While appropriately tailoring to developmental ability, adolescents should be coached by parents and healthcare providers toward the highest level of independence possible. Providers need to recognize that patients with progressive diseases or with significantly reduced expected lifespans may not have been raised by parents or providers toward independence and independent medical decision-making.
- Upon recognition that a patient may not be able to make a particular medical decision, it is essential to involve other professionals to help make that determination. If child psychiatry is available as a consultant, their insights and training can be useful in these situations. Involve these services earlier rather than later.
- Inpatient pediatric providers can discuss with parents of hospitalized teenagers with severe cognitive impairment about the importance of establishing guardianship and power of attorney before the patient's 18th birthday.
- Inpatient providers can remind outpatient providers that ensuring a power of attorney is in place is tremendously helpful should the patient need acute hospital care.
- Because of the shift in legality of communication accompanying adulthood, inpatient pediatric providers can prepare families of teenagers with chronic conditions. They can remind them that after adulthood, hospitalists will not be able to discuss the child's care with them until they have consent.
- Internal medicine providers need to listen to the parents' story too and acknowledge the range of possible emotions when their child is asked to make a difficult decision and is unable. Some parents are angry that they cannot legally make the decision for their child. Some are saddened that they, as parents, ultimately need to make the decision. It must be recognized that these can be difficult circumstances for families and that activating the power of attorney of a young adult is different than activating that of an aging parent.

Case #3

A 21-year-old male with spinal muscular atrophy (SMA) type 2 is admitted to the adult hospitalist service for influenza A. The hospitalist is comfortable with the care of patients with influenza but has not cared for a patient with SMA before and rarely cares for patients with childhood-onset illnesses. At home and at his baseline level of health, the patient's pulmonary clearance regimen includes using a vibratory vest and cough-assist device twice daily with bronchodilators, and his parents are well-versed in suctioning as needed. They have a pulse oximeter and administer oxygen by nasal cannula up to 1 L/min when ill if oxygen saturations drop below 90%. He receives bolus formula feedings and extra free water by a gastrostomy tube during the day and a slow drip feed overnight. Although the patient is currently clinically improving in terms of acute respiratory failure and infection, he is still on 3 L/min supplementary oxygen and is receiving his respiratory clearance regimen four times daily. Tube feeds were restarted at a slow continuous rate earlier today, which seems to be going well.

During the morning rounds, the patient's family states that they think the patient is ready to return home today. Both the nurses and the MD are uncomfortable with this plan since the patient continues to require supplemental oxygen and increased respiratory support from baseline, and tube feeds have not reached discharge criteria.

Discussion

This case reflects three important issues: first, the potential for gaps in knowledge of a childhood-onset condition; second, perspectives of caregiver capabilities for home care; and, third, differing ideas of how "well" a patient needs to be prior to discharge. For a patient and family experienced with caring for illness exacerbations over a child's lifetime, their comfort level with the transition back to baseline health might be far different from a healthcare provider who is unfamiliar with a condition and has more stringent discharge criteria.

Internists frequently have little training or knowledge of chronic illness management of rare childhood-onset conditions. This is especially true for diseases that, until the last 20 years, were fatal before patients reached adulthood. Although internal medicine-trained hospitalists are well-versed in common adult-onset chronic diseases and managing complex hospitalized patients, they are often "learning as they go" when caring for medically complex youth. Patients and their family members frequently know more than their physicians, particularly regarding certain treatments or approaches to specific problems that are rare in adults.

Furthermore, the internal medicine hospitalist's frame of reference for a family caregiver's ability may also be very different. For example, the skills of a parent who has amassed experience delivering medical care to their child for years can be vastly different from the skills of an adult caregiver whose spouse just suffered an acute stroke, the latter being much more commonly encountered by an adult hospitalist.

Medically complex youth and their families are often comfortable delivering many advanced forms of medical care at home. They can be comfortable titrating supplemental oxygen based on peripheral oxygen saturations, advancing tube feeds, delivering IV medications, and performing respiratory care, often including sophisticated medical devices. Pediatric hospitalists and subspecialists who have potentially cared for the family for years may be more familiar with their skill set and, as a result, may be more comfortable discharging the patient home even when the patient is not yet at his or her baseline. A more conservative approach from a less comfortable adult hospitalist can generate frustration for patients and families who feel they are ready to leave the hospital.

Potential Inpatient Transitional Care Approaches

It is important to develop strategies to overcome knowledge deficits related to uncommon conditions. Recognizing the value of patient and family experience and expertise are critical during this transition period.

- Establishing joint educational opportunities between pediatric and internal medicine providers can help bridge knowledge deficits and create an improved communication culture. Examples could include holding a joint case conference to discuss recent or anticipated complex patient cases, journal club to review clinical advances on topics relevant to both sets of providers and sharing evidence-based clinical pathways for conditions managed on both sides.
- A valuable starting point for adult hospitalists is to take advantage of the expertise that patients and families bring by asking them questions about the patient's chronic illness. Providers should spend time learning from them. Examples of questions providers may ask include, "Your child's condition is not one that we frequently care for, what do you think are the most important things I should know about caring for him?", "What are the most common reasons youth with this condition need to be hospitalized?", "Who are the providers that you consider having the most expertise in your condition?"

- Talking to the patient's previous inpatient and outpatient providers can provide pertinent, practical information about both the child's conditions and previous responses to treatment decisions.
- Adult hospitalists should become familiar with high-quality pediatric references or pediatric experts that can be sought for clinical questions about managing childhood-onset chronic conditions.
- Pediatric providers should be willing to be a resource for adult providers caring for patients with childhood-onset chronic conditions in early adulthood.
- Adult hospitalists should recognize that families of medically complex youth may provide higher levels of care at home than may be typical for adult patients. Providers should ask patients and their families what they are comfortable doing at home and what previous discharge criteria they have used during similar exacerbations. Assessing patient and family self-care skills and competencies as the patients and caregivers continue aging and care needs evolve is an important ongoing task.

Case #4

A 26-year-old female with intractable epilepsy due to being a former 25-week premature infant with severe hypoxic-ischemic encephalopathy with spastic quadriplegic cerebral palsy (gross motor function classification system V) and hydrocephalus status post ventriculoperitoneal shunt (VPS) is admitted for altered mental status. For all her previous hospitalizations, including numerous VPS malfunctions, status epilepticus, and pneumonias, she has been cared for at a large free-standing tertiary children's hospital. The nurses, therapists, and physicians know her and her family very well.

This evening, she is admitted to the children's hospital because she is lethargic compared to her baseline. In addition, her seizure frequency increased over the last several days; she's been intermittently febrile and not tolerating gastrostomy tube formula or electrolyte solution for close to 72 h. Her urine output has decreased significantly over the past 2 days, and she appears moderately dehydrated.

Just after midnight, she acutely worsens, including severe lethargy with difficulty arousing. Her team assumes she is in status epilepticus, possibly with another VPS malfunction. They prepare to give her Ativan and order a quick-sequence MRI to assess her ventricle size. A rapid response is called as the patient's vital signs become erratic, and she is transferred to the pediatric intensive care unit.

After 90 min, two rounds of Ativan and a loading dose of fosphenytoin have not improved her status. A technician is on the way to place EEG leads. Her ventricles appeared stable on her quick-sequence MRI. The ICU team orders a head CT and her imaging suggests an acute ischemic stroke. The team scrambles to organize a stroke response between the ICU, neurology, and neurosurgery.

Discussion

In contrast to case 3, this scenario highlights potential knowledge deficits of pediatric providers for clinical conditions more common in adult patients. Although many children's hospitals are well-equipped to handle emergencies experienced more frequently by adults (e.g., stroke, myocardial infarction), recognizing these conditions can still be more challenging or take longer for pediatric providers. Some children's hospitals may not have protocols in place to handle these emergencies. Even when there is a protocol, it may be used rarely and therefore be suboptimally implemented when needed.

Structural barriers may further impact services available to adult-aged patients cared for in free-standing children's hospitals. For example, appropriately sized tools, equipment, and supplies for large adults may be missing or limited. Pediatric specialists or proceduralists may become uncomfortable as patients age well into adulthood, and the relevant internal medicine providers may be unavailable. Although there is no "right answer" for when a patient should no longer be cared for in a children's hospital, at some point, it is in the patient's best interest to be cared for in an adult-oriented facility.

Potential Inpatient Transitional Care Approaches

- As noted in case 3, joint educational opportunities between pediatrics and adult providers can help bridge knowledge and communication gaps. Similarly, pediatric hospitalists should become familiar with high-quality internal medicine references and internal medicine experts that can be sought for clinical questions about adult-onset acute and chronic conditions.
- Internal medicine providers should be willing to be a resource for pediatric providers continuing to care for patients into early adulthood.
- Children's hospitals caring for adult-aged patients should have access to (1) necessary providers with relevant expertise in conditions experienced by this age group, (2) supplies and equipment appropriately sized for adults, and (3) protocols for acute conditions faced by adult-aged patients.
- Inpatient pediatric providers should set expectations with adolescents, families, and the other involved pediatric providers for when care should transition to an adult-oriented inpatient facility. Discussing these issues with the family can help explain why, although difficult, this transition is important.

Case #5

A 20-year-old woman with sickle cell disease presents to a local emergency department. Her disease has been poorly controlled during different periods of her life, resulting in avascular necrosis of both her hips and prior acute chest syndrome crises requiring pediatric intensive care unit stays when she was a teenager. Her social situation has been unstable for the past few years, with inconsistent employment and housing. She has struggled with depression and has few reliable supports. She often presents to the children's hospital when in sickle cell crisis. The children's hospital ED staff know her well and have a clear pain control regimen and admission criteria for her. When admitted, clearly delineated transfusion and plasma exchange thresholds are used to manage her disease. With these plans in place, her hospital stays have been less frequent and shorter in the past year than previously.

The hospital to which she presents this time, however, has a different electronic health record (EHR) platform than the local children's hospital. There is no access to these plans for her current providers. As a result, the ED providers undertreat her pain and she is admitted. She spends about 2 days longer than typical for her previous vaso-occlusive crisis admissions. She and her providers are frustrated with the experience.

Discussion

This case highlights information transfer challenges, the possibilities and pitfalls of EHRs, and the potentially avoidable healthcare utilization that can occur during this transition period.

Critical information needed by internal medicine providers is accumulated in the medical record throughout a patient's childhood. The degree to which this information is well-organized and accessible has tremendous implications on the care delivered during the transition. Information loss can lead to worse health outcomes and lapses in healthcare quality or safety. For example, uncommon issues such as the need for stress-dose steroids or endocarditis prophylaxis could be missed. Effective and customized contingency plans for symptoms like pain, respiratory distress, and other chronic disease management strategies may be lost. Even when new providers theoretically have access to the EHR where these care plans live, they may not be aware of them or able to find them when needed. The time it takes for new providers to hunt for and consolidate such information within the EHR can be impractical. Valuable social context impacting health can take years for a provider to understand, and the EHR is often not well-positioned to facilitate this kind of information transfer.

These realities leave receiving providers under-informed and at a disadvantage in caring for chronically ill and complex patients. At best, patients are inconvenienced and redundant tests or treatments are ordered. At worst, patients can suffer from adverse events or potentially life-threatening complications.

Potential Inpatient Transitional Care Approaches

In an ideal world, EHRs will be compatible across institutions, and documenting information relevant to the care transition from pediatric to adult providers will be efficient to construct and readily accessible. The EHR needs of inpatient and outpatient providers overlap in many ways, but there are also important distinctions. For example, inpatient providers have a more focused need to quickly understand how acute crises or chronic condition exacerbations are managed. Specific aspects of their social history can also be essential, particularly when life-changing decisions are being made during a vulnerable period.

At the same time, differences in institutional context and provider cultures across cities, states, and regions, across health systems, across disease states, etc. can make a one-size-fits-all EHR approach challenging. In the absence of a universal solution, pediatric hospitalists should work with outpatient providers to ensure a transition summary document that highlights a patient's most relevant information anticipated to impact future hospitalizations and health. As in ambulatory settings, developing such content with the patient and family is important. To the extent that these summaries can be available and follow a consistent structured format within a health system, receiving providers will learn how to more efficiently and reliably use this information.

- Work with inpatient and outpatient providers locally to determine:
  - Which types of patients or situations warrant deliberate documented inpatient transition summaries/transition plans
  - The most valuable information to be shared with future inpatient providers
  - How this information should be integrated into comprehensive transitional care plans (i.e., plans developed by outpatient or primary care providers)
  - Where, when, and, by whom this information will be assembled
  - How patient and family input will be incorporated into the plan
  - How the product will be shared with providers inside and outside the health system, as well as patients and families
- Health systems and provider groups should recognize and monitor the potentially avoidable hospital utilization and adverse events experienced by patients with chronic conditions during this transition period. Quality improvement techniques such as root cause analyses, failure modes effects analyses, and process mapping/workflow redesign should be applied to the inpatient transition process to solve problems leading to these events. A summary of strategies to improve inpatient transition is provided in Table 27.1.

Conclusion

As demonstrated by the five case scenarios, planning for inpatient transition has unique challenges that differ from those encountered in outpatient settings. We have highlighted a number of opportunities for improving inpatient transitions that can be applied today. Importantly, improving the transition process does not require a formal, institutionally endorsed effort. Rather, these changes can begin one patient at a time by simply increasing recognition and discussion of this inevitable process. Appreciating the challenges of this transition means that effective solutions will continue to emerge from a host of sources. Figure 27.1 highlights factors that may be used to evaluate system "readiness" to implement an inpatient transition program. This framework can serve as a road map for health system improvement. There are numerous opportunities for individuals and health systems to engage in quality improvement and research

Table 27.1 Summary of strategies to improve the inpatient transition

Inpatient pediatric providers	Inpatient adult providers	Both
• Remind outpatient providers to include hospital transition issues during transition planning • Develop "inpatient transition plans" for patients expected to benefit • Help families become familiar with new inpatient location before being hospitalized • Work with families and outpatient providers to establish guardianship and power of attorney, when relevant • Prepare families for the legal and culture shifts in communication practices accompanying adulthood • Set expectations with adolescents, families, and the other involved pediatric providers for when care should transition to an adult-oriented inpatient facility • Children's hospitals caring for adults should have access to (1) necessary providers with relevant expertise in conditions experienced by adults, (2) supplies and equipment appropriately sized for adults, and (3) protocols for acute conditions faced by adult-aged patients	• Listen to family and patient stories, acknowledge potential grief associated with transitioning out of children's hospitals • Recognize when young adult patients are not able to make independent medical decisions; ask for consultative support early in these situations • Identify which subspecialists (pediatric vs. adult) should be called prior to placing an inpatient consult • Identify resources and experts to bridge knowledge gaps for childhood-onset diseases • Discuss care with previous pediatric inpatient and outpatient providers • Respect the expertise and experience of families and young adults living with childhood-onset chronic conditions	• Work with hospital administrators to create a policy or guideline clarifying when youth or young adults are admitted to pediatric vs. adult units • Communicate the hospital policy or guideline with patients and outpatient providers • Become familiar with comprehensive transitional care models, such as the Six Core Elements framework • Establish joint education opportunities • Be a willing resource for expertise in childhood-onset or adult-onset conditions • Collaborate to determine (1) which patients warrant inpatient transition plans, (2) how/when the information should be shared with future providers and how it should be integrated into comprehensive transition planning, (3) how patient/family input is incorporated • Recognize and monitor potentially avoidable hospital utilization and adverse events experienced during the transition period

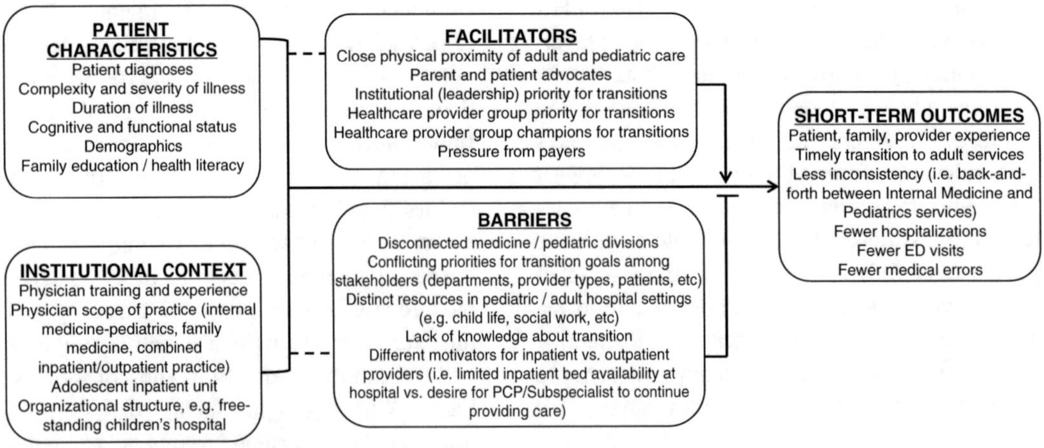

Fig. 27.1 Factors influencing pediatric to adult inpatient transition initiatives within health systems [13]

and to engage with families and advocacy groups to build a transition model which succeeds in all aspects of transition, including future hospital care.

In summary, by preparing families for changes in inpatient care, pediatricians can help manage family expectations, set their adult provider colleagues up for success, and reframe this transition from one associated with the loss of their involvement to the celebration of a major milestone in their child's life and evolution in the role of the parent as caregiver. At the same time, adult providers can succeed with an appreciation of where the young adults and their parents are coming from. Most young adults with chronic/complex conditions and/or their parent caregivers have become experts in both the patient's medical condition and its care. They possess a tremendous repository of "what works, what doesn't" and what has been tried before. Learning how to respect, recognize, and integrate that knowledge into ongoing care is a critical part of the inpatient care transfer.

References

1. Goodman DM, Hall M, Levin A, et al. Adults with chronic health conditions originating in childhood: inpatient experience in children's hospitals. Pediatrics. 2011;128(1):5–13.
2. CSHCN core system outcomes: goals for a system of care. The national survey of children with special health care needs chartbook 2009–2010. http://mchb.hrsa.gov/cshcn0910/core/co.html. Accessed 30 Nov 2016.
3. Got Transition. Center for health care transition improvement. 2016. http://www.gottransition.org/. Accessed 4 Apr 2016.
4. American Academy of Pediatrics, American Academy of Family Physicians, American College of Physicians, Transitions Clinical Report Authoring Group, Cooley WC, Sagerman PJ. Supporting the health care transition from adolescence to adulthood in the medical home. Pediatrics. 2011;128(1):182–200.
5. American Academy of Pediatrics, American Academy of Family Physicians, American College of Physicians-American Society of Internal Medicine. A consensus statement on health care transitions for young adults with special health care needs. Pediatrics. 2002;110(6 Pt 2):1304–6.
6. Bensen R, Steidtmann D, Vaks Y. A triple aim approach to transition from pediatric to adult health care for youth with special health care needs. Palo Alto, CA: Lucile Packard Foundation for Children's Health; 2014.
7. McPheeters M, Davis AM, Taylor JL, Brown RF, Potter SA, Epstein RA. Transition care for children with special health needs. Technical Brief No. 15. Rockville, MD: Agency for Healthcare Research and Quality; 2014.
8. Betz CL, Ferris ME, Woodward JF, Okumura MJ, Jan S, Wood DL. The health care transition research consortium health care transition model: a framework for research and practice. J Pediatr Rehabil Med. 2014;7(1):3–15.
9. Edwards JD, Houtrow AJ, Vasilevskis EE, Dudley RA, Okumura MJ. Multi-institutional profile of adults admitted to pediatric intensive care units. JAMA Pediatr. 2013;167(5):436–43.
10. Okumura MJ, Campbell AD, Nasr SZ, Davis MM. Inpatient health care use among adult survivors of chronic childhood illnesses in the United States. Arch Pediatr Adolesc Med. 2006;160(10):1054–60.
11. Kinnear B, O'Toole JK. Care of adults in children's hospitals: acknowledging the aging elephant in the room. JAMA Pediatr. 2015;169(12):1081–2.
12. Schor EL. Transition: changing old habits. Pediatrics. 2015;135(6):958–60.
13. Coller RJ, Ahrens S, Ehlenbach ML, Shadman KA, Chung PJ, Lotstein D, LaRocque A, Sheehy A. Transitioning from General Pediatric to Adult-Oriented Inpatient Care: National Survey of US Children's Hospitals. J Hosp Med. 2018;13(1):13–20. https://doi.org/10.12788/jhm.2923.

The International Perspective on Healthcare Transition

28

Beth E. Anderson, Swaran P. Singh, Claire Stansfield, and Kristin Liabo

Introduction

Adolescence is a period of development typically agreed to start around the age of 10 and to extend into early adulthood [1]. There are approximately 1.2 billion adolescents globally [2]. The bulk of the youth population is in low- and middle-income countries with poor access to health care [3]. In the United Kingdom (UK), young people aged 10–19 account for 11.4% of the population (equating to 7.4 million adolescents) [4]. In the United States (USA), this figure is estimated at 13.8% (42.7 million) [5]; in Canada, 11% (4 million) [6]; and in Australia, 12.2% (2.9 million) [7]. The value of engaging adolescents in positive health behaviours is well-established [3, 8, 9]. Such activity aims to mitigate negative health outcomes both for young people themselves and for any children they go on to have [2, 3]. As users of health care, adolescents are a distinct group with distinct care needs [10, 11]. While comparable cross-country data on health indicators and service use is limited [9], available figures indicate that in the U.S.A. alone, approximately three-quarters of a million young people enter adulthood with conditions that need (or are likely to need) input from health services [12]. Many of them will need their care transferred from children's to adults' health services.

This chapter focuses on health-care transition (HCT), a relatively under-researched area, in contrast to the wealth of literature on adolescence more generally. Developmental transition is referred to but only as an important element of the context for health-care transition. After summarising briefly the history of transition-specific care, we provide an overview of the extent of poor transition in high-income countries globally and an analysis of the reasons for this. We then describe how to deliver effective transition support, specifically the overarching principles of care that should apply, irrespective of the approach taken, and three emerging models of practice that have been associated with positive impacts. We conclude by identifying gaps in the literature and implications for future research and practice.

The chapter is informed by, and extends, a series of systematic reviews on supporting adolescents and young adults with special health-care needs (AYASHCN) through transitions from children's to adults' health services. The reviews

B. E. Anderson, Ph.D.
Social Care Institute for Excellence, London, UK
e-mail: beth.anderson@scie.org.uk

S. P. Singh, M.B.B.S., M.D., D.M., F.R.C.P. (✉)
University of Warwick, Coventry, UK
e-mail: s.p.singh@warwick.ac.uk

C. Stansfield, M.Sc.
University College London, London, UK
e-mail: c.stansfield@ucl.ac.uk

K. Liabo, Ph.D.
University of Exeter, Exeter, UK
e-mail: k.liabo@exeter.ac.uk

A. C. Hergenroeder, C. M. Wiemann (eds.), *Health Care Transition*,
https://doi.org/10.1007/978-3-319-72868-1_28

are complemented by a supplementary search conducted by the authors to identify recent lessons from emerging international practice.

Transition-Specific Support: A Brief History

The importance of providing age-appropriate, targeted support for adolescents moving to adults' services was first articulated in the mid-1980s at an international conference in the U.S.A. [13]. The evident gap in this provision was attributed to advancements in health care enabling more young people with childhood-onset conditions to live to adulthood [13]. This increase in life expectancy is predicted to continue across a range of chronic health conditions [14], meaning more young people will move out of paediatric care and into adults' services for long-term support. This is happening in the context of a conceptual and operational divide between children's and adults' health-care practice, the corollary of increased clinical specialisation over recent decades. The evolution of this focus on specialty-specific competence has varied from one area of medicine to another, reflecting the diversity of financial, social and political drivers on different parts of the system. Accordingly, the imperative to improve the support offered to young people with health conditions, before, during and after their move to adults' services, has been a feature of policy in a number of high-income countries over recent years [15, 16] . Such policy, however, has not led to system-level planning and provision, and poor transition care is commonplace [17].

Many young people do not experience successful transition or are simply transferred from one service to another without any introduction as to how adults' services operate and what is expected of adult patients. Fewer than 50% of young people with special health-care needs in the U.S.A. receive the support they needed at this critical stage of their care journey [18]. Poor transitions can result in significant costs to young people themselves and to the wider health economy. A recent analysis from the UK costed poorly managed transition for a young person with a lifelong condition (diabetes) at £9.94 m (equating to approximately $13.4 million) [19].

The Context for Service Transition

The multi-faceted nature of young people's transition is complicated by the fact that transition as a concept is inconsistently defined and applied. Transition (a managed process taking place over time), in practice, can be made synonymous with transfer (a discrete event at a single point in time at which responsibility for care moves from one provider to another), in spite of broad understanding in the health-care community that this is not the case [18]. As a result, young people can find themselves in the adults' service with little warning, or worse, facing a future in which there is no formal support available to them.

Transition is complicated further by the fact that it is not a process that occurs in isolation. Firstly, service transition is set against a backdrop of young people's wider developmental transition (see Chaps. 2 and 3). Adolescence is a pivotal time in a young person's life, during which they experience multiple physical, cognitive, social, emotional and behavioural changes [1]. These can be difficult to deal with, in and of themselves and can also increase risk of psychosocial or condition-specific problems [20]. There is emerging research that suggests differential maturation of the areas in the brain controlling emotional and rational aspects of development [21], which might explain that some young people start to take greater risks and be more impulsive [21] (see also Chaps. 2 and 3). It might also explain why this is a period when serious mental disorders can emerge [11]. Practitioners can therefore find it difficult, or feel insufficiently skilled, to engage this group of people—no longer treated as children, but not yet treated as adults [22]. There can also be confusion within and between services about when transition starts; that is to say, the age at which it is appropriate to begin planning for the young person's move to adult services.

Secondly, transition between support services is only one type of situational change that young people may experience around this time. Major life events taking place during late adolescence can come with significant contextual changes, for example, leaving home, starting work or going to university. Such important and potentially stressful occurrences can themselves trigger, or worsen, health conditions. Where such events involve moving from one geographical area to another, and a young person has previously been supported by services in their home area, this can pose an additional barrier to continuity of care.

Thirdly, health systems in developed countries are complex. Moving from children's to adults' services can involve navigating a confusing array of people, places and processes. There are major differences in the culture, ethos and environments of adults' services compared to children's. As a result, it is commonplace for young people and their families to feel unprepared for these changes and to find the process of change confusing and traumatic [23]. The inconsistency of health-care provision and quality across a range of services can become apparent to young people as they move across geographical, service or administrative boundaries. At worst, this can mean there is no adults' service corresponding to that available for children or that higher thresholds for adults' service entry render young people ineligible for any support after the point of transfer. This is particularly pertinent to mental health care [24, 25].

Barriers to Transition

Despite the relative profusion of transition-related policies, implementing culture change or service improvement initiatives in any health economy is difficult. This has meant that even when guidance is in place, it fails to translate into good practice [26–29]. Commissioners and practitioners have struggled to ensure young people move from children's to adults' health-care services in a streamlined way, with no gap or delay in provision.

Barriers to transition can be classified as relating to the service level or the individual level. Firstly, let us consider the service level, where lack of available provision is one of the most significant barriers; there are simply far more young people moving to adulthood with specific health-care needs than there are suitable services available to support them [30, 31]. Where there are services in place, one of the most significant factors impeding successful transition is the absence of a clear, structured transition model or pathway [32, 33]. Without this, young people and their families can feel unclear about what will happen after they leave children's services and who will support them. In addition, having a clearly communicated process in place ensures that young people are prepared for transfer, rather than this coming as a shock to them—another barrier to successful transition [34].

An additional service-level barrier to transition occurs where practitioners consider health-care support needs in isolation. Evidence on young people's perceptions of the barriers to transition consistently cites, as an example, lack of consideration given by practitioners to lifestyle changes and wider needs (including sexual health, drug and alcohol use, education, employment and social needs) [32]. As these subjects can be sensitive and complex, clinicians can find it difficult to address them with young people [16]. This problem may also be a micro-level manifestation of a macro-level barrier, specifically, poor inter-agency and intra-agency communication creating or reinforcing a silo mentality. Inefficiencies in integrated working—across both children's and adult's services and hospital and community services—are another recurring theme in the transition literature [32, 34–36]. When this service fragmentation is combined with inadequate information provision (another frequently highlighted system-level barrier), navigating the system becomes difficult [23, 32, 36, 37].

System-level barriers to effective transition relate to the culture, processes and resources in adults' services. These include lack of involvement in the planning process, lack of confidence in supporting adolescents as a distinct group and delay in initial appointments in adults' clinics [32, 37–39]. Even when AYASHCN are seen in adults' services, it can be that—for reasons of eligibility or lack of availability—they no longer have access to the same specialist expertise as they did pre-transfer [32]. The reasons for these inconsistencies are numerous including, for example, different service eligibility thresholds, incoherent service priorities or rigid service protocols (which may include clinical indicators that need to be met pre-transfer [40]) impeding individualised care [32]. These are likely to be compounded by lack of both resources and training to address the particular needs of these young adults [23, 32, 40]. By contrast, on the pre-transfer side, reluctance of children's service practitioners to hand over the AYASHCN's care, particularly when relationships are well established, has been identified as a barrier to transition [32, 36, 41]. Related to this, delays or inefficiencies in making referrals to adults' services stymie the transition process [29, 36]. There is evidence from multiple countries (the U.S.A., Canada, U.K.) that young people are invariably not referred to a specific adults' services clinician or are transferred with poor, or no, information provided to adults' services about their conditions, preferences and needs [41].

Involvement of parents in the transition process can also be a barrier to effective transition. On one hand, parents can struggle to adjust to their child's burgeoning autonomy. This can stymie practitioner efforts to encourage young people to take increasing ownership of their care [41]. On the other hand, young people can feel frustration if there is either too much focus on parents' wishes (such that they are excluded from the process) or insufficient recognition of the support they still draw from their parents [32, 37] even though they will be required to take on more responsibility for their health as part of transition.

At the individual level, certain groups of adolescents are at particularly high risk of poor (or no) transition including those who are looked after by the state [27, 42, 43], experience mental ill health [26, 42], are disabled [44], have palliative care needs, or have complex, multiple needs [45]. Opportunities to spot AYASHCN most at risk of poor transition, and intervene early, are frequently missed [46]. AYASHCN with mental health needs and developmental disabilities, among others, can face significant challenges in later life if their needs are not met during transition [31].

Overarching Good Practice Principles

A model of care can be defined as 'an integrated system of services that facilitate best practices of care' [16, p. 376]. Given that service transition takes place within the context of developmental transition and situational transition, a range of outcomes should be considered when evaluating whether any model works to deliver care in this way [14]. No single model can be identified confidently as the most successful [25, 32, 47–49]. This is attributable to a paucity of high-quality, robust research on effective approaches to transition. Many novel practice models are being developed, but this is often in isolation and/or without robustly designed evaluation of impact [50]. A number of emerging models have delivered positive impacts; examples are described later. In addition, looking across models, and in the wider literature, it is possible to identify some overarching success factors. The four key principles summarised in Table 28.1, and described thereafter, represent common features of effective approaches.

While the importance of empowering young people to make decisions about their care is beyond dispute, the extent and quality of genuine partnership work with young people varies hugely. Effective transition planning should always put the young person at the heart of all discussions and decisions about their care. This approach is both valued by AYASHCN and improves outcomes [32]. A young person-centered approach is one in which they are involved in service design, delivery and evaluation at both strategic and individual levels; the production, piloting and evaluation of transition-related materials and tools; and review of their own transition, to find out if they achieved what they wanted and needed to achieve. In working with AYASHCN in this way, practitioners should apply a strength-based philosophy. Care should

Table 28.1 Principles of effective transition support

1. Young person centred	The young person is enabled to take part in all discussions and decisions about their care. Their needs and preferences are taken into account
2. Holistic and empowering	The young person is treated as more than just their condition. Care is offered in the context of their wider life, aspirations and circumstances. They are empowered to self-manage
3. Coordinated and planned early	Transition starts around the age of 13 or 14 (at the latest) and at a time the young person can cope with and engage in it. They have a single named worker to support them throughout the process
4. Consistent and jointly owned	Responsibility for transition is shared between children's and adults' services. Young people are tracked throughout the process to ensure post-transfer follow-up actually happens

be individually focused and flexible, founded on what the AYASHCN is able to do and wants to do, rather than how they are limited by their condition [16, 32, 38, 51].

Support should address more than the health condition alone. Effective health-care transition is provided in the broader context of what it can enable the AYASHCN to achieve in their day-to-day life [32, 47]. Focusing solely on managing the health condition, or presenting a predetermined set of treatment options, can limit both the quality and experience of transition. Practitioners should draw on AYASHCN's skills and abilities and the links they have with carers, family and friends. Using these resources to best effect can help to build AYASHCN's confidence and interest in and ability to self-manage their health conditions and coordinate their own care [32, 45, 50, 52]. A strength-focused approach of this type contrasts to 'the often reactive medical model of adult health care' [22, p. 435].

Multimodal approaches that use both web- and mobile-based technologies can empower AYASHCN to self-manage their health [53]. Offering peer support, coaching and mentoring and advocacy can help AYASHCN play an active part in planning their own transition. All aspects of transition should take account of the young person's communication needs and preferences. A written record, in the form of a 'communication passport' or 'one-page profile' that the young person can share with others, can help make sure everyone providing support knows what is needed in this respect [54].

Good coordination and planning are central to any effective model of support. There is strong, consistent evidence about the benefits of a single practitioner to help AYASHCN navigate services; make the links between everyone involved in their care; provide, or tell people where they can find, advice; and arrange appointments and help young people to access them. This is a designated role rather than a job title, to be assumed by someone already providing support to the AYASHCN [54].

The timing of the transition planning relates to the difference between transition and transfer. Fictional case studies that involve timing and other aspects of HCT planning are presented in Table 28.2. Transition planning should start early, around the age of 13 or 14, and well before the physical transfer to adults' services [54]. Rather than imposing strict age thresholds, services should take account of each AYASHCN's development and the things happening in their life to make sure they are ready and able to deal with this change [41, 54]. Indeed, the importance of assessing transition readiness, as part of a coherent, comprehensive approach to transition planning, is a consistent theme in literature [14, 41]. This responds specifically to the need to recognise the range and nature of other priorities in the young person's life [39].

The number of AYASHCN lost to follow-up after transfer is a significant problem [14, 41]. To avoid transitional care being seen as someone else's responsibility [55, 56], it is critical that children's and adults' services share responsibility for pre- and post-transition support (to coordinate the actual transfer) (see Chaps. 9–12 and 16–18). In addition, it is important to track young people throughout the process to ensure post-transfer follow-up actually happens [14].

There should be systems and processes in place to prevent services losing contact with AYASHCN discharged from paediatric care. A good practice guideline in England specifies that AYASHCN should see the same health-care practitioner for the first two appointments post-transfer, and there should be proactive follow-up with those who do not attend appointments. In addition, at an early stage pre-transfer, they should be told about alternative sources of support in cases where there is no adults' service to which a young person can be referred [54].

Effective Transition Approaches

A range of promising initiatives are being implemented with some emerging evidence of benefits. Broadly, these approaches can be classified as joint working, bridging services or youth-focused support [57]. This section includes a brief summary of each, with illustrative examples from practice alongside evidence of effectiveness and cost-effectiveness.

Table 28.2 Fictional case studies: typical versus effective transition

Typical transfer transition	Effective transition, applying good practice principles
An 18-year-old male, suffering from ADHD and a mood disorder needed transition from child to adult mental health care. Having received very good clinical care from child services, the treating team could find no adult providers willing to take over care. The young man was discharged to a community counselling service who deemed him 'too complex and risky'. He was therefore left without any provision, being too complex for available community services but not 'ill enough' to be treated by adult mental health service	At a routine appointment, a paediatric nurse talked to a 16-year-old female about future transition. This was in a relaxed way, without any pressure to make decisions about transfer. Soon after this, she introduced the patient to a nurse from the adult clinic. Gradually, the young woman started having appointments with the adults' services nurse, in the paediatric department. She was then invited to visit the adults' department, when she was ready. On her visit, the adults' service nurse showed her around the department and explained how things worked. When she was nearly 18, she decided herself she was ready for transfer

Joint Working

The value of close, collaborative working between practitioners in adults' and children's services is well-evidenced [31, 34, 35, 45, 51, 58]. Shared responsibility for AYASHCN's care before and after transition is common to a number of emerging condition-specific transition models in the U.K., U.S.A., Canada and Europe (Belgium, Germany and the Netherlands) [50]. In practice, this means emphasising the importance of cross-agency collaboration at system level [16], and then translating this into strategic and operational policies, for example, by having a named responsible person at each of these levels, as well as a shared vision and jointly agreed processes and protocols [32, 35, 38, 52, 54].

Involving primary care services and staff in transition planning is emerging as an important clinical and research theme. Research from the UK, for example, indicated the importance of community-based general practitioner involvement in transition planning especially for young people with complex needs [29]. This is a best practice recommendation in the UK (England-specific) guidance [54] which may be transferable to other countries in which a similar practitioner role is a core component of community provision (such as Australia, New Zealand, Canada and much of Europe). Evidence about the detailed arrangements for primary care involvement is sparse, and, as yet, there is no definitive model of good practice in this area [48].

Bridging Service

Support from Designated Professional

A bridging service can take the form of support from a designated professional who engages the AYASHCN and their family throughout the transition process. In doing so, this worker helps the person navigate services and make decisions and provides continued support for a period after the physical handover of care. A transition coordinator of this type, who may be a professional with another job title fulfilling this role, features commonly in a number of approaches [41]. In the UK this has been recommended explicitly as good practice in national (England-specific) guidance [54]. It has been suggested that effective multi-agency integrated working can remove the need for a bridging coordinator [16]; however, it may be that an effective holistic approach includes both.

There is a small amount of evidence to highlight the potential value of nursing staff in the coordinator role, where transition takes place in community settings [59]. A recent Cochrane Review included an evaluation of a nurse-led approach to one-to-one transition support [60] and noted that this led to modest improvements in disease knowledge and self-management [49]. A retrospective U.S. cohort study of condition-specific (diabetes) outpatient clinic care found that having consistent support from the same allied health professional or clinician after transfer, as before, predicted lower hospitalisation rates [61].

Structured Transition Programme

A retrospective cohort study of a structured transition programme in Italy identified clinical and service-level benefits when compared to data prior to implementation. The intervention included support from a transition coordinator 1 year prior to transfer and after the move to adult services. In addition, the adults' service clinician was involved in transition planning, and delivered the last children's clinic appointment, and the first in the adults' clinic, jointly with the paediatric consultant. The condition-specific outcome (mean HbA1c) improved and was sustained over a year post-transfer, and attendance was higher in the structured transition group [62].

Transitions Clinics

A number of reviews have considered the effectiveness of transition clinics. The difference in the composition of these models, and the lack of rigorous trial evaluation data, renders it difficult to draw firm conclusions about clinical and cost-effectiveness [50]. There is some evidence that the components of these interventions offer the potential to improve both condition-specific outcomes [45] and the experiences of AYASHCN and their families [31] and it is possible to identify such shared features. Common to a number of condition-specific (rheumatology) transition clinics across the U.S.A., U.K., Canada and Europe, for example, are models comprising a written transition policy (with input from both children's and adults' services); shared responsibility for care before and after transfer, supported by communication of relevant information; flexible, personalised, early transition planning; a transition coordinator; and empowerment of AYASHCN through education and information [50].

One condition-specific model (renal transplant) from Canada comprises a multidisciplinary team including a social worker, support and education using email and mobile technology, regular (4–6 monthly) appointments pre-transfer at time points agreed to suit the needs of the AYASHCN, and comprehensive handover communications and 'matching' of AYASHCN to adult clinicians best suited to their needs. A retrospective cohort study attributed a number of benefits to this model including improved clinical outcomes (no death or graft loss) and, as a result, a cost saving [63].

Youth-Specific Models

Young Adult Team

A retrospective cohort study conducted in the UK found that AYASHCN supported via a dedicated multi-agency Young Adult Team experienced improved function and societal participation, compared to those who did not have access to this service [64]. This was supported by economic evidence that indicated the outcomes were not associated with increased cost.

Training Courses for Young People

A range of interventions focus on supporting AYASHCN to either increase their ability to self-manage or to engage more directly in transition planning; and this has taken different forms. A randomised controlled trial of a training course to help young people develop their health-care plan, included in a recent Cochrane Review of health-care models [49], found no evidence of impact on self-efficacy, quality of life or condition management [30]. A recent integrative review, however, highlighted that self-management training is a common feature of transition support activity across the UK, Canada and Europe and noted that empowering young people to take ownership of their health is a success factor for transition [41]. This was supported by a review of mental health-specific models [16].

Gaps in the Research

The most significant gap in the research is the lack of robust effectiveness evidence. High-quality comparative and longitudinal studies are needed to understand what works, for whom, under different circumstances (see Chap. 13). Research should also seek to understand cost-effectiveness, alongside effectiveness, and the length of time over which impacts are realised and sustained. An agreed definition of successful transition outcomes is also lacking.

There is a pressing need to provide support to practitioners working with young people on both sides of the transition divide. More research is needed on the most effective approaches to and impact of transition training for practitioners.

In summary, transition from paediatric to adult-based care is a problem shared by health-care systems across many countries, and future research on evidence-based approaches will likely benefit AYASHCN across international boundaries.

Acknowledgements The reviews informing this chapter were funded by the Department of Health and commissioned by the National Institute for Health and Care Excellence in the United Kingdom.

References

1. Hagell A, Coleman J, Brooks F. Key data on adolescence 2013. London: Association for Young People's Health; 2013.
2. World Health Organization. Adolescents: health risks and solutions. Factsheet. 2016. http://www.who.int/mediacentre/factsheets/fs345/en/.
3. Sawyer SM, Afifi RA, Bearinger LH, Blakemore SJ, Dick B, Ezeh AC, Patton GC. Adolescence: a foundation for future health. Lancet. 2012;379(9826):1630–40.
4. Office for National Statistics. Population estimates by single year of age and sex for local authorities in the UK, mid-2015. ONS. 2016.
5. U.S. Census Bureau. Annual estimates of the resident population for selected age groups by sex for the United States, States, Counties, and Puerto Rico Commonwealth and Municipios: April 1, 2010 to July 1, 2015. 2016.
6. Statistics Canada. Table 051-0001 – Estimates of population, by age group and sex for July 1, Canada, provinces and territories, annual (persons unless otherwise noted), CANSIM (database). Accessed 15 May 17.
7. Australian Bureau of Statistics. Australian demographic statistics. June Quarter 2015. 3101.0. 2015.
8. Viner RM, Barker M. Young people's health: the need for action. BMJ. 2005;330(7496):901–3.
9. Patton GC, Coffey C, Cappa C, Currie D, Riley L, Gore F, Degenhardt L, Richardson D, Astone N, Sangowawa AO, Mokdad A. Health of the world's adolescents: a synthesis of internationally comparable data. Lancet. 2012;379(9826):1665–75.
10. Sixty-fourth World Health Assembly. Resolution WHA 64.28: youth and health risks. Geneva: World Health Organization; 2011.
11. Singh SP, Winsper C. Adolescent mental health: the public health response. In: International handbook on adolescent health and development. 2017. doi: https://doi.org/10.1007/978-3-3-319-40743-2_6.
12. Scal P, Ireland M. Addressing transition to adult health care for adolescents with special health care needs. Pediatrics. 2005;115(6):1607–12.
13. Blum RW, Garell D, Hodgman CH, Jorissen TW, Okinow NA, Orr DP, Slap GB. Transition from child-centered to adult health-care systems for adolescents with chronic conditions: a position paper of the Society for Adolescent Medicine. J Adolesc Health. 1993;14(7):570–6.
14. Rachas A, Lefeuvre D, Meyer L, Faye A, Mahlaoui N, de La Rochebrochard E, Warszawski J, Durieux P. Evaluating continuity during transfer to adult care: a systematic review. Pediatrics. 2016;138(1):e20160256.
15. In UK policy, for example, this included: Department for Children, Schools and Families/Department of Health (2007) A transition guide for all services; and, Commissioning Panel for Mental Health (2012) Guidance for commissioners of mental health services for young people making the transition from child to adult mental health services.
16. Nguyen T, Embrett MG, Barr NG, Mulvale GM, Vania DK, Randall GE, Direzze B. Preventing youth from falling through the cracks between child/adolescent and adult mental health services: a systematic review of models of care. Community Ment Health J. 2017;53(4):375–82.

17. Hepburn CM, Cohen E, Bhawra J, Weiser N, Hayeems RZ, Guttmann A. Health system strategies supporting transition to adult care. Arch Dis Child. 2015;100(6):559–64.
18. Davis AM, Brown RF, Taylor JL, Epstein RA, McPheeters ML. Transition care for children with special health care needs. Pediatrics. 2014;134(5):900–8.
19. NICE. Transition from children's to adults' services for young people using health or social care services. Appendix C3 – Economic Report. London: National Institute for Health and Care Excellence; 2016.
20. Patton GC, Viner R. Pubertal transitions in health. Lancet. 2007;369(9567):1130–9.
21. Steinberg L. Risk taking in adolescence: new perspectives from brain and behavioral science. Curr Dir Psychol Sci. 2007;16(2):55–9.
22. McDonagh JE, Viner RM. Lost in transition? Between paediatric and adult services: it's time to improve the transition of adolescents from paediatric to adult services. BMJ. 2006;332(7539):435.
23. Shaw KL, Southwood TR, McDonagh JE. Developing a programme of transitional care for adolescents with juvenile idiopathic arthritis: results of a postal survey. Rheumatology. 2004;43(2):211–9.
24. Swift KD, Sayal K, Hollis C. ADHD and transitions to adult mental health services: a scoping review. Child Care Health Dev. 2014;40(6):775–86.
25. Paul M, Street C, Wheeler N, Singh SP. Transition to adult services for young people with mental health needs: a systematic review. Clin Child Psychol Psychiatry. 2015;20(3):436–57.
26. Singh SP. Transition of care from child to adult mental health services: the great divide. Curr Opin Psychiatry. 2009;22(4):386–90.
27. Beresford B, Cavet J. Transitions to adult services by disabled young people leaving out authority residential schools. Social Policy Research Unit, University of York; 2009.
28. Clarke S, Sloper P, Moran N, Cusworth L, Franklin A, Beecham J. Multi-agency transition services: greater collaboration needed to meet the priorities of young disabled people with complex needs as they move into adulthood. J Integr Care. 2011;19(5):30–40.
29. Care Quality Commission. From the pond into the sea. Children's transition to adult health services. London: Care Quality Commission; 2014.
30. Betz CL, O'Kane LS, Nehring WM, Lobo ML. Systematic review: health care transition practice service models. Nurs Outlook. 2016;64(3):229–43.
31. Bloom SR, Kuhlthau K, Van Cleave J, Knapp AA, Newacheck P, Perrin JM. Health care transition for youth with special health care needs. J Adolesc Health. 2012;51(3):213–9.
32. Kime NH, Bagnall AM, Day R. Systematic review of transition models for young people with long-term conditions: a report for NHS Diabetes. 2013.
33. Watson R, Parr JR, Joyce C, May C, Le Couteur AS. Models of transitional care for young people with complex health needs: a scoping review. Child Care Health Dev. 2011;37(6):780–91.
34. Por J, Golberg B, Lennox V, Burr P, Barrow J, Dennard L. Transition of care: health care professionals' view. J Nurs Manag. 2004;12(5):354–61.
35. Jordan L, Swerdlow P, Coates TD. Systematic review of transition from adolescent to adult care in patients with sickle cell disease. J Pediatr Hematol Oncol. 2013;35(3):165–9.
36. Mills J, Cutajar P, Jones J, Bagelkote D. Ensuring the successful transition of adolescents to adult services: Jonathan Mills and colleagues discuss findings from an audit of the referral and transfer of children with learning disabilities to services for adults. Learn Disabil Pract. 2013;16(6):26–8.
37. Beresford B, et al. Making a difference for young adult patients. Research Briefing. Bristol: Together for Short Lives; 2013.
38. Binks JA, Barden WS, Burke TA, Young NL. What do we really know about the transition to adult-centered health care? A focus on cerebral palsy and spina bifida. Arch Phys Med Rehabil. 2007;88(8):1064–73.
39. Garvey K, Wolpert H, Laffel L, Rhodes E, Wolfsdorf J, Finkelstein J. Health care transition in young adults with type 1 diabetes: barriers to timely establishment of adult diabetes care. Endocr Pract. 2013;19(6):946–52.
40. Sebastian S, Jenkins H, McCartney S, Ahmad T, Arnott I, Croft N, Russell R, Lindsay JO. The requirements and barriers to successful transition of adolescents with inflammatory bowel disease: differing perceptions from a survey of adult and paediatric gastroenterologists. J Crohn's Colitis. 2012;6(8):830–44.
41. Zhou H, Roberts P, Dhaliwal S, Della P. Transitioning adolescent and young adults with chronic disease and/or disabilities from paediatric to adult care services–an integrative review. J Clin Nurs. 2016;25(21–22):3113–30.
42. Singh SP, Paul M, Islam Z, Weaver T, Kramer T, McLaren S, Belling R, Ford T, White S, Hovish K, Harley K. Transition from CAMHS to adult mental health services (TRACK): a study of service organisation, policies, process and user and carer perspectives. London: Report for the National Institute for Health Research Service Delivery and Organisation Programme; 2010.
43. Liabo K, McKenna C, Ingold A, Roberts H. Leaving foster or residential care: a participatory study of care leavers' experiences of health and social care transitions. Child Care Health Dev. 2017;43(2):182–91.
44. Beresford B. On the road to nowhere? Young disabled people and transition. Child Care Health Dev. 2004;30(6):581–7.
45. Crowley R, Wolfe I, Lock K, McKee M. Improving the transition between paediatric and adult healthcare: a systematic review. Arch Dis Child. 2011;96(6):548–53. https://doi.org/10.1136/adc.2010.202473.
46. Butterworth S, Singh SP, Birchwood M, Islam Z, Munro ER, Vostanis P, Paul M, Khan A, Simkiss D. Transitioning care-leavers with mental health needs: 'they set you up to fail!'. Child Adolesc Mental Health. 2017;22(3):138–47.

47. Doug M, Adi Y, Williams J, Paul M, Kelly D, Petchey R, Carter YH. Transition to adult services for children and young people with palliative care needs: a systematic review. Arch Dis Child. 2011;96(1):78–84.
48. Bhawra J, Toulany A, Cohen E, Hepburn CM, Guttmann A. Primary care interventions to improve transition of youth with chronic health conditions from paediatric to adult healthcare: a systematic review. BMJ Open. 2016;6(5):e011871.
49. Campbell F, Biggs K, Aldiss SK, O'Neill PM, Clowes M, McDonagh J, While A, Gibson F. Transition of care for adolescents from paediatric services to adult health services. Cochrane Database Syst Rev. 2016;4:CD009794.
50. Clemente D, Leon L, Foster H, Minden K, Carmona L. Systematic review and critical appraisal of transitional care programmes in rheumatology. Semin Arthritis Rheum. 2016;46(3):372–9. WB Saunders
51. Watson AR. Problems and pitfalls of transition from paediatric to adult renal care. Pediatr Nephrol. 2005;20(2):113–7.
52. Allen D, Cohen D, Hood K, Robling M, Atwell C, Lane C, Lowes L, Channon S, Gillespie D, Groves S, Harvey J. Continuity of care in the transition from child to adult diabetes services: a realistic evaluation study. J Health Serv Res Policy. 2012;17(3):140–8.
53. Huang JS, Terrones L, Tompane T, Dillon L, Pian M, Gottschalk M, Norman GJ, Bartholomew LK. Preparing adolescents with chronic disease for transition to adult care: a technology program. Pediatrics. 2014;133(6):e1639–46.
54. NICE. Guideline 43: Transition from children's to adults' services for young people using health or social care services. In: National Institute for Health and Care Excellence. 2016.
55. Swift KD, Hall CL, Marimuttu V, Redstone L, Sayal K, Hollis C. Transition to adult mental health services for young people with Attention Deficit/Hyperactivity Disorder (ADHD): a qualitative analysis of their experiences. BMC Psychiatry. 2013;13(1):74.
56. Kaehne A. Transition from children and adolescent to adult mental health services for young people with intellectual disabilities: a scoping study of service organisation problems. Adv Ment Health Intellect Disabil. 2011;5(1):9–16.
57. Singh SP, Paul M, Ford T, Kramer T, Weaver T, McLaren S, Hovish K, Islam Z, Belling R, White S. Process, outcome and experience of transition from child to adult mental healthcare: multiperspective study. Br J Psychiatry. 2010;197(4):305–12.
58. Kipps S, Bahu T, Ong K, Ackland FM, Brown RS, Fox CT, Griffin NK, Knight AH, Mann NP, Neil HA, Simpson H. Current methods of transfer of young people with type 1 diabetes to adult services. Diabet Med. 2002;19(8):649–54.
59. McCallum C. Supporting young people's transition from children's to adult services in the community. Br J Community Nurs. 2017;22(1):668–74.
60. Mackie AS, Islam S, Magill-Evans J, Rankin KN, Robert C, Schuh M, Nicholas D, Muhll IV, McCrindle BW, Yasui Y, Rempel GR. Healthcare transition for youth with heart disease: a clinical trial. Heart. 2014;100(14):1113–8.
61. Nakhla M, Daneman D, To T, Paradis G, Guttmann A. Transition to adult care for youths with diabetes mellitus: findings from a universal health care system. Pediatrics. 2009;124(6):e1134–41.
62. Cadario F, Prodam F, Bellone S, Trada M, Binotti M, Allochis G, Baldelli R, Esposito S, Bona G, Aimaretti G. Transition process of patients with type 1 diabetes (T1DM) from paediatric to the adult health care service: a hospital-based approach. Clin Endocrinol. 2009;71(3):346–50.
63. Prestidge C, Romann A, Djurdjev O, Matsuda-Abedini M. Utility and cost of a renal transplant transition clinic. Pediatr Nephrol. 2012;27(2):295–302.
64. Bent N, et al. Team approach versus ad hoc health services for young people with physical disabilities: a retrospective cohort study. Lancet. 2002;360(9342):1280–6.

29 Expanding the Role of the Pharmacist

Nicola J. Gray, Jonathan Burton, Roisin Campbell, and Janet E. McDonagh

Introduction

Do you know any of the pharmacists in your place of work or the wider community? Traditionally, the pharmacy has been the "last stop" for people with chronic illness—the final place to wait for medication when the clinic visits are over. For chronic illness requiring regular medication, however, the pharmacist may be the healthcare provider with whom an individual has the most regular contact [1, 2]. Yet the pharmacist has been isolated from other providers, physically and culturally. They may have been physically separated by the nature of their practice settings—a remote retail location in the community or operating within the bounds of the hospital pharmacy. Many medical prescribers may only have interacted with the pharmacist when there is a query or potential error on a prescription, which might result in a mutually defensive exchange. This combination of factors has not historically fostered close relationships, but there are many recent developments in pharmacy and health care that herald a welcome change. For this and other reasons, reframing and expanding the role of the pharmacist in the care of adolescents and young adults with special healthcare needs (AYASHCN)—especially during transition and transfer to adult care—may offer the multidisciplinary team a new route to effective outreach and engagement with AYASHCN.

It would be misleading to suggest that the pharmacy practice described in this chapter is widespread. There is, however, increased recognition that investing in the care of AYASHCN could have a medium-term positive effect on health outcomes and healthcare costs in adulthood [3]. It seems timely to highlight real examples of isolated yet innovative pharmacy practice that could be explored by healthcare systems. Some interventions presented here are relatively close to current clinical pharmacy practice; they simply represent greater engagement with, and focus on, AYASHCN to deploy many of the skills

N. J. Gray, Ph.D. (✉)
Green Line Consulting Limited, Manchester, UK
e-mail: nicola@greenlineconsulting.co.uk

J. Burton, B.Pharm
Right Medicine Pharmacy, University of Stirling, Stirling, UK
e-mail: jonathan@rightmedicinepharmacy.com

R. Campbell, M.Sc.
Pharmacy Department, Musgrave Park Hospital, Belfast, UK
e-mail: roisin.campbell@belfasttrust.hscni.net

J. E. McDonagh, M.D.
Paediatric and Adolescent Rheumatology, Centre for Musculoskeletal Research, Faculty of Biology, Medicine and Health and NIHR Manchester Musculoskeletal Biomedical Research Centre, University of Manchester, Manchester, UK

Manchester University NHS Trust, Manchester Academic Health Science Centre, Manchester, UK
e-mail: janet.mcdonagh@manchester.ac.uk

A. C. Hergenroeder, C. M. Wiemann (eds.), *Health Care Transition*,
https://doi.org/10.1007/978-3-319-72868-1_29

that pharmacists already use every day. Others, however, may represent more significant departures from current practice that would need the commitment of pharmacy educators and healthcare policymakers to make them mainstream.

The goal of this chapter is that the reader will be able to describe the different roles a pharmacist can play in healthcare transition and to reflect upon the interface between the pharmacist, AYASHCN/family, and physician in health management during transition from pediatric- to adult-based care.

Pharmacists in Context

Most pharmacists work in retail/community (hereafter shortened to "community") or hospital settings. Most people are familiar with the retail/community setting, as the vast majority of the population are likely to have visited a pharmacy within the past year for some purpose [4]. The environment is familiar, as there are commonalities worldwide; a store front—which may be part of a large company chain or a small independent business—and any variation of health and well-being products for sale or supply. There is a team of staff, with at least one pharmacist on the premises for consultation. The last 20 years have seen increasing "upskilling" of technicians and counter assistants so that the pharmacist could be freed from the routine aspects of dispensing prescriptions and selling medicines to concentrate on more complex cases and private consultations [5]. A lack of privacy has been a concern when over-the-counter conversations take place in pharmacies [6]; as a result, many premises now have a private consultation room [5, 7].

Research has shown that people are sophisticated about their use of different community pharmacy settings; pharmacies sited within large supermarkets may attract different customers from those on a main street in a small village or town [8]. This is particularly important for adolescents and young adults (AYA) seeking services that they may not wish their parents or friends to know about; the ability to move freely among pharmacies, their ubiquity and extended opening hours, and customer-oriented systems where appointments are not usually necessary, all have the potential to help AYA access a health provider when they need a confidential service like emergency contraception or sexually transmitted infection (STI) testing [9, 10]. The lack of stigma attached to a setting where AYA could be going in to purchase cosmetics or hair products means that the pharmacy offers unique and complementary opportunities to offer healthcare advice to AYA and their families.

Hospital pharmacists have been expanding their patient-facing role since the 1980s [11]. Pharmacists visit wards and monitor the drug therapy of inpatients. Many AYASHCN are seen in ambulatory clinics, however, so the pharmacist may not see outpatients beyond their dispensing role. A literature review and engagement with key informants in projects exploring the role of the pharmacist in the care of AYA with juvenile arthritis [12, 13] showed that innovation is happening. Pharmacists with independent prescribing qualifications, for example, are prescribing methotrexate in some rheumatology clinics, and pharmacists are running their own clinics for AYA including demonstration of injecting technique. Thus pharmacists in both community and hospital settings have the potential to give greater support to young people and families, but their role in the care of AYA with chronic illness is currently under-researched.

In countries such as the UK, New Zealand, and the U.S.A., pharmacists are going beyond supplying medicines to offer services to patients that involve in-depth discussions of their medication use. Pharmacists in the U.S.A. coined the term "pharmaceutical care" [14], which has been adopted by the profession globally; other country-specific terms include "medication therapy management" (MTM, U.S.A.) and "medicines optimization" (MO, England).

Pharmacists report a lack of training and confidence in engaging with young people [1, 15]. Some community pharmacy staff, moreover, are unsure whether their adult-focused services should be offered to AYA, especially minors [16]. UK pharmacists, however, may be gaining confidence from providing public health services to young people. In a small study, almost two-thirds (62.2%) of the 143 community pharmacists surveyed felt "reasonably confident" about engaging with young people, and a significant minority (30.1%) felt "very confident" [15]. This study of UK community pharmacists reported significant self-reported engagement with young people. While approximately half of these pharmacists reported dispensing prescriptions "often" and providing public health services "often" for young people aged 13–19 (53.8% and 45.4%, respectively), only 5.2% reported doing cognitive services like medication review "often" with this age group.

The shift from parental management of a chronic illness during early childhood to eventual shared and/or self-management during adolescence [17] is a major component of transitional care [18]. In an international Delphi study, discussion about self-management with AYA and their family was the third most important indication of successful transition [19]. Medication management has been identified by AYASHCN themselves as important [20]. How this is addressed within the clinical setting—and how effective such interventions are—is not clear and seems to vary across different subspecialties [21, 22]. In a study of parents of AYASHCN with arthritis, for example, Scal et al. [23] reported they were significantly less likely to have had discussions about self-management compared to parents of AYASHCN with diabetes. A medical case note audit study in the rheumatology clinics at a large UK pediatric hospital revealed that documentation of self-medication practices was present only in the minority of medical case notes. Moreover, the identification and recording in the notes of a community pharmacy that the family wished to use were rare [24].

Getting the Medication Right

Pharmaceutical care has been defined as a process that "includes the determination of the drug needs for a given individual and the provision not only of the drug required but also the necessary services (before, during or after treatment) to assure optimally safe and effective therapy. It includes a feedback mechanism as a means of facilitating continuity of care by those who provide it" [25]. Hepler and Strand [26] included an orientation toward outcomes in their later definition: "Responsible provision of drug therapy for the purpose of achieving definite outcomes that improve a patient's quality of life." What is implicit within the concept of pharmaceutical care is the safe supply of the correct medication for an individual, from which all other opportunities flow. As a core duty, the pharmacist must be able to help AYASHCN to maintain a consistent supply of medication before and during transfer of care; otherwise, any attempt to move the conversation beyond supply problems will be fruitless.

AYASHCN may need special pediatric formulations of medication during adolescence, but as they transfer to adult care, they may be expected to change to traditional adult products. AYA are likely to need reassurance that any change in product will not result in breakthrough symptoms, which would be particularly acute, for example, in AYASHCN with epilepsy. The palatability of tablet formulations may also need extra counselling and reassurance. Pharmacists in community and hospital settings have the potential to help AYASHCN and families cope with those changes.

There is merit in finding a local community pharmacy where an empathetic pharmacist can be enlisted as part of the extended multidisciplinary team. For example, AYASHCN could embark on a series of mystery shopping episodes in order to choose their preferred community pharmacy provider.

Promoting Healthcare Knowledge and Skills Among AYA

Knowledge and skills were one of five factors associated with successful transition in a meta-summary of the qualitative research literature [27]. The wide range of knowledge and skills required by a young person to take over the care of their conditions during adolescence and the transition process, including medication-related activities, have been highlighted in various conditions [18, 28] and are included in the numerous transition readiness measures currently being developed [29] (see Table 29.1). Moreover, a Delphi study identified medication knowledge and adherence to medication as two of the ten agreed outcomes for a successful transition [35].

Information about prescription medication may be obtained from a wide range of sources. Many providers will readily think about online information when considering AYASHCN, but we must not overlook the potential to provide written and spoken advice within consultations. A dispensing pharmacist has the advantage that the medication item itself that they hand to the patient contains information, both on the packaging and on the leaflet inside the packaging. Arguably an underused resource, the information leaflet in the box is often seen as complex—there to fulfil the pharmaceutical company's regulatory obligations, rather than being truly useful to the user.

Pharmacists are skilled in interpreting scientific information about medication, and there are other examples of pharmacist-led information initiatives. There is a UK website called "HeadMeds" http://www.headmeds.org.uk/ which was created by the charity Young Minds where pharmacists translated scientific jargon about medication for mental health problems into a format that would help AYA to consider the benefits and harms of prescribed medication. AYA were engaged at the start of the process to identify concerns about which they would want information, and there were two AYA medication users on the project advisory group. Medication-related concerns included efficacy, side effects, and possible withdrawal effects. The website also tackles concomitant use with illicit drugs, effects on concentration for schoolwork, whether the substance is banned for athletes, and effects on relationships and fertility. The website combines frank information about the properties of mental health medication with the real-life stories of AYASHCN.

Conversations with UK community pharmacists [36] about their engagement with AYASHCN who have chronic illness revealed situations where AYASHCN came to their local pharmacy with information that they had found on the Internet about health and medication. It was seen as an excellent opportunity to open a discussion with that medicine user, which the pharmacists felt was not as likely to happen with older people. The pharmacist felt able to help them to critically appraise the information found. Adolescent rheumatology research in this area strongly supported a role for the pharmacist—in both hospital and

Table 29.1 Reference to medication-related activities in selected transition readiness questionnaires

Readiness questionnaire name	Reference	Example of medication management item/s
Readiness for transition questionnaire	Gilleland et al. [30]	Taking medication daily as prescribed Calling in or ordering refills
Transition Q	Klassen et al. [31]	I am in charge of taking any medicine that I need I drop off or pick up my prescriptions when I need medicine
Transition readiness assessment questionnaire TRAQ	Sawicki et al. [32]	Do you take medications correctly and on your own? Do you reorder medications before they run out? Do you fill a prescription if you need to? Do you pay or arrange payments for your medications?
University of North Carolina TRxANSITION scale	Ferris et al. [33]	Do you usually remember to take your medicines on your own? Does someone usually have to remind you to take your medicines? Do you call in your prescription refills yourself? Do you usually pick up refills from the pharmacy yourself?
Self-management skills assessment guide	Williams et al. [34]	I know the names of my medications, what they do and how to buy them I prepare/take my own medications/treatments as required I keep track of my healthcare visits, treatment plan, and medications

community settings—in the sharing of websites and apps with AYA about chronic illness and medication [13], echoing previous research [37].

Maximizing Adherence

It is asserted that adherence to medication for chronic illness is worse among adolescents than for younger children or adults [38, 39]. The challenge for the multidisciplinary team is how to keep AYA and their families motivated to maintain their treatment regimen through this developmental period of great change [40]. A review of the barriers to adherence has reflected on the significant contribution of simply forgetting to take medication among AYA [41], echoed by other illness-specific studies, e.g., Koster et al. for asthma [42]. This is not constructed as an act of rebellion, or intentional nonadherence, but simply the precedence of other life activities. A number of commentators on adherence and transition have noted the potential for pharmacists to construct plans with AYA and to identify cues in their daily routine that can be linked to medication-taking [38, 43, 44].

Prescription Medication Systems

Pharmacists, particularly those in community settings, are generalist healthcare providers who see the breadth of health and well-being concerns of their local community. They help people to navigate the healthcare system; they intimately understand the procedures for ordering refill prescriptions and the different funding mechanisms for medication in their jurisdiction. In our research, pharmacists and hospital-based rheumatology staff felt strongly that pharmacists could help AYASHCN who need long-term medication to build their health literacy skills [13] (see Table 29.2). These may include:

- Timely ordering of refill requests from prescribers
- Liaising with the pharmacy to preorder stock if the medication is unusual or costly
- Finding the best way to fund their medication, in terms of exemptions for certain chronic illnesses, prepayment plans or co-payments according to their local healthcare system

This last point is particularly important for AYA in transition. During this time of late adolescence/early adulthood, the funding mechanism for medication may change. Automatic enrollment in a parent's insurance plan may be coming to an end, or an automatic age exemption from payment, as a minor, may no longer apply. Conversely, a new job may carry its own coverage and healthcare entitlements—the pharmacist is experienced in these matters and thus well-placed to help AYASHCN to navigate the system and avoid any lapse in coverage and treatment.

Self-Management of Minor Illness

Another area where the development of health literacy skills is valuable is the treatment of self-limiting illnesses such as coughs and colds. If AYASHCN have a chronic illness, the minor illness remedies held by their families in the home may not be suitable for them; an example would be the use of the nonsteroidal anti-inflammatory agent ibuprofen for dysmenorrhea by AYASHCN living with asthma. Pharmacists can advise AYASHCN about the best treatments for common ailments that will not interact with their prescription medication nor aggravate an underlying condition, empowering them to self-manage common ailments safely. When AYASHCN move out of the family home to attend college or start work, this may coincide with the time that they transfer to adult services. Previous work by our team with college students showed that they had reduced their reliance on their parents or caregivers because they were no longer physically present to advise them or physically give them medication. These AYA reported that they had come to recognize the local community pharmacist as an accessible source of advice, particularly for common ailments [45].

Table 29.2 Results of the pharmacists' role prioritization activity in multidisciplinary discussion groups [13]

Current/future role	Priority score
Community pharmacists help young people to develop their general healthcare skills, e.g., prescription refills, getting free prescriptions	4.78
Information supplied by hospital pharmacists at discharge goes directly to a nominated community pharmacist as well as the GP (General Practitioner - primary care physician)	4.71[b]
Community pharmacists can build long-term relationships with young people and families	4.71[b]
Pharmacists share information with young people about apps and websites that support adherence and give information about JIA (Juvenile Idiopathic Arthritis)	4.57[b]
Hospital pharmacists are included in MDT (multidisciplinary team) sessions for rheumatology patients	4.44
Pharmacists develop specialist expertise in pediatric/adolescent rheumatology	4.44
Pharmacists develop specialist expertise in young people's medication use for other long-term conditions (asthma, diabetes)	4.44
Pharmacists provide educational sessions for the multidisciplinary rheumatology team about medicines optimization	4.43[b]
Community pharmacists can support young people and families in medication-taking	4.33
Pharmacists facilitate young people's self-advocacy skills (e.g., decision-making, effective communication, disclosure)	4.29[b]
Hospital pharmacists can build long-term relationships with young people and families	4.14[b]
Hospital pharmacists do continuing professional development sessions for community pharmacists about JIA medicines	4.11
Pharmacists support transition services for young people going into adult rheumatology care	4.00[b]
Pharmacists develop better skills in communicating with young people and parents	3.89
Rheumatology team members do continuing professional development sessions for community pharmacists about JIA medicines	3.88[a]
Pharmacists work with home delivery companies to optimize medication supply	3.78
Pharmacists are advocates for young people with JIA and challenge prescribing decisions	3.75[a]
Pharmacists can be directly available to young people and parents/carers by email or telephone	3.71[b]
Hospital pharmacists can do clinics in the hospital for young people with JIA	3.67
Young people with JIA carry a card to signal their condition and their ability to collect their own prescriptions	3.63[a]
Pharmacists do medication review for young people with JIA	3.56
Pharmacists need to develop better skills in confidentiality and consent for young people	3.22
Pharmacists need to develop better skills in safeguarding for young people	3.11
Community pharmacists coordinate supply of JIA medication for young people	2.89
Hospital pharmacists do clinics in the community for young people with JIA	2.22

Priority mean scores are reported to two decimal places—data averaged from nine multidisciplinary groups. [a]Eight groups and [b]seven groups—some groups did not complete ranking for all roles. 1 was low priority for future development and 5 was high

This table is reprinted from the Journal of Adolescent Health, Vol 60(2), Gray NJ, Shaw KL, Smith FJ, Burton J, Prescott J, Roberts R, Terry D, McDonagh JE, The role of pharmacists in caring for young people with chronic illness, pp. 219–225, Copyright 2017, with permission from Elsevier

Theory into Practice: Expanding the Role of the Pharmacist

A review of the relevant literature shows significant pharmacist inclusion and innovation within AYA health teams to expand the role of the pharmacist (see Table 29.3). Studies across different clinical specialties show the inclusion of a clinical pharmacist in the hospital team [30, 56, 61]. Our work in the UK has shown differing levels of engagement, from a pharmacist who can be contacted by telephone for queries through to having prescribing rights to adjust maintenance therapies in clinic [36].

There has been significant international work done to describe, and then promote or accredit, the attributes of young people friendly services [3, 62, 63]. A study of their applicability to community pharmacy services concluded that they would be applicable to that setting [64], but their

Table 29.3 Examples of pharmacist involvement (actual and potential) in AYASHCN care for chronic illness

Chronic illness	Authors, year of publication, country	Nature of actual or recommended pharmacist involvement and/or transition-relevant pharmacy-related tasks
ADHD	Adamou and Bowers 2011 UK [46]	Authors remarked that the lack of clinical pharmacy involvement with child/adolescent mental health teams might be responsible for poor adherence to guidance, resulting in under-dosing of stimulants and AYA being severely symptomatic—recommended clinical pharmacy input
Asthma	Bynum et al. 2001 U.S.A. [47]	Reported on an initiative in rural Arkansas where telepharmacy counselling of AYA using inhalers showed more improvement in inhaler technique than the control group
	Shah et al. 2008 Australia [48]	Outreach initiative in rural community schools for 11-year-old students by local community pharmacists
	Ducharme et al. 2011 Canada [49]	Reported on the implementation of written action plans (WAP) for AYA with asthma in the emergency room, which improved patient adherence and asthma control. Suggested that the WAP would help pharmacists to reinforce medical recommendations
Cancer	Hollis and Morgan 2001 UK [50]	Recommended that the treatment and supportive care team for AYA with cancer should include a pharmacist who specializes in pediatric oncology
	Hord et al. 2014 U.S.A. [51]	An AAP statement "that the pediatric hematologist/oncologist must be assisted by skilled pharmacists who specialize in pediatric oncology"
Congenital heart disease	Moceri et al. 2015 France/Belgium/UK [52]	The authors reflected that "patients with stable CHD may not require long-term medications; thus, they are less exposed to the health system. CHD young adult patients may not benefit from the pharmacist assistance to help them in the healthcare pathway and deliver therapeutic education. This might partly explain the high percentage of loss of follow-up in CHD"
Diabetes	Gay et al. 2006 France [2]	Local pharmacists provided telecare to AYA with diabetes. No significant improvement was seen in their glycemic control, but there were system challenges that could be changed to improve the situation. The authors assert that pharmacists could have a valuable role because of their accessibility. They suggest better connection between pharmacists and the healthcare team, creating a pharmacist-hospital network for training and the use of software for sharing data with physicians
Epilepsy	Jurasek et al. 2010 Canada [53]	The authors describe the development and implementation of an AYA epilepsy transition clinic and assert the importance for AYA to know how to refill prescriptions and how to fund medication for epilepsy
HIV	Wiener et al. 2007 U.S.A. [54]	The authors of this study reflected that effective transition interventions would need to focus on equipping AYASHCN with the skills and knowledge to understand their disease and medications, and how to access a pharmacy and refills, among other healthcare-related tasks
	Tulloch et al. 2014 Thailand [55]	In the Thai Pediatric Antiretroviral Programme, services are provided from a "one-stop clinic" where AYA have consultations with a nurse, pediatrician, pharmacist, and social worker
	Campbell et al. 2010 UK [56]	AYA who are HIV positive attend a transition program which is led by clinical psychologists and an HIV clinical nurse specialist but includes contributions from a specialist pharmacist, specialist midwife, a drama specialist, and the local young peoples' sexual health team

(continued)

Table 29.3 (continued)

Chronic illness	Authors, year of publication, country	Nature of actual or recommended pharmacist involvement and/or transition-relevant pharmacy-related tasks
Inflammatory bowel disease	Fishman et al. 2010 U.S.A. [57]	The authors contend that older adolescents must develop the skills and confidence to interact independently within the clinic and pharmacy settings
Juvenile arthritis	McDonagh 2008 UK [18]	A proposed knowledge and skills framework for transition includes several pharmacy-related tasks including knowledge of the therapy regime and any impact on sexual and reproductive health as well as interactions with drugs and alcohol
	Lawson et al. 2011 U.S.A. [58]	In a U.S.A. study considering transition readiness, pharmacy-related tasks considered included ones which improved with age, e.g., the ability to fill prescriptions, and some which didn't, e.g., taking medications as prescribed.
	Hilderson D 2016 Belgium [59]	Medication adherence issues were a core component and secondary outcome measure in a current trial of a brief transition intervention although preliminary results did not reveal an improvement in adherence
Mental health	Jabbal 2010 Canada [60]	The author suggests a scenario where the pharmacist is able to have independent consultations with AYA and families, during which they can identify medication-related problems, formulate care plans and prescribe medication in their own right
Sickle cell disease	Cerns et al. 2013 U.S.A. [61]	AYA in transition are seen by a multidisciplinary team. The adolescent-focused team includes the clinical nurse specialist, nurse manager, physicians, social workers, case managers, and pharmacists. The adult multidisciplinary group includes a physician, pharmacist, social worker, and case manager among others
Transplantation	Gilleland et al. 2012 U.S.A. [30]	The context of an adolescent kidney transplant transition clinic (AKTTC) at a large pediatric transplant center is described. "The patients have individual interactions with members of a multidisciplinary healthcare team, including a transplant coordinator, social worker, psychologist, clinical pharmacist, and pediatric nephrologist. At each clinic visit, the multidisciplinary healthcare team assesses and encourages medication adherence and knowledge, healthcare responsibility, psychosocial adjustment, and avoidance of risk behaviors."
	Prestidge et al. 2012 Canada [44]	The authors describe the utility and cost of a renal transplant transition clinic. They found that the clinic was economically feasible and resulted in patient and allograft survival. "Behavioural strategies commonly used by our pharmacist include teaching patients to use pill boxes, watch and cell-phone alarms as medication reminders and linking medication-taking to cues in their daily routine"
General	Staples and Bravender 2002 U.S.A. [38] Dean et al. 2010 Australia [43] Prestidge et al. 2012 Canada [44]	These papers have noted the potential for pharmacists to construct plans with AYA and to identify cues in their daily routine that can be linked to medication-taking, to optimize adherence and facilitate transition

adoption by pharmacies remains rare. One of the reasons that community pharmacists give for a lack of direct engagement with AYA is that their parents tend to collect refills, limiting opportunities for building rapport [13].

These possible roles for pharmacists will be illustrated in context through two vignettes—one from the perspective of a community pharmacist and the other from a hospital-based pharmacist.

Vignette 1: The Hospital Pharmacist—Supporting AYA with Juvenile Arthritis [*Contributed by Roisìn Campbell*]

Katie first came to the Pediatric Rheumatology Unit as a quiet 13-year-old girl who clearly had evidence of long-standing polyarticular juvenile idiopathic arthritis (JIA) involving several large and small joints which had been missed in primary care. Katie and her parents were introduced to the members of the multidisciplinary team including the pharmacist and underwent a full assessment by the multidisciplinary team. A course of oral prednisolone was initiated to gain control over her long-standing inflammation, to be followed by methotrexate. Steroids can be a frightening concept to a young person and/or their parents, so it was important to put the low dose in context and to provide a steroid warning card. After discussion with Katie and the rheumatologist, the pharmacist found a suitable preparation and regimen of oral prednisolone which would both alleviate the symptoms and control the inflammation while limiting unwanted toxicity.

As they came to terms with the diagnosis, it was decided that Katie and her parents were too overloaded with information about the diagnosis to begin the counselling for methotrexate at the first visit. The pharmacist provided them with written information regarding methotrexate, her contact email address and direct telephone number and made arrangements for them to return a few days later to discuss it further.

Working together, the nurse specialist discussed the necessary blood monitoring arrangements, while the pharmacist focused on potential benefits and side effects, when to give methotrexate or withhold it and when to seek advice and from whom. A copy of information given was also sent to their family physician, with whom Katie and her parents were encouraged to discuss the treatment plan.

Katie responded well to the oral prednisolone with reduction in swelling and stiffness. Katie initially took the methotrexate easily and then began to refuse it saying she didn't like the taste of it. Strategies were given to make it more palatable: ice pops to numb the tongue before and after, placing methotrexate in tooth kind juice, and taking peanut butter before and afterward. However, Katie began to develop anticipatory vomiting on the day the medication was due, unresponsive to antiemetics 2 h before methotrexate. Katie returned to the ward, having missed several doses of methotrexate due to vomiting, and her joints were beginning to flare. At this stage the decision was made to switch to subcutaneous methotrexate.

Katie attended the Joint Nurse Specialist/Pharmacist subcutaneous methotrexate clinic where she underwent a structured training program and after two supervised injections was 'going solo' at home. She was encouraged to use her cell phone to set reminders for when to take her injections and to use the calendar to book her own blood monitoring appointments with the clinic.

Katie managed to adhere well to subcutaneous methotrexate until around the age of 15 years. This is a challenging age for any adolescent but can be particularly difficult if they have a chronic illness and are required to take medication even when they feel well. From pharmacy records, it was clear that Katie was no longer adherent, and when the pharmacist contacted her, she said that nausea was becoming a major issue. Katie attended the Joint Pharmacist/Specialist Nurse Clinic, and it became evident that Katie was having difficulties accepting her diagnosis and was unsure of her future.

At subsequent visits, Katie was seen independently of her parents to further address these difficulties. As part of routine psychosocial screening, other generic health issues were addressed using a non-judgmental approach including the interaction of alcohol with methotrexate and the importance of using effective contraception when sexually active. Following the discussion of the latter, Katie emailed the pharmacist the next day with specific questions regarding the impact of her disease and therapy on future fertility.

Once Katie accepted her condition, found her voice, and took control of her treatment plan, she was encouraged to utilize all these skills to prepare for adult services including attendance at appointments by herself, ensuring she contacted individual members of the team when she was in difficulty and reinforcing education about her medication, so her decision-making was informed. At the time of transfer, the pharmacist ensured continuity of supply of drug prescription until handover to the adult team and pharmacy was confirmed. The hospital pharmacist asked Katie if she and her family had a community pharmacy that they used regularly. They did have one, so the community pharmacist there—with Katie's permission—was briefed about the situation, and Katie made an arrangement to visit so that they could start to build a relationship.

Vignette 2: The Community Pharmacist—Supporting AYA with Depression [*Contributed by Jonathan Burton*]

Robert was an 18-year-old high school student who came to the pharmacy seeking advice regarding "feeling tired" on a regular basis. It was November, and he concluded that it was probably due to the time of year and the fact that he had had several recent viral infections. "Tired all the time" can be a sign of underlying mental health issues and, after introducing himself and having a brief welcoming chat at the counter, the community pharmacist invited Robert to talk further about his symptoms in the private pharmacy consulting room, and he accepted.

As well as exploring the physical nature of his tiredness, the pharmacist asked about sleep habits and more generally about his studies and high school life. A picture emerged of sleep disturbance, study worries, and a feeling of distance from his friends. The pharmacist explained how depressive illness might be a contributing factor in his feeling unwell and that he should not be shy about speaking to his doctor about this, as such feelings are common and help is available. Robert agreed to make an appointment with his primary care doctor in the next few days and admitted that he was worried about feeling low but did not like the thought of being put on antidepressants. The pharmacist explained that medication was one option and if his doctor did recommend medication then he could return to speak to the pharmacist in more depth about his concerns.

Two weeks later Robert presented in the pharmacy with a prescription for a 2-week supply of sertraline 50 mg tablets, one to be taken daily. As this was a new prescription for an antidepressant, the pharmacist invited him to discuss his prescription in private including the main features of his new medication, such as possible side effects and how long the medication may take to work.

After checking that Robert had another clinic appointment lined up, which was scheduled for 2 weeks after the first prescription, the pharmacist arranged a 1-week telephone follow-up so they could discuss how his first few days taking the sertraline were going. At the time of follow-up, Robert disclosed that he had found it difficult to tolerate the sertraline, so it was agreed that he would take the dose early in the day—with or after breakfast—to minimize stomach upset. The pharmacist reassured him that this side effect is usually short-lived. After this the pharmacist continued to see Robert with his refills every month or two, and they would occasionally take the opportunity to have a brief chat regarding his progress on the sertraline treatment, which was increased to 100 mg daily after a few weeks.

Within a few months, Robert had started his studies at a local college and had moved out of the family home to live on campus. His care was being transferred from his adolescent medicine team to a psychiatric provider near the college. The pharmacist asked him if he had questions about his health and medication resulting from the change in his life. He was concerned about mixing alcohol with the medication and of any potential impact on sexual performance, as Robert had recently started a new relationship. He was anxious that the medication would have a negative impact on his sexual health and social life. The pharmacist asked again about sleep and advised on good sleep hygiene in his new environment. Robert had been offered talking therapies but was on a waiting list, so the pharmacist advised speaking to the college student support department as well as his new provider. Commentators from the UK have noted that "transition in mental health [services] appears to be equally, if not more, problematic than in physical health settings." [65]. The pharmacist ensured he was still covered for services and medication on his parental insurance. Robert told his new provider which pharmacy he used for his refills and gave them contact details for any queries that may arise. The pharmacist spoke to Robert's clinic nurse about his prescription, so that the refills would not be interrupted.

The following spring, the pharmacist once again took the opportunity to speak in private to Robert when he came for his refill, knowing exam season was looming and that this can be a difficult time for college students, especially those with a history of mental health problems. He seemed to be coping well and reported being happy with his studies as well as enjoying spending time with his friends and his girlfriend in particular. He asked the pharmacist when he might be able to stop the sertraline as he really did feel better and whether this was safe to do as he had heard horror stories about withdrawal symptoms. The pharmacist could refute popular myths and offer reassurance but also advised that he would probably need to continue his treatment for a few more months. The pharmacist encouraged him to discuss an exit strategy with his psychiatric team at his next clinic visit, as a reduction in dosage might be the first step to take. The pharmacist recommended some good, credible mental health information websites to Robert to read at his leisure after the consultation.

Reflection on the Expanding Role of the Pharmacist

These vignettes show common and contrasting themes. In both settings, the pharmacist develops a long-term relationship with the adolescent and checks in with them at important milestones regarding their medication. Their goal was to gradually broach different topics in their conversations, sensing when information overload is a danger and tailoring information to different stages of expertise. Both pharmacists used technology to supplement their spoken advice. They also responded to developing and new concerns as the AYA moved through adolescence, when their life context changed. They revisited their advice and education at intervals, recognizing that advancing cognitive development would open up new opportunities to talk to AYA about long-term medication benefit and harm. Both pharmacists recognized that AYA might have concerns about alcohol and sexual health and took a holistic view of health and well-being.

The main contrasts were that the hospital pharmacist was integrated into the multidisciplinary team, working in the same place as other clinicians, able to access medical information, and having their own prescribing rights. The community pharmacist relied more on patient report and had to empower the patient to ask a doctor for further help if medication was needed. The community pharmacist could support Robert indefinitely across the transition period, whereas the hospital pharmacist had to end her relationship with Katie just after the transfer to adult services.

We noted at the beginning of the chapter that some of the roles we would describe would be close to current practice and that some would be more aspirational. Most of the activities taking place in both vignettes are traditional pharmacy roles—ensuring a consistent supply of medication and offering counselling. The more holistic focus on AYASHCN and their concerns, however, is an extension of the pharmacist's skill, and some extra training may be needed. We also recognize that time and workload in the pharmacy environment may not currently allow long consultations with AYASHCN, but we are confident that growing recognition of the investment needed in adolescent health care—and its long-term future benefits for health systems—may help organizations to think differently about their resources. In this way we can realize the triple dividend cited by the Lancet Commission on Adolescent Health and Wellbeing—"benefits for adolescents now, their future adult lives and for their children" [3].

In the hospital-based scenario, there was notable innovation as the pharmacist was teaching injection technique in a multidisciplinary clinic. Hospital-based and community-based pharmacists each have the potential to support AYASHCN and can contribute their medication expertise to the multidisciplinary team in increasingly innovative ways. Recognition of this potential by the specialist multidisciplinary team may result in hitherto underused resources being available to empower and support AYA before, during, and after transition.

In early to mid-adolescence, parents are invaluable partners in medication management, but pharmacists must facilitate independent activities as young adulthood approaches. This includes practical system-dependent activities, such as ordering refills, and consultation-based medication review activities to help AYA to understand how to elicit and consider the benefit and harms of medication in order to be an active decision-maker. We noted earlier in the chapter, for example, that parents were more likely to collect refills than AYA; transition programs should encourage AYA to find an empathetic local pharmacist and start an independent conversation.

Concluding Remarks

Major components of the knowledge and skills framework for AYASHCN during transition from child- to adult-centered services address health and medication management. Pharmacists, whether in hospital or community settings, have the expertise to contribute significantly to this framework. Such expertise needs to be acknowledged and utilized by both their colleagues in multidisciplinary hospital-based teams and the young people themselves. This acknowledgement can be readily integrated into transition planning practices. Core principles of adolescent health, particularly around biopsychosocial development [66] and youth friendly service provision [62], should be included within the core training of pharmacists to enable them to deliver this care to AYASHCN in a developmentally appropriate manner particularly at times of transition, irrespective of setting. By so doing, pharmacists will, alongside their colleagues in multidisciplinary teams, potentially improve health outcomes for the increasing numbers of adolescents and young adults with special healthcare needs.

Acknowledgement The authors would like to thank Dr Heather Schumann, Clinical Pharmacist at Sutter Health in Northern California, for reviewing this chapter.

References

1. Conard LAE, Fortenberry JD, Blythe MJ, Orr DP. Pharmacists' attitudes toward and practices with adolescents. Arch Pediatr Adolesc Med. 2003;157:361–5.
2. Gay CL, Chapuis F, Bendelac N, Tixier F, Treppoz S, Nicolino M. Reinforced follow-up for children and adolescents with type 1 diabetes and inadequate glycaemic control: a randomized controlled trial intervention via the local pharmacist and telecare. Diabetes Metab. 2006;32:159–65.
3. Patton GC, Sawyer SM, Santelli JS, Ross DA, Afifi R, Allen NB, Arora M, Azzopardi P, Baldwin W, Bonell C, Kakuma R. Our future: a lancet commission on adolescent health and wellbeing. Lancet. 2016;387:2423–78.
4. Todd A, Copeland A, Husband A, Kasim A, Bambra C. The positive pharmacy care law: an area-level analysis of the relationship between community pharmacy distribution, urbanity and social deprivation in England. BMJ Open. 2014;4(8):e005764.
5. Gardner J, Oftebro R. Pharmacist partners in the care of children and adolescents. Arch Pediatr Adolesc Med. 2003;157:317–8.
6. Bednarczyk RA, Nadeau JA, Davis CF, McCarthy A, Hussain S, Martiniano R, Lodise T, Zeolla MM, Coles FB, McNutt LA. Privacy in the pharmacy environment: analysis of observations from inside the pharmacy. J Am Pharm Assoc. 2010;50:362–7.
7. Anderson C, Blenkinsopp A, Armstrong M. Feedback from community pharmacy users on the contribution of community pharmacy to improving the public's health: a systematic review of the peer reviewed and non-peer reviewed literature 1990–2002. Health Expect. 2004;7:191–202.
8. Royal Pharmaceutical Society of Great Britain. Community pharmacy: the choice is yours. Access to and usage of community pharmacies—the customer's view. London: RPSGB; 1996.
9. Tilson EC, Sanchez V, Ford CL, Smurzynski M, Leone PA, Fox KK, Irwin K, Miller WC. Barriers to asymptomatic screening and other STD services for adolescents and young adults: focus group discussions. BMC Public Health. 2004;4:21.
10. Anderson C, Blenkinsopp A. Community pharmacy supply of emergency hormonal contraception: a struc-

tured literature review of international evidence. Hum Reprod. 2006;21(1):272–84.
11. Calvert RT. Clinical pharmacy-a hospital perspective. Br J Clin Pharmacol. 1999;47:231–8.
12. Gray NJ, McDonagh JE, Harvey K, Prescott J, Shaw KL, Smith FJ, Stephenson R, Terry D, Fleck K, Roberts R. Arthriting: exploring the relationship between identity and medicines use, and to identify the contribution of medicines and pharmacy services, for the care of young people with arthritis. Final report. PRUK: London; 2013.
13. Gray NJ, Shaw KL, Smith FJ, Burton J, Prescott J, Roberts R, Terry D, McDonagh JE. The role of pharmacists in caring for young people with chronic illness. J Adolesc Health. 2017;60(2):219–25.
14. Hepler CD. Clinical pharmacy, pharmaceutical care, and the quality of drug therapy. Pharmacotherapy. 2004;24(11):1491–8.
15. Gray NJ, Prescott J. Community pharmacists' engagement with young people aged 13–19 years. Int J Pharm Pract. 2013;21(Suppl 2):128.
16. Horsfield E, Kelly F, Sheridan J, Stewart J, Clark T. Could community pharmacies help to improve youth health? Service availability and views of pharmacy personnel in New Zealand. Int J Public Health. 2014;59(5):789–98.
17. Kieckhefer GM, Trahms CM. Supporting development of children with chronic conditions: from compliance toward shared management. Pediatr Nurs. 2000;26:354–63.
18. McDonagh JE. Young people first – juvenile idiopathic arthritis second. Transitional care in rheumatology. Arthritis Care Res. 2008;59:1162–70.
19. Suris JC, Akre C. Key elements for, and indicators of, a successful transition: an international Delphi study. J Adolesc Health. 2015;56(6):612–8.
20. Tong A, Jones J, Craig JC, Singh-Grewal D. Children's experiences of living with juvenile idiopathic arthritis: a thematic synthesis of qualitative studies. Arthritis Care Res. 2012;64(9):1392–404.
21. Fredericks EM, Dore-Stites D, Well A, Magee JC, Freed GL, Shieck V, James Lopez M. Assessment of transition readiness skills and adherence in pediatric liver transplant recipients. Pediatr Transplant. 2010;14(8):944–53.
22. Gray WN, Holbrook E, Morgan PJ, Saeed SA, Denson LA, Hommel KA. Transition readiness skills acquisition in adolescents and young adults with inflammatory bowel disease: findings from integrating assessment into clinical practice. Inflamm Bowel Dis. 2015;21(5):1125–31.
23. Scal P, Horvath K, Garwick A. Preparing for adulthood: healthcare transition counselling for youth with arthritis. Arthritis Rheum. 2009;30:52–7.
24. McDonagh JE, Shaw KL, Stephenson R, Gray NJ. Are they ready and do we know they are ready? Documentation of medicine management tasks in an adolescent rheumatology clinic. Rheumatology. 2014;53(Suppl 3):iii10.
25. Brodie DC, Parish PA, Poston JW. Societal needs for drugs and drug related services. Am J Pharm Educ. 1980;44:276–8.
26. Hepler CD, Strand LM. Opportunities and responsibilities in pharmaceutical care. Am J Pharm Educ. 1989;53(suppl):S7–15.
27. Lugasi T, Achille M, Stevenson M. Patients' perspective on factors that facilitate transition from child-centered to adult-centered health care: a theory integrated metasummary of quantitative and qualitative studies. J Adolesc Health. 2011;48(5):429–40.
28. Hait E, Arnold JH, Fishman LN. Educate, communicate, anticipate-practical recommendations for transitioning adolescents with IBD to adult health care. Inflamm Bowel Dis. 2006;12(1):70–3.
29. Stinson J, Kohut SA, Spiegel L, White M, Gill N, Colbourne G, Sigurdson S, Duffy KW, Tucker L, Stringer E, Hazel B, Hochman J, Reiss J, Kaufman M. A systematic review of transition readiness and transfer satisfaction measures for adolescents with chronic illness. Int J Adolesc Med Health. 2014;26(2):159–74.
30. Gilleland J, Amaral S, Mee L, Blount R. Getting ready to leave: transition readiness in adolescent kidney transplant recipients. J Pediatr Psychol. 2012;37(1):85–96.
31. Klassen AF, Grant C, Barr R, Brill H, Kraus de Camargo O, Ronen GM, Samaan MC, Mondal T, Cano SJ, Schlatman A, Tsangaris E. Development and validation of a generic scale for use in transition programmes to measure self-management skills in adolescents with chronic health conditions: the TRANSITION-Q. Child Care Health Dev. 2015;41(4):547–58.
32. Sawicki GS, Lukens-Bull K, Yin X, Demars N, Huang IC, Livingood W, Reiss J, Wood D. Measuring the transition readiness of youth with special healthcare needs: validation of the TRAQ—transition readiness assessment questionnaire. J Pediatr Psychol. 2011;36(2):160–71. https://doi.org/10.1093/jpepsy/jsp128.
33. Ferris ME, Harward DH, Bickford K, Layton JB, Ferris MT, Hogan SL, Gipson DS, McCoy LP, Hooper SR. A clinical tool to measure the components of health-care transition from pediatric care to adult care: the UNC TRxANSITION scale. Ren Fail. 2012;34(6):744–53.
34. Williams TS, Sherman EMS, Mah JK, Blackman M, Latter J, Mohammed I, Slick DJ, Thornton N. Measurement of medical self-management and transition readiness among Canadian adolescents with special health care needs. Int J Child Adolesc Health. 2010;3:1–9.
35. Fair C, Cuttance J, Sharma N, et al. International and interdisciplinary identification of health care transition outcomes. JAMA Pediatr. 2016;170(3):205–11.
36. Gray NJ, McDonagh JE, Barker C, Burton J, Campbell R, Prescott J, Shaw KL, Smith FJ, Terry D. Exploring the perceived and potential medicines optimisation role of pharmacy for young people with long-term conditions, through the case study of juvenile arthritis. Final report. PRUK: London; 2016.
37. Wytiaz RM, Lee HM, Odukoya OK. Smart phone apps: an innovative approach to improving Pediatric medication adherence. Innov Pharm. 2015;6(4):4.
38. Staples B, Bravender T. Drug compliance in adolescents. Pediatr Drugs. 2002;4(8):503–13.

39. Costello I, Wong IC, Nunn AJ. A literature review to identify interventions to improve the use of medicines in children. Child Care Health Dev. 2004;30(6):647–65.
40. McGrady ME, Ryan JL, Gutiérrez-Colina AM, Fredericks EM, Towner EK, Pai AL. The impact of effective paediatric adherence promotion interventions: systematic review and meta-analysis. Child Care Health Dev. 2015;41(6):789–802.
41. Hanghøj S, Boisen KA. Self-reported barriers to medication adherence among chronically ill adolescents: a systematic review. J Adolesc Health. 2014;54(2):121–38.
42. Koster ES, Philbert D, de Vries TW, van Dijk L, Bouvy ML. "I just forget to take it": asthma self-management needs and preferences in adolescents. J Asthma. 2015;52(8):831–7.
43. Dean AJ, Walters J, Hall A. A systematic review of interventions to enhance medication adherence in children and adolescents with chronic illness. Arch Dis Child. 2010;95(9):717–23.
44. Prestidge C, Romann A, Djurdjev O, Matsuda-Abedini M. Utility and cost of a renal transplant transition clinic. Pediatr Nephrol. 2012;27(2):295–302.
45. Gray NJ, Gardner H, Cantrill JA, Noyce PR. Mummy will make it better: influence on the product choices of young adults in the UK when buying over-the-counter medicines. Int J Customer Relationship Manage. 2000;1:79–86.
46. Adamou M, Bowers S. Dose of methylphenidate during service transition for adults with ADHD. Ther Adv Psychopharmacol. 2011;1(3):71–5.
47. Bynum A, Hopkins D, Thomas A, Copeland N, Irwin C. The effect of telepharmacy counseling on metered-dose inhaler technique among adolescents with asthma in rural Arkansas. Telemed J E Health. 2001;7(3):207–17.
48. Shah S, Taylor S, Kritikos V, Bosnic-Anticevich SZ, Saini B, Krass I, Armour C. Innovative asthma health promotion by rural community pharmacists: a feasibility study. Health Promot J Austr. 2005;16(1):69.
49. Ducharme FM, Zemek RL, Chalut D, McGillivray D, Noya FJ, Resendes S, Khomenko L, Rouleau R, Zhang X. Written action plan in pediatric emergency room improves asthma prescribing, adherence, and control. Am J Respir Crit Care Med. 2011;183(2):195–203.
50. Hollis R, Morgan S. The adolescent with cancer—at the edge of no-man's land. Lancet Oncol. 2001;2(1):43–8.
51. Hord J, Feig S, Crouch G, Hale G, Mueller B, Rogers Z, Shearer P, Werner E. Standards for pediatric cancer centers. Pediatrics. 2014;134(2):410–4.
52. Moceri P, Goossens E, Hascoet S, Checler C, Bonello B, Ferrari E, Acar P, Fraisse A. From adolescents to adults with congenital heart disease: the role of transition. Eur J Pediatr. 2015;174(7):847–54.
53. Jurasek L, Ray L, Quigley D. Development and implementation of an adolescent epilepsy transition clinic. J Neurosci Nurs. 2010;42(4):181–9.
54. Wiener L, Battles H, Ryder C, Zobel M. Transition from a pediatric HIV intramural clinical research program to adolescent and adult community-based care services: assessing transition readiness. Soc Work Health Care. 2007;46(1):1–9.
55. Tulloch O, Theobald S, Ananworanich J, Chasombat S, Kosalaraksa P, Jirawattanapisal T, Lakonphon S, Lumbiganon P, Taegtmeyer M. From transmission to transition: lessons learnt from the Thai paediatric antiretroviral programme. PLoS One. 2014;9(6): e99061.
56. Campbell T, Beer H, Wilkins R, Sherlock E, Merrett A, Griffiths J. "I look forward. I feel insecure but I am ok with it". The experience of young HIV+ people attending transition preparation events: a qualitative investigation. AIDS Care. 2010;22(2):263–9.
57. Fishman LN, Barendse RM, Hait E, Burdick C, Arnold J. Self-management of older adolescents with inflammatory bowel disease: a pilot study of behavior and knowledge as prelude to transition. Clin Pediatr. 2010;49(12):1129–33.
58. Lawson EF, Hersh AO, Applebaum MA, Yelin EH, Okumura MJ, von Scheven E. Self-management skills in adolescents with chronic rheumatic disease: a cross-sectional survey. Pediatr Rheumatol Online J. 2011;9(1):35.
59. Hilderson D, Moons P, Van der Elst K, Luyckx K, Wouters C, Westhovens R. The clinical impact of a brief transition programme for young people with juvenile idiopathic arthritis: results of the DON'T RETARD project. Rheumatology. 2016;55(1):133–42.
60. Jabbal R. Pharmacist prescribing: improving access to care in mental health. [commentary]. J Can Acad Child Adolesc Psychiatry. 2010;19(1):3.
61. Cerns S, McCracken C, Rich C. Optimizing adolescent transition to adult care for sickle cell disease. Medsurg Nurs. 2013;22(4):255.
62. Ambresin AE, Bennett K, Patton GC, Sanci LA, Sawyer SM. Assessment of youth-friendly health care: a systematic review of indicators drawn from young people's perspectives. J Adolesc Health. 2013;52(6):670–81.
63. Hargreaves DS, McDonagh JE, Viner RM. Validation of You're welcome quality criteria for adolescent health services using data from national inpatient surveys in England. J Adolesc Health. 2013;52(1):50–7.
64. Alsaleh F, Smith FJ, Rigby E, Gray NJ. Applying the 'You're welcome' youth-friendly service criteria to community pharmacy in the UK. J Pharm Health Serv Res. 2016;7(1):71–9.
65. Singh SP, Tuomainen H. Transition from child to adult mental health services: needs, barriers, experiences and new models of care. World Psychiatry. 2015;14(3):358–61.
66. Bennett D, MacKenzie RG. Normal psychosocial development in adolescence. In: Steinbeck K, Kohn M, editors. A clinical handbook in adolescent medicine: a guide for health professionals who work with adolescents and young adults. Singapore: World Scientific; 2013. p. 27–40.

Legal Issues: Guardianship and Supportive Decision Making

30

Beth Sufian, James Passamano, and Amy Sopchak

Guardianship

General Nature of Guardianship

Guardianship of an adult is sometimes necessary to assist an adult who has become unable to care for himself or unable to manage his financial matters. An adult, regardless of the extent of his illness or injury, is presumed by the law to be competent to make decisions and has the right to exercise his decision-making authority regarding his person, money and property. The law protects an individual's right to exercise decision-making authority until a court finds evidence of incapacity and creates a guardianship over the person, his property or both.

Disclaimer
The following information is general in nature and is not meant to be legal advice regarding a specific situation. Nothing in this chapter should be considered as legal advice regarding a specific individual's situation. The Law changes frequently and the information in this chapter may have changed between the time it was drafted and the time the chapter was published. Please consult with an attorney for specific advice regarding your situation.

B. Sufian, J.D. (✉) • J. Passamano, J.D.
A. Sopchak, J.D.
Sufian and Passamano, LLP, Houston, TX, USA
e-mail: bsufian@sufianpassamano.com; jpassamano@sufianpassamano.com; asopchak@sufianpassamano.com

Guardianship fundamentally alters an individual's basic decision-making authority. In a guardianship, the authority to make decisions is removed from the disabled person, who is usually called a "Ward." The decision-making authority is reassigned to another person, who is called the "guardian" or the "conservator".[1]

Types of Guardianship

A guardianship may be a guardianship of the person or a guardian of the estate. These may be either full or partial guardianships, and may be either permanent or temporary.[2]

Guardianship of the Person

A guardianship of the person is a form of guardianship that grants to the guardian the authority to make personal decisions regarding the Ward, but not the authority to make decisions about the person's property. In a full guardianship of the person, the Guardian is granted authority over all aspects of the Ward's personal life, including medical and psychiatric care, where the Ward lives, with whom the Ward may associate, where and when the Ward may travel, the personal privileges the Ward may exercise (such using a cell

[1] Tex Estates Code Ann. § 1001.001 (2016).
[2] Tex Estates Code Ann. § 1002.012 (2016).

A. C. Hergenroeder, C. M. Wiemann (eds.), *Health Care Transition*,
https://doi.org/10.1007/978-3-319-72868-1_30

phone, accessing the internet, driving a car, voting, marrying, etc.), and all other aspects of the Wards' personal life.

A guardianship of the person need not be a full guardianship. A guardianship of the person may be only a partial guardianship of the person. In a partial guardianship of the person, the court may specify the particular decision-making authority given to the guardian and the guardian's authority to make decisions is limited to the authority specified by the court. Usually, when an individual retains some capacity to make personal choices, the guardian of the person makes major decisions about living arrangements, medical care, psychiatric care and other major personal decisions, but leaves minor personal decisions to the individual.

Guardianship of the Estate

A guardian of the estate is a form of guardianship that grants the guardian decision-making authority over the disabled person's money, property and other financial matters. A guardian of the estate is typically responsible for paying bills from the Ward's resources, managing the Ward's money and assets, investing the Ward's money, buying and selling property, and making other decisions related to the Ward's property interests.

A guardian of the estate may be a full guardianship, encompassing all aspects of an individual's money and property. A guardian of the estate may also be limited with the guardian authorized to exercise decision-making authority only over particular assets, such as an investment account or bank account. In a limited guardian of the estate, any power not granted to the guardian is retained by the Ward. The Ward continues to have decision-making capacity for any financial decision that is not specifically granted to the guardian during the guardianship.[3]

Duration of Guardianship

Most Guardianships are established when a disabled individual has a permanent or degenerative impairment that limits his ability to make decisions on his own. Once a guardianship is established by a court, it remains effective until the court modifies or terminates the guardianship.

In some states, guardianships must be renewed with evidence of an on-going disability. If not renewed, then the guardianship is allowed to expire. Because guardianship is a matter of state law, each state has its own rules governing when a guardianship will lapse or expire.

Occasionally, the condition or circumstances that justify establishing a guardianship are temporary in nature. In such cases, the court may establish a temporary guardianship that exists for a specified duration or expires at a particular event. A temporary guardianship may be extended if evidence shows that the reasons for the guardianship persist.[4]

Guardianship Legal Process

When Guardianship Is Appropriate

Generally, guardianship is appropriate when a person is substantially unable to manage his personal or financial affairs because of a physical or mental impairment. Guardianship is a matter of state law and each state has its own formulation of when a guardianship is appropriate and what evidence is required to show that an individual cannot manage his own affairs. However, the evidence necessary to create a guardianship requires more than merely evidence that the person has a diagnosis of a physical or mental impairment. Guardianship also requires more than just evidence that the person engages in foolish behaviors or makes bad decisions. The evidence must show that the individual lacks the capacity to make sound judgments regarding his person, his property or both. However, guardianship is not an appropriate means of solving all problems. Guardianship cannot change the behavior or attitudes of the Ward. A guardian cannot force a Ward to take medications. Because guardianship alters an individual's

[3] Tex Estates Code Ann. §§ 1101.151–1101.152; 1151.001(2016).

[4] Tex Estates Code Ann. § 1202.001 (2016).

authority to make decisions about himself and his property it can only be accomplished through a court proceeding.

Creating a Guardianship

Requires Action by a Court

Guardianship is an involved legal process that typically requires the services of an attorney, both for the person seeking to establish the guardianship and for the Ward—especially when the Ward does not voluntarily give up his decision-making authority. A family may attempt to represent themselves in a guardianship proceeding, but it is a complex area of law with many subtleties. A family is more likely to achieve its desired result with the assistance of an experienced lawyer.

Some law schools may have legal programs that offer representation at no cost to those in need of guardianship. Some local or state Bar Associations may have programs that offer free legal assistance with guardianship proceedings.

Evidence About the Individual's Condition and Circumstances

Guardianship proceedings require the proposed guardian and Ward to appear in court and provide testimony and other evidence stating the reasons that a guardianship is appropriate under the circumstances.

The court will also require medical evidence from a physician who has examined the disabled person and who is able to certify that the person has a physical or mental impairment and can testify about how that impairment affects the person's ability to care for himself, make personal decisions, and manage his property. The physician may be required to provide a specific assessment of the individual's capabilities, including whether the person can make decisions, vote, drive an automobile, marry or make other decisions regarding themselves. The specific facts about which a physician must testify in a guardianship proceeding depend on state law.[5]

Appointment of a Guardian

If the court determines that a guardianship is appropriate, it will appoint a person to act as the guardian for the ward. The guardian can be a family member, an unrelated person, or even a public agency or private institution. Any person serving as a guardian must affirmatively accept the appointment, be qualified under law, and themselves be capable of performing the duties of a guardian. Naturally, a parent or other family relation serving as a guardian is most common, but others can serve as a guardian as well.[6]

Duties of a Guardian

In addition to making decisions and managing the affairs of his ward, a guardian is obliged to perform administrative functions. Because the court that creates a guardianship retains continuing supervisory authority, the guardian must periodically report to the court the status of the Ward and provide an accounting of personal income, assets, expenses and any other information required by the court. Also, some actions by the guardian require prior approval by the court.[7]

Time Line for Guardianship Decisions

Decisions about pursuing guardianship do not have to made before a person turns 18 years of age. Before the age of 18, the parent or legal guardian can make decisions for the child. Once a child turns 18 years of age the law assumes the young adult is able to make his own decisions. Some parents may want to gather information about guardianship prior to their child reaching the age of 18. However, the guardianship process cannot start until after the child has reached the age of 18. There is no time limit for filing for guardianship. There is no requirement that guard-

[5]Tex Estates Code Ann. §§ 1101.101, 1101.103 (2016).
[6]*See generally* Tex Estates Code Ann. Ch. 1104.
[7]Tex Estates Code Ann. §§ 1151.051, 1151.101 (2016).

ianship proceedings start right after the 18th birthday. Many years can pass and if guardianship is necessary later there is no problem with starting proceedings at the time of need.

Some parents who have a child who is severely limited in his ability to make decisions due to an intellectual disability may want to initiate guardianship proceedings shortly after the child turns 18 years of age. Often the parents are best positioned to be the young adult's guardian.

Some hospitals may make it difficult for the parents to make medical decisions without proof of guardianship. However, other hospitals and medical practices may allow the parent to make medical decisions as the young adult's surrogate without a guardianship. When the young adult is transitioning to a new medical practice for care it is important to ask the medial team if guardianship is necessary for the parent to make medical decisions for the young adult who is transitioning.

A young adult who has a disability and is able to make decisions for himself does not need a guardianship simply because he has a disability. The decision of whether a guardianship is necessary is mainly driven by the young adult's inability to make decisions and the possibility healthcare providers will require a guardianship in order to allow the parent to make medical decisions for the young adult. However, less restrictive alternatives to guardianship are available and should also be considered by the young adult and his family members. The medial team should become familiar with these less restrictive alternatives.

Alternatives to Guardianship

Guardianship is a substantial restriction on an individual's independence and self-determination and so some advocates advise establishing a guardianship only when there is not a less restrictive option. There is research that shows guardianship can cause some people to feel helpless, hopeless and more self-critical. Consequently, some disability advocates suggest that alternatives to guardianship should be considered and understood before guardianship is pursued. Individuals with disabilities have different needs. While guardianship may be appropriate for some people a less restrictive arrangement may be better for others.

Several alternatives to guardianship are appropriate when an individual merely needs assistance and support in exercising his own decision-making capacity.[8]

Power of Attorney

Medical Power of Attorney

A medical Power of attorney is an assignment of decision-making authority from the disabled person to another person. The assignment must occur when the person making the assignment has the capacity to make decisions, and cannot be made after the disabled person becomes incapacitated. Typically, a medical Power of attorney is granted to a spouse, parent or other trusted person.

The person assigning the power to make medical decisions is called the "principal" and the person who is making the decisions is called the "agent." Under a medical power of attorney, the agent has the authority to make medical decisions for the principal after the principal becomes incapacitated and unable to make decisions for himself. A medical power of attorney becomes effective when signed by the principal, delivered to the agent, and accepted by the agent. The medical power of attorney continues to be effective until it is revoked or when it expires at a time stated in the document. The agent's authority to make medical decisions for the principal begins when the principal's attending physician certifies in writing that the principal is unable to make healthcare decisions on his own.

A medical power of attorney has several limitations. First, a medical power of attorney can only be executed when the principal is competent to make decisions. A medical power of attorney cannot be established at a time when the principal is incapacitated, incompetent or otherwise inca-

[8] Tex Estates Code Ann. § 1002.0015 (2016).

pable of making decisions. Also, the principal can object to healthcare decisions made by the agent even after he is certified to be incompetent. No treatment may be given or withheld over the objection of the principal, even when a valid medical power of attorney is in place.

Furthermore, an agent exercising a medical power of attorney may not consent to certain medical procedures, such as commitment to a mental health facility, convulsive therapy, psycho-surgery, abortion or withholding comfort care.[9]

Durable Power of Attorney

A durable power of attorney, like a medical power of attorney, is a principal's assignment to an agent of the authority to make decisions. However, a durable power of attorney is limited to the assignment of decision-making authority regarding money, assets and property. Durable powers of attorney are very flexible. Durable powers of attorney can grant some powers to the agent, while the principal retains all others. A power of attorney can be limited to specific actions, such as managing property, maintaining a bank account, or managing other financial accounts.

A durable power of attorney may either be effective immediately upon execution, even if the principal retains competency to act for himself. A durable power of attorney may be arranged such that the agent only has the power to act on behalf of the principal after the principal becomes incapacitated and unable to act for himself.[10]

Representative Payee

Another alternative to guardianship may be a representative payee who has authority to handle the Social Security benefits a person receives based on his disability. A representative payee is a person appointed to receive and manage a person's Social Security Disability Insurance (SSDI) benefits or Supplemental Security Income (SSI) benefits for anyone who cannot manage or direct the management of the benefits by himself. A medical provider must submit evidence and paperwork to Social Security that supports a finding the person who receives Social Security benefits is not able to manage his Social Security benefit. It is often difficult to remove the representative payee so the decision to appoint a representative payee should be made after careful consideration. The representative payee should be trustworthy and act in the best interest of the young adult with a disability.

A representative payee's duties are to use the Social Security benefits to pay for the current and future needs of the Social Security beneficiary, and properly save any benefits not needed to meet current needs according to the asset rules set out by Social Security. In 2017 individuals who receive SSI benefits can only have $2000 in assets if the person is single. The representative payee should make sure he understands the SSI rules regarding assets. If the representative payee saves too much money for the young adult the young adult will lose his SSI benefits and his Medicaid benefits.

A representative payee must also keep records of expenses. The Social Security Administration can (and frequently does) request representative payees provide an accounting of how he used or saved the Social Security benefits. If a person only needs help managing his Social Security benefits but is able to make other decisions related to his daily living and healthcare decisions, having a Social Security representative payee who handles the Social Security benefits is a good option.

Shared Decision-Making Authority[11]

Supportive Decision Making Agreements

Supportive decision making agreements are an alternative to guardianship. The Texas Legislature was the first state to enact a Supportive Decision Making statute in 2015. The Supportive Decision Making statute creates a process for supporting and accommodating an adult with a disability and is intended to enable the adult to make life decisions without impeding his self-determination. The purpose of supportive deci-

[9] Tex Health & Safety Code Ann. § 166.152 (2016).

[10] *See generally* Tex Estates Code Ann. Ch. 751 (2016).

[11] *See generally* Tex Estates Code Ann. Ch. 1357 (2016).

sion making agreements is to provide assistance to a disabled adult in making decisions about where to live, what services and medical care to receive, where to work and other decisions, while at the same time preserving the individuals independence.

Who Is Involved in a Supportive Decision Making Agreement

Supported Individual

Supportive Decision Making Agreements are appropriate for any individual 18 years of age or older with a disability. For the purpose of supportive decision making agreements, "disability" is broadly defined as any physical or mental impairment that substantially limits a major life activity. However, the disabled individual must still have sufficient mental capacity to agree to a supportive decision making agreement. If the individual with a disability lacks decision making capacity, then he lacks the capacity to form a supportive decision making agreement and a supportive decision making agreement would not be appropriate.

Supporter

The law does not place any restrictions on who may become a supporter. Obviously, the supporter must be someone who the individual with a disability trusts and who is willing to assume the obligations of a supporter described in the agreement. Typically, the supporter is a family member or trusted friend.

The supporter's role is to assist the adult with a disability in understanding options, responsibilities and consequences of the decision he is making. The supporter also helps the disabled person in accessing, obtaining, understanding and using information relevant to the decision, such as medical records, mental health records, financial information, educational records and other information. The supporter also has an important role in aiding communications with third parties about the disabled person's decisions.

Duty of Confidentiality

Because the supporter will have access to private information, the statute imposes on the supporter a duty to keep information confidential and keep it safe from any unauthorized access, use or disclosure. Also, a supportive decision-making agreement creates a confidential relationship between the supporter and the disabled adult. Consequently, a supporter may be liable to the disabled individual for the breach of the confidential relationship.

Contents of a Supportive Decision-Making Agreement

The form of a supportive decision-making agreement is flexible. The statute provides a sample agreement, but no particular form is required. Any form of agreement will be sufficient provided the document substantially complies with the statute.

To be effective, the parties must voluntarily sign the agreement either in the presence of two witnesses who are 14 years of age or older, or under oath before a notary public.

Duration of Supportive Decision-Making Agreements

Because a supportive decision-making agreement is essentially an at will contract, it can be terminated whenever the adult with a disability or the supporter elect to do so. A supportive decision-making agreement may also specify when it will terminate. Agreements may also be terminated if the adult with a disability has been abused, neglected or exploited by the supporter.

Supportive Decision-Making Agreements Do Not Preclude the Use of Other Alternatives to Guardianship

A supportive decision-making agreement can be used in conjunction with other alternatives to guardianships, such as a medical power of attorney or Social Security representative payee.

Supportive Decision Making Agreement Compared to Guardianship and Compared to Power of Attorney

Comparison to Guardianship

A supportive decision making agreement is different from guardianship because it is a voluntary arrangement between the disabled person and his supporter. It does not require court approval nor on-going court supervision like a guardianship.

The scope of a supportive decision making agreement is flexible and is determined by the adult with a disability. The adult decides what support is needed and the supporter agrees to provide assistance only regarding those matters.

Comparison to Power of Attorney

Like a power of attorney, a supportive decision making agreement is informal and does not require a court proceeding. Unlike a power of attorney, the disabled adult does not assign his ability to make decisions to someone else. Rather, the disabled adult retains decision making authority. The person named in the supportive decision making agreement does not make decisions for the disabled person, but provides substantial assistance in making decisions.

Fiduciary Duties

A significant difference between a supportive decision making agreement and guardianship or a power of attorney is that the supporter is not a fiduciary of the disabled adult.

Guardianships and powers of attorney involve a fiduciary relationship. By law, a fiduciary duty exists between a guardian and a ward in a guardianship, and between a principal and an agent in a power of attorney relationship. A fiduciary has the duty to act in good faith, with loyalty and without conflicts of interest. A supportive decision-making agreement does not create a fiduciary relationship and therefore the supporter does not owe a duty of good faith and loyalty to the disabled adult.

Preference for Supportive Decision Making Agreement or Power of Attorney

There are some advocates who do not think guardianship is appropriate for anyone with a disability. These advocates are strong proponents of supportive decision making agreements. Since there is no need to hire an attorney or have a court proceeding when entering into a supportive decision making agreement this can be a good option for those who cannot afford to hire legal counsel and cannot find low or no cost representation.

Options Available

There are some in the medical and legal profession who may indicate that people with certain cognitive limitations must have a guardianship and cannot use supportive decision making agreements or powers of attorney. However, many in the disability community argue that anyone can use a supportive decision making agreement or power of attorney. For example, some may say that a person who cannot speak must have a guardianship. However, this is not true as long as the person has some ability to make decisions and communicate those decisions. Some individuals with significant cognitive disabilities are still able to make some decisions for themselves and these individuals may be best served with supportive decision making instead of guardianship.

People with disabilities, their family members and healthcare providers should be informed and understand the different options available to them and chose the best option.

Footnotes

Please note Guardianship and Shared Decision Making Statuses are governed by state law. The Footnotes for this Chapter refer to Texas State law. The Guardianship laws and Shared Decision Making law in Texas are similar to laws in other states. However, there may be some variation among state law in this area.

31 Transitioning Adolescents and Young Adults with Medical Complexity

Mary R. Ciccarelli

Introduction

Children with medical complexity (CMC) are a small subset of the population of children who must age from pediatric to adult systems of care. Children with special healthcare needs (CSHCN) account for 18% of the pediatric population; CMC are estimated to account for 0.5–1% of children. While there is no clear definition of CMC, four cardinal domains have been proposed by the Children's Hospital Association to characterize this population, including chronic, severe health conditions, substantial health service needs, major functional limitations, and high health resource utilization [1]. An analysis from 2005 through 2007 identified 0.67% of children in Ontario, Canada, who were identified as CMC; of these, 65.6% had single-organ chronic conditions, 6.7% had multi-organ conditions, 27.6% had neurologic impairment, and 11.8% were technology dependent [2]. The Canadian Provincial Council for Maternal Child Health convened a Transition to Adult Healthcare Services Work Group in February 2012. Along with recommendations for all children, they identified a subgroup of youth requiring a more intense approach to transition, perhaps even a lifelong approach. This group included youth who are medically fragile, those with very rare conditions for which there is not a readily identified adult provider, and those with serious mental illness [3]. This chapter will therefore focus specifically on complex transition of care to include youth with rare or multiple chronic conditions, with significant neurocognitive and/or mental health impairments and/or technology dependence.

M. R. Ciccarelli, M.D.
Indiana University School of Medicine, Indianapolis, IN, USA
e-mail: mciccare@iupui.edu

Defining the Care of Children with Medical Complexity

The CMC from the Ontario analysis saw a median of 13 outpatient physicians and 6 distinct subspecialists. Their healthcare costs accounted for almost one-third of child health spending. Thirty-six percent received home care services. Their 30-day readmission rates spanned 12.6–23.7%. The care of these children has been described by primary care providers to require many layers of additional clinical work, such as polypharmacy, medical devices, rare and/or unfamiliar diagnoses, and a large number of specialists [4]. Hospitalists similarly report that CMC have intensive hospital- and/or community-based service needs, including polypharmacy, technology, and/or home care, and are at risk for frequent and/or prolonged hospitalizations [5].

A. C. Hergenroeder, C. M. Wiemann (eds.), *Health Care Transition*,
https://doi.org/10.1007/978-3-319-72868-1_31

In 2012, the Lucile Packard Foundation described the stages of adjustment experienced by children and families living with chronic conditions: (1) pre-diagnosis, (2) crisis diagnosis and treatment, (3) reentry, (4) "new normal" maintenance and complications, (5) preparation for transition, and (6) "hitting the transition wall" [6]. This transition wall can be described as the series of barriers which block the transfer and receipt of continuous and comprehensive care to meet anticipated adult needs. Well-planned preparation for transition should be designed to alleviate the proverbial hitting of a wall. Pre-transition, the families of CMC continue to experience concerns about poorly informed decision-making, poor information, fragmented and uncoordinated health management, reactive rather than proactive care management, over-medicalization, and inadequate caregiver support [1]. There are often mismatches in the child/youth's needs and the availability or access to resources that are amplified as the CMC prepares to move to adult services. Gaps between needs and available resources are often magnified by situations where families function less effectively as their own advocates. Cultural, environmental, and psychological factors can impact self-advocacy skills. Those who tend to act more submissively or compliant in their clinician-family partnership may be unlikely to speak up and ask for more [6]. When a comprehensive needs assessment is systematically performed for individuals with disabilities, unmet needs are commonly identified [7]. Fragmentations in care and limitations in self-advocacy both contribute to these unmet needs.

Key Policies Around Transition

Policies for CMC transition should employ basic requirements for the transition of all youth and supplement these with the specific needs related to complex medical care. Transition, as a core outcome for CSHCN defined by the Maternal and Child Health Bureau (MCHB), sets the expectation that youth receive the services necessary to make transitions to all aspects of adult life, in order to participate in adult healthcare, work, and experience the independence of adult life. MCHB measures success in healthcare transition (HCT) as having health insurance, a usual source or provider of adult healthcare, receiving preventive services, and having no delayed or unmet healthcare needs [8]. These goals are germane for CMC with the addition of transition goals to (1) maximize current function and (2) provide proactive rather than reactive care in order to prevent or reduce the impact of secondary conditions [9, 10]. The Institute of Medicine's 2007 report, "The Future of Disability in America," focused on the transition of young people with disabilities from pediatric to adult healthcare services [11]. This report highlighted that successful healthcare transitions for young people with serious disabilities depend on public policies to support access to health insurance, assistive technologies, personal care services, housing, vocational training, and/or postsecondary education and income support, as well as public policies that support nondiscrimination in employment and the physical accessibility of transportation and public spaces. Some of these services are within the scope of clinical medicine, while others require collaboration across other agencies and organizations.

Concepts in Chronic Condition Management

In 1996, Wagner already proposed that successful models of care for those with chronic conditions share common features, including (1) the use of explicit plans and protocols; (2) the reorganization of practices to meet the needs of patients who require more time, a broader array of services, and closer follow-up; (3) systematic attention to patient information needs and behavioral changes; (4) ready access to necessary expertise; and (5) supportive information systems [12]. The IOM report recommended that improvements in the transition of youth with disabilities into adult healthcare systems would require support for coordinated care, transition planning, and use of integrated electronic medical records and would also benefit from an expansion of chronic care training in pediatric and adult medicine residencies [11].

Care Coordination

The processes needed to facilitate a proactive, organized transition from pediatric to adult health systems appropriate for CMC should promote self-navigation across the system by the activated young adult or his/her caregivers, with additional supports from health systems or community organizations to complement the patient and family's strengths and weaknesses. These additional transition needs can be provided as a specific type of care coordination, in which the patient's complex care activities are deliberately organized between participants (including the patient). Complex, high-utilizing patients require more than health system navigation information and healthcare utilization oversight as found in the services sometimes available through payer and institutional navigators or care managers. Effectively organizing care involves the marshalling of personnel and resources to carry out the required patient care along with the exchange of valuable information to the participating team [13]. Care coordination for children with developmental disabilities has demonstrated shorter hospitalization average lengths of stay and lower hospital charges [14]. Care coordinators best suited to CMC transition services have experience and/or training in the specific skills commonly required. These include an understanding of healthcare financing (particularly Medicaid programs for individuals with disabilities), a familiarity with the variations in the scope of practice across pediatric and adult specialists and systems of care, and a versatility with community-based disability organizations and their availability to support patients and families. Legal supports are also often needed to ascertain decision-making capacity and the level of support which may be needed as the youth grows to the age of majority. Paratransit transportation system access, home equipment and home care services, and sources of caregiver respite and support are all integral to the function and well-being of CMC and their families. With this broad array of necessary skills, transition coordinators for CMC need a combination of nursing and social work skills [15]. In addition, clinical input into complex treatment plans may require a higher level of clinician support as has been described in the Indiana transition programs and other projects for CMC, such as the Milwaukee program [15, 16]. The U Special Kids in Minnesota and Special Care Clinic in Colorado programs utilize nurses, pediatric nurse practitioners, social workers, secretaries, and pediatricians who collaborate with specialists [17, 18].

Shared Plans of Care

A document commonly referred to as the shared plan of care guides the patient and caregiver with a clear point of contact to the health system and promotes sharing of critical information across the care team. By principle, it should be a comprehensive, integrated, concise, and user-friendly summary of relevant information. It should facilitate a better shared overview and agreement of the patient's needs and treatment to all of the engaged providers within the home and the healthcare system and thereby help to avoid errors, gaps, and duplication in services. The medical summary component details young adult/family demographics, care team members and contacts, current medical treatments, and a synthesized concise historical summary. The plan contains negotiated actions which are the steps that need to next be taken to move forward in reaching desired personal and clinical goals and are ideally described with planning of desired timelines and identified responsibilities and accountabilities [19]. U Special Kids distributes its final document to the patient, decision-maker, group home agency, residential supervisor, hospital ward, emergency department, and medical home team [17].

Protective Factors and Unique Challenges for Transition in Children with Medical Complexity

Once the preliminary steps of developing the team of professionals to lead and deliver medically complex transition services have been identified and a method for creation and delivery of a shared plan of care has been created, the specific tasks of tracking, assessing, and planning transition may be addressed. Got Transition recommends that tracking start at age 13–14 years. Assessments and planning need to consider the routine needs of all youth moving toward adult life and then account for the specific protective and risky situations that accompany CMC.

There are a larger number of issues that make transition for CMC more complex and less safe than the HCT of youth with less complex chronic conditions, but there are also a few protectors. Table 31.1 identifies both the risks and protective factors to the transition of youth with medical complexity to guide our further discussion.

The majority of young adults aged 21–25 with disabilities live with their families, rather than independently; 16% of those with multiple disabilities and 17% of those with autism live independently [20]. Residing in the same home as caregivers is a potential benefit when the home has been accommodated to fit the person's disability needs and caregivers are familiar with the person's needs and trained in their care. Caregivers can help mitigate gaps in care and suboptimal treatment adherence associated with increased morbidity, long-term complications, hospitalizations, and need for urgent interventions. One of the most significant risk factors for gaps at transfer is having missed appointments while still in pediatric care [21]. Residing with parents also creates opportunity for ongoing oversight of medication administration; parental supervision is a significant protective factor for treatment adherence in teens [22]. Although one-third of U.S. young adults aged 19–26 were uninsured in 2006 [23], youth with disabilities are likely to have sustained insurance eligibility through multiple possible avenues and are not at the same risk to experience the gaps in insurance that occur more often in young adults without disabilities. In addition to Medicaid disability program eligibility, young adults may also be eligible for sustained coverage as disabled dependents through parents' employer coverage. Dependents who receive Social Security Disability Income through a retired, disabled, or deceased parent can also become eligible for Medicare.

In order to retain young adults with CMC successfully in their family homes, as is desired by most families, it is necessary to provide for needed community, family, and financial resources and address means to ease the emotional burden of the family [24].

Table 31.1 Protective factors and unique challenges associated with HCT for individuals with medical complexity

Protective factors
• Continuity of prepared caregivers • Continuity of living setting • Continuity of insurance coverage through disability programs
Unique challenges
• Adjustment of existing pediatric care plan for new adult status • Decision-making supports and best interest of the person • Creation of care team with prepared adult providers • Inpatient/outpatient service accommodations • Home and community adaptations and supports • Caregiver needs in training and respite • Special billing and coding issues

Unique Challenges Associated with Medical Complexity

Changes Related to Adult Status

As youth age and grow and their bodies achieve physical adult maturation, one of the first preparations for adult care is to adjust the existing pediatric care plan to meet the person's new adult status with respect to physiological, psychological, social, and emotional needs. The nutrition for maintenance of adult weight is different compared to the growth calories of childhood. Adult supplemental formulas are adjusted to have the correct recommended daily allowances for adults. However, not all adult-aged patients with medical complexity are adult size. Home care agencies may be able to help the care team with dietician support to establish nutritional goals. Adult-sized patients also require different lifting and transferring supports than children. As family caregivers age themselves, they may also need additional help with lifting. Appropriate home care personnel, equipment, and home modifications may be needed to promote safety for the patient and caregivers.

Attainment of adult physical size also includes pubertal maturation. Many families caring for CMC feel anxious or ill prepared for the physical, psychological, and social changes associated with puberty. Aspects of puberty and sexuality include sex education, pubertal maturation, hygiene, privacy, sexual feelings, masturbation, personal relationships, intimacy, contraception and sterilization, and parenthood [25]. The healthcare team, including transition specialists, can assist families in navigating these issues and needs. Addressing both the youth and caregivers' educational needs and whether to intervene in rates of pubertal development and growth requires individualized attention to each individual's case. Whether their disabilities are physical, intellectual, or mixed, young adults need assistance to express their own personal developing adult voice while carefully balancing definitions of "best interest" and safety as well as the long-term consequences into adult life of any interventions [26].

Advance Care Planning

Despite a perceived need expressed by providers and families for pediatric advance care planning for CMC, several barriers impede its implementation [27]. In the adult care system, all adults, even those with significant disabilities and limited capacity, should be encouraged to participate in advance care planning to the extent their abilities allow. Special attention should be provided to quality of life values and care preferences of the person with disability [28]. If these conversations do not happen while still in pediatric care, it creates an additional complication at transition for the new adult providers to broach advance care planning prior to the establishment of trusting relationships with the patient and caregivers.

Sharing Information Across the Medical Neighborhood

Many institutions are working toward the use of electronic shared plans of care, but these tools are not yet broadly implemented. Without a clear summary of a patient's current state, pertinent history, and current care goals, it is very difficult to design next steps in transfers of care. CMC have complex needs, long medication lists, and use technology in their care, by definition. New providers are better able to assume care when they understand how the current plan evolved and how it is designed to meet the person's current needs and goals. Standardizing and sharing protocols, such as feeding tube management guidelines, along with care coordination also improves care [29]. Proactive, prepared emergency plans created for CMC have been shown to improve care when the person presents in crisis [30].

Individuals who require complex, continuous care frequently require services from multiple providers and settings that often operate independently from each other, leading to potential safety risks [25]. Finding ways to tie together this care neighborhood is one of the important tasks of transition for CMC. Youth and young adults with neurocognitive disabilities report perceptions of the lack of access to healthcare, lack of knowledge in adult health professionals, and personal lack of information and uncertainty regarding the transition process. Their suggested solutions are early provision of detailed information and more extensive support throughout the clinical transition process [31].

While some pediatric specialists might recommend that a mirror image of the pediatric care team be replicated in the adult system, this is not always indicated. More ideally, the young adults' current needs should direct the makeup of the adult care team. The scopes of practice of pediatric and adult health systems are not identical (see Chap. 15). For example, adults with attention deficit disorder are more likely to involve a prescribing psychiatrist for their care team than children with the same condition, and children with hypertension are more likely to have a pediatric nephrologist than adults with this condition.

Complex care programs located at the tertiary children's hospital are typically most familiar with adult specialists at a nearby adult tertiary facility. However, families who travel long distances to the tertiary sites for pediatric care may be interested in available adult subspecialty options closer to home. Also, tertiary care centers often need the assistance of local providers for knowledge of community resources and the geographical spread of adult subspecialists. There are, however, conditions which are more likely to need the tertiary care of the university setting. For example, adults with hydrocephalus often need continuous access to expert surgical and medical providers. One approach to adult care is an integrated team of pediatric and adult medical and surgical specialists [32]. This can include an integrated team of primary care providers (pediatricians, internists, and medicine-pediatrics) who care for children through adults, with facilitated access to subspecialists, as needed, from neurology, rehabilitation, genetics, urology, neurosurgery, and orthopedics.

Decisions around who should lead the adult care team are not always straightforward. The primary care provider and specialist who oversee the patient's principle disability may both have significant roles, as transition or adult system care coordinators. Regular cross-team communication is critical. Care is improved when this communication is bidirectional with different members of the care team listening, expressing opinions, and offering flexibility in treatment decisions [33]. Most family medicine and internists do not yet have integrated training around congenital conditions in their residency experiences. They recognize that a super-specialist with adolescent training would be helpful during the bridging period, and for patients with self-care limitations, they also value the persistent involvement of parents in care [34]. Medicine pediatric physicians are often identified as potential providers of this service; however, given their relatively small numbers, they cannot be the sole solution. Questions about how new adult providers should be prepared still need further attention to develop the appropriate answers.

Accommodations in Clinical Settings

Once providers are identified, accommodations needed for office visits should be discussed. Nurses recognize the need to be familiar with the expanded needs of patients with intellectual disability. They recommend incorporating contextual and practical elements to ensure the security of these patients [35]. Patients with limitations in neurologic, cognitive, and/or speech functions may not have the ability to appropriately sense, interpret, and/or communicate their bodily needs and functions. Caregivers and care teams must become familiar with how the individual patient expresses sensations and symptoms of illness and demonstrates pain. Sensory integration alterations may interfere with the patient's ability to effectively interpret their own positional discomfort, sleepiness, thirst, hunger, and the need to void. Proactive use of instruments such as the DisDAT tool is useful for recognizing the changes in a patient's characteristics when feeling calm and relaxed versus stressed or in pain [36]. A significant subgroup of adults with intellectual disabilities have emotional dysregulation and may exhibit challenging behaviors in clinical settings. Aggression, self-injury, elopement, and sexually explicit behaviors are the types of disruptions that can occur. Challenging behaviors are often initiated as a means to communicate an unmet need, which can be physical, psychological, emotional, social, or environmental in nature. It is important for care teams to understand the communication methods that each patient uses. Shared plans of care should indicate patients who utilize adapted sign language, yes/no indicators, or pictorial or electronic systems. In addition, updated behavior plans that describe triggers and alternatives can assist with activity suggestions for distracting or calming the patient. Adult providers may not be familiar with the spectrum of mental and behavioral healthcare teams who are available to provide further assistance. In addition to psychologists, psychiatrists, and counselors, a few additional examples include behavioral, habilitative, music, and recreational therapists. These services are usually supported through home- and community-based services through Medicaid.

The CMC population of patients has increased hospitalization risk, and their unique needs around hospitalization should be identified and documented. Young adults with medical complexity are not uniformly "adult" in size. Those under 50 kg, in particular, may not fit safely in the equipment available in adult facilities. They are also not best treated with routine "adult" doses of medications and supplies. Adjustments must be made for the safety in their care. Nursing skills in working with smaller patients as well as adult patients who may need behavioral supports during hospitalization must be addressed within adult facilities. Some patients struggle to cooperate with frightening or potentially painful procedures and may benefit from the help of extra personnel for support or even appropriate utilization of conscious sedation for blood drawing or other procedures. Retaining patients who are interpreted to have more "pediatric" behaviors in pediatric facilities is one possible option. In an analysis from 30 children's hospitals, about 3% of the inpatient service were transitional and adult patients [37]. However, the reciprocal is also true that pediatric facilities are not as facile in the care of adult diagnoses that can occur in this population, including pregnancy, myocardial ischemia, or cerebral vascular accidents. Hospitals or health systems with both pediatric and adult units can use the skills of their pediatric and adult teams to reciprocally help each other with these issues.

Resources Beyond the Healthcare System

CMC often exit secondary education services, including therapies they received in educational settings, around the time of their healthcare transition. Youth with non-asthmatic chronic illnesses are noted to be significantly less likely to complete high school or be employed. Exiting from the school environment can lead to significant social isolation with associated secondary physical and mental health comorbidities. New scheduled day activities (such as higher education, employment, or adult day programming) are not always readily available, feasible, or planned. Vocational rehabilitative programs are an important resource at this juncture. Transportation can become a significant barrier. Larger communities often have paratransit options, while more rural settings may not. Community participation (getting out of the house) in some capacity is a recommended goal for all young adults with disabilities. Transition coordinators need familiarity with navigating existing community supports for persons with disabilities, such as paratransit, adaptive recreational opportunities, and community organizations.

Youth with non-asthmatic chronic illnesses are also more likely to receive public assistance than youth without chronic illness or with asthma [38]. Public assistance through Social Security Insurance (SSI) has a change in eligibility at the person's eighteenth birthday, so it is important to include this intitial application or reapplication as one of the many transition activities for CMC (see Chap. 8). In the majority of states, the application for SSI is linked to Medicaid as well.

Decision-Making Supports

Young adults with significant disabilities may have limits in their decision-making capacity. Early in transition preparation, the ability to develop one's skills as a decision-maker should be encouraged by promoting opportunities through childhood to practice making decisions. Disability advocates encourage that each person should be afforded the highest level of self-advocacy and personal decision-making they can manage. The spectrum of supports that a person may utilize, from least to most restrictive, are verbal assistance or an actual contract for decision-making support from another person to formal power of attorney and court-appointed limited to full guardianship (see Chap. 30). Psychoeducational or neuropsychological evaluations performed by the school or health system can be quite helpful in reviewing a person's prior demonstration of intelligence, school achievement, and adaptive and executive function. These results can inform the process of planning for more training in decision-making and the establishment of legal decision-making supports. Youth who have limits to their capacity but no identified spokesperson or support person to assist them are particularly vulnerable at transition and should be noted as particularly high risk in a registry of CMC. One example of this situation is the foster child with cognitive or mental health limits who is aging out of supports without an existing, effective adult social support system.

Ongoing Needs for Caregivers

Caregivers of CMC experience physical, emotional, and functional health stressors, which can impact their ability to provide long-term care for their children [39]. Under half of CMC move from their family's home into other living settings (college dormitories, group homes, independent living) at the time of transition. These young adults need to find living situations with appropriate physical accommodations to meet their needs. They also need to find caregivers who can assist in their care. Young adults or their spokesperson must know the young adults' needs well enough to advocate for the physical accommodations and the caregiver training needed to provide for their necessary ongoing care. Assessing a potential living arrangement for adequacy, safety, and accessibility includes looking at the structure for ease of mobility, bathroom safety, temperature stability, electrical and water needs, and road accessibility, including snow removal. Assessment of the local community may include proximity of a home care agency, ambulance access, medical supply vendors, a pharmacy, and community support groups [40]. Young adults and families must remember that Medicaid funding is state based and therefore services in other states may vary from what they are currently accustomed to receive.

Youth who plan to remain with their family caregivers may experience few changes in their home setting and caregiver team during the transition process. However, changes that accompany the aging of parents of CMC can cause concerns or anxiety regarding their ongoing ability to meet the physical and emotional demands of providing care to their CMC. It is a delicate dance as a child becomes an adult, to move from being the managing parent of a child with disabilities to the invited consultant and support person for an adult with disabilities. This dance is particularly difficult when the parent still serves as the child's caregiver. Adults with disabilities, like all humans, have an innate need for some freedoms and a sense of self. Parents struggle with the balance between providing enough support and supervision versus affording an increase in freedom. As caregivers, they might be accustomed to doing things their own way and now feel challenged or uncomfortable if their child wants to make a decision to explore or use other methods of care.

While most parents approach caretaking with the best interests of their CMC at heart, occasionally, parents may be acting from a perspective that may not fully appreciate their child's actual abilities, limitations, or potentials and thereby are at risk to set goals that don't optimize that child's future. On those occasions, it may be beneficial for the health team to assist in stretching the parents' view of the situation. For example, caregivers may be so focused on surviving amid the day-to-day needs of their child that they are not yet taking steps to envision a future adult life vision or plan for their child. If they are struggling in preparing their child for changes that may occur in adult life, the transition team can assist in opening up a dialogue about these future possibilities. Parents may themselves become unwell physically or mentally and unable to fully care for their CMC. Then they may need help with creating a proactive plan around their potential loss of ability to serve as caregivers. As previously mentioned, issues surrounding sexuality can be a source of discomfort or conflict between the adolescent or young adult CMC and parent. Parents may also experience disincentives to maximize certain aspects of health. For example, children who are dependent for transfers and continence care need to maintain a healthy weight even though that means being heavier in transfer. They may need to get enough water for hydration even if that means there will be more diaper changes. In extreme circumstances, dangerous health beliefs or actual neglect and abuse can become an issue of concern on behalf of the incapacitated patients at the hands of either family caregivers or paid caregiving staff. Adult healthcare providers do not have as much experience with overseeing the safety of patients who are dependent on proxy decision-makers and caregivers. Reporting concerns to adult protective service programs is a duty of the members of the healthcare team, and therefore familiarity with surveillance for neglect and abuse must be a part of the care team's training and skills.

Payment for Care Services

Current payment models for CMC via fee-for-service programs have not covered the cost of care, especially care coordination and other non-billable services. Options for feasible payment models for this complex transition care require collaboration with Medicaid agencies and should consider raising fee-for-service payments, providing compensation for non-face-to-face care, and upfront payments for care management (see Chap. 23) [9]. Finding individuals who have the skills for care coordination in this unique population is also a challenge. Trained professionals who have previous experience with this population are more effective than new graduates with little life experience [15]. Coverage for services also can change when moving from pediatric to adult billing definitions and codes. Occupational, physical, and speech therapy are more liberally funded for children who are still on the 18-year developmental trajectory of childhood. In adult life, typically there needs to be evidence of forward progress in order to sustain these types of therapy services. Mental health service payment requires adult diagnostic codes that are not the same as those used in childhood, therefore requiring use of appropriate and potentially new codes at the changeover to the new provider.

Systematizing the Process of Transition Planning for Youth with Medical Complexity

Table 31.2 outlines categories of actionable items that may need attention during the transition of youth with medical complexity. Each of these 12 categories may have one or more actionable items in the transition process for CMC. Healthcare financing (1) must be maintained in a continuous fashion while also maximizing applications to eligible special services. Rather than moving the entire healthcare team (2) at one time, transfers of different specialists can ideally be scheduled in a staggered manner so that relationships with some pediatric providers continue during the bridging period. This will enable youth and caregivers to sustain confidence in their team while they are getting to know each of the new adult providers. This staggering can also promote communication between old pediatric and new adult providers, to help with any questions regarding the current treatment plans, health status, and goals. Mental health (3) is listed as a separate category to emphasize its importance for all CMC, in terms of both the increased risk for mental health conditions in youth with medical complexity and their need to develop functional stress management and coping skills in order to better adhere to their increased treatment demands. Most CMC will benefit from the identification and cultivation of sources of care coordination (4), either within health systems, payer organizations, or community agencies. Further stratification of level of care coordination needs should address both physiological and psychosocial and environmental issues. Attention to health habits (5) addresses the individual's abilities to meet their own needs in terms of nutrition, physical activity, sleep, and hygiene. It recognizes that the adult healthcare team and home caregivers must become aligned regarding how these basic needs will be met in an adapted manner to accommodate

Table 31.2 Transition categories for youth with medical complexity

1. Healthcare financing
2. Healthcare team
3. Mental/behavior health
4. Care coordination support
5. Health habits
6. Self-management
7. Decision-making and advance care
8. Family/caregiver needs
9. Home living needs
10. School/work
11. Community participation
12. Transportation

special needs and risks. For example, a family may have learned to use a soft mechanical diet for their CMC for years without having been instructed to do that or formally diagnosed with a specific swallowing diagnosis. It is valuable to recognize this natural development of accommodations as either a person's preference or, in fact, true swallowing dysfunction and future possible risk. Addressing the person's current state and developmental or stretch goals in self-management (6) is the next area for review. Formal transition readiness assessments (see Chap. 13) can be used to assess current transition preparation status and help establish educational goals [41]. Decision-making (7) and capacity from the legal perspective and advance care planning are categories which often benefit from identification of needs and actions to prepare for the future. Medical legal partnerships are helpful in developing the skills that the transition team may need in meeting legal concerns around eligible services, appropriate accommodations, and future planning.

Family/caregiver needs (8), home living arrangements (9), community participation and activities across education and employment (10), as well as recreation (11) and transportation (12) to these activities are specific areas for discussion and attention.

Resources to Enhance the Healthcare Transition

Easing the transition of CMC requires access to individuals who are experts in assisting youth and families across these 12 categories. Social workers, school-based transition teams, and workforce services are all potential helpful sources of support through transition. There are national and state resources which provide planning and support systems to assist families across these additional categories. Developmental Disabilities Services (DDS) agencies exist in each state to provide services to persons with intellectual disabilities. The U.S. Developmental Disabilities Act establishes state resources, which include State Councils on Developmental Disabilities, University Centers for Excellence in Developmental Disabilities (UCEDDs), and legal Protection and Advocacy Systems (P&As). Centers for independent living (CIL) are cross-disability, consumer-controlled, nonresidential nonprofit community agencies that are designed and operated by individuals with disabilities and provide an array of independent living services. Area agencies on aging and disability (AAA) are public or private nonprofit agencies that are designated, like CILs, to be responsible for a specific geographic area, in order to address the needs of persons with disabilities and older persons. They coordinate and offer services to help these consumers to remain in their homes, if that is their preference. All three types of organizations, DDSs, CILs, and AAAs, are important resources for individuals with disabilities and their families before, during, and after the transition to adult life.

Summary

Youth with medical complexity, by virtue of their higher utilization of healthcare services, need enhanced preparation and supports to successfully negotiate the transition from pediatric to adult health systems. Use of a framework of categories of services (Table 31.2) to assist in organizing this process is recommended. Implementation of skilled care coordinators and collaboration with community and state organizations can assist youth and families, as well as the various healthcare teams who serve them, in maintaining continuous and safe care for these youth throughout their life course.

References

1. Berry JG, Agrawal RK, Cohen E, et al. The landscape of medical care for children with medical complexity Children's Hospital Association, Overland Park, KS, 2013. www.childrenshospitals.net.
2. Cohen E, Berry J, Camacho X, Math M, Anderson G, Wodchis W, Guttmann A. Patterns and costs of health care use of children with medical complexity. Pediatrics. 2012;130:e1463–70.

3. Canadian Provincial Council for Maternal Child Health Transition to Adult Healthcare Services Work Group (2013). Transition: a framework for supporting children and youth with chronic and complex care needs as they move to adult services. http://www.pcmch.on.ca/health-care-providers/paediatric-care/pcmch-strategies-and-initiatives/transition-to-adult-healthcare-services/.
4. Foster CC, Mangione-Smith R, Simon TD. Caring for children with medical complexity: perspectives of primary care providers. J Pediatr. 2017;182:275–282.e4.
5. Srivastava R, Stone BL, Murphy NA. Hospitalist care of the medically complex child. Pediatr Clin North Am. 2005;52(4):1165–87.
6. Lucile Packard Foundation for Children's Health (2012). Report: Six models for understanding how families experience the system of care for children with special health care needs: an Ethnographic approach. http://www.lpfch/cshcn.org. Accessed May 2017.
7. Baxter H, Lowe K, Houston H, Jones G, Felce D, Kerr M. Previously unidentified morbidity in patients with intellectual disability. Br J Gen Pract. 2006;56(523):93–8.
8. Oswald DP, Gilles DL, Cannady MS, Wanzel DB, Willis JH, Bodurtha JN. Youth with special health care needs: transition to adult health care services. Matern Child Health J. 2013;17(10):1744–52.
9. Kuo DZ, Houtrow AJ. Council on children with disabilities. Recognition and management of medical complexity. Pediatrics. 2016;138(6):e1–13.
10. Linroth R. Meeting the needs of young people and adults with childhood-onset conditions: Gillette Lifetime Specialty Healthcare. Dev Med Child Neurol. 2009;51(Suppl 4):174–7.
11. Institute of Medicine. The future of disability in America. Washington DC: National Academies Press; 2007.
12. Bodenheimer T, Wagner E, Grumbach K. Improving primary care for patients with chronic illness: the chronic care model. JAMA. 2002;288:1775–9.
13. Shojania KG, McDonald KM, Wachter RM, Owens DK, editors. 2007. Closing the quality gap: a critical analysis of quality improvement strategies. AHRQ Publication No. 04(07)-0051-7.
14. Criscione T, Walsh KK, Kastner TA. An evaluation of care coordination in controlling inpatient hospital utilization of people with developmental disabilities. Ment Retard. 1995;33(6):364–73.
15. Ciccarelli MR, Gladstone EB, Armstrong Richardson EA. Implementation of a transdisciplinary team for the transition support of medically and socially complex youth. J Pediatr Nurs. 2015;30(5):661–7.
16. Gordon JB, Colby HH, Bartelt T, Jablonski D, Krauthoefer ML, Havens P. A tertiary care-primary care partnership model for medically complex and fragile children and youth with special health care needs. Arch Pediatr Adolesc Med. 2007;161(10):937–44.
17. Kelly AM, Kratz B, Bielski M, Rinehart PM. Implementing transitions for youth with complex chronic conditions using the medical home model. Pediatrics. 2002;110(6):1322–7.
18. Berman S, Rannie M, Moore L, Elias E, Dryer LJ, Jones MD. Utilization and costs for children who have special health care needs and are enrolled in a hospital-based comprehensive primary care clinic. Pediatrics. 2005;115(6):e637–42.
19. McAllister JW. 2014. Achieving a shared plan of care with children and youth with special health care needs. www.lpfch.org/sites/default/files/field/publications/achieving_a_shared_plan_of_care_full.pdf.
20. National Longitudinal Survey of Youth 79 (Report release 2/9/11) National Longitudinal Surveys: Bureau of Labor Statistics, Washington DC.
21. Goossens E, Bovijn L, Gewillig M, Budts W, Moons P. Predictors of care gaps in adolescents with complex chronic condition transitioning to adulthood. Pediatrics. 2016;137(4):e20152413.
22. Fredericks EM. Nonadherence and the transition to adulthood. Liver Transpl. 2009;15(Suppl 2):S63–9.
23. Holahan J, Kenney G. 2008. Health insurance coverage of young adults: issues and broader considerations. Timely analysis of immediate health policy issues. Urban Institute.
24. Llewellyn G, Dunn P, Fante M, Turnbull L, Grace R. Family factors influencing out-of-home placement decisions. J Intellect Disabil Res. 1999;43(pt 3):219–33.
25. Institute of Medicine. Crossing the quality chasm: a new health system of the 21st century. Washington, DC: National Academies Press; 2001.
26. Cuskelly M, Bryde R. Attitudes towards the sexuality of adults with an intellectual disability: parents, support staff, and a community sample. J Intellect Dev Disabil. 2004;29(3):255–64.
27. Butler GE, Beadle EA. Manipulating growth and puberty in those with severe disability: when is it justified? Arch Dis Child. 2007;92(7):567–8.
28. Lotz JD, Jox RJ, Borasio GD, Führer M. Pediatric advance care planning from the perspective of health care professionals: a qualitative interview study. Palliat Med. 2015;29(3):212–22.
29. Stein GL, Kerwin J. Disability perspectives on health care planning and decision-making. J Palliat Med. 2010;13(9):1059–64.
30. Abraham G, Fehr J, Ahmad F, Jeffe DB, Copper T, Yu F, White AJ, Auerbach M, Schnadower D. Emergency information forms for children with medical complexity: a simulation study. Pediatrics. 2016;138(2):e2.
31. Young NL, Barden WS, Mills WA, Burke TA, Law M, Boydell K. Transition to adult-oriented health care: perspectives of youth and adults with complex physical disabilities. Phys Occup Ther Pediatr. 2009;29(4):345–61.
32. Simon TD, Lamb S, Murphy NA, Hom B, Walker ML, Clark EB. Who will care for me next? Transitioning to adulthood with hydrocephalus. Pediatrics. 2009;124(5):1431–7.

33. Nurock M, Sadovnikoff N, Gewertz B. 2017. Leadership for complex care: the ship's ballast in troubled waters. Catalyst, N Engl J Med Leadership Blog.
34. Peter NG, Forke CM, Ginsburg KR, Schwarz DF. Transition from pediatric to adult care: internists' perspectives. Pediatrics. 2009;123(2):417–23.
35. Ndengeyingoma A, Ruel J. Nurses' representations of caring for intellectually disabled patients and perceived needs to ensure quality care. J Clin Nurs. 2016;25(21–22):3199–208.
36. Regnard C, Reynolds J, Watson B, Matthews D, Gibson L, Clarke C. Understanding distress in people with severe communication difficulties: developing and assessing the Disability Distress Assessment Tool (DisDAT). J Intellect Disabil Res. 2007;51(Pt 4):277–92.
37. Goodman DM, Hal M, Levin A, Watson RS, Williams RG, Shah SS, Slonim AD. Adults with chronic health conditions originating in childhood: inpatient experience in children's hospitals. Pediatrics. 2011;128(1):5–13.
38. Maslow GR, Haydon AA, Ford CA, Halpern CT. Young adult outcomes of children growing up with chronic illness: an analysis of the national longitudinal study of adolescent health. Arch Pediatr Adolesc Med. 2011;165(3):256–61.
39. Murphy N, Christian B. Disability in children and young adults: the unintended consequences. Arch Pediatr Adolesc Med. 2007;161(10):930–2.
40. Elias ER, Murphy NA, Council on Children with Disabilities. Home care of children and youth with complex health care needs and technology dependencies. Pediatrics. 2012;129(5):996–1005.
41. Wood DL, Sawicki GS, Miller MD, Smotherman C, Lukens-Bull K, Livingood WC, Ferris M, Kraemer DF. The transition readiness assessment questionnaire (TRAQ): its factor structure, reliability, and validity. Acad Pediatr. 2014;14(4):415–22.

Transitioning Youth with Intellectual and Developmental Disabilities

32

Laura Pickler and Janet Hess

Introduction

According to the American Association on Intellectual and Developmental Disabilities, an intellectual disability is characterized by significant limitations in both intellectual and adaptive functioning that occurs prior to 18 years of age [1]. Standardized testing is typically required for both intellectual ability and adaptive skills in order to make this diagnosis. The individual's culture and primary language and abilities of the individual's peer group are also considered. Strengths are often noted in an assessment and used in crafting a plan for supports that should be expected to improve overall functioning in life. In this chapter it will be assumed that people with intellectual and developmental disabilities (IDD) represent a heterogeneous population with a wide set of needs that could include co-occurring medical conditions, but these may not always be present.

L. Pickler, M.D., M.P.H (✉)
Family Medicine and Clinical Genetics,
University of Colorado, Children's Hospital Colorado,
Aurora, CO, USA
e-mail: Laura.Pickler@childrenscolorado.org

J. Hess, Dr.P.H.
Department of Pediatrics, Morsani College of Medicine,
University of South Florida,
Tampa, FL, USA
e-mail: jhess@health.usf.edu

Transition from pediatric to adult care for adolescents and young adults (AYA) with IDD is a multifaceted process that has many components, all aimed at maximizing independence and self-advocacy in the areas of health and wellness. People with IDD have unique needs and considerations that can make the process challenging, rewarding, and sometimes simply different from other youth. Examples are modifications in office procedures, physical examination approach, adaptive communication strategies, and a focus on families or caregivers that is not generally needed with other transitioning youth. Clinicians and other health-care professionals involved in this part of a young person's life can feel confident that they are making a significant difference in quality of life and well-being for their patients when they acknowledge the differences of this patient population. This chapter will attempt to delineate these differences as well as provide examples and suggestions for how to improve interrelated systems that impact the success of the process within the context of the individual and the communities where they reside.

Youth with IDD need a carefully planned transition to adulthood, as they have unique health-care needs when compared to the general population. They are more likely to have comorbid conditions, such as dysphagia, chronic constipation, osteoporosis, hearing impairment, visual impairment, epilepsy, gastroesophageal reflux, thyroid dysfunction, and psychiatric

A. C. Hergenroeder, C. M. Wiemann (eds.), *Health Care Transition*,
https://doi.org/10.1007/978-3-319-72868-1_32

concerns [2]. AYA with IDD are more likely than age-matched peers to be treated with multiple medications including psychotropic agents, although they are less likely to have a psychiatrist managing their psychopharmacologic medications [3, 4]. One study reported only 24% of adults with IDD on psychotropic medications had received psychiatric consultation [5]. Models of care for transition planning for youth with IDD have been at the forefront of professional society meetings [6].

Despite the increased interest and need for transition, only 41% of youth with special health-care needs receive transition planning [7]. AYA with IDD were even less likely to receive transition planning [7–11], which may lead to disparities in preventive care [5]. Only 34% of young women with IDD received cervical and 42% received breast cancer screenings [12]. Only 34% of young adults with IDD reported being routinely screened for colorectal cancers [13]. The lack of needed screenings could be considered reflective of discomfort among health-care providers, the absence of medical homes for adults with IDD, and a failure in the transition process.

Service Systems that Support People with IDD

Important steps have been taken in recent years to address the needs and status of people with IDD across the lifespan. The State Title V programs, Medicaid, the Affordable Care Act (ACA), Social Security/Supplemental Security Income (SSI), Medicare, and civil rights laws like the Americans with Disabilities Act (ADA) and the Individuals with Disabilities Education Act (IDEA) are critical for persons with IDD, providing benefits, supports, and civil rights protections for their health and well-being [14]. However, service systems are largely siloed and uncoordinated and can be difficult to access. Some systems are set up to provide direct services to people with IDD; others serve as gateways to needed services and supports. We describe here some key systems that aid transition among AYA with IDD.

Children and youth with IDD are covered from birth under the broad authority of the Social Security Act of 1935. The Title V of the Social Security Act provides funding to state maternal and child health (MCH) programs, which serve 44 million women and children in the U.S.A. [15]. In 1989, the Maternal and Child Health Bureau (MCHB) outlined the need to develop population-based systems of care for Children and Youth with Special Health-Care Needs (CYSHCN) that are family-centered, community-based, coordinated, and culturally competent. Today, in order to receive federal funds, each state must submit an annual standardized application to the MCHB for the Title V Maternal and Child Health Block Grant Program. Through a comprehensive process that identifies all potential MCH priorities, states and territories conduct surveys and analyze data to determine where they can have the most impact and need the most resources to address local MCH problems and challenges. A formula is used to determine funding allocations based on population size and need [16]. Virtually all states use these grants to fund programs that provide care coordination for CYSHCN, as well as diagnostic medical services and treatments. This includes making sure children have access to programs by providing transportation, translation, and other services.

In 2016, 15 national performance measures (NPMs) were selected to guide a major transformation process in the Title V Program, including one on transition: *Increase the percentage of adolescents with and without special health care needs who receive services necessary to make transitions to adult care.* A total of 32 state Title V agencies subsequently selected transition as a NPM for their 5-year action plan. Those plans included a variety of evidence-informed transition strategies and interventions, such as the Six Core Elements for practice improvement, consumer and health-care professional education, and interagency transition planning [17]. The National Survey of Children's Health (NSCH), sponsored by the MCHB and redesigned for initial data release in 2017, will measure annually national and state transition performance among youth with and without special health-care needs ages 12 through 17. Detailed information about NPM performance is available through the Child and Adolescent Health Measurement Initiative [18].

Another significant piece of legislation is Section 504 of the Rehabilitation Act of 1973, which complements provisions in the Social Security Act [19]. These Acts and their revisions dictate SSI benefits, which many people with IDD receive. Whereas child eligibility is based on a functional assessment, and impairment in two or more life areas is required to qualify, adult eligibility is based on the ability to work. Many young adults with IDD will remain eligible under the adult rules but some may not. As such, reapplication for SSI benefits at age 18 is a critical transition process for this population (see Chap. 8).

Schools also play a pivotal role in shaping transition to adulthood for AYA with IDD. IDEA of 2004 states that a primary objective of special education is to "further education, employment, and independent living" [20]. The law requires schools to provide an Individualized Education Program (IEP) to each student with a disability and mandates transition activities. By age 16, the IEP must contain a statement of needed transition services along with a coordinated set of activities that promotes movement from school to post-school life, including postsecondary education, vocational training, adult services, independent living, and/or community participation. Each year the IEP team must develop, confirm, or update these goals and services [21]. For students with chronic medical conditions, Individualized Healthcare Plans (IHPs) help address items such as daily medication, nutritional needs, and instructions for medical emergencies during the school day.

The Developmental Disabilities Assistance and Bill of Rights Act (DD Act), authorized in 1963 and last reauthorized in 2000, provides a number of programs to support individuals with IDD, such as the State Councils on Developmental Disabilities and University Centers for Excellence in Developmental Disabilities (UCEDDs) Education, Research, and Service [22]. The Administration on Developmental Disabilities (ADD) is the federal agency responsible for implementation and administration of the DD Act.

Most recently, growth in the Medicaid program has shifted the system of supports for people with IDD from one that is funded predominantly by state funds to one that is funded predominantly by Medicaid—with joint federal and state funding [22]. Home and Community-Based Services (HCBS) Waivers are Medicaid programs that provide services in the home for persons who would otherwise require institutional care in a hospital or nursing facility. Without waiver services being delivered in the community, some AYA with IDD might not be able to live at home or receive needed supports in the workplace. Waivers provide specific services over and above those in the general Medicaid adult benefits package and are targeted to persons who demonstrate the need for a high level of care. Services typically include items such as personal care assistance, companion services, transportation, therapy, behavioral support, skilled nursing, durable medical equipment, and supported employment services. A care coordinator is assigned to the Medicaid waiver enrollee to assist with access to community services. There is significant variation across states in Medicaid waiver eligibility, and enrollment is typically capped; that is, once enrollment reaches a specified number or dollar threshold, waiting lists are created [23, 24].

Patient Preparation

Vignette 1

AH is a 19-year-old woman with autism spectrum disorder and intellectual disability brought in by her mother for a routine health maintenance visit. She has been doing well, and transition to adulthood-related milestones has been discussed for the last several years. Despite AH's cognitive and communication limitations, she has been included in transition-related discussions over time utilizing assistive technologies. Her mother is employed by a local community service agency and has counseled other families as they encounter transition-related issues on a wide variety of topics, including medical transition. Guardianship has been obtained and AH's mother is her medical decision-maker. AH has several health-related issues that require consideration. Her family are Jehovah's Witnesses and have declined blood transfusions. This became an issue in the past when AH swallowed a caustic substance at school that caused significant damage to her esophagus and limited swallowing of all solid foods and liquids for a period of time. Several surgeries were required to place a gastrostomy tube and reconstruct her esophagus. While she has fully recovered from this episode of illness, she will occasionally develop strictures in her esophagus that require dilation evidenced by increasing difficulty with swallowing solid foods. Today you discuss transfer to an adult practice with AH and her mother. You anticipated this conversation would go smoothly when you prepared for the visit because AH is doing well and her mother is considered a transition expert in the community. As you launch into a transfer discussion, suggesting a well-prepared adult practice, AH's mother bursts into tears. She cannot believe that, after all they have been through, a transfer would be considered so early. What went wrong? What do you do next?

This case example illustrates a number of key points when considering transition and transfer for patients with intellectual disabilities. First is the importance of health maintenance over time as an opportunity to build relationships, discuss transition concepts gradually, and understand family strengths. This case may have proceeded differently if the provider had accurately assessed the parent's readiness to discuss a transfer of care. People with IDD have many transitions in their lives from early childhood through adulthood as they progress from early intervention services through school systems. Frequently, strengths and contributions of young adults with IDD are overlooked due to perceived lack of ability to understand and participate in the process. It should not be expected for youth with IDD and their families to make transfers quickly [25, 26].

Youth with IDD have indicated that the relationship with their medical provider involves considerable trust. A transfer should not be forced based on chronological age but instead facilitated when preparation has been adequate for everyone involved—the provider, the family, and the young adult [27]. Many resources available to facilitate transition are grounded in assumptions about the cognitive ability of the young adult. The relationship that a clinician has with his or her patient is an essential component to deciding how to adapt currently available tools so that the young person has maximal ability to participate meaningfully. Accessing neuropsychological test results during the time of transitioning may also help clinicians understand how to communicate best with their patients and maximally involve them in the transition process.

There has been increasing acknowledgment of the need for guidance specific to working with patients with IDD. In 2016, a collaborative effort among the American College of Physicians, the American Academy of Pediatrics, and the American Academy of Family Physicians resulted in the development of useful tool kits available online [28]. These resources are free and can be accessed using the link provided in our references. Altman et al. [29] have provided a useful timeline for youth with disabilities to guide transition. Using their model, one might consider a logical time for transfer to an adult provider in the early 20s as opposed to late teens, as might be considered for typical youth.

Another important consideration is to not focus exclusively on the IDD diagnosis but to also give attention to other aspects of the past medical history that may be currently resolved but will require ongoing management. The provision of care within a medical home is complex. Multiple items on a problem list may be managed in primary care with periodic help from specialists, or specialists may take the lead requiring increased care coordination in primary care to avoid duplications or gaps in care. AH's case illustrates just such a situation. Ideally the pediatric provider would specify the management plan and additional physicians that need to be involved now and in the future. This is especially important if a pediatric specialist is involved only periodically since the need for intervention may not come for several years. The following questions should be addressed prior to transfer to a new adult provider: Does the family establish care with a new adult specialist now while asymptomatic? Do they wait until there is a problem and then go to the ED with comprehensive notes? How does the primary care clinician facilitate participation of specialists in a transfer to colleagues? Are there differences in how care is organized in adult settings that would be important to explore so that patients and families are not faced with an emergency to navigate on their own? The answers to these questions will be specific to individual communities, medical systems, and insurance restrictions in place at the time of transfer. Best practices have been proposed to ease the burden of care coordination and improve collaboration and co-management between primary and specialty cares [30, 31].

Addressing the Needs of the Family

Germane to any discussion of patient preparation for transition is a recognition of the role and needs of parents and caregivers. This is especially true among the IDD population, where the demands are typically long term and different from caring for someone with fewer physical and behavioral health issues. The pervasive and often complex needs of patients with IDD can follow an unpredictable course, requiring an extensive variety and range of caring activities [32]. A parent's sense of duty, concern over loss of control, fear of the unknown, and wariness at the possibility of a child with IDD leaving home can contribute to a significant emotional impact [33]. As a result, entry to adulthood is just as challenging for families as it is for the AYA with IDD, perhaps more so.

In this case, AH's mother is presumably better equipped than most in planning for transition, given her professional role in counseling other families. Her emotional response to a discussion about actual transfer of care for her daughter was surprising to the provider. Certainly, the reality of leaving a supportive, trusting relationship with her child's pediatric provider was distressing to her. She was also confronting a final step in "letting go" of her daughter's childhood and allowing AH to step into the adult world. Beyond these unnerving tasks, a multitude of factors may create concerns for caregivers like AH's mother.

Up to this point, the adolescent's life has often been orchestrated by parents. Reaching the age of majority (18 years in most states and jurisdictions) means an individual has the right and responsibility to make certain legal choices about finances, education, and health care. Some young adults with IDD need support in making meaningful legal decisions. While several levels of decision-making assistance are available based on individual capacity, guardianship has been established in this case, and AH's mother is her medical decision-maker. An alternative, newer approach for considering the legal capacity of persons with IDD is called supportive decision-making (see Chap. 30). This model starts with the premise that everyone, even those with the most significant disabilities, has the ability to make his or her own decisions, though some people need more support than others. Members of a person's support network (informal and/or formal) can provide information and advice to help the individual with decision-making. With supportive decision-making, the person with IDD is the primary decision-maker; there is no hierarchy of capacity, only varying levels of support [34, 35]. As parents age, their ability to coordinate and provide care will diminish. In AH's case, transfer of guardianship from AH's mother will need to be addressed at some point in the future.

Further, in-home support from other family members can vary drastically over time. For example, siblings who may have been helpful in a caregiving role may move out of the family home to establish their own life trajectories. Similarly, grandparents who may have assisted are becoming care recipients themselves. Parents may be approaching their own retirement age, yet their caregiving role can remain as demanding and, in some cases, more demanding than ever. For some, these changes coincide with an escalation in problematic behaviors exhibited by the individual with IDD, with the behaviors becoming increasingly more difficult to manage as the adolescent matures to an adult height and weight [36].

Also pertinent to this case are the family's religious and cultural beliefs. As Jehovah's

Witnesses, AH and her family had experienced the medical impact of declining blood transfusions. Providers should ensure that the family's values and preferences are considered and honored throughout the process. For example, cultures vary dramatically in the way they approach sexual health. Given the high risk for individuals with IDD to be sexually abused and/or inappropriately act on their sexual impulses [37], caregivers and providers need to be prepared for the expression of sexual feelings and desires among AYA with IDD as they mature.

The issue that creates the most fear and anxiety among families of individuals with IDD is planning for life after the caregiver has died. Common questions are as follows: Where will they live? Do they have the skills they need to live without me? Will they be well supported? Will they have friends and be happy or will they be socially isolated? Will they have a good life? [36]. As AH's mother has counseled other parents, these concerns can be somewhat ameliorated by starting early with development of a person-centered future plan, integrating it with the health-care transition plan (which may already address key social and adult service items), and updating it regularly to focus on the patient's preferences and desires. The planning process can help identify the skills, resources, and services needed to optimize the individual's quality of life over the lifespan, including housing and community living options (e.g., family home, group home, intermediate care facility), eligibility and access to public benefits (e.g., Social Security/SSI, Medicaid HCBS waivers), education and employment (e.g., vocational rehabilitation), and long-term financial security (e.g., special needs trust, state-sponsored savings accounts for people with disabilities). Acquisition of self-management skills is integral to maximizing personal independence and self-determination in adulthood. Because individuals with IDD often require directed instruction, specific learning strategies (e.g., modeling, role play, visual cues), and frequent practice in order to master self-care skills, it is critical for plans to include developmentally appropriate learning opportunities.

Any of these issues, along with others outlined in Table 32.1, could have contributed to the visceral response exhibited by AH's mother during the office visit. It is also possible that she neglected or underestimated her own need for emotional and physical support. Despite her extensive knowledge about the transition process, was she adequately prepared with coping strategies to counteract the stressors of daily caregiving and to prevent burnout? Health professionals involved in the provision of care to AYA with IDD can assist parents and caregivers by encouraging them to use formal and informal supports—such as respite care, support groups, social networks, and stress management training—and reminding them to pay attention to their own health needs. Though we have focused here on the challenges facing parents and caregivers during transition, many embrace their role, finding it an extremely rewarding endeavor that brings purpose to their lives. Given the complex and ever-evolving dynamics of family relationships, transition preparation should be proactive, deliberate, and attentive to the health and well-being of both AYA with IDD and their caregivers.

Provider Education and Training

Vignette 2

Dr. Z is a pediatrician in a busy metropolitan practice. She has a number of young adults with intellectual disabilities whom she has cared for since they were babies and has begun to think about transition-related quality improvement activities for her practice. While she is comfortable with most aspects of their care, issues of sexuality, resources for adults in the community, and routine examination and screening for adults have not been part of her professional training. She is concerned that she may miss something that could be handled proactively by a clinician trained in adult medicine. She has yet to identify a partner in adult medicine who is interested in her patients. She wants someone with the medical knowledge necessary to care for adults while also understanding the special considerations her patients need, such as more time for appointments, communicating

Table 32.1 Adult-living issues and resources for AYA with IDD and caregivers as they prepare for transition

Issue	Application to transition	Resources[a]
Self-management	Acquisition of skills to maximize self-reliance and self-determination, including communication, self-advocacy, time management, and organization	Videos, brochures, and lesson plans available at http://healthytransitionsny.org, www.floridahats.org/for-youth-families, http://hscj.ufl.edu/jaxhats/Videos.aspx
Role of caregivers	Gradual transfer of responsibility and control from parent/caregiver to patient; role of siblings may evolve	Series of videos available at www.pacer.org/transition/video
Behavioral health	Change or escalation in problematic behaviors that may require different treatment approaches	Anxiety and depression facts sheets for people with IDD available at http://flfcic.fmhi.usf.edu/program-areas/health.html Referral to psychiatrist and/or behavioral health professional may be needed during this time
Sexuality	Developmentally appropriate instruction to build healthy relationships; prevent sexual abuse, inappropriate displays, unplanned pregnancy, sexually transmitted disease	Sexuality Across the Lifespan for Children and Adolescents with IDD, http://flfcic.fmhi.usf.edu/program-areas/health.html
Oral health	People with IDD often have poorer oral health and oral hygiene than those without and may require special dental care	Practical dental care strategies, www.nidcr.nih.gov/OralHealth/Topics/DevelopmentalDisabilities/PracticalOralCarePeopleIntellectualDisability.htm#OralHealthProblems
Independent living	Access to services and resources for residential housing, transportation, assistive technology, recreation, socialization	Medicaid HCBS Waivers; Centers for Independent Living (CILs); local ARC programs
Decision-making	Levels of decision support range from least restrictive (durable powers of attorney) to most restrictive (guardianship) alternatives	Legal aid, pro bono legal services, State Bar organizations: video from Nemours at www.youtube.com/watch?v=CpvIyfiRjRM&feature=youtu.be
Education and employment	Postsecondary programs and services for college experiences, work training, and range of employment options	Vocational Rehabilitation; Medicaid HCBS Waivers; Transition and Post-Secondary Programs for Students with Intellectual Disabilities (TPSID), www.thinkcollege.net
Financial security	Access to public benefits and protection of assets across the lifespan	Social Security/SSI, special needs trusts

[a]Many additional resources are listed on websites such as the Autism Speaks Transition Tool Kit at www.autismspeaks.org, www.aucd.org, www.thearc.org, and www.gottransition.org

with care givers, and modified exams to ensure comfort and full participation. She worries about polypharmacy in her patients, especially with regard to behavior management, since medications may have unintended side effects of decreasing functional skills needed for independence. She seeks someone from her local disability advocacy association to present at her practice to guide her and the office staff in helping their young adult patients move toward adulthood.

A core factor in the successful transition from pediatric to adult medical care is collaboration among clinicians. Even for the most savvy young adults, transfers of care involve risk for many reasons. Patients may not fully understand the new system and how to get their needs met, leading to unnecessary hospitalizations, medication errors, gaps in care, and use of the emergency department as a default when things go wrong [38]. Physicians and other clinicians have a responsibility to ensure that their contribution to the transition/transfer process is met. Clinicians who care for adults and children still have significant roles in transition. All of the transition competencies that have been published pertaining to transition for this group apply with the exception of transfers of care to new providers. For patients who see a number of providers, some may change while others will not. The practice responsible for care coordination will have the task of organizing which providers are involved and their role throughout the transition process. This section will focus on specific aspects of provider preparation that are unique to caring for patients with IDD. Table 32.2 is a summary of items to consider.

Adequate preparation of health-care professionals to care for individuals impacted by intellectual disability is needed. University Centers for Excellence in Developmental Disabilities (UCEDDs) were established in 1963 and "have worked towards a shared vision that foresees a nation in which all Americans, including Americans with disabilities, participate fully in their communities" [39]. Their core functions include service provision (including technical assistance, community education, and direct services), research, and information dissemination. UCEDDs have focused on preservice training for health-care professionals. There are resources available through partners in each state that can be accessed for health profession students in multiple disciplines.

Table 32.2 Considerations for pediatric and adult clinicians as they prepare AYASHCN for transition

• Foster health literacy and independence among parents and patients to develop skills that translate well between pediatric and adult health-care settings
• Proactively prepare for transfers to coordinate labs, procedures under anesthesia, and specialty referrals that are easily done in pediatric settings. If problematic behaviors are present, consider a referral to a psychiatrist to review the role of medication vs behavioral management strategies in these situations
• Communicate with other team members about a planned transfer, with regular reminders
• Think about important facts to be included in a transfer note to adult providers, including religious preference, choices around sexuality, strategies for a successful office visit, aggressive behaviors that may have been noted and triggers for these behaviors, and advanced directives
• Address issues with office staff who are not comfortable with patients who have IDD. Training may be needed to recognize troubling behaviors and to know how to enact a safety plan if aggression occurs
• Assess whether or not staff are familiar with how to refer to community resources such as understanding options for access to transportation, employment, and housing
• Develop an understanding from the patient perspective about the potentially intense feeling of loss in leaving pediatrics, and learn how to be supportive and understanding during the process of establishing adult care
• Articulate the differences in culture between pediatric and adult medicine so that patients and families understand expectations prior to transfer
• Build in office flexibility when interacting with caregivers/families of adults with IDD to account for variances in the degree of caregiver involvement in decision-making and communication
• Assess and improve, if necessary, skills to communicate effectively with persons with IDD, including familiarity with alternative communication/assistive technologies

Medical education has not been at the forefront of training providers to care for people with IDD, although nursing has made specific training for this patient population a priority [40]. There are a number of barriers that help explain this. Most importantly, the breadth and scope of medical curricula subject matter make focused work in this subject area challenging. Recently there has been interest in integration of specific developmental disability content into existing medical student curricula. Efforts are being led by the National Curriculum Initiative in Developmental Medicine (NCIDM), in partnership with the American Academy of Developmental Medicine and Dentistry (AADMD), Special Olympics International (SOI), and Alliance for Disability in Health Care Education. Postgraduate education does not have the same level of focused resources, although there are examples of excellent programs implemented in residencies around the country.

This chapter is not a comprehensive resource to guide curriculum development effort; however Table 32.3 summarizes important provider preparation activities specific to the care of patients with IDD. The integration of a young adult with IDD into an adult practice also deserves specific mention. Table 32.4 summarizes the Got Transition best practice recommendations for all young adults completing a transfer in care and should be also used for patients with IDD and their families.

Table 32.3 Summary of suggested IDD-specific training content

• Provide patient-centered care as it relates to people with IDD
• Avoid making assumptions about functional skills based on cognitive test results
• Learn how to document functional and behavioral status at baseline so that changes can be recognized
• Learn how behaviors may be communicative about physical health status
• Always talk to the patient and not just the caregiver
• Become familiar with the Americans with Disabilities Act and implement best practices
• Address sexuality and reproductive health at routine intervals
• Avoid polypharmacy
• Learn how to modify physical examination skills, if needed, to account for differences in attention, sensory sensitivity, and physical mobility

Table 32.4 Tips for integrating transition-age patients with IDD into adult-oriented clinical practice

Staff training	Pre-visit	During visit	Post-visit
Arrange in-service to discuss: – “People-first” language – Supported decision-making – IDD life challenges	Review the Six Core Elements	Speak directly to patient	Consider more frequent office visits
Identify office champion	Request patient records and condition information from pediatric provider	Identify caregiver(s) and role(s)	Consider follow-up phone call to review plan of care
		Identify legal decision-maker; if needed, secure patient approval to share HIPAA-protected information with specified caregivers/family members	
Elicit feedback from patients with IDD	Identify communication status and need for special accommodations	Provide orientation to office/practice	Follow up with pediatric provider; request “reverse consultations”
	Schedule adequate visit time	Provide same standard of care as “typical” patient	Elicit feedback after first visit from both patient and caregiver
		Implement the Six Core Elements	
		Pay special attention to identification of appropriate adult specialists	

Source: Adapted from Cooley and Cheetham, Got Transition, The National Alliance to Advance Adolescent Health, 2015, http://www.gottransition.org/resourceGet.cfm?id=367

Clinical Implications

People with disabilities are generally healthy, and one should not expect a decline in health and function over time to be more than that experienced by the general population. Therefore, clinicians must have an index of suspicion for such conditions, which may have onset in late adolescence or adulthood or be insidiously progressive. Conditions may include progression of pathology or impairment, either through complications or through the aging process. There is a need for health-care clinicians to adopt a health and wellness paradigm for patients with IDD rather than waiting for illness/injury to occur. If a patient has a known underlying diagnosis, this information may be utilized to guide medical evaluation and screenings during the transition process.

While physical health may be the predominant focus of many medical visits, behavioral health is just as important. It is estimated that 20–40% of children and youth with IDD need support in order to manage self-injurious, disruptive, destructive behavior or behaviors linked to psychiatric disturbances [41, 42]. Despite the prevalence of behavioral health needs, most medical providers feel poorly equipped to meet these needs. Many communities experience shortages of behavioral health providers. The additional expertise and training needed to comprehensively manage mental health challenges in the IDD population are even more scarce. The importance of management of behaviors cannot be understated for the individual's quality of life and the safety of others. A young adult's choices for where, how, and with whom they spend their time may be heavily influenced by how their behavior is understood and managed.

Aberrant behavior can be due to many factors including attempts at communication, response to confusing signals, self-stimulatory behaviors, or sensory drive. They can be repetitive, stereotypical, self-injurious, or an exaggerated or unusual expression of emotion. It is important to not prematurely attribute such behaviors to emerging mental illness or blame all behaviors on the intellectual disability. Initial evaluation of problem behaviors requires the recognition of antecedents and consequences, context, and timing. The onset, frequency, and duration of the behavior are important to note. The provider will need to determine if the problem is situational or pervasive. Is there a temporal relationship to activities of daily living or tasks requiring higher demands of attention and effort? Are other medications or supplements contributing to the incidence of the behavior? The presence of psychological stressors, which can include transition-related activities, can be a trigger for escalating problems.

Once a comprehensive behavioral history has been performed, the clinician must explore whether an underlying medical condition exists to help explain the behavior. A review of systems approach is suggested as one way to organize such an evaluation. Be sure to include inspection of the mouth and teeth as pathology is often present in individuals who do not tolerate routine dental care without sedation. Growth charts allow for detection of weight loss or gain and laboratory or radiographic evaluation may be needed. When communication is impaired, the clinician should not hesitate to order additional tests even when these are not deemed necessary for the general population. If sedation is needed for these tests, this presents an opportunity for less well-tolerated exams to take place simultaneously, such as comprehensive dental, eye, hearing, or pelvic evaluation.

There is no one best approach to treatment for young adults with IDD who present with behavioral disorders. A general hierarchy has been suggested that considers the least invasive strategy first in an effort to minimize medications and restore the patients to their most independent level of functioning [43]. Start with a review of all medications and supplements that could cause behavioral issues via direct mechanism of action or side effect. If a psychiatric medication is indicated, look critically at the medication list to avoid polypharmacy. A behavioral approach is suggested first. Environmental modifications may be helpful. In that successful interventions in the environment will hinge on having an accurate history, consider going back to review the behavioral history to be sure no details have been missed. If the behaviors are not well controlled, despite best efforts at behavioral or environmental modification, consider other psychiatric conditions. Medications may be used for symptom management or for the treatment of psychiatric illness. Collaboration with a psychiatrist may be needed. If the community is fortunate to have professionals trained in behavioral modification with experience treating patients with IDD, these professionals may also be tapped as partners.

As recently as 10 years ago, the cause for intellectual disability was unknown in most cases. Young adults coming of age today may bring much more information to their medical providers in the form of genetic test results than was previously possible. In many cases, this information leads to greater efficiency and effectiveness in health-care provision due to having an accurate diagnosis. The provision of accurate information, including natural history and recurrence risks, hinges on the underlying cause. Screening for commonly co-occurring comorbidities can be directed by knowing the genetic syndrome involved. There are an increasing number of conditions that have published management recommendations that may prove helpful for clinicians. The reader is directed to the GeneReviews (https://www.ncbi.nlm.nih.gov) published by the National Center for Biotechnology Information to search for information on specific clinical conditions. At the time of this writing, the GeneReviews has published 687 peer-reviewed chapters intended to be clinically relevant management resources for practicing clinicians.

While busy clinicians need online tools to help focus intervention for specific patients, the opportunity to discuss community-specific strategies and resources can be helpful. One major barrier for practicing pediatric clinicians with interest in transferring patients to adult providers is knowing how to access partners. Community education events facilitate the formation of these relationships and meet the clinician's need for continuing education. The role for public health in this activity is an opportunity for states to explore.

Adults with IDD should receive the same quality health care and have the same opportunities for normal development throughout their lifetimes. Decisions regarding health and life should be person-centered whenever possible. The individual with IDD and their family should continue to be active partners in the interdisciplinary team. Preventative health guidelines should be followed except when specific guidelines for specific conditions exist. More information is needed to describe the health and life experiences of adults with specific conditions resulting in IDD.

Cross-System Collaboration

The complex needs of individuals with IDD will necessitate access to many systems throughout their lives. Acknowledging the lack of integration of these systems, policy makers and professionals have stressed the importance of adopting broad-based partnerships across systems to ensure successful transition to adulthood [44]. In 2013, the AUCD published a report to promote a coordinated, interdisciplinary transition planning process for AYA with IDD [45]. In 2015, the Federal Partners in Transition Workgroup, comprised of representatives from the Departments of Education, Health and Human Services, and Labor and the Social Security Administration, outlined five overarching strategies to enhance interagency coordination and improve outcomes for students with disabilities [44]. In their *2020 Plan*, the Workgroup highlighted the need for agencies to work collaboratively to prepare AYA and provide services for health-care management, high school graduation, postsecondary education, vocational training, and/or employment. Initiatives such as the Youth Transitions Collaborative and National Youth Transitions Center [46] and briefs like *A Young Person's Guide to Health Care Transition*, published by the National Collaborative on Workforce and Disability for Youth [47], further the goals set forth in the *2020 Plan*.

The integration of federally mandated educational transition planning (e.g., IDEA) and healthcare transition planning has important implications for AYA with IDD. By including health-care self-management and health literacy activities in classroom instruction, IEPs, and IHPs, educators can better meet their mandate to prepare students for postsecondary life, work, and independent living. Special education classes generally offer a comfortable and safe learning environment in which students with disabilities up to age 22 can model and practice new skills. There is evidence that schools provide an effective setting for other psychosocial and behavioral interventions such as prevention of drug, alcohol, and tobacco use [48]. For students with IDD, directed instruction and frequent practice in a school setting can provide critical learning opportunities that they might not experience otherwise.

Concurrently, health-care providers can offer more than the expected health forms for school participation and services. Physicians working with schools can provide valuable inputs to the student's educational team, including providing diagnostic/behavioral consultation and advocating for appropriate programming. No matter how much team building is accomplished, there will likely be an attitude of the "consultant as outsider" when providing advice to schools or other organized entities. It is important to recognize that while a medical provider can offer suggestions, others within the education team will be responsible for adopting and implementing those recommendations [49].

A number of programs have been developed to promote increased collaboration between education and health care. Research-based classroom curricula that teach secondary and postsecondary students with disabilities about health-care transition are available to schools [50], including some designed especially for low-literacy students with IDD [51, 52]. There are web-based training programs for teachers and school administrators that provide guidance for integrating health-care self-management skills in IEPs, IHPs, and classroom instruction [53–55]. The University of Florida has developed a certificate program for graduate students and professionals interested in bringing health-care providers and educators together to help youth with special health-care needs manage their health, navigate the adult health-care system, and self-advocate for their health needs [56]. To help facilitate adoption of a collaborative transition planning model, consideration should be given to increased utilization of teleconferencing technologies for joint meetings (e.g., telehealth platforms) and the development of a single, validated transition preparation and planning tool that can be promoted widely and integrated across organizations. Table 32.5 below lists some cross-system resources currently available to assist AYA, families, and professionals.

Conclusion

People with intellectual and developmental disabilities represent a varied population in their level of functioning and medical needs. This presents a refreshing challenge to providers who welcome the opportunity to build their skills while also working with patients for whom they can make a significant difference in their quality of life. This chapter has highlighted rewards and challenges inherent in working with this patient population. The fragmented systems that must be navigated are often frustrating. Clinicians are in a position to significantly advocate for streamlining resources, which can lead to better efficiency and ease of use for patients and their families. Our hope is that the resources provided, especially the websites that can be referenced over time, will provide guidance not readily available outside IDD-specific training programs.

Transition can be a time of vulnerability for both patients and families. The chosen vignettes in this chapter highlight common, real-life scenarios to illustrate road blocks that frequently derail well-intended efforts. Solutions are suggested; however, the relationship a clinician has with his/her patient and family members is the cornerstone upon which successful transition plans hinge. Without reciprocal trust and partnership between patients, clinicians, and their families, one should not expect for transition into adulthood to be a time of celebrating great accomplishment. Clinicians working primarily with adults often have a steep learning curve

Table 32.5 Cross-system transition resources for AYA with IDD

System	Resource	Description
Workforce	Youth Transitions Collaborative and National Youth Transitions Center (NYTC), www.thenytc.org	The Collaborative is a group of 45 organizations nationally that provide resources and advocacy to help AYA with disabilities as they enter adulthood and the workforce. NYTC, located in Washington, DC, coordinates the efforts of the Collaborative and provides office/conference space for member organizations
	A Young Person's Guide to Health Care Transition, www.ncwd-youth.info/health-care-transition-guide	A 16-page brief targeted to AYA with disabilities; topics include moving to adult health care, living a healthy lifestyle, and paying for health care
Education	*My Health Care*, www.cpalms.org/project/my_health_care.aspx	A classroom curriculum for students and adults with IDD, designed to improve health literacy, communication, and self-advocacy; uses the GLADD (Give-Listen-Ask-Decide-Do) teaching model, embedded video, and adaptive tools
	What's Health Got To Do with Transition? http://health.usf.edu/medicine/pediatrics/ad_med/resources	A classroom curriculum for secondary students with SHCN or disabilities; encompasses preparation for entry to adult systems of care, decision-making, understanding rights and responsibilities as young adults, and better managing their lives
	Healthy Transitions, http://healthytransitionsny.org	Health-care transition skills, tools, guides, videos, and classroom lesson plans for AYA with IDD
	Health Transition Planning and the Individualized Education Program (IEP), www.pacer.org/transition/learning-center/health/planning-and-iep.asp	Guidance on integrating health-care transition goals and activities in IEPs, from the Pacer's National Center on Transition and Employment
	Health Care Transition in the School Setting: A Training Program for Educators, www.floridahats.org/secondary-post-secondary-education	Web-based modules for teachers and administrators; provides knowledge and tools to integrate health-related activities into school curricula and IEPs, from the Florida Health and Transition Services
	Health and the Transition to Adulthood, www.youtube.com/watch?v=EVbG56T1IJM&feature=youtu.be	Webinar provides information and tools for incorporating health goals into IEPs and transition plans, webinar from the Chapter of the American Academy of Pediatrics
	Graduate Certificate in Education and Health Care Transition https://education.ufl.edu/education-healthcare-transition	An integrated approach to health-care transition for education and health-care students and professionals, from the University of Florida

and fewer resources to support the integration of young adults into their practices. Establishing new trusting partnerships with families takes time. Opportunity exists for community organizations, including public health systems, to collaborate with adult providers in order to develop and support best practices that ensure success for all youth. Systems will need to be evaluated and integrated in order to leverage the greatest impact. While the costs in terms of time and effort need consideration, investment should be seen as an improvement for all patients and their families, not just for youth with IDD.

References

1. Schalock RL, Borthwick-Duffy SA, Bradley VJ, Buntinx WH, Coulter DL, Craig EM, et al. Intellectual disability: definition, classification, and systems of supports. 11th ed. Washington, DC: American Association on Intellectual and Developmental Disabilities; 2010.
2. Coppus A. People with intellectual disability: what do we know about adulthood and life expectancy? Dev Disabil Res Rev. 2013;18(1):6–16. https://doi.org/10.1002/ddrr.1123.
3. Hermans H, Evenhuis H. Multimorbidity in older adults with intellectual disabilities. Res Dev Disabil. 2014;35(4):776–83. https://doi.org/10.1016/j.ridd.2014.01.022.

4. Wee L, Koh G, Auyong L, Cheong AL, Myo TT, Lin J, Lim EM, Tan SX, Sundaramurthy S, Koh CW, Ramakrishnan P, Aariyapillai-Rajagopal R, Vaidynathan-Selvamuthu H, Khin MM. The medical, functional and social challenges faced by older adults with intellectual disability. Ann Acad Med Singapore. 2013;42(7):338–49.
5. Lewis M. The quality of health care for adults with developmental disabilities. Public Health Rep. 2002;117(2):174–84. https://doi.org/10.1093/phr/117.2.174.
6. Dietz IC, Armstrong-Brine MM. Evaluation of current transition models for youth with developmental disabilities (DD) aging out of pediatric practice. Presented at Society for Developmental and Behavioral Pediatrics 2015 Annual Meeting, Las Vegas, NV, 3 Oct 2015.
7. McManus M, Pollack L, Cooley W, McAllister J, Lotstein D, Strickland B, Mann M. Current status of transition preparation among youth with special needs in the United States. Pediatrics. 2013;131(6):1090–7. https://doi.org/10.1542/peds.2012-3050.
8. Cheak-Zamora N, Yang X, Farmer J, Clark M. Disparities in transition planning for youth with autism spectrum disorder. Pediatrics. 2013;131(3):447–54. https://doi.org/10.1542/peds.2012-1572.
9. Jensen K, Davis M. Health care in adults with down syndrome: a longitudinal cohort study. J Intellect Disabil Res. 2012;57(10):947–58. https://doi.org/10.1111/j.1365-2788.2012.01589.x.
10. Kuhlthau K, Delahaye J, Erickson-Warfield M, Shui A, Crossman M, van der Weerd E. Health care transition services for youth with autism spectrum disorders: perspectives of caregivers. Pediatrics. 2016;137(Supplement):S158–66. https://doi.org/10.1542/peds.2015-2851n.
11. Roux A, Shattuck P, Rast J, Rava J, Anderson K. National autism indicators report: transition into young adulthood. Philadelphia, PA: Life Course Outcomes Research Program, A.J. Drexel Autism Institute, Drexel University, 2015.
12. Cobigo V, Ouellette-Kuntz H, Balogh R, Rose R, Dababnah S. Are cervical and breast cancer screening programmes equitable? The case of women with intellectual and developmental disabilities. J Intellect Disabil Res. 2013;57(5):478–88. https://doi.org/10.1111/jir.12035.
13. Deroche C, McDermott S, Mann J, Hardin J. Colorectal cancer screening adherence in selected disabilities over 10 years. Am J Prev Med. 2017;52(6):735–41. https://doi.org/10.1016/j.amepre.2017.01.005.
14. The Arc. www.thearc.org. Accessed 14 May 2017.
15. Association of Maternal & Child Health Programs. www.amchp.org. Accessed 13 May 2017.
16. Celebrating the legacy, shaping the future: 75 years of state and federal partnership to improve maternal and child health. Association of Maternal & Child Health Programs. 2010. www.amchp.org/AboutTitleV/Documents/Celebrating-the-Legacy.pdf. Accessed 15 May 2017.
17. McManus M, Beck D. Transition to adult health care and state title V program directions: a review of 2017 block grant applications. Washington, DC: Got Transition, The National Alliance to Advance Adolescent Health, March 2017. www.gottransition.org/resourceGet.cfm?id=431. Accessed 14 May 2017.
18. Data Resource Center for Child and Adolescent Health. http://childhealthdata.org/learn/NSCH. Accessed 15 May 2017.
19. United States Department of Labor, U.S. Code 701, Title 29. www.dol.gov/oasam/regs/statutes/sec504.htm. Accessed 7 August 2017.
20. U.S. Code 1400 Chapter 33 (d) (1) (A). www.law.cornell.edu/uscode/text/20/1400. Accessed 16 May 2017.
21. Antosh AA, Blair M, Edwards K, Goode T, Hewitt A, Izzo M, et al. A collaborative interagency, interdisciplinary approach to transition from adolescence to adulthood. Association of University Centers on Disabilities. April 2013. www.ncset.org/publications/viewdesc.asp?id=423. Accessed 12 May 2017.
22. National Council on Disability. www.ncd.gov/publications/2011/Feb142011#toc1. Accessed 16 May 2017.
23. Wood D, Edwards LR, Hennen B. Health care transition. In: Rubin IL, Merrick J, Greydanus DE, Patel DR, editors. Health care for people with intellectual and developmental disabilities across the lifespan. Switzerland: Springer; 2016. p. 219–28.
24. Smith G, O'Keefe J, Carpenter L, Doty P, Kennedy G, Burwell B, et al. Understanding medicaid home and community services: a primer. Department of Health and Human Services: Washington, D.C; 2000.
25. Reiss J, Gibson R, Walker L. Health care transition: youth, family and provider perspectives. Pediatrics. 2005;115:112–20.
26. Krahn GL, Hammond L, Turner A. A cascade of disparities: health and health care access for people with intellectual disabilities. Ment Retard Dev Disabil Res Rev. 2006;12:70–82.
27. Pickler L, Kellar-Guenther Y, Goldson E. Barriers for pediatric patients with intellectual disabilities transitioning to adult medical care. Int J Child Adol Healt. 2011;3(4):575–84.
28. Health Readiness Assessment for Patients With Intellectual Disabilities. https://www.acponline.org/system/files/documents/clinical_information/high_value_care/clinician_resources/pediatric_adult_care_transitions/gim_dd/idd_transitions_tools.pdf. Accessed 5 June 2017.
29. Altman S, O'Connor S, Anapolsky E, Sexton L. Federal and state benefits for transition aged youth. J Pediatric Rehab Med. 2014;7(1):71–7. https://doi.org/10.3233/PRM-140270.
30. Stille CJ. Communication, co-management and collaborative care for children and youth with special health care needs. Pediatr Ann. 2009;38(9):498–504.
31. Pollard RQ, Betts WR, Carroll JK, Waxmonsky JA, Barnett S, deGruy FV, et al. Integrating primary care and behavioral health with four special populations: children with special needs, with serious mental

illness, refugees, and deaf people. Am Psychol. 2014;69(4):377–87.
32. Raina P, O'Donnell M, Schwellnus H, Rosenbaum P, King G, Brehaut J, et al. Caregiving process and caregiver burden: conceptual models to guide research and practice. BMC Pediatr. 2005;4:1.
33. Acharya K, Schindler A, Heller T. Aging: demographics, trajectories and health system issues. In: Rubin IL, Merrick J, Greydanus DE, Patel DR, editors. Health care for people with intellectual and developmental disabilities across the lifespan. Switzerland: Springer; 2016. p. 1423–32.
34. Sarkar T. Guardianship and alternatives: decision-making options. In: Rubin IL, Merrick J, Greydanus DE, Patel DR, editors. Health care for people with intellectual and developmental disabilities across the lifespan. Switzerland: Springer; 2016. p. 1960–80.
35. Dinerstein RD. Implementing legal capacity under Article 12 of the UN Convention on the Rights of Persons with Disabilities: the difficult road from guardianship to supported decision-making. Hum Rights Brief. 2012;2:8–12.
36. Perkins EA, Hewitt A. Coping with caregiver stress. In: Rubin IL, Merrick J, Greydanus DE, Patel DR, editors. Health care for people with intellectual and developmental disabilities across the lifespan. Switzerland: Springer; 2016. p. 2165–83.
37. Furey E. Sexual abuse of adults with mental retardation: who and where. Ment Retard. 1994;32(3):173–80.
38. Devernay M, Ecosse E, Coste J, Carel JC. Determinants of medical care for young women with Turner syndrome. J Clin Endocrinol Metab. 2009;94(9):3408–13. https://doi.org/10.1210/jc.2009-0495.
39. Association of University Centers on Disabilities. http://www.aucd.org. Accessed 5 June 2017.
40. Smeltzer S, Dolen MA, Robinson-Smith G, Zimmerman,V. Integration of disability-related content in nursing curricula. Nurs Educ Perspect 2005, 26(4):210–216.
41. National Association for the Dually Diagnosed. http://thenadd.org/resources/information-on-dual-diagnosis-2. Accessed 21 July 2017.
42. National Core Indicators Data Brief. https://www.nationalcoreindicators.org. Accessed 21 July 2017.
43. Ageranioti-Belanger S, Brunet S, D'Anjou G, Tellier G, Boivin J, Gauthier M. Behaviour disorders in children with an intellectual disability. Paediatr Child Healt. 2012;17(2):84–8.
44. Federal Partners in Transition Workgroup. The 2020 federal youth transition plan: a federal interagency strategy. 2015. http://youth.gov/feature-article/federal-partners-transition. Accessed 11 June 2017.
45. Association of University Centers on Disabilities. A collaborative interagency, interdisciplinary approach to transition from adolescence to adulthood. 2013. www.aucd.org/docs/publications/transition2013_full_sm2.pdf. Accessed 8 June 2017.
46. Youth Transitions Collaborative and National Youth Transitions Center. www.thenytc.org/. 2017. Accessed 12 June 2017.
47. National Collaborative on Workforce and Disability for Youth. A young person's guide to health care transition. 2016. www.ncwd-youth.info/sites/default/files/Young-Persons-Guide-to-Health-Care-Transition.pdf. Accessed 5 June 2017.
48. Botvin GJ, Kantor LW. Preventing alcohol and tobacco use through life skills training. Alcohol Res Health. 2000;24(4):250–7.
49. Stein S, Stohmeier C, Barthold CH. Working with children and working with schools. In: Rubin IL, Merrick J, Greydanus DE, Patel DR, editors. Health care for people with intellectual and developmental disabilities across the lifespan. Switzerland: Springer; 2016. p. 1645–54.
50. Hess J, Straub D. Brief report: preliminary findings from a pilot health care transition education intervention for adolescents and young adults with special health care needs. Jour Ped Psych. 2011;36(2):172–8. https://doi.org/10.1093/jpepsy/jsq091.
51. Hess J, Slaski P, James L, Reiss J, Miller GR. My health care: health literacy, communication and self-advocacy instruction for persons with developmental or intellectual disabilities. Florida Developmental Disabilities Council, Inc., and University of South Florida. 2016. www.cpalms.org/project/my_health_care.aspx. Accessed 15 June 2017.
52. New York State Developmental Disabilities Planning Council: healthy transitions, moving from pediatric to adult health care. http://healthytransitionsny.org. Accessed 15 June 2017.
53. PACER'S National Parent Center on Transition and Employment. Health transition planning and the individualized education program. 2017. www.pacer.org/transition/learning-center/health/planning-and-iep.asp. Accessed 16 June 2017.
54. Illinois Chapter of the American Academy of Pediatrics and University of Illinois at Chicago Specialized Care for Children, Integrated Services Committee: health and the transition to adulthood: building the foundation for success. 2013. www.youtube.com/watch?v=EVbG56T1IJM&feature=youtu.be. Accessed 14 June 2017.
55. Bargeron J, Hess J, Reiss J. Health care transition in the school setting: a training program for educators [online curriculum]. Florida Health and Transition Services, Florida Department of Health. 2017. www.floridahats.org/secondary-post-secondary-education. Accessed 15 June 2017.
56. University of Florida Interdisciplinary Collaborative on Health Care and Education Transition: education and health care transition graduate certificate. https://education.ufl.edu/education-healthcare-transition. Accessed 14 June 2017.

33 Palliative Care in Adolescents and Young Adults with Special Healthcare Needs

Jill Ann Jarrell, Ellen Roy Elias, and Tammy I. Kang

Introduction to Palliative Care

Case 1: Roxana

Roxana is an 18-year-old female with cystic fibrosis who is several years post-lung transplant with chronic rejection and who is admitted to the pediatric hospital with acute-on-chronic respiratory failure and malnutrition requiring high settings on noninvasive positive pressure ventilation and total parenteral nutrition. Besides her severe dyspnea and anxiety, Roxana has myriad psychosocial stressors including divorced parents who do not get along and who each consider themselves to be the "main caregiver and decision-maker" for Roxana. Before hospitalization, Roxana was in the midst of transition to an adult Cystic Fibrosis Center.

Palliative care issues for Roxana include:

- *Distressing symptoms including dyspnea and anxiety*
- *Psychosocial stressors*
- *Care coordination between pediatric and adult providers*
- *Complex medical decision-making with progressive illness and multiple potential decision-makers including the patient and each of her parents*
- *Need for advance care planning*

The pediatric pulmonary team manages her respiratory support, secretion control, and nutrition, while the palliative care team initiates opioids for her dyspnea with good effect. Over the weeks that she is in the hospital, the palliative care social worker, chaplain, and bereavement specialist are able to establish a therapeutic alliance with Roxana and discuss advance care planning with her. She does not want

J. A. Jarrell, M.D., M.P.H. (✉)
T. I. Kang, M.D., M.S.C.E.
Section of Pediatric Palliative Care, Department of Pediatrics, Baylor College of Medicine, Texas Children's Hospital, Pavilion for Women, Houston, TX, USA
e-mail: jajarrel@texaschildrens.org; tikang@texaschildrens.org

E. R. Elias, M.D.
Departments of Pediatrics and Genetics, University of Colorado School of Medicine, Special Care Clinic, Children's Hospital Colorado, Aurora, CO, USA
e-mail: Ellen.Elias@childrenscolorado.org

A. C. Hergenroeder, C. M. Wiemann (eds.), *Health Care Transition*,
https://doi.org/10.1007/978-3-319-72868-1_33

to go home as she feels she will upset the parent to whose house she does not go and she does not want to be intubated, despite her mother insisting that she "shouldn't give up." The healthcare teams are able to document her wishes with Voicing my Choices and help her communicate them to her family.

Roxana's condition deteriorates soon thereafter and she dies comfortably in an inpatient hospice unit. The family was grateful for the mediation and to have a written document of Roxana's final thoughts and wishes.

This case highlights how palliative care may benefit adolescents and young adults with special healthcare needs (AYASHCN) in transition through its interdisciplinary team and approach to care and focus on elucidating patient and family values and goals and enhanced communication strategies.

Definition

Palliative care is an approach to caring for patients and families facing life-threatening illnesses that focuses on improving quality of life through prevention and relief of suffering that is physical, psychosocial, emotional, and spiritual [1]. Palliative care focuses on mitigating the pain and other distressing symptoms; aiding the patient and family with education, coping, grief, and bereavement; and assisting the patient, family, and healthcare team with elucidating patient and family values and goals, communication, complex medical decision-making, and advance care planning.

Indications for Palliative Care

Palliative care is for patients at any age and at any stage of illness, whether that illness is curable, chronic, or life-threatening. Patients do not have to be at the end of life to receive palliative care.

Table 33.1 Indications for palliative care

Medical	Pain management Other symptom management (e.g., dyspnea, agitation, secretions, nausea) Prognostication End-of-life management
Psychosocial-spiritual	Communication (e.g., elucidating patient and familial goals of care) Coping Grief Bereavement
System-based	Complex medical decision-making (e.g., deciding on technology implementation) Advance care planning Transitions of care (e.g., hospice referral) Care coordination

Multiple national healthcare organizations including the American Academy of Pediatrics, the Institute of Medicine, the National Quality Forum, and the National Institutes of Health have identified palliative and end-of-life care as national priorities with a focus on integrating palliative care into the care of patients with chronic, advanced illnesses [2–4].

There are no specific diagnoses that necessitate palliative care involvement; rather patients with many diseases in varying stages can have palliative care needs. It is important to note that many studies have highlighted children who could benefit from palliative care including those with neuromuscular disorders, congenital anomalies, and cystic fibrosis. Many of these diseases carry life expectancies well into adulthood [5–7]. Table 33.1 lists some common indications for palliative care referral, but is not exhaustive.

Provision of Palliative Care

Every medical provider should provide palliative care to the extent of his/her abilities and comfort. *Primary palliative care* refers to basic skills and competencies required of all healthcare providers in basic aspects of palliative care relevant to complex chronic illness, including pain management,

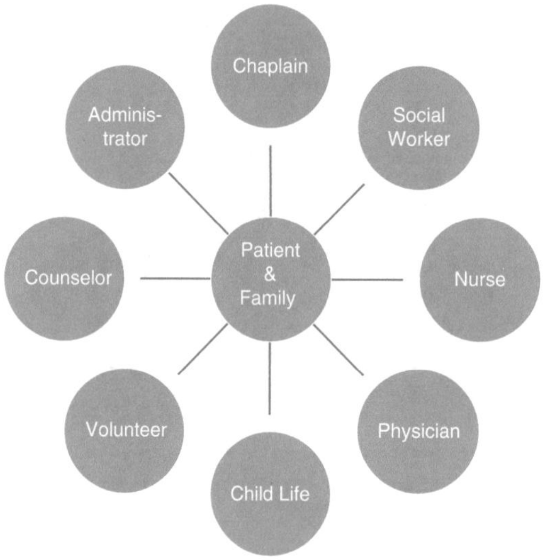

Fig. 33.1 Palliative care interdisciplinary team with the patient and family at its center

communicating difficult news, and advance care planning.

Referral to a specialist or center for palliative care should occur when the limit of the primary provider has been reached. Higher levels of palliative care are commonly accomplished through an interdisciplinary team comprised of nursing, social work, child life, chaplaincy, counselors, volunteers, administrators, and physicians with the patient and family at its center (Fig. 33.1).

Primary palliative care should take place in the context of every patient-provider relationship, regardless of place. Specialty palliative care can take place in the hospital, post-acute facility, outpatient setting, or at home [8].

Timing of Palliative Care

Early implementation of palliative care can improve patients' symptom control, decrease healthcare utilization, and prolong life [9, 10]. The components of palliative care should be offered at the time of diagnosis of a life-threatening condition and continue throughout the course of the illness, whether the outcome is cure or death. Palliative care can be provided alone or alongside efforts to cure illness and/or prolong life, as appropriate and desired [3].

Role of Palliative Care as AYASHCN Transition from Pediatric to Adult Care

Population

Over one quarter of adolescents and young adults (AYA) have a special healthcare need and approximately 700,000 adolescents transfer to adult-based care per year [11, 12] translating into millions of AYA in the United States with a chronic condition who are currently transitioning to adult-based care [13]. Of this population, an unknown but significant proportion may benefit from palliative care.

Addressing Physical Needs

In transition, there can be many providers and teams with different areas of focus so that some needs of the AYASHCNs may be overlooked. Primary and subspecialty adult providers may not be knowledgeable about or comfortable with symptom assessment and palliative care treatment, particularly if pediatric methods of assessment and treatment are warranted, or with unique symptom management strategies such as integrative medicine techniques (see Case #2). Palliative care teams are expert in assessing and treating distressing symptoms associated with chronic illness such as pain, dystonia, dyspnea, secretions, anxiety, and agitation in developmentally appropriate and holistic ways.

Many AYASHCN may be technology dependent due to their underlying disease process. Palliative care teams can assist in technology procurement and management and decision-making related to technology implementation, particularly as patients transition from pediatric- to adult-based care when resources may be in flux as discussed in Case 2.

Case 2: Deborah

Deborah is a 21-year-old female with a connective tissue disorder, chronic pain, GI dysmotility necessitating chronic intravenous nutrition, visceral hyperalgesia, dysautonomia, progressive weakness, and anxiety. She is cognitively intact but reliant on her parents for care, support, and transportation. As she transitions to an adult primary care physician, gastroenterologist, and neurologist, her pediatric palliative care team remains intimately involved in her care to assist with her chronic pain and anxiety. Specifically, she requires pediatric pain assessment tools such as pictorial self-reports and behavioral/observational assessments. Deborah is on large methadone and gabapentin doses and does well with music therapy and aromatherapy as adjuvants for pain and anxiety. Her adult-based care team is unfamiliar with these assessment techniques, large medication doses, and how to incorporate integrative medicine and appreciates the palliative care guidance and education. The palliative care team is also able to assist with transitioning her durable medical equipment and home nursing agencies to ones that are adult-based and educating these homecare teams them on the unique aspects of Deborah's care.

Complex Medical Decision-Making

Some AYASHCNs are cognitively impaired or have insufficient coping and decision-making skills requiring help and/or support with complex medical decision-making and advance care planning.

Complex medical decision-making is the collaborative process by which patients, families, and healthcare teams make decisions regarding specific aspects of care including if and when to implement assistive technology (tracheostomy, ventilator support, gastrostomy, etc.), certain medications, and therapies as well as overall direction of care. This process can be emotionally difficult for patients, families, and healthcare providers. Palliative care teams can help elucidate patient and family goals of care and align them with healthcare team recommendations through shared decision-making [14, 15] (see Fig. 33.2).

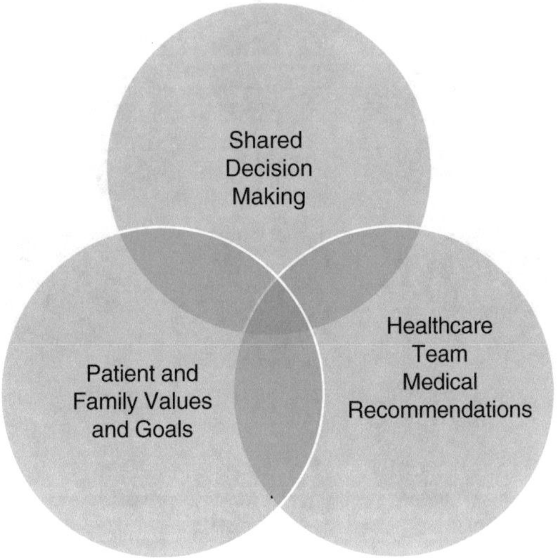

Fig. 33.2 Shared decision-making is the alignment of patient and family values and goals with healthcare team's medical recommendations

These decision-making processes can be complicated during transition when the patient has more legal responsibility but may lack insight or emotional ability to fully participate in decision-making. Often parents have been the primary medical decision-makers, and transitioning decisions to the patient can be difficult for all parties [15, 16]. Pediatric palliative care teams are expert in developmentally appropriate communication with patients and can help navigate these discussions with families and healthcare teams. Adult palliative care teams may lack experience in these areas and may need to consult with pediatric colleagues or psychosocial team members to assess patients' ability and readiness for decision-making.

Advance Care Planning

Advance care planning (ACP) is the process that clarifies an individual's wishes regarding their care in the event of illness or death. An advance directive (AD), sometimes referred to as a living will, refers to the document(s) that contain the wishes of the patient. ACP gives guidance to family members, friends, and healthcare providers in what can be a difficult time or situation. Additionally, it can provide patients with a sense of control and peace regarding their future health care. ACP is not just for sick or dying people. All adults, emancipated minors, and children with chronic illnesses are encouraged to have conversations about and documentation of their wishes. Some advance directives, such as an "Out of Hospital Do Not Resuscitate" and "Physician Orders for Life-Sustaining Treatment", are for patients with serious illness or frailty.

There are several types of advance directives (Table 33.2), which vary by state. It is important to be aware of the advance directives specific to the state in which an individual lives or seeks care. Some patients have advance directives in multiple states (see chap. 30).

In most situations, ACP documents can be accessed and completed in the privacy of ones' own home or in a physician's office. Physicians can play an important role in initiating and guiding the ACP process by making it a routine part of care for all patients, which is revisited regularly to explore any changes a patient may have in his or her wishes. One does not need a legal expert to facilitate advance care planning or to complete advance directives.

The verification of ACP documentation also varies by state. Some states require two witnesses, some require notarization, and others require both witnesses and notarization.

Social workers often have access to ACP forms. Useful Internet resources for obtaining state-specific advance care planning information and paperwork include www.caringinfo.org and individual states' Departments of Aging and Disability. State-specific organ donor registries and forms can be accessed via http//donatelife.net.

Voicing My Choices (www.agingwithdignity.org/voicing-my-choices.php) is an ACP guide designed for AYA patients to help them communicate their end-of-life preferences to family, caregivers, and friends developed through research with AYA with cancer and HIV infection [9, 17].

Table 33.2 Types and descriptions of advance directives

Directive to physicians	Provides direction for inpatient care in the event of a sudden, severe illness and inability to participate in decision-making; typically differentiates between aggressive and comfort care; recommended for general population
Medical power of attorney	Designates surrogate or proxy for medical decision-making in the event of inability to participate in decision-making; recommended for general population
Out of Hospital or prehospital Do Not Resuscitate (OOH DNR)	Provides direction to emergency response teams for giving or withholding cardiopulmonary resuscitation; recommended for patients with serious illness or frailty, for whom a healthcare professional would not be surprised if they died within 1 year
Directive for Mental Health	Provides direction for inpatient treatment of mental health conditions regarding medications and restraints if unable to participate in decision-making; recommended for general population
Organ donation	Provides direction for organ and/or tissue donation; recommended for general population
Statutory durable power of attorney	Designates surrogate or proxy for medical decision-making in the event of inability to participate in decision-making; recommended for general population
Physician Orders for Life-Sustaining Treatment (POLST)	Provides direction to healthcare providers across the continuum of care for giving or withholding cardiopulmonary resuscitation as well as other treatments such as antibiotics or nutrition; recommended for patients with serious illness or frailty, for whom a healthcare professional would not be surprised if they died within 1 year

Recommendations for ACP from this research include that ACP be [15]:

- Introduced by a trusted member of the healthcare team
- Done when the AYA's health is relatively stable
- Incorporate documentation that is done gradually, addressing the AYA's concerns at the time
- Supported by a healthcare professional for decisions regarding life support even when the patient's wish is to complete documents on their own
- Completed if possible for younger patients even though the documents have no legal status for patients younger than 18
- Shared with providers to give insight into preferences

Addressing Family Needs

Many families of AYASHCN have centered their lives around the patient and the patient's care. Many parents find their identity in their AYASHCN, and there can be difficulty in letting the patient assume goal setting and decision-making responsibility.

The caregiver is the expert in their AYASHCN; this expertise can be threatened during transition when providers and institutions are changing and the caregiver expertise is not recognized. Palliative care is often solely associated with end of life resulting in a variety of emotions for the parent or caregiver, and, because of different perspectives on what palliative care means, there may be discord among family members and between the family and the healthcare team.

Siblings are impacted by AYASHCN receiving palliative care during transition as there may be disruption in the family's routine by new clinic visits, healthcare providers, or hospice in the home. Siblings will have questions, thoughts, or fears about advancing illness or death of their sibling.

Family members should be asked about these coping issues by their healthcare team, provided intervention and/or support and guided toward appropriate resources outside the providers' domain. Case #3 illustrates some of these points.

Case 3: Ben

Ben is a 26-year-old male with a mitochondrial disorder, moderate intellectual disabilities, and blindness. He is non-ambulatory, fed via a combination of oral and gastrostomy nutrition, and has a tracheostomy with ventilator support at night and when ill. His parents have found it difficult to accept his disabilities, which have been slowly progressive over time, and have declined to pursue guardianship despite encouragement to do so. The palliative care team at the pediatric hospital where he has been cared for all his life has been working with the family to communicate his changing prognosis, cope with their anticipatory grief, continue guardianship discussions, and also assist Ben in understanding his illness and articulating his wishes regarding care in a developmentally appropriate manor.

Addressing Provider-Related Issues

Pediatric healthcare teams and providers are often unable to care for AYASHCN into adulthood. Adult healthcare teams and providers can be unfamiliar with aspects of pediatric diseases and treatments, such as medication dosing and equipment needs. Adult healthcare teams and providers are sometimes ill-equipped to assess and address the psychosocial and familial issues such as patient decision-making and familial coping mentioned above.

Generally speaking, pediatric hospices are unique entities that are expert in caring for AYASHCN but do not have the licensure or certification to continue to care for them into adulthood. Adult hospices are usually unfamiliar with pediatric disease processes and treatment, as outlined above, and should maintain a connection with a pediatric palliative care provider for assistance with pediatric-specific issues [18].

Addressing Systems-Based Issues

Pediatric hospitals and palliative care programs are often not prepared to care for AYAs with terminal conditions due to lack of provider education, staff training, and institutional policies [19, 20]. Adult providers and institutions may be similarly lacking in infrastructure and resources to effectively treat this population. Education methods are needed to equip healthcare providers to provide competent, confident, and compassionate palliative care to AYASHCN during transition to adult-based care [21].

Hospice

Definition

Hospice is a collection of services provided at the end of life.

Eligibility

In the United States, hospice is a benefit for individuals who are terminally ill and have a life expectancy of less than 6 months if their underlying disease runs its normal course. It is available to those who are eligible for Medicare Part A. Medicaid provides a hospice benefit to terminally ill patients in most states and territories, although the individual eligibility criteria and services provided vary by state. The Department of Veterans Affairs, most private insurance plans, HMOs, and other managed care organizations also provide a hospice benefit.

Patients who live beyond their expected 6-month prognosis may be recertified and continue hospice if their physician assesses them as having progressive clinical decline and ongoing hospice needs.

Services

Hospice beneficiaries are entitled to multiple services that can be provided at home, in a custodial care setting, or in a free-standing hospice unit. These services include nursing; physician; counseling; social, spiritual, and family support; short-term inpatient care; medical supplies and equipment; medications; home health aide; homemaker; physical therapy; occupational therapy; and speech-language pathology. Hospice continues to support the family with bereavement services for approximately 1 year after the patient has died.

When Hospice Is Not Sufficient

Many patients and families have needs and desires that exceed what hospice can provide and require additional nursing, personal care services, therapy services, and familial support. These needs can be met through placing the hospice patient in custodial care or by acquiring additional services in the home setting via private duty nursing, home health care, or paid personal caregiver.

Concurrent Care

As part of the Patient Protection and Affordable Care Act of 2010, terminally ill individuals who are 21 years of age or younger and who are enrolled in a Medicaid or state Children's Health Insurance Plan (CHIP) may concurrently receive hospice care and curative care related to their terminal health condition.

The concurrent care model allows patients and families to continue therapeutic and supportive relationships with primary care and subspecialty providers with whom they have often had long-standing alliances.

Medicare beneficiaries can also receive concurrent care with primary and subspecialty providers while receiving hospice. However, the services must be separate and distinct in documentation and billing. The hospice physician and services bill for the terminal diagnosis and related symptoms under Medicare Part A, while the physician and services providing the concurrent care must address and treat non-hospice diagnoses and bill under Medicare Part B.

Insurance

Children with special healthcare needs in the United States are eligible for a multitude of benefits under private insurers and government-sponsored programs, for example, the concurrent care provision afforded to children receiving the Medicaid hospice benefit. Due to this provision of the ACA, children can receive hospice services along with disease-modifying or curative treatment. This benefit does not extend to adults under the hospice benefit and could lead to a breach in medical care and psychosocial support in the period of transition from pediatric- to adult-based care.

There are other changes that take place in children's insurance coverage as they become adults, ranging from staying on their parents' insurance to losing eligibility for certain waivers that can make the transition period challenging to navigate from a palliative care perspective. AYASHCNs are an extremely vulnerable population to shifts in federal and state healthcare policy that affect their access to palliative care.

Case 4: Melissa

Melissa is an 18-year-old girl with congenital arthrogryposis who has severe neuromuscular scoliosis and restrictive lung disease with respiratory failure on a home tracheostomy with ventilator. She lives several hours away from the medical center and sees many pediatric subspecialists monthly. Her older sister died of the same disorder at age 20, and her parents are consumed with the role of caregiver for Melissa. Despite her medical challenges, she has maintained social relationships and completed high school with home schooling.

Melissa is having more discomfort with the long ambulance rides to and from the medical center several times per month and wants to have more care at or near home, but her parents are fearful to completely sever their relationships with the physicians who have known Melissa her entire life. A pulmonologist, family practitioner, and adult hospice are found to help care for Melissa at home, but they need a fair amount of assistance in navigating unfamiliar equipment, medication dosing, nutritional recommendations, and working with her very assertive and directive parents. The pediatric palliative care team stays involved by calling into weekly hospice care conferences and communicating with mom and her care teams. Melissa and her family are able to visit their pediatric subspecialists and care team periodically under the concurrent care provision for children on Medicaid receiving hospice services aiding in the gradual transition to adult-based care.

Summary

Palliative care can be an important adjunct for AYASHCN transitioning from pediatric- to adult-based care. Specifically, palliative care may be useful in assessing and managing symptoms; facilitating communication between patients, families, and providers as family and care team roles change; aiding in complex medical decision-making and advance care planning; and coordinating care with hospice and other healthcare entities.

References

1. World Health Organization. WHO definition of palliative care
2. Ferrell B, et al. The national agenda for quality palliative care: the National Consensus Project and the National Quality Forum. J Pain Symptom Manage. 2007;33(6):737–44.
3. American Academy of Pediatrics. Section on hospice and palliative medicine. June 2016. http://www2.aap.org/sections/palliative/.
4. Tulsky JA. Improving quality of care for serious illness: findings and recommendations of the Institute of Medicine report on dying in America. JAMA Intern Med. 2015;175(5):840–1.

5. Ajayi TA, et al. Palliative care teams as advocates for adults with sickle cell disease. J Palliat Med. 2016;19(2):195–201.
6. Kazmerski TM, et al. Advance care planning in adolescents with cystic fibrosis: a quality improvement project. Pediatr Pulmonol. 2016;51(12):1304–10.
7. Lyon ME, et al. A randomized clinical trial of adolescents with HIV/AIDS: pediatric advance care planning. AIDS Care. 2017;29:1–10.
8. Quill TE, Abernethy AP. Generalist plus specialist palliative care—creating a more sustainable model. N Engl J Med. 2013;368(13):1173–5.
9. Temel JS, et al. Early palliative care for patients with metastatic non-small-cell lung cancer. N Engl J Med. 2010;363(8):733–42.
10. Zimmermann C, et al. Early palliative care for patients with advanced cancer: a cluster-randomised controlled trial. Lancet. 2014;383(9930):1721–30.
11. 2011–2012 NSCH: Child health indicator and subgroups SAS codebook, Version 1.0, in 12 National Survey of Children's Health. Child and Adolescent Health Measurement Initiative (CAHMI). 2013
12. Health, T.N.A.t.A.A. From prevalence data from the National Health Interview Survey and the Substance Abuse and Mental Health Services Administratio006E
13. White PH, McManus M. Facilitating the transition from pediatric-oriented to adult-oriented primary care. In: Care of adults with chronic childhood conditions. Switzerland: Springer; 2016.
14. Rosenberg AR, et al. Ethics, emotions, and the skills of talking about progressing disease with terminally ill adolescents: a review. JAMA Pediatr. 2016;170(12):1216–23.
15. Wiener L, et al. Allowing adolescents and young adults to plan their end-of-life care. Pediatrics. 2012;130(5):897–905.
16. Haydock R. Transition must balance young people's autonomy and support for families. Nurs Child Young People. 2014;26(3):13.
17. Voicing my choices. www.agingwithdignity.org/voicing-my-choices.php
18. Kirk S, Fraser C. Hospice support and the transition to adult services and adulthood for young people with life-limiting conditions and their families: a qualitative study. Palliat Med. 2014;28(4):342–52.
19. Humphrey L, Dell ML. Identifying the unique aspects of adolescent and young adult palliative care: a case study to propel programmatic changes in pediatric hospitals. Semin Pediatr Neurol. 2015;22(3):166–71.
20. Kaal SE, et al. Experiences of parents and general practitioners with end-of-life care in adolescents and young adults with cancer. J Adolesc Young Adult Oncol. 2016;5(1):64–8.
21. Wiener L, et al. Threading the cloak: palliative care education for care providers of adolescents and young adults with cancer. Clin Oncol Adolesc Young Adults. 2015;5:1–18.

Healthcare Transitions and Dental Care

34

Kimberly Espinoza

Dental Needs of Youth and Young Adults with Special Healthcare Needs

Oral health across the life span is essential to overall health and quality of life. Dental caries, a process involving demineralization of tooth structure caused by biofilm, can lead to cavitation of teeth, oral pain, infection, and even death if left untreated. Periodontitis (gum disease) is the leading contributor to tooth loss. Access to appropriate preventive care and treatment of oral diseases is essential to maintaining oral health. Unfortunately, patients with special healthcare needs of all ages experience disparities in access to oral health care, and this is complicated by the transition to adult-based services.

Dental care is the greatest unmet healthcare need among children with special healthcare needs (CSHCN), surpassing unmet needs for mental healthcare, medical specialty care, occupational and physical therapy, and prescription medications [1]. An estimated 8.9% of CSHCN need but do not receive dental care compared to approximately 5% of children without special needs (CWOSN) [1]. Studies reveal differing levels of unmet need among CSHCN when further classified based on severity and complexity. The level of unmet need arises to 20% for those severely affected by their condition and drops to 5% for those not affected by their condition, the same rate seen in CWOSN [1]. When examining unmet need by diagnosis, children with cerebral palsy, Down syndrome, intellectual disability, and autism experience higher rates of unmet need compared to other CSHCN [2, 3]. For example, children with Down syndrome have the highest unmet need by diagnosis at 14.7% and children with asthma the lowest at 8.6% [1]. Overall, when looking at caries rates, those with developmental disabilities have similar rates of caries compared to the general population, but higher rates of untreated caries [4]. Studies of Special Olympics athletes found untreated caries rates between 28% and 30% [5, 6]. Adults with intellectual and developmental disabilities had a similar rate of untreated caries at 32.2% [7]. Unfortunately, untreated caries is only one manifestation of unmet dental preventive and treatment needs in this population.

Oral pain and periodontitis are two other major concerns for individuals with special healthcare needs. Oral pain is prevalent in both children and adults with special healthcare needs. A study of CSHCN revealed that 19% of those severely affected by their condition experienced a toothache in the last 6 months compared to 10% of CWOSN [1]. For adults, approximately 13% of Special Olympics athletes had oral pain at the

K. Espinoza, D.D.S., M.P.H.
Department of Oral Medicine, University of Washington School of Dentistry, Seattle, WA, USA
e-mail: kmespino@uw.edu

A. C. Hergenroeder, C. M. Wiemann (eds.), *Health Care Transition*,
https://doi.org/10.1007/978-3-319-72868-1_34

time of screening during Special Olympics games [5, 6]. Periodontitis also occurs in much higher rates among those with developmental disabilities, with one study showing a rate of 80.3% in this population [7]. Dental hygiene problems, linked to periodontitis, are one of the top ten limiting secondary conditions for those with developmental disabilities [8].

Disparities in oral health are linked not only to diagnosis but to income and access to dental insurance as well. Unmet dental needs among CSHCN rise to 29.4% among those who are uninsured or have lapses in insurance [1]. For CSHCN below 100% of the federal poverty level, 17.6% experience unmet dental needs. Poor and low-income CSHCN severely affected by their condition have 13.4 times the odds of having unmet dental needs compared to high-income CSHCN not affected by their condition [1]. Disparities seen in other populations are also likely to occur among those with special healthcare needs, such as disparities by race and ethnicity and rural versus urban status.

Barriers to Accessing Dental Care During the Transition Years

Unmet dental needs among CSHCN stem from a variety of reasons. Among CSHCN with unmet dental needs, approximately one third of their parents cited the dentist being unwilling to treat their child as a reason for their lack of routine care [9]. Twenty percent of parents of CSHCN had difficulty finding a dentist willing to treat their child [3]. Three quarters of this group stated this difficulty sometimes or often prevented them from taking their child to the dentist. Parents of children with autism reported that the most common reason for not having a regular dental provider was inability to find a dentist willing to treat their child [10]. This evidence for dentists' reluctance to treat patients with special healthcare needs extends beyond parental perceptions.

Dentists themselves note they may be hesitant to treat patients with special healthcare needs. Only 18% of dental school students reported they would definitely be willing to treat patients with intellectual disability in their future practices [11]. Moreover, one study found three out of four dental students did not feel competent to care for patients with developmental disabilities, while another study found 60% had little or no confidence treating patients with intellectual disabilities [12, 13]. In practice, few general dentists treat patients with special needs. Only 10% of general dentists report treating patients with cerebral palsy, intellectual disabilities, or medical complexity often or very often [14]. Pediatric dentists are much more likely to treat patients with special needs, with up to 95% reporting they treat this population [15]. While one study showed 71% of pediatric dentists continue to see patients beyond age 21, pediatric dentistry is an age-defined specialty limited to children [15]. Few pediatric dentists treat patients significantly beyond young adulthood. When pediatric dentists aid in the transition of patients from pediatric to general practice, they encounter a major barrier in finding a dentist who is willing to treat their patients with special needs [16].

Two main factors significantly affect access to care during the transition years: the dental education system and the dental care financial system. General dentists typically practice immediately after completing dental school or after a postdoctoral residency in general dentistry. Dental school accreditation standards require only that the dental student can assess the treatment needs of patients with special needs [17]. The Commission on Dental Accreditation implemented this standard as recently as 2004. Prior to that for many years there were no accreditation standards related to patients with special needs in the predoctoral curriculum [18].

Even with the current standard, dental students are not required to be able to treat this population. The same holds for dental hygiene schools. In general dentistry residency programs, the accreditation standard requires that the resident assesses, diagnoses, and plans treatment for patients with special needs (Table 34.1) [17]. Again, no requirement exists for residents to be competent in the actual treatment of this population.

The dental school curriculum is typically rigorous, and school administrators cite limited time

Table 34.1 Commission on dental accreditation predoctoral standard 2-24 regarding the assessment of patients with special needs

Graduates *must* be competent in assessing the treatment needs of patients with special needs
Intent:
An appropriate patient pool should be available to provide experiences that may include patients whose medical, physical, psychological, or social situations make it necessary to consider a wide range of assessment and care options. The assessment should emphasize the importance of non-dental considerations. These individuals include, but are not limited to, people with developmental disabilities, cognitive impairment, complex medical problems, significant physical limitations, and the vulnerable elderly. Clinical instruction and experience with the patients with special needs should include instruction in proper communication techniques and assessing the treatment needs compatible with the special need.

in the curriculum as a barrier to incorporating education in the treatment of patients with special needs. Fifty percent of dental school deans felt education in special care dentistry was not a high priority in the curriculum [12]. Even when it is a high priority, students at the predoctoral level are learning to improve their speed with basic clinical skills. Many patients with special needs require a provider who is able to complete a procedure quickly and competently. Some advanced facilitation techniques are beyond the skill of even the top dental students.

Pediatric dentistry is the only dental specialty with accreditation standards that mandate the treatment of patients with special needs [19]. Pediatric dentists have advanced training in the provision of care for CSHCN. However, given that pediatric dentistry is an age-defined specialty, when individuals with special needs age out of pediatric practice, they often have nowhere to go.

The other major factor that impacts access to adolescents and young adults with special healthcare needs (AYASHCN) during the transition years is changes in child versus adult Medicaid benefits. The majority of adults with developmental disabilities rely on Medicaid for healthcare coverage [20]. Dental care is considered an "essential health benefit" for children, whether or not the child has a special healthcare need [21]. As it is an "essential health benefit," dental coverage must be included under state Medicaid plans for children. Children who qualify for Medicaid services will have dental benefits under Medicaid. However, dental care is not considered an "essential health benefit" for adults. It is up to each state to determine if dental benefits will be included among other Medicaid benefits for adults. As of 2015, 18 states offered emergency-only or no dental coverage to adult Medicaid recipients, 17 states offered coverage for 1–4 dental services only, and 15 states offered coverage for 5 or more dental services [22]. State-by-state coverage for adult Medicaid dental benefits also varies over time. Between 2003 and 2014, 20 states moved between these coverage categories, while even more states changed specific services offered [22]. In addition to having the discretion to provide dental coverage to their adult Medicaid population, states can also choose whether or not to offer more dental benefits for adults with developmental disabilities compared to other adults. For example, both Washington and New Mexico offer more fluoride services for adults with developmental disabilities compared to adults without developmental disabilities. Finally, even if a state offers adult dental Medicaid benefits, states use different fee schedules for children versus adults. Adult Medicaid dental reimbursement is on average 40.7% of the typical reimbursement for private insurance [23]. States can also choose to increase reimbursement rates for treating patients with developmental disabilities. For example, the New Mexico Special Needs Dental Program allows increased reimbursement under Medicaid for the treatment of patients with developmental disabilities and is linked to provider training in the care of patients with special needs.

Specific Challenges for Those with Intellectual and Developmental Disabilities

To explore the challenges faced by those with intellectual and developmental disabilities in maintaining oral health, this section outlines the determinants of oral health using biopsychosocial

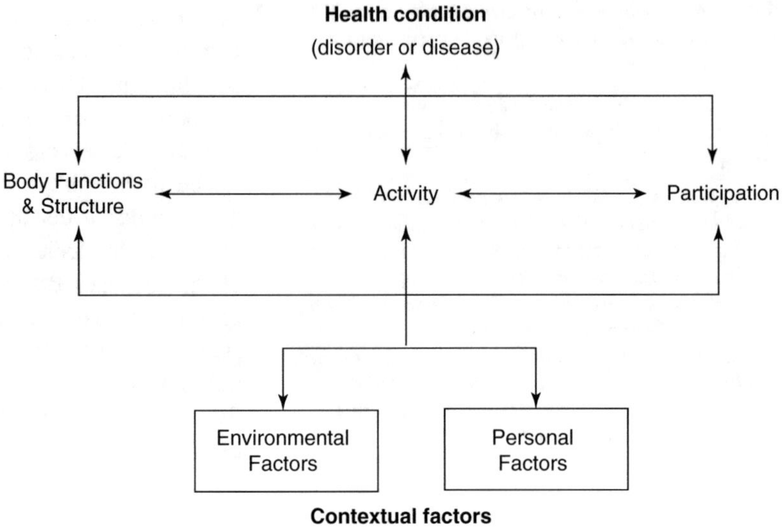

Fig. 34.1 World Health Organization model of disability. The model shows the interplay between health condition, body functions and structures, activity, participation, and environmental and personal factors

and socioecologic frameworks. The World Health Organization International Classification of Functioning (WHO ICF) is a biopsychosocial model that examines the interplay of medical conditions with the environment and personal factors to paint a picture of the overall disability and functioning of an individual (Fig. 34.1) [24]. When considering patients' barriers to oral health, it is important to examine how diagnoses and environmental factors interact to impact functioning.

Body Functions and Structures

The structure and function of the oral cavity and perioral region can highly affect one's ability to receive oral care, such as brushing and flossing, or dental care. An example seen in patients with developmental disabilities includes manifestations of the hypoplastic midface that occur in individuals with Down syndrome. Patients with Down syndrome are likely to have a smaller, narrower palatal form (roof of the mouth), a relatively larger tongue, oral hypotonia, and a hyper-gag reflex, all of which can complicate access to the oral cavity [25]. Those requiring sedation or general anesthesia may have increased risk due to sleep apnea or difficult airway access. Individuals with Down syndrome also have much higher rates of periodontitis [26]. This can manifest early, in some cases in the teen years. This is at least partially due to slower neutrophil chemotaxis and phagocytosis and increased inflammatory mediators involved in periodontal disease. When combined with the on average smaller tooth roots seen in Down syndrome, young adults are at risk for early tooth loss.

Individuals with cerebral palsy, a movement disorder that can affect oral movements, often have difficulty tolerating dental care. Cerebral palsy can result in hypertonia or hypotonia and involuntary head, arm, and body movements. This can lead to difficulty accessing the oral cavity, risk of injury from dental instruments, and chronic injury to teeth from bruxism (tooth grinding). Additionally, growth and development under conditions of high or low muscle tone or frequent involuntary oral movements can result in atypical jaw form and malocclusion.

People with cerebral palsy and Down syndrome may have oropharyngeal dysphagia, a swallowing disorder that can lead to the risk of aspiration pneumonia, especially in patients who aspirate thin liquids. When oral hygiene is poor, this increases the risk for aspiration pneumonia due to bacterial pathogens in dental plaque [27]. Water used in a dental procedure along with saliva represent thin liquids that can be difficult to tolerate for many patients with developmental conditions, especially when keeping the mouth open and leaning back in a dental chair. Some patients with a severe aspiration risk or oral aversion may use a feeding tube for nutrition. In these cases the individual does not conduct normal chewing activities, resulting in increased calcification of dental plaque, sometimes covering the entire tooth surface in several-millimeter-thick deposits. The combinations of these factors can make dental cleaning appointments more difficult for patients to tolerate.

Other developmental conditions can affect the structure of the oral cavity, such as syndromes involving the orofacial region. Conditions such as intellectual disability, autism, or ADHD can affect the ability to lie down and stay still in a dental chair. Additionally, some patients with developmental disabilities have limitations in their ability to brush their own teeth or the ability to accept tooth brushing from a caregiver if needed. Other areas of concern include prescription medications and medical complexity. Many medications taken by patients with developmental disabilities can have oral manifestations. Seizure medications can result in gingival enlargement, and a multitude of medications can result in dry mouth, a significant risk factor in developing dental caries. Conditions that result in medical complexity can affect overall oral health as well as ability to safely receive certain dental treatments, such as oral surgical procedures, prescription medications, sedation, and general anesthesia.

Activities and Participation

As noted above, conditions related to body functions and structures can decrease the ability to perform certain activities, such as oral hygiene, as well as decrease the ability to participate in routine dental care. Resistance to oral care is another challenge oral health providers and direct support staff may experience with AYASHCN who have developmental disabilities. This can occur due to the inability to understand the reasons for care, oral aversion, dental anxiety, or a history of negative dental experiences, among other reasons. The impact of resistance to dental care changes as people age from early childhood to adulthood. With a history of positive experiences and desensitization to dental care during the pediatric years, a patient who had difficulty cooperating for dental care as a child may have learned to fully participate in dental care during adolescence and adulthood. The consequences of resistance during a dental appointment, such as attempting to hit a dental provider or grab at sharp dental instruments that were placed in the oral cavity, are much different for a small child compared to a large adult.

Participation in the dental appointment can also be limited when there is a communication disorder. If the patient is not able to clearly communicate health needs, understand healthcare messages, communicate oral pain, or discuss their medical history, it can make it difficult for the dental provider to meet their dental needs. Some AYASHCN who have developmental disabilities may have significant difficulty understanding the risks and benefits of procedures as well as treatment alternatives. Access to dental care can be further limited by the individual's ability to schedule their own appointments and arrange for their own transportation to receive dental care. Difficulty accessing dental care and oral hygiene care, however, is not solely a consequence of the impact of the individual's diagnosis or their physical, medical, intellectual, or emotional conditions and functioning. Environmental factors also play a role.

Environmental and Personal Factors

Environmental factors play a significant role in the ability of AYASHCN to access dental care. These environmental factors are examined further using the socioecologic framework for the determinants of health, which classifies determinants of health into various levels, from individual factors to environmental factors.

Individual Factors

Individual risk factors for oral disease include factors related to functioning as discussed previously as well as nutritional factors, substance use, and other health-related behaviors such as tooth brushing and flossing. Poor oral hygiene can stem from structural and functional issues, discussed previously, as well as the motivation of the patient to perform oral hygiene. Many individuals with developmental disabilities have a high sugar, high acidic diet which can contribute to the development of dental caries. When a high sugar, high acidic diet combines with poor oral hygiene and dry mouth due to medications, the risk of dental caries is considerably higher. Additionally, there is a high rate of vitamin and mineral deficiencies in individuals with developmental disabilities [28]. Some of the causes of this include oral aversion, a highly restricted diet, and oropharyngeal dysphagia. An example of a nutritional deficiency resulting in oral manifestations is described in the vignette, below. Smoking, a known risk factor for oral cancer as well as periodontitis, does occur in this population. Those with mild to moderate intellectual disabilities have a higher risk of smoking than those with severe intellectual disabilities [29].

Nutrition Vignette

The mother of a 24-year-old nonverbal female with autism called a special care dental clinic for an emergency appointment on a Monday due to "bleeding gums." The patient received a same-day appointment and was found to have severely swollen, bleeding, purple gingiva beginning to detach from the teeth. This was an unusual presentation, and the patient was referred for urgent medical evaluation due to a high suspicion of oral cancer. The physician scheduled an evaluation appointment for the patient on Friday afternoon. On Friday morning, the patient awoke lethargic and pale. The mother took the patient to the emergency room and the patient was diagnosed with severe anemia. The physician that was to evaluate the patient for oral cancer visited the patient while she was in the emergency department. After further workup, it was determined that the patient actually had scurvy, a nutritional deficiency due to severe vitamin C deficiency. The patient's limited diet contributed to this condition, which originally presented with only oral manifestations. (*Some of the patient details have been changed for privacy.*)

Relationships and Living Conditions

Many individuals with developmental disabilities require the support of caregivers into adulthood. An individual who is not able to brush their own teeth requires the assistance of a caregiver, whether that person is a family member or paid support staff. A process of deinstitutionalization began in the 1970s, resulting in most individuals who were living in state-run institutions retuning to community settings, with families or in small group homes. An individual living in a group home setting may receive services from paid support staff who perform a variety of caregiving services, including oral hygiene services. The person who performs oral hygiene services for one individual may change frequently, with temporary hours, mobility within the caregiving organization, and turnover into other fields of work [30]. In many cases, the individuals responsible for performing oral hygiene services for their clients are not the same individuals who are responsible for transporting them to dental appointments. This complicates the ability of dentists and dental hygienists to provide appropriate oral hygiene instructions to the patient and caregiver. Additionally, paid support staff typically have limited training in providing oral hygiene for another individual, and many find tooth brushing, and to a greater extent flossing, to be difficult [31]. When AYASHCN rely on a caregiver to manage their oral health needs, the caregiver's oral health literacy plays a key role in the individual's own oral health. This may include performing daily oral care, making dental appointments, transporting patients to dental appointments, recognizing urgent dental needs, or making decisions related to diet for the individual.

A major factor in dental care transition for patients with developmental disabilities is the change in legal status from childhood to adulthood. For many patients this means having legal independence in medical decision-making for the first time. However, some adults with developmental disabilities are unable to understand treatment proposals, risks, benefits, and alternatives. In these cases, the individual will require some form of supported decision-making or surrogate decision-making (see Chap. 30). The question of who will make treatment decisions is not always examined prior to adulthood for patients with intellectual and developmental disabilities. This can present a great barrier to care and makes obtaining consent for dental procedures difficult or impossible for some patients.

Unlike routine medical care, routine dental care is often surgical in nature, uses sharp instruments, and often results in irreversible procedures (removing tooth structure or entire teeth). The simple signing of a consent form does not indicate informed consent, and the provider must determine that the patient is able to understand the risks, benefits, and alternatives. For some procedures this is simple, such as for an examination. For other procedures this is more complex, such as deciding between a root canal and an extraction or electing to do a procedure with a risk of serious complications. In cases where a patient requires general anesthesia in an operating room or medical immobilization for clinical care, the stakes are even higher for having an appropriate consent process in place.

Institutional Factors

Institutions that impact the oral health of AYASHCN include state-run institutions, private caregiving organizations, and public and private dental schools, among others. State-run institutions and caregiving organizations may have policies and procedures that promote or inhibit a person's oral health. While most state-run institutions have closed, some remain. Prior to closing, many institutions had dental practices located in their facilities. As institutions closed, the need for dental care in the community for patients with more complex special needs quickly rose. Individual caregiving agencies and group homes must find dental care for their residents in the community, where access to care is lacking. Within group homes, policies and procedures may exist regarding tooth brushing that impact oral health. This includes defining what qualifies as tooth brushing resistance, how caregiving staff may support patients with tooth brushing, and when to stop if a client resists tooth brushing.

Dental schools represent another form of institution that impacts the oral health of AYASHCN. Dental school accreditation requirements include that dental school graduates can assess the needs of patients with special needs, but do not require that they are able to treat them. Dental schools can decide how much clinical experience and didactic education students have in relation to the care of patients with special needs, including patients with developmental disabilities. Dentists are more likely to be comfortable treating patients with developmental disabilities if their dental school education prepared them to do so [13]. Some studies have shown that half of dental students had clinical training with patients with intellectual and developmental disabilities while in dental school [12, 13]. Another study showed that seventy-five percent of dental students had no experience with patients with intellectual disability, cerebral palsy, or the medically complex while in dental school [14]. The dental school accreditation standard now includes an intent statement added in 2013 to specify that dental schools should have a diverse patient pool consisting of patients with special needs, including patients with developmental disabilities [17]. However, the majority of dentists practicing today graduated under older accreditation standards.

Policy and Societal Factors

The Americans with Disabilities Act (ADA) mandates that dental providers, along with other healthcare providers, do not discriminate against patients with disabilities in their practices [32]. A seminal case testing the ADA through the U.S. Supreme Court was Bragdon v. Abbott [33]. This case involved a dentist treating a patient with asymptomatic HIV. The dentist told the patient he would treat her, however, only in the operating room. The dentist lost this case and it was emphasized that asymptomatic HIV was a disability under the ADA. The profession of dentistry has a legal and societal obligation to meet the needs of the public, including those with special healthcare needs. Yet many dentists intend not to treat patients with particular disabilities, such as intellectual disability [11]. Dentists are advised not to exclude patients with particular diagnoses from their practices and to assure that each patient is evaluated for their ability to tolerate and cooperate with care, their need for advanced care techniques, and the provider's skill in employing the advanced care techniques needed.

Ableism is the pervasive oppression of people with disabilities at individual, institutional, and societal levels. Ableism manifests on the individual level when providers choose not to care for patients with disabilities when they have the capacity to provide appropriate care. It occurs when people with disabilities are stigmatized and when providers make generalizations about an individual based on their disability label as opposed to examining them as an individual. On institutional levels, ableism is manifested by a dental education system that lacks an accredited pathway for advanced education in the care of adults with disabilities. On a societal level ableism is manifested by lack of access to care for people with disabilities as well as a healthcare financing system that makes dental care unaffordable or inaccessible for this population.

AYASHCN encounter financial difficulties related to obtaining dental care. One of the primary reasons given for unmet dental care needs is the cost of dental care, reported by 25% of parents of CSHCN with unmet dental needs. Lack of dental insurance is another reason given by 22% [1]. The majority of individuals with developmental disabilities qualify for Medicaid services [20]. A major barrier to transition from pediatric to adult dental services is the difference between pediatric and adult Medicaid coverage, with adult coverage being up to the discretion of the state. Even when adult dental Medicaid benefits are provided, reimbursement rates remain low [23]. Dentist participation in the Medicaid program is limited, and patients often have difficulty accessing a dental Medicaid provider. A number of states have undergone Medicaid reform with varying levels of success in recruiting more providers to the Medicaid system and increasing the number of Medicaid recipients who received care [34]. Some states offer additional reimbursement or cover additional services for the treatment of patients with developmental disabilities, although this is not consistent across states [35].

Models to Train the Next Workforce of Providers

To adequately prepare the next workforce of dental providers, changes should happen at predoctoral and postdoctoral levels as well as within dental hygiene and dental assisting programs. In the absence of stronger accreditation standards, predoctoral, dental hygiene, and dental assisting programs should assure that students are competent to care for patients with special needs who require limited facilitation techniques. Advanced training programs should be promoted that train providers in the care of patients with advanced facilitation techniques. This can include specialty status, residency, fellowship, or advanced continuing education programs. There is currently no specialty in special care dentistry in the United States. In the early 2000s, specialties in special care dentistry were formed in several countries, specifically Brazil, Australia, New Zealand, and the United Kingdom [36]. The process to designate a dental specialty in the United States is long and complicated. The Special Care Dentistry Association (SCDA) set up a task force to investigate the possibly of an accredited residency training program in special care dentistry [37]. The SCDA also offers continuing education at annual meetings and through online content, as well as fellowship status for dentists and dental hygienists, and board certification through the American Board of Special Care Dentistry. The advantages and disadvantages of these various training pathways are outlined in Table 34.2. A multi-tiered approach is the most likely to be successful. One example of a program (UW DECOD) that has sought to do this is described, after Table 34.2.

An example of a training program in special care dentistry is the University of Washington Dental Education in the Care of Persons with Disabilities (DECOD) Program (described below). This program aims to improve access to care by providing direct services and training

Table 34.2 Training pathways to develop dental workforce in special care dentistry

Training pathway	Advantages	Disadvantages
Predoctoral dental, dental hygiene, and dental assisting programs: Increase/improve training in dental schools, dental hygiene schools, and dental assisting schools	Reach the largest number of future dentists, dental hygienists, and dental assistants	Limited time within dental school curriculum, would not be able to learn advanced techniques, schools can continue to meet minimal standards if so desired
Specialty in special care dentistry: Designate special care dentistry as a specialty in the United States	Raise profile of special care dentistry as a profession, create awareness among dental students of advanced training opportunities	Complicated process, concern about general dentists referring patients that don't need specialty-level care
Special care dentistry residency: Create a CODA accredited residency in special care dentistry	Raise profile of special care dentistry as a profession, create awareness among dental students of advanced training opportunities	Complicated process, although less complicated than creating a specialty
General dentistry residency: Provide special care dentistry emphasis within existing advanced general training residency programs	May fit well into some existing programs, either as component in first postgraduate year or emphasis in second postgraduate year	Limited time in residency curriculum, residency program buy-in required
Special care dentistry fellowship training: Provide fellowship training programs to practicing dentists, dental hygienists, and dental assistants	Easier to set up than a residency program	May be shorter term, no accreditation standards
Continuing education in special care dentistry: Promote continuing education in special care dentistry	Accessible to general dentists by attending meetings or through online education	CE offerings are limited, generally not hands-on
SCDA fellowship status: Promote SCDA fellowship in special care dentistry	SCDA already offers designation for fellowship and dental hygiene fellowship in special care dentistry and gives recognition to those practicing special care dentistry	Not an educational pathway
ABSCD board certification: Promote board certification in special care dentistry	Designation of expertise in special care dentistry, may satisfy board certification requirement to work in some hospital-based programs	Not an educational pathway

multiple levels of learners to meet the needs of patients with developmental and acquired disabilities.

UW DECOD

The DECOD Program provides clinical training in the care of patients with developmental and acquired disabilities for dental students, dental hygiene students, residents, and practicing dentists, dental hygienists, and dental assistants. The DECOD Program aims to train all dental graduates to provide care for patients with disabilities. The program also aims to train select providers in the advanced care of patients with disabilities. The clinic provides over 6000 patient visits per year, primarily to adults with developmental disabilities. At the predoctoral level, an introductory lecture and patient care experience is given during the first year, a longer didactic course occurs in the second year, case-based written portfolios and student-led presentations occur in the third year, and a final written portfolio occurs in the fourth year. The bulk of clinical instruction occurs in the third and fourth years. Dental students attend 8–10 clinical sessions during their third year and complete a 3.5-day clinical rotation during their fourth year at the DECOD Clinic. During this time they learn how to assess new patients, determine their need for facilitation techniques, obtain consent appropriately, and provide routine care for patients using basic facilitation techniques. The program also coordinates with multiple dental hygiene schools to give dental hygiene students experience in treating patients with developmental disabilities. Residents and fellows of the DECOD program learn to provide care to patients using both basic and advanced facilitation techniques. The DECOD Program uses the International Association of Disability and Oral Health Predoctoral and Postdoctoral curricula as a guide for the objectives of the educational programs. These curricula are readily available for other programs looking to advance dental education in this area [38, 39].

Summary

Dental needs are more likely to be unmet than other healthcare needs for AYASHCN. These unmet dental needs are magnified when an individual is severely affected by their condition, is more medically complex, experiences poverty, experiences insurance lapses, or has a developmental disability and is going through transition to adult-based care. Multiple factors affect the oral health of AYASHCN, and these can be examined using the WHO ICF and socioecologic frameworks. Dentists' unwillingness to treat is a major contributor to this problem. Reasons for this include minimal accreditation standards and limited experience in dental school, resulting in decreased comfort in providing care. Pathways for addressing these barriers include expanding dental education at the predoctoral level and creating advanced training programs to meet the needs of those requiring advanced care. Addressing the larger determinants of health, including those related to the financing of healthcare and the exclusion of people with disabilities from the dental health care system, will also be essential.

References

1. Lewis CW. Dental care and children with special health care needs: a population-based perspective. Acad Pediatr. 2009;9(6):420–6.
2. Iida H, Lewis C, Zhou C, Novak L, Grembowski D. Dental care needs, use and expenditures among U.S. children with and without special health care needs. JADA. 2010;141(1):79–88.
3. Nelson LP, Getzin A, Graham D, Zhou J, Wagle EM, McQuiston J, McLaughlin S, Govind A, Sadof M, Huntington NL. Unmet dental needs and barriers to care for children with significant special health care needs. Pediatr Dent. 2011;33(1):29–36.
4. Anders PL, Davis EL. Oral health of patients with intellectual disabilities: a systematic review. Spec Care Dentist. 2010;30(3):110–7.
5. Reid C, Chenette R, Macek MD. Special Olympics: the oral health status of U.S. athletes compared with international athletes. Spec Care Dentist. 2003; 23(6):230–3.
6. Reid C, Chenette R, Macek MD. Prevalence and predictors of untreated caries and oral pain among Special Olympics athletes. Spec Care Dentist. 2003;23(4):139–42.
7. Morgan JP, Minihan PM, Stark PC, Finkleman MD, Yantsides KE, Park A, Nobles CJ, Tao W, Must A. The oral health status of 4,732 adults with intellectual and developmental disabilities. J Am Dent Assoc. 2012;143(3):838–46.
8. Traci MA, Seekins T, Szalda-Petree A, Ravesloot C. Assessing secondary conditions among adults with developmental disabilities: a preliminary study. Ment Retard. 2002;40(2):119–31.
9. Al Agili DE, Roseman J, Pass MA, Thornton JB, Chavers LS. Access to care in Alabama for children with special needs: parents' perspectives. JADA. 2004;135(4):490–5.
10. Brickhouse TH, Farrington FH, Best AM, Ellsworth CW. Barriers to dental care for children in Virginia with autism spectrum disorders. J Dent Child. 2009;76(3):188–93.
11. Baumeister SE, Davidson PL, Carreon DC, Nakazono TT, Gutierrez JJ, Andersen RM. What influences dental students to serve special care patients? Spec Care Dentist. 2007;27(1):15–22.
12. Holder M, Waldman HB, Hood H. Preparing health professionals to provide care to individuals with disabilities. Int J Oral Sci. 2009;1(2):66–71.
13. Wolff AJ, Waldman HB, Milano M, Perlman SP. Dental students' experiences with and attitudes toward people with mental retardation. JADA. 2004;135: 353–7.
14. Casamassimo PS, Seale S, Ruehs K. General dentists' perceptions of educational and treatment issues affect-

ing access to care for children with special health care needs. J Dent Educ. 2004;68(1):23–8.
15. Nowak AJ. Patients with special health care needs in pediatric dental practices. Pediatr Dent. 2002;24(3):227–8.
16. Nowak AJ, Casamassimo PS, Slayton RL. Facilitating the transition of patients with special health care needs from pediatric to adult oral health care. J Am Dent Assoc. 2010;141(11):1351–6.
17. CODA. Accreditation Standards for Dental Education Programs. Commission on Dental Education Accreditation. 2016. http://www.ada.org/en/coda/current-accreditation-standards.
18. Thierer T, Meyerowitz C. Education of dentists in the treatment of patients with special needs. J Calif Dent Assoc. 2005;33(9):723–9.
19. CODA. Accreditation Standards for Advanced Specialty Education Programs in Pediatric Dentistry. Commission on Dental Accreditation. 2016. http://www.ada.org/en/coda/current-accreditation-standards.
20. Ervin DA, Merrick J. Intellectual and developmental disability: healthcare financing. Front Public Health. 2014;2:1–3.
21. CMMS. Essential Health Benefits. U.S. Centers for Medicare & Medicaid Services. https://www.healthcare.gov/glossary/essential-health-benefits/.
22. MACPAC. Report to congress on Medicaid and CHIP. Chapter 2: Medicaid coverage of dental benefits for adults. 2015:23–53. https://www.macpac.gov/publication/coverage-of-medicaid-dental-benefits-for-adults-3/.
23. Nasseh K, Vujicic M, Yarbrough C. A ten-year, state-by-state, analysis of Medicaid fee-for-service reimbursement rates for dental care services. 2014. ADA Health Policy Institute Research Brief.
24. International Classification of Functioning, Disability, and Health: ICF. Geneva:World Health Organization; 2001.
25. Mubayrik AB. The dental needs and treatment of patients with Down syndrome. Dent Clin N Am. 2016;60(3):613–26.
26. Morgan J. Why is periodontal disease more prevalent in people with Down syndrome? Spec Care Dent. 2007;27(5):196–201.
27. Barnes CM. Dental hygiene intervention to prevent nosocomial pneumonias. J Evid Based Dent Pract. 2014;14S:103–14.
28. Humphries K, Traci MA, Seekins T. Nutrition and adults with intellectual or developmental disabilities: systematic literature review results. Intellect Dev Disabil. 2009;47(3):163–85.
29. Steinberg ML, Heimlich L, Williams JM. Tobacco use among individuals with intellectual or developmental disabilities: a brief review. Intellect Dev Disabil. 2009;47(3):197–207.
30. Bogenschutz MD, Hewitt A, Nord D, Hepperlen R. Direct support workforce supporting individuals with IDD: current wages, benefits, and stability. Intellect Dev Disabil. 2014;52(5):317–29.
31. Minihan PM, Morgan JP, Park A, Yantsides KE, Nobles CI, Finkelman MD, Stark PC, Must A. At-home oral care for adults with developmental disabilities: a survey of caregivers. J Am Dent Assoc. 2014;145(10):1018–25.
32. Americans with disabilities act of 1990. Pub. L. 101-336. 26 July 1990. 104 Stat 328.
33. U.S. Supreme Court. Bragdon v. Abbott West Supreme Court report. 1998;118:2196–2218.
34. California HealthCare Foundation. Increasing access to dental care in Medicaid: does raising provider rates work? Issue Brief. 2008.
35. McGinn-Shapiro M. Medicaid coverage of adult dental services. State Health Policy Monitor. 2008. www.nashp.org/Files/shpmonitor_adultdental.pdf.
36. Mugayar L, Hebling E. Special care dentistry: a new specialty in Brazil. Spec Care Dentist. 2007; 27(6):232–5.
37. Hicks J, Vishwanat L, Perry M, Messura J, Dee K. SCDA task force on a special care dentistry residency. Spec Care Dentist. 2016;36(4):201–12.
38. IADH. Undergraduate Curriculum in Special Care Dentistry. International Association of Disability & Oral Health. 2012. http://iadh.org/wp-content/uploads/2013/09/iADH-Curriculum-in-SCD-ENGLISH-NEW-LOGO-1672013.pdf.
39. IADH. Special Care Dentistry Postgraduate Curriculum Guidance. International Association for Disability & Oral Health. 2014. http://iadh.org/wp-content/uploads/2014/10/iADH-post-graduate-curriculum-2014.pdf.

Part VIII

Models of Healthcare Transition Programs

A Successful Healthcare Transition Program in a Hospital Setting

35

Khush Amaria and Miriam Kaufman

History

The Hospital for Sick Children (SickKids) is a tertiary pediatric hospital in Toronto with an upper age limit of 17. In the mid-1980s, a program began for adolescents with chronic health conditions and/or disabilities. This program offered a regular adolescent health presence in chronic illness clinics, as well as inpatient and outpatient consultation. By the end of the 1980s, it was recognized that youth with special healthcare needs (YSHCN) leaving pediatric care often felt as though they were falling off a cliff and, indeed, were often lost in adult follow-up. In response, the first transition planning intervention at SickKids—an eight-session psychoeducational group called "On the Move"—was designed and implemented. While a hospital-wide program was envisioned, it could not be established without administrative support. SickKids' YSHCN therefore experienced lapses in care when entering the adult system.

K. Amaria, Ph.D., C.Psych. (✉)
Division of Adolescent Medicine and Department of Psychology, Good 2 Go Transition Program, Hospital for Sick Children, Toronto, ON, Canada
e-mail: Khush.amaria@sickkids.ca

M. Kaufman, B.S.N., M.D.
Division of Adolescent Medicine, Good 2 Go Transition Program, Hospital for Sick Children, Toronto, ON, Canada

In the early 2000s the OnTrac program in British Columbia was developed. This included readiness checklists and a group process to promote self-management and self-efficacy. However, SickKids staff reported being overwhelmed by trying to implement such a program with limited protected time or guidance.

A full-day symposium for pediatric and adult providers, held in Toronto, was provided to broaden the awareness of healthcare transition (HCT) to include issues beyond the transfer of medical care and to bring together key players to plan a transition program for SickKids. The proposed model for establishing the program was Kieckhefer's Shared Management Model [1]. Over 75 people attended, including pediatric and adult providers, and YSHCN and caregivers. A three-page summary of these proceedings became a reference document to guide further planning of a hospital-wide program (see Table 35.1).

In 2004, a Teen Clinic Advance Practice Nurse (APN) was providing individual transition care along with her clinical duties. She spearheaded a plan for transition using a program logic model (see Fig. 35.1). By 2005, a full-time HCT APN was hired. Importantly, this was hard funding—not a pilot program or tied to research dollars.

In 2006, the Good 2 Go Transition Program (Good 2 Go) was funded with dedicated time for part-time clinical nurse specialist and physician. Easy-to-use resources and tools for patients and healthcare providers that supported transition

A. C. Hergenroeder, C. M. Wiemann (eds.), *Health Care Transition*,
https://doi.org/10.1007/978-3-319-72868-1_35

Table 35.1 Issues in the transition of youth with chronic illness/disability symposium (2004) summary of small groups

Successes

- Disease-specific, specialty programs that transfer patients to adult teams with which they have a close relationship
- Disease-specific associations link children, adolescents, and parents with young adults and staff from the adult programs
- Hospital for Sick Children (HSC) programs where an "adult" practitioner conducts clinics at HSC as a vehicle for transition and other shared care arrangements
- HSC programs that offer "transition days"
- HSC programs/clusters that offer developmental workshops (self-esteem, teasing, psychosexual development)
- Oncology program has a province-wide, after-care program that provides adolescents with a passport outlining medical history
- Resources at CHIP give information that helps teens lead a normal life

Barriers

- Lack of systemic processes and standards for transition
- Attitudinal issues
  - We want to "own" the care plan, not give up control
  - Attached to our patients, hard to let go
- HSC transition programs are program specific and isolated
  - Disease-specific, but many patients cared for in several programs, not always clear who is taking primary responsibility
  - Lack/limited sharing of resources among specialty programs
  - We don't know who offers what
  - Most information is not written down, but the process is known by the staff implementing
  - Not multidisciplinary in nature
- Developing, implementing, and evaluating a transition program are labor-/resource-intensive
  - Currently, programs that work well are supported by one committed individual. The program then becomes dependent on that one person, usually a nurse
- Having a set age (18) for transfer of care may not be developmentally appropriate for some adolescents. There are little flexibility and limited support to address the developmental needs of children and adolescents with chronic illness
  - At the time we need to promote independence, we tend to "coddle" them instead
  - Some adolescents may require more support, while other adolescents may be emotionally and developmentally prepared to transfer by an earlier age
- There is usually no individual transition plan
- We have created a culture of dependency
- The role of parents is not well-articulated
  - Do we promote learned helplessness?
  - Are we too paternalistic?
- There is limited attention/emphasis to patients/families with cultural diversity and the impact of culture on the role of the family in health and illness.
- There may be problems in identifying an adult center for the patient (i.e., no one interested in the disease, if few patients survive into adulthood…)
- Patients and families may not want to go to specific centers
- Lack of connections with family practitioners who could provide continuity of care throughout the time of transition
- Adult programs are perceived to be less likely to support developmental, educational, vocational, and sexual issues

Goals

- HSC goals
  - An integrated, hospital-wide, multidisciplinary approach to transition

Clearly differentiates transition as a process and the transfer of care as an event. The transition process should begin early and not weeks or months prior to the event

Starts early, with a shared management approach from time of entry into HSC system

Take into consideration unique context of chronic illness, with some teens having lifelong involvement at HSC and others much more recent, those whose conditions are disabling…

Culturally-sensitive

Career/vocational focus

Collaborative with adult system

Table 35.1 (continued)

- Goals for the adolescent
  - Safe young adults accessing care appropriately in the adult healthcare system
  - Successful adult who has met developmental tasks of adolescence and is leading as normal a life as possible
  - Low levels of anxiety regarding transfer to adult system
- Goals for the parent
  - To foster an adult relationship with their teen that allows the teen to take primary responsibility for their healthcare
  - To support them in an important time of loss
  - To facilitate parental "letting-go"

Strategies

- HSC survey/needs assessment to determine
  - Existing transition efforts
  - Key contacts/opinion leaders within programs
  - Educational needs of the staff
- Survey of adult counterparts [needs assessment] to determine
  - Details of existing transition efforts or programs
  - Key contacts/opinion leaders
  - Educational needs of staff
  - Identification of recent "alumni" of the pediatric program who might be mentors
- Parent and youth survey to determine
  - Developmental needs
  - Educational requirements
  - Vocational planning needs
  - Sexual health and education needs
- Develop a shared management approach to be implemented in early childhood with all patients with a chronic illness. Additional contact with Gail Kieckhefer for information/training in this approach.
- Convene an advisory group of
  - Healthcare professionals across the pediatric-adult continuum, including key individuals who can serve as consultants/mentors
  - Youth
  - Parents
- Develop partnerships with adult facilities and identify resources and programs in the adult sector
- Improve quality of information transfer and access by
  - Creating a file or journal that a teen can carry into new setting
  - Including copies of letters from clinic assessments and admissions
  - Exploring opportunities for adult providers to access HSC file electronically
  - Implementing tele-health conferencing with adult colleagues
- Identify a "transition planner" for each program (similar to discharge planner role)
- Career/vocational center, perhaps in conjunction with HRDC
- Education component for staff, including:
  - In services/rounds for individual programs
  - Transition newsletter
  - Annual transition day for pediatric and adult staff to focus on clinical practice, education, and research
- Online resource manual for healthcare professionals
  - Services, agencies, and societies
  - Internet resources
- Education component for teens and families
  - Peer support groups
  - Psychoeducational groups (On the Move model, OnTrac model)
  - Wellness/resiliency models [health promotion]
  - Mentorship (provides advantages for both mentors and mentees)
  - Written and online resources (collaborate with Ability OnLIne)
  - Consider developing a model that is fun and engaging, perhaps using a navigation/adventure metaphor
- Yearly review of patients who are turning 17 to insure that transition issues are being dealt with (format to be adapted to needs of individual programs)
- Transition checklists on charts to be completed yearly starting at age 12
- Use Bloorview MacMillan [note: now Holland Bloorview Kids Rehab] as a resource as they are already addressing transition planning and transfer more formally.

(continued)

Table 35.1 (continued)

Summary of Recommendations The Hospital for Sick Children cares for a large number of young people every year. Although some have a brief encounter with illness and the hospital, many others stay in the system for their entire adolescence. Some of these teens have illnesses that would have been fatal during childhood until quite recently. Every year large numbers of patients turn 18 and are transferred to the adult system. (About 4000 visits per month are made to HSC by 16–18 year olds.) Some of these teens undergo a systematic process of transition that prepares them (and their parents) for the adult system (with its unique culture) as well as providing some preparation for other aspects of adult life with a chronic illness or disability. But the vast majority of teens "graduating" from HSC do not benefit from such a program
A hospital-wide initiative is needed, with a central program that can provide planning, support, consultation, evaluation, and education. Ideally, this program would be coordinated by a full-time advanced practice nurse, with some administrative support and a part-time physician. A full-time research assistant would be invaluable in including a research and evaluative component as services are being planned
The first job of the team would be to liaise with HSC and adult programs to determine more exactly what already exists and to survey parents and teens about their transition needs. It is clear that success of a hospital-wide program will depend on a great degree of flexibility—there are big differences in the needs of patients, numbers of patients transitioned (from less than ten a year in some areas to hundreds in others) and resources within programs
Specific ideas for this team include providing psychoeducation groups, promoting shared management, facilitating yearly reviews in every program of teens who will be transferred in the next year, arranging adult mentors, planning with adult subspecialty programs, offering vocational planning (perhaps in conjunction with HRDC), and creating resources and an annual transition symposium for pediatric and adult providers

Note *HSC* SickKids

planning, including MyHealth Passport, the MyHealth 3-Sentence Summary, and a revision of a timeline for parents, were developed. Continuing education for healthcare providers about adolescent development, chronic illness management, and summaries of the transition literature were provided.

In parallel, a hospital-wide consultation service to support individuals, programs, and/or directors and managers in incorporating HCT into their clinical practice was pivotal. The most important element of the early days of starting a transition program was to provide this consultation to all who requested it. These strategies were employed to help change the culture of care at SickKids to support youth in their transition through development and into adult care.

In the next few years, Good 2 Go grew to 2.5 full-time personnel and was identified as a leading practice by Accreditation Canada. After five years a new team leader was identified and tasked with program development and evaluation. In hindsight, evaluation methods should have been systematically present from the outset. The original program logic model was expanded, and the first version of the Good 2 Go Transition Program Resource Manual (described further below) was created. The rest of this chapter is dedicated to describing these elements and next steps for Good 2 Go.

As written in 2005, the aims of the Good 2 Go Transition Program were:

1. To prepare youth with chronic health conditions and their families to transition from SickKids to the adult healthcare system, in a timely fashion, by participating in a comprehensive, consistent, developmentally appropriate, coordinated, transition program
2. To assist individual programs in providing comprehensive, consistent transition services to youth and their families

The program supported a paradigm shift in the culture at SickKids to embrace transition thinking and develop transition practices in order to improve long-term health of children and adolescents with chronic conditions and special healthcare needs. Achieving the aims required a broad approach wherein program activities were placed in a framework with clear expected outcomes.

Program Logic Model for SickKids Transition Program
***November 2005* Created by Laurie Horricks RN, MN and Miriam Kaufman MD**

The Problem

Lack of formalized hospital-wide approach to the transition of HSC patients to adult care system

The Information

Implement an evidence-based, formalized hospital-wide transition program to meet the needs of youth and their families.

The Goal

To prepare youth with chronic health conditions and their families to transition from SickKids to the adult health care system, in a timely fashion, by participating in a comprehensive, consistent, developmentally -appropriate, coordinated, transition program.
To assist individual programs in providing comprehensive, consistent transition services to youth and their families.

Objectives

1. Infuse transition thinking into the culture at SickKids
2. Adopt the Shared Management Model as a care delivery model
3. Alter clinical practices to support transition efforts
4. Provide direct transition services to adolescents and their families
5. Identify and secure ongoing funding for the transition program
6. Engage in research and add to the current literature on transition

Enabling excellence in Transition

- "Growing Up" timeline poster in clinic waiting areas and on SickKids website
- "Growing Up" timeline handouts available to families in all clinics

Adolescent Medicine will:
1) assist programs in:
a) Adopting the Shared Management model of care delivery
b) Identifying "Transition Champions"
2) customize/individualize transition materials:
a) Transition checklists (Getting Started, Almost There, On My Way)
b) Two-year intensive pre graduation package and program.
c) Health Passport
Transition Rounds every 2 months, with speakers' case presentations

Provision of Transition Services

- Adolescent Medicine to provide direct transition services:
a) psycho-educational groups for both youth and parents
b) Individual interventions for high risk adolescents
c) Creating individual transition plans for high risk youth
d) Provision of adolescent health care (contraception, reproductive counseling, substance use, body image…) through Teen Clinic
e) Web based "My Health Passport"
f) transition website with interactive, educational games, information, links
g) Speak/lead workshops at Transition Days held by individual programs.

Research

1) Perceptions of Transitional Care Needs and Experiences in Paediatric Heart Transplantation—Data collection starting 01/05
2) According to Adult Rheumatolgists: What skills do teens need to navigate the adult system successfully? – Data collection staring 01/06
3) Use of My Health Passport by Adolescents Approaching Transfer to Adult Care. (Proposal to be written by 03/05)
4) Evaluation of Transition Website (will depend on funding sources)
5) Evaluation of Hospital-Wide Transition Program—proposal to be developed in early 2006
6) Readiness for Change tool development – 09/06
7) Survey of current transition practices within Sick Kids – 12/05 to 03/06

Outcomes

- The Shared Management Model of care will be adopted by all programs
- Transition thinking infused into SickKids culture and will become embedded throughout clinical practice
- Increased understanding and awareness of the importance of transition processes in all programs.
- Individual programs will be prepared to offer transition programming to all patients
- Decreased fear and anxiety of youth and parents.
- Improved preparedness of youth and their families for participating in adult system.
- Timely transition of care of all patients.
- Dissemination of research knowledge

Fig. 35.1 Program logic model for SickKids' transition program

Key Components

In 2011 our activities were organized into five service domains. Currently, Good 2 Go includes 2.35 FTE across three personnel. Our primary processes are outlined below:

1. *Direct clinical care of patients and families.* The program provides assessment and transition-related interventions as part of our Good 2 Go Transition Clinic to YSHCN and their families. The clinic accepts referrals from all healthcare providers, including patients with complex transition needs. Clinic staff serve as experts in transition planning and work in conjunction with patients' healthcare teams.
2. *Education and knowledge broker* activities include traditional educational events and workshops to SickKids' staff and their community adult partners on the key components of HCT care. This includes understanding providers' roles in transfer and transition planning and available supporting resources to implement plans. Good 2 Go staff members provide direct education to pediatric patients and their families on transition preparation using game-like activities such as Jenga or Jeopardy. Animations about goal setting, the MyHealth 3-Sentence Summary, and other transition topics are available on YouTube (http://bit.ly/2q3yYfC). Good 2 Go staff also present at local, national, and international conferences. The Good 2 Go website (www.sickkids.ca/good2go) includes resources and information for anyone who can access.
3. *Resource and tool development* service leads the development of tools and resources for patients and healthcare providers designed to be modified and/or embedded to meet specific patient and program needs.
4. *Program development support and consultation.* Good 2 Go uses a "bottom-up" approach—responding to the needs, requests and calls from partners within the hospital. Rarely is a "top-down" model of telling programs or clinics what to do taken. This has allowed us to be cheerleaders, matchmakers, and collaborators in our consulting role, facilitating programs in integrating the resources and tools that have the best chance (or evidence) to support their patients' transition needs. Healthcare providers are matched with other healthcare providers with similar patient populations working on the same transition problems, supporting the development of partnerships with community and adult healthcare sites to provide continuous smooth transfers for patients and families. Good 2 Go team members have served as experts in transition programming to multi-organizational and government level panels/councils developing transition guidelines and best practices (e.g., [2, 3]).
5. *Research and evaluation* activities include planning and implementing evaluation studies of HCT initiatives/tools and transition programs within SickKids and collaborating hospital and community settings.

Program Outcomes and Defining Success

Defining success of the program led to the development of Good 2 Go's resource manual. The resource manual includes descriptions of our past and current activities and related outcomes. We adopted a modified version of Betz and Smith (2011) description of healthcare transition planning outcomes to build our early framework for success [2]. At the time of the first edition in 2012, the push for more cohesive and consistent transition outcome studies and framework were not yet developed [e.g., 4, 5]. The focus was on the impact of Good 2 Go's transition activities in four areas: (1) the learning and acquisition of self-management skills, (2) health-related or disease-specific outcomes, (3) biopsychosocial (and developmental) elements, and (4) process/program components.

As the day-to-day activities of the Good 2 Go Transition Program overlapped across the five service domains, so did the projected outcomes. For example, Good 2 Go supported the development of an intervention we call the transfer clinic. The transfer clinic is loosely defined as an event that involves dedicated time in a clinic to discuss the transition process and pragmatically prepare for the upcoming move to adult healthcare with patients of a specific condition around the age of 17. The elements are customized to the specific condition and include orientation to an adult care site or healthcare provider. Good 2 Go provides guidelines to healthcare providers on how to operate (i.e., tips and planning strategies), transition-focused patient care during transfer clinics, and leads the evaluation (as a quality improvement project) on the patient impact in real-time (post-clinic) and follow-up (post-transfer).

This event is an example of how all four areas of impact/outcomes can be addressed. Patients who attended a transfer clinic report being better prepared, more knowledgeable, and less worried about transfer to adult care (i.e., focus on biopsychosocial elements and learning and acquisition of self-management outcomes). A year after transfer, subsets of patients followed up report feeling well prepared by the transfer clinic and experienced lower nonadherence rates [6] (i.e., health-related or disease-specific outcomes). The growth of the transfer clinic across SickKids is manifest as starting with one transfer clinic in 2009. In 2017, 14 ambulatory programs are offering transfer clinics—that means 14 plus new collaborations with adult clinics. Support of new programs continues through enabling frontline staff to feel empowered to lead transition initiatives. Some programs continue to need less hands-on support from our program over time (i.e., process/ program components). The transfer clinic guidelines are widely disseminated within SickKids and other institutes to allow others to improve with each round and avoid reinventing the wheel. Our model was identified as leading practice through Accreditation Canada (http://bit.ly/2pl64c7) in 2015.

Vignette

Kalee was a patient of the Hospital for Sick Children (SickKids) since before birth. During her mother's pregnancy, Kalee was found to have hypoplastic left heart syndrome. Kalee and her mother were followed by the cardiology program for 18 years.

As expected, most of the initial teaching about her heart condition took place shortly after Kalee's birth and was directed at her parents. Kalee often described SickKids, and the cardiology clinic, as her second home. During her early years as a young child, she made friends with each of the clowns, hung out with the child life specialists, and even attended the Teddy Bear Heart Function Clinics each year. As she began adolescence, she would attend Marnie's Lounge on her own, between appointments when she came for day-long visits, and even attended camps for teens with chronic heart conditions.

Kalee, and her parents, reported being sad about leaving SickKids as her 18th birthday approached, even though Kalee felt she'd outgrown the Hospital for Sick Children. They recognized that Kalee would continue to need lifelong care, and because of the transition planning that took place throughout her 18 years at SickKids, Kalee was ready for the transfer. Most of her transition interventions were subtle and integrated into the care she and her family received. Shortly after she was diagnosed, her mom was introduced to the Help Them Grow… so They're Good 2 Go Timeline to help her envision Kalee growing up to be independent. The timeline stressed that even though Kalee was born with a special healthcare need, she would still be a regular kid in many ways. The timeline provided Kalee's mom with some ideas of ways to teach Kalee about her medical needs, as well as understand general developmental expectations.

Kalee and her mom made her first MyHealth Passport when she entered kindergarten. It was a way for Kalee to let her teachers know about her health condition—she was very proud to give her teachers a copy on the first day of school each year. By the time she was 7, Kalee was able to tell people the name of her condition and make some choices about her healthcare (e.g., which arm to take a blood pressure reading). When she turned 10, her cardiology nurse began spending a few minutes in a solo interaction with Kalee at every visit, to allow Kalee to practice speaking up for herself. By the time she was an adolescent, she was used to answering questions on her own.

In her early adolescent years, Kalee attended the Good 2 Go Transition Clinic for an assessment of her transition needs, as she began to report some worries about leaving SickKids. She completed an assessment, including a summary of her transition readiness which helped identify her HCT needs—Kalee's anxiety was about her lifelong care needs and prognosis. Together with her clinic nurse, she filled in her knowledge gaps, while the Good 2 Go clinic staff taught her to practice some of the skills she would need in adult care. This included learning how to use the MyHealth 3-Sentence Summary at every clinic visit. She even updated her own MyHealth Passport with the help of her mom.

Around age 15, Kalee also attended a cardiology family education event, where members of the Good 2 Go Transition Program played Transition Jeopardy with all the adolescents, and she learned about some of the key differences between pediatric and adult healthcare systems. At 17, she attended a transfer education clinic during which she learned more about what to expect at her adult cardiology program and even met a young adult graduate who went through a similar transfer. She went on a tour of the adult clinic to learn where to go at her first adult appointment. Before she left, Kalee was provided with some resources on Planning Your Future, with specific information on how to prepare for university with a chronic health condition. Finally, as Kalee approached 18, her cardiology clinic team celebrated her graduation, providing her with a copy of her discharge note, transfer checklist, and a graduation certificate with everyone's signatures. Each of these tools and moments in her care at SickKids prepared Kalee, and her parents, for her entry into adult care. She knows her transition will continue even after transfer, and she's Good 2 Go.

Facilitators for Success

The success and sustainability of the Good 2 Go Program is due to multiple factors: financial support by SickKids leadership to pay for personnel, to provide these individuals with creative freedom to meet the transition needs of patients, to develop and distribute tools, and to provide training and mentorship to current staff, new staff, and inter-professional trainees. There was a rigorous feedback loop between Good 2 Go patient and family alumni, each contributed ideas and compliments, and then shared their experiences to improve the program. Finally, enthusiasm and the cohesion of the core team members over the years have been invaluable.

Innovations in Action

The transition program strives to remain innovative by keeping up with the literature and exchanging ideas with other professionals doing HCT work. Promoting the adoption of our resources (rather than reinventing the wheel) and asking for permission to use others' ideas lead to the rapid spread of best practices. It has also been important that the program does not always take leadership of local groups aiming to improve transition quality. For example, Good 2 Go chooses to *contribute to* a network of professionals (in downtown Toronto's adult hospitals) who are interested in transitions and the emerging adult, rather than leading or taking responsibility for the group's function and goals.

Program practices have been described through peer-reviewed publications, an example being the THRxEADS interview model, in that transitions-related questions are added to the traditional HEADS interview for YSHCN [7]. Others practices have been shared, without a formal evaluation, such as MyHealth 3-Sentence Summary (the idea that adolescents can learn to present their health history to a new healthcare provider in the same way that medical trainees present to their supervisors). Validation of these processes is needed.

We worked with an inpatient unit for several years to establish robust transition interventions. This started with kidney and liver transplant patients and has spread to other populations. The most recent addition is evening groups that employ some of our more fun techniques (Transition Jeopardy, Transition Jenga, Kahoot). The feedback has been excellent and the nurses on this ward now feel comfortable leading the groups without help. It would be wonderful to be able to use a simulation lab to help patients go through situations they will encounter in the adult healthcare system. However, simulations are expensive. Instead, we are introducing quasi-simulation called the alien test. We ask patients, "If your parents were kidnapped by aliens, what would you do to get more medications before you have taken all the ones you have?" We then help them, with prompts, work through this process, with the critical steps being knowledge of medication names and doses, recognition of refills, prescriber of refills, pharmacy contact information, transportation to pharmacy, and payment. In a quality improvement project using this tool, patients all needed at least one prompt. On the whole, they felt more confident about getting their medications. We were able to engage a medical resident to take this idea on as part of a 1-month research project to evaluate if the alien test could work. More importantly, this example emphasizes how we work to influence the next generation of medical practitioners to become transition leaders.

Next Steps

Our immediate plans are to disseminate two smartphone apps in the next year, to get the word out about our hospital's new transition policy, and to continue creating resources and programs for young people and families with the biggest transition obstacles including those with complex medical issues that, up until recently, have been exclusively pediatrics issues or for young people with autism and other developmental delays. There are challenges ahead. Every year at budget time, we worry that transition will be seen as last year's issue, or not as important as some other program, and that we will experience a major and massive cut to our program. We work hard to prove our worth to our institution on a regular basis to keep funding available. We know that we are still far from our goal of having every one of our patients fully prepared to leave our hospital by age 18, but we move closer every day. Table 35.2 contains tips for starting and sustaining a transition program and Table 35.3 contains favorite innovations, impacts, and moments from the Good 2 Go Program.

Table 35.2 Tips for a starting and sustaining a transition program (lessons learned)

• Embrace new people—gaps in personnel are challenging, yet, often new great people and ideas join the HCT team—even if just temporary. The same goes for students, trainees, and mentorship opportunities
• It's ok to toot your own horn—if you are doing great transition-related work, spread the word so that others can learn from your successes (and failures) along the way
• Collaborate on ideas and don't think you can do it all alone. Let others lead projects, even if you are the expert—everyone is the expert in something.
• Small things count and small wins add up. Even if you want to change everything, start with something small
• Have dedicated time to recoup as a team and frequently. While each team member will have their pet project, everyone needs to work together
• Be creative, be a kid, have fun, and keep it positive. Every game can become a transition game. Celebrate achievements of patients (and providers) along the way with graduation ceremonies, certificates, and thank you cards!
• When starting to work with a new program, engage as large a group as possible and continue being totally inclusive (both staff and families), rather than investing in only supporting one champion. If that champion leaves, so can all the work and great changes

Table 35.3 Favorite innovations, impacts, and moments

• In 2012, Good 2 Go celebrated its 5-year anniversary celebration with a day-long symposium. We nominated five transition champions, including our very own Miriam Kaufman, to her surprise
• The contacts, collaborations, and matchmaking that have happened over the years between pediatric and adult healthcare providers
• Leading others to be champions
• Awarded funding to support the further development of our transition fun platform in an inpatient unit and sharing it with our transition colleagues at the chronic illness and disability conference in Houston 2016
• Good 2 Go contributed as experts to various provincial and national guidelines, position statements, and clinical pathways. The development of the first Canadian national guidelines for transition from pediatric to adult healthcare for youth with special healthcare needs (https://goo.gl/oUDPZz) was a great feat in 2016 (i.e., [3])
• The first quasi-simulation alien test was executed as a quality improvement study with promising results and presented at congress for International Pediatric Transplant Association in 2017
• Expanding and building our network of collaborators to include community programs and government organizations. This supports the release of our newest documents for families, specifically for parents of youth with complex care needs, and emerging adults entitled Planning Your Future (www.sickkids.ca/planningmyfuture)

References

1. Kieckhefer GM, Trahms CM. Supporting development of children with chronic conditions: from compliance toward shared management. Pediatr Nurs. 2000;26(4):354–63.
2. Betz C, Smith K. Measuring health care transition planning outcomes: challenges and issues. Int J Child Adolesc health. 2011;3(4):463–72.
3. Guideline Development Group, CAPHC National Transitions Community of Practice (2016). A guideline for transition from paediatric to adult health care for youth with special health care needs: a national approach. https://goo.gl/oUDPZz.
4. Prior M, McManus M, White P, Davidson L. Measuring the "Triple Aim" in transition care: a systematic review. Pediatrics. 2014;134(6):e1648–61. https://doi.org/10.1542/peds.2014-1704.
5. Suris J-C, Akre C. Key elements for, and indicators of, a successful transition: an international delphi study. J Adolesc Health. 2014;56(6):612–8.
6. McQuillan RF, Toulany A, Kaufman M, Schiff JR. Benefits of a transfer clinic in adolescent and young adult kidney transplant patients. Can J Kidney Health Dis. 2015;2(1):45. https://doi.org/10.1186/s40697-015-0081-6.
7. Chadi N, Amaria K, Kaufman M. Expand your HEADS, follow the THRxEADS! Paediatrics & Child Health. 2017;22(8):23–5. https://doi.org/10.1093/pch/pxw0075.

36 Different Healthcare Transition Models

Cecily L. Betz

Introduction

Beginning nearly three decades ago, the changing survival rates of children diagnosed with special healthcare needs (CSHCN) and disabilities were forecasted to bring about significant changes in the care models to meet their service needs [1]. In response, experimental models of care were developed to support this new generation of CSHCN who were growing into adulthood [2]. Since then, the tentative stages of early service development have progressed at an accelerated pace with the development, implementation, and testing of HCT service models [3–7]. Currently, limited evidence exists regarding interventions to effect successful HCT outcomes; however, a growing body of research and consensus opinion are available to guide the development of models considered to exemplify best practices [8–14].

This chapter will begin with an examination of the recommended structural components to include in the development of healthcare transition service models. Service components of HCT models of care that have been described in the literature will be presented. A discussion of the processes involved with HCT, which are based upon the frameworks of HCT care reported in the literature, will follow. Depending on the service model, the process of service delivery differs in terms of the selection and integration of structural components. A discussion of the expected and proposed outcomes of HCT care will be presented, and the chapter will conclude with an analysis of the current state of model development.

Key Structural Components of Different Models

To date, position statements authored by the major pediatric professional organizations have provided the guidance for the early development of HCT service models [8–11, 13, 14]. Although there is widespread recognition of the limitations of the HCT models given their preliminary stages of development, there is an emerging body of evidence to support the inclusion of structural components as integral to this service model evolvement. The key HCT structural components that will be discussed are the Adoption of HCT Guidelines/Protocol of Care, Period of Preparation, Transfer/Transition Readiness Assessment, Care Coordination, Healthcare Transition Coordinator, Medical Summary, Healthcare Transition Plan, Ongoing Instructional and Self-Management Support, and Evaluation of Outcomes. These structural components often require adaptation to

C. L. Betz, Ph.D., R.N.
Department of Pediatrics, University of Southern California (USC), Keck School of Medicine, Los Angeles, CA, USA

USC University Center for Excellence in Developmental Disabilities, Children's Hospital Los Angeles, Los Angeles, CA, USA
e-mail: cbetz@chla.usc.edu

A. C. Hergenroeder, C. M. Wiemann (eds.), *Health Care Transition*,
https://doi.org/10.1007/978-3-319-72868-1_36

appropriately meet the needs of specific diagnostic groups of adolescents and young adults with special healthcare needs (AYASHCN) [6, 15].

Adoption of HCT Guidelines/Protocol of Care. Ideally, the guidelines or protocol of HCT services to be delivered over the program preparation period serves as the template for implementation. Position statements authored by specialty organizations (i.e., American Academy of Pediatrics, Society of Pediatric Nurses) are available for guidance in the development of a program-specific service for a diagnostic group of AYASHCN or for institutional-wide policies and procedures as presented in Table 36.1 [9, 10]. Other resources for HCT pro-

Table 36.1 Resources to consult for the development of HCT protocols/clinical guidelines

Resource	Description	Key structural elements
Clinical Report-Supporting the Health Care Transition from Adolescence to Adulthood in the Medical Home (AAP, 2012)	Depicts an algorithm to assist pediatricians with the development of guidelines/protocol that can be adapted to their programmatic needs	• Initiate HCT plan at age 12 years • Start HCT planning at age 14 years • HCT is individualized and written based upon identified needs beginning at age 14 and expanded as needed • Plan is reviewed regularly and updated • Readiness assessments are conducted • Transfer of care occurs when pediatric eligibility terminates
2016 Society of Pediatric Nurses Transition Position Statement	Provides a framework for the development of a HCT protocol, which is nursing-focused based upon an interdisciplinary model of care	• *Extended HCT preparation (age 12)*: This preparation involves nurses and interdisciplinary colleagues with the expertise in the comprehensive biopsychosocial needs of all adolescents as they move from pediatric-focused care to emerging adult and adult provider systems • *Transfer of care period*: The process of execution will begin prior to the transition to adult care, and the intensity of the execution process will increase as plans progress • *Post healthcare transition/transfer of care*: Although pediatric nurses do not generally provide direct care for young adults following the transfer of care, there are several important considerations to be addressed following the transfer to adult care to ensure successful outcomes
Six Core Elements of Health Care Transition 2.0	Provides a framework for guidance to assist with the development of a HCT service program	• Transition policy • Transition tracking and monitoring • Transition readiness • Transition planning • Transfer of care • Transfer completion
6 Key elements and 1 Indicator (Suris & Are, 2015)	Provide guidance with the development of HCT service models in terms of conceptualizing the components of the service model to foster the successful HCT	• Patient not lost to follow-up (indicator) • Assuring a good coordination between pediatric and adult professionals (key element) • Starting planning transition at an early age (key element) • Discussing with patient and family about self-management (key element) • Including young person's views and preferences to the planning of transition (key element) • If developmentally appropriate, seeing the adolescent alone at least for part of the consultation (key element) • Identifying an adult provider willing to take on the young patient before transfer (key element)

gram development found in Table 36.1 include the Six Core Elements of Health Care Transition 2.0 [16] and the HCT framework developed by Suris and Akre that identifies six key elements and indicators considered essential for a HCT program and demonstrative of its success [12].

Period of Preparation. All HCT service models incorporate a period of preparation. The service interval for HCT preparation depends on the structural components and the process of the model design. Some models concentrate on the transfer of care with a short-term focus compared to those whose focus is more divergent, that is, directed toward other facets of healthcare transition planning. Examples of the latter include the *Movin On Up*, *Center for Youth and Adults with Conditions of Childhood* model, and a transitional program for youth with juvenile idiopathic arthritis [17–21]. Pediatric professional organizations recommend that the preparation period be initiated in early adolescence, between the ages of 12 and 14 years [9, 10]. One model suggests initiation of HCT planning at nearly 10 years of age [17]. Programs with longer preparation periods incorporate a life span approach extending from early adolescence to emerging adulthood. Preparation programs that emphasize the transfer of care are less focused on other developmental considerations and are generally 2 years or less in duration [3–7, 22, 23].

Transfer/Transition Readiness Assessment. For many AYASHCN who receive specialty care in a pediatric medical center, there is an inevitable future date wherein interdisciplinary services are terminated as insurance coverage ends. Termination of insurance plan eligibility varies, with public insurance coverage ending between 18 and 21 years of age and private insurance coverage ending at age 26 (see Chaps. 8, 23, 24, and 25). Hospital policies concerning the termination of the provision of care for AYASHCN who lose insurance may differ among selected specialty care departments within the same institution.

Some programs use age as the determining factor for transfer timing, typically between 18 and 21 years; other programs transfer care based upon significant life events, such as marriage or pregnancy, that legally enable younger adolescents who have not yet reached the state's age of majority to become the decision-maker [3–5, 11]. Other programs recommend the transfer to adult care based on a more comprehensive approach that involves formalized assessment of readiness and/or determination of the AYASHCN's maturity [14, 24–26]. Various readiness assessment tools available are described in Chap. 13. These measures are generally used to evaluate areas in which greater transition preparation is needed. Some experts have advocated for HCT planning to begin early in adolescence for those with complex medical needs such as AYASHCN with severe seizures or spina bifida, wherein the meaning of readiness does not infer an immediacy or soon-to-be-anticipated transfer of care [3, 17, 27] but rather a long-term process of knowledge and skill attainment [3, 17, 27]. The ultimate goal of all HCT preparation programs, whatever the model, is to facilitate the AYASHCN's adaptation to a new system of care and transition into a stage of development with higher-order competencies to function as independently and productively as possible [24].

Transition readiness refers to a defined set of generic and fundamental skills/knowledge that AYASHCN should possess prior to transferring to adult care such as making physician appointments, knowing the names of medications, and communicating with their healthcare providers. An important element of the transfer of care is the identification of self-management skills and knowledge that the AYA may still need to learn to be as self-sufficient and self-reliant as possible [8–10].

Self-management, which is the ability to manage the tasks associated with the daily care needs of the AYASHCN, is an essential self-care competency that must be achieved. The self-management skills and knowledge needed to be as feasibly independent as possible will be dependent on the level of involvement of the SHCN, the type of SHCN, and the functional capacity of the AYA, which includes cognitive level of functioning and gross and fine motor skills. Healthcare self-management not only involves the most fundamental tasks associated with daily management of the condition but also the array of competencies needed to be a health-literate and health-competent consumer [17].

A number of condition-specific self-management tools to assess self-management knowledge and skills exist (see Chap. 13 for a more thorough description of available measures). For example, the Epilepsy Self-Management Scale (ESMS), with established psychometric properties, measures epilepsy self-management [28, 29]. The Adolescent/Young Adult Self-Management and Independence Scale II with demonstrated reliability and validity has been used with adolescents and emerging adults (ages 12–25 years) with spina bifida to measure self-management as it pertains to their condition and independent living [30, 31]. Tools measuring self-management knowledge and skills of AYA with type 1 diabetes, HIV, and arthritis have been reported [32–34].

Instruction enables AYA with SHCN to become more informed and competent as healthcare consumers, which is pivotal to functioning as independently and productively as possible as adults [35]. For parents, preparatory instruction not only provides them with the HCT knowledge and skill building they may need to be effective advocates but also to be a navigator for their son or daughter [36].

Care Coordination. As the Agency for Healthcare Research and Quality states: "Care coordination involves deliberately organizing patient care activities and sharing information among all of the participants concerned with a patient's care to achieve safer and more effective care" [37]. Care coordination, which can be provided by any discipline, is essential to the provision of comprehensive HCT services. Community-based pediatric care based upon a medical home model provides care coordination services (Table 36.1; see also Chap. 26). Beginning with their diagnosis, most AYASHCN require services from an interdisciplinary team. This requires care coordination, which intensifies during HCT planning and transfer. A HCT coordinator is pivotal to ensure the uninterrupted transfer of care and referrals to community-based systems of care for AYASHCN [7, 9, 10, 19, 20, 27, 38–41] (see Table 36.2). Care coordination activities include (a) continuous assessment of needs, (b) reevaluation of services provided based on emerging needs, (c) facilitating communication among team members and among team members and AYASHCN and their parents/guardians, (d) ensuring referrals are completed, (e) providing ongoing instructional and self-management support, and (f) serving as an informational resource.

Healthcare Transition Coordinator. The HCT coordinator [3, 5, 10, 17, 20, 25, 38–40, 42, 43] is

Table 36.2 Role responsibilities of healthcare transition coordinator

• Serves as the lead for the development of the HCT policy
• Ensures team members are cognizant and supportive of HCT policy
• Identifies the needs for HCT program materials/resources
• Designates (when possible) individuals responsible for creating resources; assists with the development of resources
• Coordinates the assessment of transition readiness
• Coordinates the ongoing assessment of self-management knowledge and skills
• Serves as the lead for healthcare transition planning
• Facilitates the development of the written healthcare transition plan
• Formulates with team members realistic timeframe for goal achievement
• Continuously monitors needs for HCT services and supports
• Serves as the liaison/contact person for the AYA with SHCN and family pertaining to HCT
• Updates the HCT Plan as needed
• Implements a plan to evaluate the outcomes of care
• Serves as the liaison among HCT team members to facilitate communication pertaining to changes in AYA status; scheduling
• Facilitates care coordination that involves clinical, biopsychosocial, and educational needs
• Facilitates service referrals to transition and adult agencies; systems of care
• Facilitates the transfer of care procedure
• Ensures that each AYA whose care is transferred has medical summary
• Works with financial administrator to obtain reimbursement for services
• Develops and implements quality improvement projects to assess outcomes of services [6, 8, 15, 36]

responsible for coordinating the clinical evaluations and recommendations of HCT team members into a HCT plan of care that integrates diverse perspectives and input based upon the needs of the AYASHCN and family. The HCT coordinator is typically responsible for ensuring that referrals for services and supports are made, identified needs for instruction are provided, and benchmarks achieved or to be achieved are noted [17, 26, 43]. To illustrate, in a patient with spina bifida who is also obese, the physical therapist recommends increasing physical activities and exercise and offers a listing of community-based adaptive sports and exercise programs. The dietician's recommendations pertain to workable weight management strategies the AYA and family have discussed. The HCT coordinator will ensure that (a) PT has provided the AYA and parent with the list of available community-based programs and has reviewed the offerings listed with them, (b) the AYA and parent are encouraged to contact the clinic office if obstacles are encountered with contacting these programs, (c) PT follows up with the AYA and parent as to the recommendation made during the previous clinic visit, adjustments are made as needed, (d) the dietician provides contact information should questions/issues arise, and (e) dietician is scheduled to follow up with the status of weight management goals. The HCT coordinator serves as the primary team member responsible for monitoring and updating the plan, as needed.

Importantly, the HCT coordinator serves as the liaison to the AYA and family for issues encountered during the planning process, informational needs, and requests for additional service referrals. The HCT coordinator is viewed as the designated resource for the transfer of care, access to transition, and adult-related services as well as the conduit for questions pertaining to interdisciplinary and interagency services and supports. Updates on AYA and family issues and benchmarks of achievement are noted by the HCT coordinator and transmitted to other team members for updates and possible informational input to relay back to the AYA and family. A listing of HCT coordinator positional responsibilities is presented in Table 36.2.

Medical Summary. A transition medical summary is a concise synopsis of the AYA's medical history and current plan of care for the receiving adult provider/team members [5, 9–11, 14, 25]. An informative medical summary contains the following content: (a) diagnosis and its date of confirmation; (b) condition severity and level of involvement based upon provider's estimate/predetermined criteria; (c) comorbidities; (d) previous surgeries including type(s) and date(s); (e) previous ED visits including reasons and dates; (f) previous hospitalizations including reason (s) and date (s); (g) history of complication(s)/relapse(s); (h) medications, dosage, frequency, and administration mode; (i) daily treatments required for management (i.e., catheterization, postural drainage); (j) use of assistive devices (i.e., braces); (k) special diets, use of formulas, and total parental nutrition; (l) allergies; (m) measurements (i.e., BMI); (n) vital signs; and (o) contact information of HCT coordinator and members of pediatric team. A number of medical summary formats are available (see Table 36.3).

Healthcare Transition Plan. The HCT plan serves as a road map during preparation for HCT (described below). The plan begins with an assessment of needs and future plans, which then guides the development of the plan [9, 10, 17, 26]. Depending on the scope of services provided in the HCT program, those that focus on the transfer of care will formulate plans with AYA and, as appropriate, other family members. Identification of the adult primary and specialty providers who have the expertise and experience to provide the necessary services to the AYASHCN is a priority. Depending on the transfer structure arrangements, such as a joint HCT service clinic, the HCT plan may include details as to the coordination of joint care management (see *Pediatric-Adult Provider Transfer Models of Care*, below).

The plan should include maintaining or acquiring access to a health insurance plan that meets the AYASHCN's needs. Prior to the transfer of care, arrangements for supplies and durable medical equipment vendors should be made. Requisitions for durable medical equipment, i.e., wheelchairs, assistive devices (i.e., walkers,

Table 36.3 Examples of medical summaries

Medical summaries	
American College of Rheumatology	Medical Summary and Emergency Care Plan: Juvenile Idiopathic Arthritis https://www.rheumatology.org/Portals/0/Files/Medical-Summary-JIA.pdf
American College of Rheumatology	Medical Summary and Emergency Care Plan: Systemic Lupus Erythematosus (SLE) https://www.rheumatology.org/Portals/0/Files/Medical-Summary-SLE.pdf
Carolina Health and Transition (CHAT)	Alliance of Disability Advocates, Center for Independent Living, Raleigh, North Carolina http://sys.mahec.net/media/brochures/youth_guide.pdf
Got Transition?	Sample Medical Summary and Emergency Care Plan Six Core Elements of Health Care Transition 2.0 http://www.gottransition.org/resourceGet.cfm?id=227
Healthcare Information and Management Systems Society (HIMSS). Type I and Type II diabetes ©2012	Clinical Summary for New Health Care Team http://s3.amazonaws.com/rdcms-himss/files/production/public/HIMSSorg/Content/files/SampleFormClinicalSummaryTransitionNewHealthCareTeam.pdf
MyHealth Passport	SickKids Hospital website https://www.sickkids.ca/myhealthpassport/

crutches), and braces, may be needed to avert unnecessary delays in obtaining replacements if the equipment is no longer usable.

HCT programs that are more comprehensive incorporate other transitions to future planning, including postsecondary education/training; job development and placement; community living planning such as housing, civic responsibilities, public transportation, and recreational programs; and social relationships and programs. Additional content on the process involved with comprehensive models of care is presented in the section entitled *Comprehensive Model of Care*.

Ongoing Instruction, Self-management, and Support. The discussion begins with instructional needs for parents and AYASHCN and then self-management as it intensifies during HCT planning and concludes with the use of transition readiness assessments.

Parental support can be provided to caregivers as they undergo the process of role and responsibility changes [9, 10, 36]. The parent's role as the person responsible for the care and/or oversight of their children's care evolves to a role of relinquishing some or all of their parental caregiving responsibilities [44–48]. Surveys have identified parent learning needs pertaining to transition and adult-related services and programs that their children will eventually access in order to be better informed and helpful to their children [36, 49]. Although reaching out to parents has been identified as a component of care, scant efforts to provide programmatic support during the HCT process have been identified [36, 50, 51].

In studies exploring AYA's instructional needs, issues pertaining to information about the transition process, the availability of adult services, and the additional information about their condition have been identified by AYA [35]. Although, HCT programs report instructional assistance provided to AYASHCN, it is unclear as to the type, scope, and effectiveness of instruction provided. Preparatory instruction for AYA has been identified as an area of need to be addressed in HCT programs. Although recommendations have been suggested in terms of peer support programs to assist AYA during this period of HCT, few have been implemented and validated [35, 44, 52, 53].

Key Processes that Define Different Models

There are two predominant HCT delivery models: the transfer vs. transition models. The transfer model has a narrow focus: the transfer of care from pediatric to adult healthcare systems, including primary and specialty care. The transition model is broader in scope. Its aim is to not only facilitate the transfer of care to the adult healthcare system but to address the other domains of emerging adulthood. Recently published systematic reviews have noted that most studies examining HCT models of care have focused primarily on the transfer of care to adult providers [1, 3, 12, 21, 22, 27, 56].

Comprehensive Model of Care. A framework of several HCT service models reported is based upon a comprehensive model of care [4–7, 54]. These models incorporate a broader perspective: facilitating the transfer of care and transition to adulthood. The HCT preparation period of comprehensive models of care is usually longer; it may extend from early adolescence to emerging adulthood, distinguishing the transfer of care as an event in contrast to the process of healthcare transition planning [3, 5, 6].

Comprehensive models of care are based upon a life span approach that addresses the biopsychosocial and developmental needs of AYASHCN. A comprehensive HCT model acknowledges that AYASHCN needs permeate all aspects of living and, therefore, require attention to other domains including educational, employment, social, and community living [15, 54].

The scope and breadth of comprehensive service models are dependent upon the resources and support within the healthcare setting and in the community of choice of the AYASHCN and their family. For example, the scope of interdisciplinary (ID) services in a tertiary level pediatric healthcare setting will differ from services in a rural setting. There may be limited job training and employment opportunities for AYASHCN in rural compared to urban settings. Other alternatives can be considered such as local volunteer experiences, informal networking with family and friends, as well as online training programs.

Initiation of a comprehensive HCT program takes time and can be done incrementally. The development of the capacity to provide comprehensive services is a process requiring ongoing time and effort. The development of a HCT program plan that includes the framework for implementation with benchmarks to be achieved as identified in the tables of this chapter will ultimately facilitate the achievement of its mission and goal.

Based upon a comprehensive HCT approach, self-management instruction is not solely focused on the fundamental tasks and knowledge required for daily SHCN care. Self-management instruction attends to other lived experiences that the AYASHCN encounter that are affected by the chronic condition. For example, instruction on acquiring the health-related accommodations needed in the educational settings is provided to ensure the student receives the support needed to perform academically [11].

Instruction about the provision of health-related accommodations in schools includes advocacy training for parents/guardians and AYASHCN about obtaining needed health-related accommodations. The HCT coordinator would review the adolescent's current IEP or 504 plan in terms of what is currently being provided and what may be needed. Also, the HCT coordinator would be expected to provide instruction to the AYASHCN and parents/guardians about the student's legal rights and protections pertaining to receiving additional services and supports at school as illustrated in the case example at the end of the chapter.

Comprehensive models of care continuously explore AYASHCN needs for advocacy, service and support referrals, and instruction as it pertains to their lived experiences and future planning. For example, youth employment could be explored at age 16 years. Participation in youth employment programs is associated with positive psychosocial outcomes [55, 56]. Additionally youth employment programs provide AYASHCN with preparatory job training and experiences in a supportive and supervised environment as the students will be trained by job coaches who, in many instances, will be coordinating these efforts with school personnel. HCT coordinators are in an ideal position given their understanding of the health-related services and supports needed for employment purposes to make referrals to youth employment programs that include these job training and placement experiences.

Other activities related to employment options include counseling AYA on their rights and protections as an interview applicant to address issues of disclosure concerning their condition. Anticipatory guidance can be provided about employment issues concerning provision of workplace accommodations, workplace resources, and dealing with coworkers and supervisors. These long-term recommendations enhance AYA efforts to obtain employment.

These selected examples of services provided illustrate the scope and depth of HCT planning offered in comprehensive models of care. The extent to which comprehensive services can be provided will depend on the resources available not only within the healthcare setting but also within the community itself.

Pediatric-Adult Provider Transfer Models of Care. There are differences between the pediatric and adult systems of healthcare, including the family-centered model in pediatrics compared to patient-centered model in adult care [26, 57]. For additional content on the service delivery differences between these two systems of care, refer to Chap. 15.

Training and clinical practice concerns pertaining to the provision of care during HCT have been identified in studies of pediatric and adult providers. Pediatricians and adult providers identify the limitations of their training for AYASHCN and hence their hesitancy to provide services to this growing population [57]. Pediatricians identify gaps in their training and clinical practice pertaining to HCT planning best practices.

The competencies and comfort level of adult providers to provide care to AYASHCN have been described [58]. Furthermore, adult providers have AYASHCN referred to them as ill-prepared healthcare consumers [59].

The limitations of knowledge and clinical acumen of providers of both systems of care are not confined to provision of primary and specialty care services. It also involves knowledge of community resources and other health-related services such as therapy, durable equipment and medical supply vendors, and disability advocacy organizations. It also involves knowledge of when to confer with interdisciplinary colleagues to initiate referrals for services and adult community-based agencies that can provide assistance for psychosocial development and the competencies associated with the emerging adult [26, 60, 61]. Capacity building of providers on both ends of the bridge of two very different service models is needed to improve care [26].

The goal of the transfer of care process is to eliminate the potential for discontinuity with the provision of care and to ensure the receiving primary care and specialty adult providers are receptive, professionally competent, and well informed about the AYA's past medical history and treatment needs [4, 11, 15]. The importance of the transfer of care has been emphasized in position statements of pediatric, pediatric and adult consensus, and interdisciplinary organizations. The transfer of care to an adult system of healthcare is the centerpiece of the healthcare transition model. The methodology of implementing the transfer event has been operationalized differently in various models reported. Table 36.4 displays different models for the transfer of care.

These transfers of care models include shared service with both the pediatric and adult providers for a time-limited interval [11, 25], occurring in the pediatric setting pre-transfer or post-transfer in the adult setting [62]. A variation of the formal joint service model is combined meetings with pediatric and adult providers including AYA with SHCN and parents present [28]. Some programs have shared services pre- and post-transfer in both settings [23, 63]. A comparable model has been developed involving nurses from the pediatric and adult teams who provide joint services to AYA with epilepsy [64]. An expansion of the medically-oriented shared services is the "joint working" collaboration involving pediatric and adult care providers from various service systems of care-interagency colleagues with whom one is not accustomed to working (i.e., job developers and rehabilitation specialists) [64].

Another model is the intermediate transfer from pediatrics to an adolescent/young adult clinic prior to final transfer to adult services [32, 65, 66]. Other models locate adult providers on a

Table 36.4 Transfer of care models

Program	Providers involved	Transfer protocol
Cadario et al. (2009)	HCT coordinator; pediatric and adult endocrinologists	1. Joint pediatric and adult endocrinologist last visit in pediatric care 2. Summary report given to AYA and adult MD 3. Joint pediatric and adult endocrinologist first visit in adult care
Hankins et al. (2012)	Pediatric hematology nurse case manager	1. Tour of adult clinic and meet members of adult hematology team 2. Lunch with pediatric team to discuss issues pertaining to transfer of care and transition 3. RN case manager schedules appointment with hematology adult services
Hazel et al. (2010)	Nursing	1. Transfer letter sent to adult rheumatologist 2. Youth (between 17 and 19 years of age) are responsible for making appointment 3. Nursing monitors until transfer is complete
Holmes-Walker et al. (2007)	HCT coordinator (diabetes educator)	1. Transfer of care from pediatric to young adult clinic (YAC) prior to final transfer to adult services 2. YAC based in adult hospital 3. Telephone reminders 4. Missed appointments rebooked 5. After hours telephonic support
Pyatak et al. (2017)	Pediatric and young adult case managers (public health background)	1. Transfer from pediatric clinic to young adult diabetes clinic (up to 30 years of age) 2. Received reminder calls for clinic visits and follow-ups pertaining to clinic attendance
Steinbeck et al. (2015)	HCT coordinator	1. Provided hard copy and flash drive of transfer information including adult providers, diabetes resources; letter of referral 2. Scheduled appointment with adult provider 3. Structured series of calls to follow up on adult appointment
Vanelli et al. (2004)	Pediatric and adult MDs	1. Information about the forthcoming transfer of care provided at 18 years and older 2. 1st joint peds/adult visit in pediatric care 3. 2nd joint peds/adult visit in adult care

less formalized basis [8–10, 14, 25] wherein the AYA is referred to the adult provider without any prior contact. In one transfer program, the AYA is expected to assume the responsibility for making the appointment [67], whereas in another model, the HCT coordinator is responsible for coordinating the transfer of care [68].

There is general agreement that transfer of care should be a formalized and structured process [4, 11]. An important feature, although not always possible, is to have ongoing professional communication between the transfer teams based upon mutual commitment and collaboration [15]. Effective channels of communication are predicated on forming partnerships with providers in the community, which requires additional time and effort between service centers/providers. However, the pediatric-adult partnerships described here can be more difficult for larger medical centers that draw populations of AYASHCN from larger catchment areas. In these situations, an emerging adult may live far beyond the catchment area of the pediatric medical center, and forming professional linkages with adult providers in their community may be difficult for the pediatric specialty program. In other circumstances, the emerging adult may move to another state to attend college or for employment, economic, or social reasons, creating additional challenges to locating adult primary and specialty care providers.

HCT Program Outcomes

The measurement of HCT program outcomes has been a challenge. The majority of outcomes reported are service-oriented rather than

AYA-oriented. Additionally, examination of the outcomes associated with HCT has been predominately focused on those associated with the transfer event such as clinic attendance, avoidable emergency department visits, and hospitalizations [6, 69, 70].

HCT outcomes are categorized into two primary types: disease specific and non-disease specific [6]. As several systematic reviews of the literature demonstrate, the predominant outcome type reported to date is disease-specific [3, 66], including biomedical measures and use of clinical services, such as hospitalization rates and emergency department use. Non-disease outcomes include demographic data (i.e., race, age, gender) and psychosocial variables (patient activation, self-efficacy, employment, postsecondary enrollment) and those related to the transfer of care event (i.e., age of transfer, AYA self-report, clinic attendance, rates of retention).

Examples of biomedical indices used to measure HCT outcomes include A1C levels [32, 71], tacrolimus levels [42], and other indices of health status such as blood pressure and adverse consequences of congenital adrenal hyperplasia [72]. Transition outcomes suggested for monitoring adolescents with hemophilia are bleeding episodes, joint functioning, and adherence to factor replacement regimen [73]. Several studies reporting on the transfer of care of AYA with solid transplants have examined transplant loss and rejection as HCT outcomes [74, 75]. The biomedical indices serve as proxy measurements of adherence behaviors and uninterrupted access to adult care [3, 6, 42, 69]. Examination of disease-specific outcomes has limitations as the findings may not be generalizable.

Outcomes with generic focus have more applicability [3, 69]. The most frequently studied non-condition indices are clinic attendance [6], patient satisfaction [21, 42, 76, 77], and quality of life [6, 42, 78]. Few studies have examined outcomes associated with postsecondary education, employment, housing, or rates of marriage/partnerships with significant others [69, 79, 80] due in part to the emphasis on the transfer of care [3, 6, 80]. The paucity of research investigating psychosocial outcomes is due in part to the lack of theoretical frameworks used as the basis for the study [2, 3, 12, 16, 66, 81, 82]. There is also a lack of consistency with the time intervals selected to measure the outcomes of HCT services. A recent systematic review reported that measurement of study outcomes ranged from 3 to 24 months [4]. However, many challenges exist with tracking AYASHCN into other systems of care, and include loss to follow-up, assignment of new identifiers that prohibit tracking, and the costs associated with long-term tracking [4, 6].

Limitations of the Science

Limitations of the aforementioned research include:

- Lack of rigorous designs as few randomized control designs were cited [3–6, 70, 80, 81].
- Small convenience samples with insufficient power for analysis [4].
- A lack of consistency with the operationalization of the construct of transfer of care.
- Insufficient details provided about the interventions make it difficult to understand intervention effects [3–6, 70, 80, 81] and synthesize findings across studies [26].
- Few intervention models incorporate technology; unlike previous generations, this generation of AYASHCN is accustomed to and often prefers it [15].

Also noted was the testing of the models themselves as the interventions were complex and were not adequately tested. Each of the studies reviewed incorporated multidimensional interventions that were not sufficiently tested as to program effects [4, 70]. Most of the reviews on the transfer of care focus on specialty care; few have explored the transfer of primary care [4]. Even fewer studies have explored issues pertaining to other populations of youth such as those with mental health problems [26, 80]. Importantly, the use of measurements that are reliable and valid has not been consistently evident in the studies conducted as reported in the HCT systematic reviews [3–6, 70, 83] nor has the time frame for evaluating outcomes [6].

Future studies will need to address the issues and limitations identified to create the evidence needed for HCT intervention models. The reviews and critical analyses provide a guide to designing more rigorous and methodologically sound research needed to advance the field of practice and science.

Case Example

David and his mother come to the Spina Bifida Clinic several months after his corrective bilateral foot surgery as he has been followed postoperatively in the orthopedic clinic by the orthopedic surgeon. During his recovery period, he has been homeschooled as he was to stay off his feet. The HCT coordinator meets with David and his mother to monitor how his postoperative recovery is progressing as well as the academic and health-related accommodations he is currently receiving while being homeschooled.

Prior to his foot surgery, the HCT coordinator had conferred with David and his mother about the forthcoming accommodations he would need while recuperating at home. The HCT coordinator reminded them that the school is required to provide the academic accommodations he needs in order to keep up with his schoolwork. The HCT coordinator explained the accommodations David would need during his postoperative recovery while at home: (a) home visits by one of the high school teachers assigned to work with students who have homeschooling and (b) provision of classroom assignments and the tutoring needed from the homeschool teacher to keep up with the classwork. David and his mother are advised to consult with the 504 coordinator at his high school to formulate the plans needed. Additionally, they were advised to contact the HCT coordinator in the event they encountered any problems.

During the first Spina Bifida Clinic appointment following his surgery, David and his mother are asked how his homeschool program progressed as he recovered postoperatively at home. David replied that now that he was back at school, he was working hard to "catch up" with his course work and "bring up" his grades. When queried about these statements, his mother replied that a homeschool teacher was not available to tutor David on his academics. In turn, David said that he had problems keeping up with his classes. David indicated that he was confident that he could "pull up his grades" to his former GPA average. As the HCT coordinator heard this recounting of his current academic challenges, David and his mother were reminded of the rights and protections that were afforded to him with having a 504 plan.

A plan was devised to enable David and his mother to participate in discussions with school personnel about the accommodations that David currently needed. The accommodations included the following plans: (a) access to academic tutoring in the classes wherein his grades were not equivalent to his typical academic performance, (b) additional time to complete his makeup work for each of the classes without academic penalty, (c) extra time initially for test-taking for examinations in his classes, and (d) academic advisement pertaining to his current GPA and strategies for raising up his GPA.

As this case example illustrates, David's needs for healthcare support extend beyond the typical confines of the clinical setting. David's lived experience with spina bifida coupled with his current stage of development and lifestyle extends into the school and community setting, wherein he lives, learns, and grows.

This case example describes a prototype of an AYASHCN lifestyle situation that is often experienced as reported in national surveys and research studies. Situations as described here can have enduring effects that last a lifetime such as school failure, due in part to the inadequate and/or lack of appropriate resources and supports that AYASHCN need in the other domains of their life. A HCT coordinator and members of the HCT team, sensitive to the lived experience of AYASHCN, can do much to promote the provision of needed resources and referrals.

Conclusion

This chapter presented a detailed discussion of the HCT models currently used in practice and tested empirically. This examination included a discussion of the key structural components and the distinguishing processes of various HCT intervention models. A discussion of the HCT outcomes was provided. This chapter concluded with the limitations associated with the state of the science as it is hindered by the designs and methods that are insufficient to generate the evidence needed to identify effective models of HCT care that will serve to improve outcomes for AYASHCN. Although the science of the field is a representative of the emerging field, much progress has been made within the last decade. Many more studies, thoughtful commentaries, and systematic reviews are strong evidence of the growth of the field. Given this backdrop of growth and development, it is likely more substantive evidence will be forthcoming to foster the implementation of effective HCT models of care.

References

1. Magrab PR, Miller HEC, editors. Surgeon's General's Conference: growing up and getting medical care: youth with special health care needs. A summary of conference proceedings. 1989 March 13–15. Jekyll Island, Georgia: National Center for Networking Community Based Services. Georgetown University Child Development Center; 1989.
2. Betz CL. Transition of adolescents with special health care needs: review and analysis of the literature. Issues Compr Pediatr Nurs. 2004;27:179–240.
3. Betz CL, O'Kane LS, Nehring WM, Lobo ML. Systematic review: health care transition practice service models. Nurs Outlook 2016;64(3):229–243. PubMed
4. Chu PY, Maslow GR, von Isenburg M, Chung RJ. Systematic review of the impact of transition interventions for adolescents with chronic illness on transfer from pediatric to adult healthcare. J Pediatr Nurs. 2015;30(5):e19–e27. PubMed Pubmed Central PMCID: NIHMS710745.
5. Bloom SR, Kuhlthau K, Van Cleave J, Knapp AA, Newacheck P, Perrin JM. Health care transition for youth with special health care needs. J Adolesc Health 2012;51(3):213–219. PubMed English.
6. Coyne B, Hallowell SC, Thompson M. Measurable outcomes after transfer from pediatric to adult providers in youth with chronic illness. J Adolesc Health 2017;60(1):3–16. PubMed
7. Binks JA, Barden WS, Burke TA, Young NL. What do we really know about the transition to adult-centered health care? A focus on cerebral palsy and spina bifida. Arch Phys Med Rehabil. 2007;88(8):1064–73.
8. American Academy of Pediatrics American Academy of Family Practice, & American College of Physicians-American Society of Internal Medicine. A consensus statement on health care transitions for young adults with special health care needs. Pediatrics. 2002;110(6 Pt 2):1304–6.
9. American Academy of Pediatrics, American Academy of Family Practice, American College of Physicians, Transitions Clinical Report Authoring G, Cooley WC, Sagerman PJ Supporting the health care transition from adolescence to adulthood in the medical home. Pediatrics 2011;128(1):182–200. PubMed
10. Society of Pediatric Nurses. SPN position statement: transition of pediatric patients into adult care. Chicago, Illinois: Society of Pediatric Nurses; 2016. p. 9.
11. Ludvigsson JF, Agreus L, Ciacci C, Crowe SE, Geller MG, Green PH, et al. Transition from childhood to adulthood in coeliac disease: the Prague consensus report. Gut 2016;65(8):1242–1251. PubMed
12. Suris JC, Akre C. Key elements for, and indicators of, a successful transition: an international Delphi study. J Adolesc Health 2015;56(6):612–618. PubMed
13. Rosen DS, Blum RW, Britto M, Sawyer SM, Siegel DM. Transition to adult health care for adolescents and young adults with chronic conditions. J Adolesc Health. 2003;33(4):309–11.
14. Baldassano R, Ferry G, Griffiths A, Mack D, Markowitz J, Winter H. Transition of the patient with inflammatory bowel disease from pediatric to adult care: recommendations of the North American Society for Pediatric Gastroenterology, Hepatology and Nutrition. J Pediatr Gastroenterol Nutr. 2002;34(3):245–8.
15. Geerlings RP, Aldenkamp AP, de With PH, Zinger S, Gottmer-Welschen LM, de Louw AJ. Transition to adult medical care for adolescents with epilepsy. Epilepsy Behav 2015;44:127–135. PubMed
16. McManus M, White P, Pirtle R, Hancock C, Ablan M, Corona-Parra R. Incorporating the six core elements of health care transition into a medicaid managed care plan: lessons learned from a pilot project. J Pediatr Nurs. 2015;30(5):700–13.
17. Betz CL, Smith KA, Van Speybroeck A, Hernandez FV, Jacobs RA. Movin' on up: an innovative nurse-led interdisciplinary health care transition program. J Pediatr Health Care 2016;30(4):323–338. PubMed
18. Bridgett M, Abrahamson G, Ho J. Transition, it's more than just an event: supporting young people with type 1 diabetes. J Pediatr Nurs. 2015;30(5):e11–e4.
19. Ciccarelli MR, Gladstone EB, Armstrong Richardson EAJ. Implementation of a transdisciplinary team for the transition support of medically and socially complex youth. J Pediatr Nurs. 2015;30(5):661–7.
20. Woodward JF, Swigonski NL, Ciccarelli MR. Assessing the health, functional characteristics, and health needs of youth attending a noncategorical transition support program. J Adolesc Health 2012;51(3):272–278. PubMed English.
21. McDonagh JE, Shaw KL, Southwood TR. Growing up and moving on in rheumatology: development

and preliminary evaluation of a transitional care programme for a multicentre cohort of adolescents with juvenile idiopathic arthritis. J Child Health Care 2006;10(1):22–42. .PubMed English.
22. Dabadie A, Troadec F, Heresbach D, Siproudhis L, Pagenault M, Bretagne JF. Transition of patients with inflammatory bowel disease from pediatric to adult care. Gastroenterol Clin Biol. 2008;32(5 Pt 1):451–9.
23. Vanelli M, Caronna S, Adinolfi B, Chiari G, Gugliotta M, Arsenio L. Effectiveness of an uninterrupted procedure to transfer adolescents with Type 1 diabetes from the paediatric to the adult clinic held in the same hospital: eight-year experience with the parma protocol. Diabetes Nutr Metab 2004;17(5):304–308. PubMed
24. Bhawra J, Toulany A, Cohen E, Moore Hepburn C, Guttmann A. Primary care interventions to improve transition of youth with chronic health conditions from paediatric to adult healthcare: a systematic review. BMJ Open 2016;6(5):e011871. PubMed
25. Bollegala N, Nguyen GC. Transitioning the adolescent with IBD from pediatric to adult care: a review of the literature. Gastroenterology Research & Practice 2015;2015:853530. PubMed
26. Embrett MG, Randall GE, Longo CJ, Nguyen T, Mulvale G. Effectiveness of health system services and programs for youth to adult transitions in mental health care: a systematic review of academic literature. Adm Policy Ment Health 2016;43(2):259–269. PubMed
27. Peter NG, Forke CM, Ginsburg KR, Schwarz DF. Transition from pediatric to adult care: internists' perspectives. Pediatrics. 2009;123(2):417–23.
28. DiIorio C, Shafer PO, Letz R, Henry TR, Schomer DL, Yeager K. Behavioral, social, and affective factors associated with self-efficacy for self-management among people with epilepsy. Epilepsy Behav. 2006;9(1):158–63.
29. DiIorio C, Osborne Shafer P, Letz R, Henry T, Schomer DL, Yeager K. The association of stigma with self-management and perceptions of health care among adults with epilepsy. Epilepsy Behav. 2003;4(3):259–67.
30. Sawin KJ, Brei T, Holmbeck G. The development of the adolescent\young adult self-management and independence scale-AMIS II: psychometric data. 2017.
31. Sawin, KJ, Bellin, M, Woodward, J,Brei, T. Self-management in spina bifida: a synthesis in literature. Paper presented at the Third World Congress on Spina Bifida Research and Care; 2017 March 16–19; San Diego, CA
32. Holmes-Walker DJ, Llewellyn AC, Farrell KA. transition care programme which improves diabetes control and reduces hospital admission rates in young adults with Type 1 diabetes aged 15–25 years. Diabet Med. 2007;24(7):764–9.
33. Smith GM, Lewis VR, Whitworth E, Gold DT, Thornburg CD. Growing up with sickle cell disease: a pilot study of a transition program for adolescents with sickle cell disease. J Pediatr Hematol Oncol 2011;33(5):379–382. PubMed
34. Wiener LS, Kohrt B, Battles HB, Pao M. The HIV experience: youth identified barriers for transitioning from pediatric to adult care. J Pediatr Psychol. 2011;36(2):141–54.
35. Betz CL, Lobo ML, Nehring WM, Bui K. Voices not heard: a systematic review of adolescents' and emerging adults' perspectives of health care transition. Nurs Outlook 2013;61(5):311–336. PubMed
36. Betz CL, Nehring WM, Lobo ML. Transition needs of parents of adolescents and emerging adults with special health care needs and disabilities. J Fam Nurs 2015;21(3):362–412. PubMed
37. Agency for Healthcare Quality and Research. Care Coordination Rockville, MD: Agency for Healthcare Research and Quality. 2016 [updated July 2016; cited 15 October 2017]. http://www.ahrq.gov/professionals/prevention-chronic-care/improve/coordination/index.html.
38. Blomquist K, Brown G, Peersen A, Presler E. Transitioning to independence: challenges for young people with disabilities and their caregivers. Orthop Nurs. 1998;17(3):27–35.
39. Blomquist KB. Healthy and ready to work: Kentucky: incorporating transition into a state program for children with special health care needs. Pediatr Nurs 2006;32(6):515–528. PubMed
40. Lerret SM, Menendez J, Weckwerth J, Lokar J, Mitchell J, Alonso EM. Essential components of transition to adult transplant services: the transplant coordinators' perspective. Prog Transplant 2012;22(3):252–258. PubMed
41. Rogers K, Zeni MB. Systematic review of medical home models to promote transitions to primary adult health care for adolescents living with autism spectrum disorder. Worldviews Evid Based Nurs 2015;12(2):98–107. PubMed
42. Annunziato RA, Baisley MC, Arrato N, Barton C, Henderling F, Arnon R, et al. Strangers headed to a strange land? A pilot study of using a transition coordinator to improve transfer from pediatric to adult services. J Pediatr 2013;163(6):1628–1633. PubMed
43. Betz CL, Redcay G. Dimensions of the transition service coordinator role. J Soc Pediatr Nurs 2005;10(2):49–59. PubMed
44. Jivanjee P, Kruzich J. Supports for young people with mental health conditions and their families in the transition years: youth and family voices. Best Prac Ment Health. 2011;7:115–33.
45. Jivanjee P, Kruzich JM, Gordon LJ. The age of uncertainty: parent perspectives on the transition of young people with mental health difficulties to adulthood. J Child Fam Stud. 2009;18:435–46.
46. Kieckhefer GM, Trahms CM, Churchill SS, Simpson JN. Measuring parent-child shared management of chronic illness. Pediatr Nurs. 2009;35(2):101–8.
47. Kieckhefer GM, Trahms CM. Supporting development of children with chronic conditions: from compliance toward shared management. Pediatr Nurs 2000;26(4):354–363. PubMed

48. Stinson JN, Toomey PC, Stevens BJ, Kagan S, Duffy CM, Huber A, et al. Asking the experts: exploring the self-management needs of adolescents with arthritis. [see comment]. Arthritis Rheum. 2008;59(1):65–72.
49. Heath G, Farre A, Shaw K. Parenting a child with chronic illness as they transition into adulthood: a systematic review and thematic synthesis of parents' experiences. Patient Educ Couns 2017;100(1):76–92. PubMed
50. Andreoni KA, Forbes R, Andreoni RM, Phillips G, Stewart H, Ferris M. Age-related kidney transplant outcomes: health disparities amplified in adolescence. JAMA Intern Med 2013;173(16):1524–1532. PubMed English.
51. Allen D, Channon S, Lowes L, Atwell C, Lane C. Behind the scenes: the changing roles of parents in the transition from child to adult diabetes service. Diabet Med 2011;28(8):994–1000. PubMed
52. Hess JS, Straub DM. Brief report: preliminary findings from a pilot health care transition education intervention for adolescents and young adults with special health care needs. J Pediatr Psychol 2010;36(2):172–178. PubMed
53. Scott L, Vallis M, Charette M, Murray A, Latta R. Transition of care: researching the needs of young adults with type 1 diabetes. Can J Diabetes. 2005;29:203–10.
54. Betz CL, Ferris ME, Woodward JF, Okumura MJ, Jan S, Wood DL. The health care transition research consortium health care transition model: a framework for research and practice. J Pediatr Rehabil Med 2014;7(1):3–15. PubMed
55. Ihara ES, Wolf-Branigin M, White P. Quality of life and life skill baseline measures of urban adolescents with disabilities. Soc Work Public Health 2012;27(7):658–670. PubMed English.
56. Yorkery B, Test DW. Improving educational outcomes and post-school success for students with disabilities. N C Med J 2009;70(6):542–544. PubMed
57. Rosen D. Between two worlds: bridging the cultures of child health and adult medicine. J Adolesc Health 1995;17(1):10–16. PubMed
58. Okumura MJ, Heisler M, Davis MM, Cabana MD, Demonner S, Kerr EA. Comfort of general internists and general pediatricians in providing care for young adults with chronic illnesses of childhood. J Gen Intern Med 2008;23(10):1621–1627. PubMed
59. Nehring WM, Betz CL, Lobo ML. Uncharted territory: systematic review of providers' roles, understanding, and views pertaining to health care transition. J Pediatr Nurs 2015;30(5):732–747. PubMed
60. Arnett JJ. Emerging adulthood. a theory of development from the late teens through the twenties. Am Psychol. 2000;55(5):469–80.
61. Arnett JJ, Tanner JL. Emerging adults in America. Coming of age in the 21st century. American Psychological Association: Washington, D.C; 2006.
62. Camfield P, Camfield C, Pohlmann-Eden B. Transition from pediatric to adult epilepsy care: a difficult process marked by medical and social crisis. Epilepsy Currents 2012;12(Suppl 3):13–21. PubMed
63. Cadario F, Prodam F, Bellone S, Trada M, Binotti M, Trada M, et al. Transition process of patients with type 1 diabetes (T1DM) from paediatric to the adult health care service: a hospital-based approach. Clin Endocrinol (Oxf) 2009;71(3):346–350. PubMed
64. Jurasek L, Ray L, Quigley D. Development and implementation of an adolescent epilepsy transition clinic. J Neurosci Nurs 2010;42(4):181–189. PubMed
65. Pyatak EA, Carandang K, Vigen C, Blanchard J, Sequeira PA, Wood JR, et al. Resilient, Empowered, Active Living with Diabetes (REAL Diabetes) study: methodology and baseline characteristics of a randomized controlled trial evaluating an occupation-based diabetes management intervention for young adults. Contemp Clin Trials 2017;54:8–17. PubMed
66. Wafa S, Nakhla M. Improving the transition from pediatric to adult diabetes healthcare: a literature review. Can J Diabetes 2015;39(6):520–528. PubMed
67. Hazel E, Zhang X, Duffy CM, Campillo S. High rates of unsuccessful transfer to adult care among young adults with juvenile idiopathic arthritis. Pediatr Dent 2010;8:2. PubMed
68. Steinbeck KS, Shrewsbury VA, Harvey V, Mikler K, Donaghue KC, Craig ME, et al. A pilot randomized controlled trial of a post-discharge program to support emerging adults with type 1 diabetes mellitus transition from pediatric to adult care. Pediatr Diabetes 2015;16(8):634–639. PubMed
69. Betz CL, Smith K. Measuring health care transition planning outcomes: challenges and issues. Int J Child Adolesc Health. 2010;3:463–72.
70. Le Roux E, Mellerio H, Guilmin-Crepon S, Gottot S, Jacquin P, Boulkedid R, et al. Methodology used in comparative studies assessing programmes of transition from paediatrics to adult care programmes: a systematic review. BMJ Open 2017;7(1):e012338. PubMed
71. Kipps S, Bahu T, Ong K, Ackland FM, Brown RS, Fox CT, et al. Current methods of transfer of young people with Type 1 diabetes to adult services. Diabet Med. 2002;19(8):649–54.
72. Gleeson H, Turner G. Transition to adult services. Arch Dis Child Educ Pract Ed 2012;97(3):86–92. PubMed English.
73. Bolton-Maggs PH. Transition of care from paediatric to adult services in haematology. Arch Dis Child. 2007;92(9):797–801.
74. Harden PN, Walsh G, Bandler N, Bradley S, Lonsdale D, Taylor J, et al. Bridging the gap: an integrated paediatric to adult clinical service for young adults with kidney failure. BMJ 2012;344:e3718. PubMed English.
75. Watson AR. Non-compliance and transfer from paediatric to adult transplant unit. Pediatr Nephrol. 2000;14(6):469–72.
76. Shaw KL, Southwood TR, McDonagh JE, British Society of Paediatric and Adolescent Rheumatology.

Development and preliminary validation of the 'Mind the Gap' scale to assess satisfaction with transitional health care among adolescents with juvenile idiopathic arthritis. Child Care Health Dev. 2007;33(4):380–8.
77. Shaw KL, Southwood TR, McDonagh JE, British Society of Paediatric and Adolescent Rheumatology. Young people's satisfaction of transitional care in adolescent rheumatology in the UK. Child Care Health Dev. 2007;33(4):368–79.
78. Reid GJ, Irvine MJ, McCrindle BW, Sananes R, Ritvo PG, Siu SC, et al. Prevalence and correlates of successful transfer from pediatric to adult health care among a cohort of young adults with complex congenital heart defects. Pediatrics. 2004;113(3 Pt 1):e197–205.
79. Betz CL, Redcay G. An exploratory study of future plans and extracurricular activities of transition-age youth and young adults. Issues Compr Pediatr Nurs. 2005;28(1):33–61.
80. Di Rezze B, Nguyen T, Mulvale G, Barr NG, Longo CJ, Randall GE. A scoping review of evaluated interventions addressing developmental transitions for youth with mental health disorders. Child Care Health Dev 2016;42(2):176–187. PubMed
81. Prior M, McManus M, White P, Davidson L. Measuring the "triple aim" in transition care: a systematic review. Pediatrics 2014;134(6):e1648–e1661. PubMed
82. Institute for Healthcare Improvement (IHI). IHI triple aim initiative. Better care for individuals, better health for populations, and lower per capita costs (n.d.) [cited 2017 April 15]. http://www.ihi.org/engage/initiatives/TripleAim/Pages/default.aspx.
83. Sheehan AM, While AE, Coyne I The experiences and impact of transition from child to adult healthcare services for young people with Type 1 diabetes: a systematic review. Diabet Med 2015;32(4):440–458. PubMed

Part IX

Conclusions

37 Conclusions

Constance M. Wiemann and Albert C. Hergenroeder

The natural history of most childhood onset conditions has improved over the past 40 years so that 90% of AYASHCN will live into adulthood. For some conditions, for example, congenital heart disease and cystic fibrosis, there are more adults than minors. However, the resources invested in treating pediatric conditions have not been matched by improvements in methods to successfully transition AYASHCN into adult-based care. The same sort of ingenuity, perseverance, and investments to enhance the diagnosis and treatment of child-onset conditions must be applied to improving HCT.

The chapter authors in this textbook are providers, payors, AYASHCN, and families with extensive HCT experience. Given the quality of the chapter contributions, there is cause for optimism; the collective experience of these frontline workers suggests we are not that far from developing best practices.

The framework for transitioning from pediatric to adult health care includes preparation, transfer, and engagement on the adult side. Within this framework, HCT models need to be developed and tested with the understanding that there will not be one solution that applies to all settings and conditions. Each will need to recognize the young adult's brain maturation and the accompanying behavioral manifestations across diseases with their own natural history as well as the impact of the AYASHCN's immediate environment and broader societal systems of care. Those AYASHCN with supportive families and access to care are more likely to successfully transition into adulthood; those with the most complicated conditions and from the lowest socioeconomic status do not fare as well. Definitions of successful HCT are needed, as determined by AYASHCN and their families, providers, and key constituents in the healthcare systems that care for AYASHCN.

Our collective ability to develop and implement evidence-based HCT programs hinges on access to appropriate services. Healthcare access is being threatened by proposed cuts to Medicaid and other publicly funded insurance programs in the United States and the erosion of protection that AYASHCN currently have against discrimination in the insurance market for those with preexisting conditions. Although the limitations of medical insurance in the United States are associated with increased morbidity and mortality for AYASHCN, improving medical insurance coverage alone will not solve all HCT-related problems, as problems also exist in single-payer systems such as those in Canada and Europe. Several chapters suggest different reimbursement models that could go a long way toward better care coordination to improve HCT outcomes.

C. M. Wiemann, Ph.D. • A. C. Hergenroeder, M.D. (✉)
Section of Adolescent Medicine and Sports Medicine, Department of Pediatrics, Baylor College of Medicine, Texas Children's Hospital, Houston, TX, USA
e-mail: alberth@bcm.edu

A. C. Hergenroeder, C. M. Wiemann (eds.), *Health Care Transition*,
https://doi.org/10.1007/978-3-319-72868-1_37

There has been increasing research to develop evidence-based HCT methods. Innovations are evolving such as the role of the medical home and the role of pharmacists in improving HCT processes and outcomes. There is optimism based on increasing research conducted in the field of HCT and the publications of HCT guidelines by professional societies. However, the field will only improve on the basis of rigorous evaluation of methods and guidelines.

We have come a long way yet there is much more to be done. The progress that has been made in HCT over the last two decades should empower us to conquer the challenges that lie ahead. To do so will be to build on the medical accomplishments of diagnosing and treating pediatric-onset conditions of the last century and honor the heroism of AYASHCN and their families to extend their quality of life into adulthood.

Appendix*

Example Inpatient Transition Planning Assessment

Patient or Caregiver to answer

Date:

Demographics

Patient: Prefers to be called:

MR# DOB: Age: Sex:

Primary Caregiver(s): Guardianship:

Language/Learning Considerations: Individualized Education Plan Y/N (contact):

Employment/School: DME Provider:

Clinical Information

2-line Clinical Summary (incl functional status)

What inpatient and outpatient providers know you best (Why)?

Admission Pattern (Main reasons for hospital admissions)

Typical Discharge Criteria

Nutrition Considerations

Activity Considerations

Primary Supports and Resources

What level of care can the family deliver at home (e.g. medical devices)?

Symptom Management/Intervention Plan (e.g. pain plan)

Transition Planning and Readiness

Patient's Transition Readiness Assessment

Competency Y/N Patient's comfort with medical decision making

Caregiver comfort with patient's medical decision making

Verbal Release Y/N My Chart Y/N Code Status Advance Directive Y/N

Have you transitioned to an Adult PCP (if no, has anyone discussed)?

Have you transitioned to Adult Subspecialists (if no, has anyone discussed)?

Anticipated Insurance Issues

Other Anticipated Transition/Adult Care Issues

Which of your providers do you want at the transition planning meeting?

*This Appendix belongs to chapter 27.

A. C. Hergenroeder, C. M. Wiemann (eds.), *Health Care Transition*,
https://doi.org/10.1007/978-3-319-72868-1

What's important to me

(to be completed by patient and primary caregivers)

Inpatient Transition Plan Recommendations

To be completed after transition meeting with providers and family

TK is a 22 year old male with a history of complex congenital heart disease, hypoxic encephalopathy leading to severe spastic quadriplegic cerebral palsy, epilepsy, enteral tube feeding, and is completely dependent for his care. He needs cardiac anesthesia and has prolonged recovery from sedation. He has chronic lung disease, likely due to chronic microaspiration, and is frequently hospitalized from respiratory-related problems.

Important Background / Context:

- TK was cognitively and developmentally healthy until preschool. He had an ischemic brain injury related to a relatively minor hospital procedure, and this led to many of his current co-morbidities. This occurred during a hospitalization and while his father was at work. His father has tremendous guilt that he did not raise his discomfort with having the procedure done while he was not present. This pivotal event has since shaped everything about his approach to TK's care since that time.

Primary Care Provider → Dr. Booker (family medicine), not changing primary care from pediatric to adult care
Subspecialty Providers → Dr. Bledsoe (pediatric cardiology), Dr. Stone (pediatric neurology), Dr. Tompkins (physical medicine and rehabilitation), Dr. Cherney (pediatric gastroenterology)

TRANSITION PLAN RECOMMENDATIONS		SETTING (INPT, OUTPT?)	OWNER	TIMELINE
ISSUE	PLAN			
1. Negative experience during adult hospitalization a. Felt a lack of compassion and abruptness from staff	1. Future hospitalizations in J6 (possible backup being F2). a. Nurse managers will coordinate b. If full, they will frequently move patients 2. Place FYI about this plan in chart 3. Aim for admissions to H1 or H4 services a. Better continuity with NP / PA and non-teaching 4. Limit additional providers when possible to avoid precipitating anxiety	Inpatient	Jack Keyes (nurse manager) and Dr. James (adult hospitalist)	1 month
2. Parent readiness	1. Next visit, ask parents "what needs to happen to help them feel more ready"	Outpatient and Inpatient	Social work, Dr. Booker (primary care) and Dr. James (adult hospitalist)	Next visit – 2 months
3. Guardianship not completed	1. Discuss at next primary care visit 2. Share internet resources 3. Work with SW to see if options to help pay for guardianship process	Outpatient	Dr. Booker (primary care)	Next visit – 2 months
4. Costs / insurance	1. Ensure receiving disability, SSI	Outpatient	Social work	Now
5. Discharge criteria a. Has home oxygen – family prefers to be discharged and wean oxygen at home if otherwise improving b. Caregivers feels high level of confidence delivering all cares to TK	1. Caregivers knows TK very well and are technically very skilled – home with oxygen is very reasonable as long as illness trajectory improving a. Maximum flow rate 2 L/min by nasal cannula 2. Adjusting feeding at home is not a problem 3. Discuss with past providers if any question / disagreement – Dr. Bledsoe (cardiology), Dr. Booker (primary care), etc	Inpatient	Adult hospitalist services (Dr. James lead) and subspecialists	Ongoing
6. Unclear which subspecialists to consult when hospitalized	1. Dr. Booker (primary care) to discuss with family and providers 2. Identify timeline for <u>if and when</u> subspecialists will transition to adult subspecialists. 3. Identify which (adult or pediatric) subspecialists should be consulted for issues when hospitalized	Outpatient	Dr. Booker (primary care)	Next visit – 2 months

Index

A. C. Hergenroeder, C. M. Wiemann (eds.), *Health Care Transition*,
https://doi.org/10.1007/978-3-319-72868-1

Printed in the United States
By Bookmasters